Atlas of Uniportal Video Assisted Thoracic Surgery

Diego Gonzalez-Rivas • Calvin Sze Hang Ng
Gaetano Rocco • Thomas A. D'Amico
Editors

Atlas of Uniportal Video Assisted Thoracic Surgery

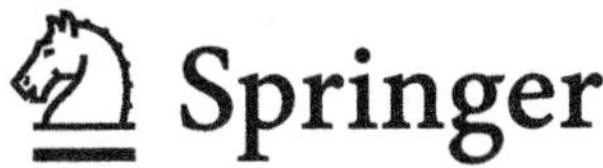

Editors
Diego Gonzalez-Rivas
Department of Thoracic Surgery
Shanghai Pulmonary Hospital
Tongji University School of Medicine
Shanghai, China

Department of Thoracic Surgery and Minimally Invasive Thoracic Surgery Unit (UCTMI),
Coruña University Hospital
Coruña, Spain

Gaetano Rocco
Service of Thoracic Surgery
Department of Surgery Memorial Sloan Kettering Cancer Center
New York, NY
USA

Calvin Sze Hang Ng
Division of Cardiothoracic Surgery
Department of Surgery
Prince of Wales Hospital
The Chinese University of Hong Kong
Hong Kong SAR
China

Thomas A. D'Amico
Gary Hock Endowed Professor of Surgery
Duke University Medical Center
Durham, NC
USA

ISBN 978-981-13-2603-5 ISBN 978-981-13-2604-2 (eBook)
https://doi.org/10.1007/978-981-13-2604-2

Library of Congress Control Number: 2019934469

This Springer imprint is published by the registered company Springer Nature Singapore Pte Ltd.
The registered company address is: 152 Beach Road, #21-01/04 Gateway East, Singapore 189721, Singapore

Contents

Part I General Aspects & Background

The Evolution of Video Assisted Thoracic Surgery 3
Alan D. L. Sihoe

The New Era of Uniportal VATS 17
Peter Sze Yuen Yu and Calvin S. H. Ng

Room Set Up and Instrumentation 23
Mahmoud Ismail

Anaesthesia for Uniportal VATS 29
Sonia Alvarado, César Bonome, and Diego Gonzalez-Rivas

Geometric Considerations in Uniportal VATS 33
Luca Bertolaccini

Modified Uniportal Approach 39
H. Volkan Kara, Stafford S. Balderson, and Thomas A. D'Amico

Part II Uniportal VATS in Pleural and Mediastinal Diseases

Uniportal Video-Assisted Thoracoscopic Surgery for the Management of Pleural Effusions, Empyema and Pleural Biopsy 47
Marco Scarci, Fabrizio Minervini, and Gaetano Rocco

Uniportal Approach to Pericardial Window and Sympathectomy 51
Simon C. Y. Chow and Calvin S. H. Ng

Uniport Anterior Mediastinal Surgery 59
Ching Feng Wu and Diego Gonzalez-Rivas

Uniportal Posterior Mediastinal Surgery 67
Luis Angel Hernandez-Arenas, Yang Yang, Zhu Yu-Ming, Gening Jiang, and Diego Gonzalez-Rivas

Subxiphoid Mediastinal Resections 73
Takashi Suda

Part III Parenchymal Lung Diseases

Uniportal Treatment for Spontaneous Pneumothorax 83
Alessandro Brunelli and Cecilia Pompili

Uniportal Bullectomy for Emphysematous Bullous Lung Disease 87
Fernando Vannucci

Hookwire Localization of Pulmonary Nodules in Uniportal VATS 95
Ze-Rui Zhao and Calvin S. H. Ng

Intraoperative Ultrasound Guidance in Pulmonary Nodule Localization in Uniportal VATS 101
Gaetano Rocco, Raffaele Rocco, and Marco Scarci

Videoendoscopic Uniportal Resection of Solitary Peripheral Lung Nodule 103
Marco Scarci, Fabrizio Minervini, and Gaetano Rocco

Part IV Uniportal Major Lung Resections

Right Lower Lobe 109
Eva Fieira Costa, María Delgado Roel, and Marina Paradela de la Morena

Left Lower Lobe Resection 115
Hyun Koo Kim and Kook Nam Han

Right Middle Lobe 121
Miao Lin and Li Jie Tan

Uniportal Video-Assisted Thoracoscopic Right Upper Lobectomy 123
Diego Gonzalez-Rivas and Marina Paradela de la Morena

Uniportal Right Upper Lobectomy 129
Heron Andrade, Arthur Vieira, and Paula Ugalde Figueroa

Left Upper Lobectomy 135
Chengwu Liu and Lunxu Liu

Left VATS Upper Lobectomy 141
Marco Scarci, Benedetta Bedetti, Luca Bertolaccini, Ilaria Righi, Davide Patrini, and Roberto Crisci

Uniportal Video-Assisted Thoracoscopic Segmentectomy 145
Dong Xie, Konstantinos Marios Soultanis, Xuefei Hu, and Yuming Zhu

Segmental Resection 151
Hyun Koo Kim and Kook Nam Han

Left Uniportal VATS Pneumonectomy 165
Peter Sze Yuen Yu and Calvin S. H. Ng

Right Pneumonectomy 169
Mercedes de la Torre, Eva Mª Fieira, and Marina Paradela

Uniportal Lymphadenectomy 175
Maria Delgado Roel, Eva Fieira Costa, Marina Paradela De La Morena, Diego Gonzalez-Rivas, Ricardo Fernandez Prado, Juan Pablo Ovalle Granados, and Mercedes De La Torre Bravos

Part V Advanced Uniportal Techniques

Uniportal Video-Assisted Thoracoscopic Sleeve Resections 183
Diego Gonzalez-Rivas, Jiang Lei, and Dmitrii Sekhniaidze

Sleeve Resection 199
Hyun Koo Kim and Kook Nam Han

Tracheal and Carina Resection/Reconstruction 205
Guilin Peng, Wei Wang, Minzhang Guo, Hui Pan, and Jianxing He

Uniportal VATS Chest Wall and Diaphragm Resection and Reconstruction 213
Diego Gonzalez-Rivas

Troubleshooting: Management of Bleeding 223
Ricardo Fernandez Prado, Juan Pablo Ovalle Granados, Luis Fernandez Vago, Eva Maria Fieira Costa, Marina Paradela De La Morena, Maria Delgado Roel, Diego Gonzalez-Rivas, and Mercedes De La Torre Bravos

Uniportal Minimally Invasive Esophagectomy 227
Sun-Moa Yang and Jang-Ming Lee

Part VI The Future of Uniportal VATS

Non-intubated Uniportal VATS Major Pulmonary Resections 237
Diego Gonzalez-Rivas, Sonia Alvarado, and César Bonome

Subxiphoid Uniportal Video-Assisted Thoracoscopic Surgery 245
Diego Gonzalez-Rivas, Firas Abu Akar, and Jiang Lei

Natural-Orifice Uniport VATS for Lung Resection 259
Ming-Ju Hsieh, Yen Chu, Yi-Cheng Wu, Chieng-Ying Liu, Tzu-Ping Chen, Yin-Kai Chao, Ching-Yang Wu, Chi-Ju Yeh, Po-Jen Ko, and Yun-Hen Liu

Natural Orifice Transluminal Endoscopic Surgery (NOTES) Uniportal VATS for Sympathectomy 263
Weisheng Chen

Image-Guided Uniportal VATS in the Hybrid Operating Room 269
Ze-Rui Zhao and Calvin S. H. Ng

Development of 3D VATS 279
Jun Liu, Jingpei Li, Yidong Wang, Fengling Lai, Wei Wang, Guilin Peng, Zhihua Guo, Jiaxi He, Fei Cui, Shuben Li, and Jianxing He

Future Development and Technologies 283
Zheng Li and Calvin S. H. Ng

Part I

General Aspects & Background

The Evolution of Video Assisted Thoracic Surgery

Alan D. L. Sihoe

Evolution: The Cornerstone of Surgical Progress

Surgery is not a static entity, but a constantly evolving discipline. It adapts itself in response to changing patient needs, emergence of new technologies, and developments in medical knowledge.

The importance of this aspect of surgery is exemplified by the story of Video Assisted Thoracic Surgery (VATS). Since its first appearance in the early 1990s, VATS has been demonstrated to significantly reduce pain, hasten recovery, minimize complications, and improve post-operative quality of life for patients requiring Thoracic Surgery when compared to traditional open thoracotomy [1–4]. Conventional three-port VATS has become established as the preferred approach for almost every general thoracic operation today.

However, far from resting on their laurels, VATS surgeons have continued to strive for better outcomes for their patients. By innovating, improvising and incorporation of new technologies, they have brought forth a range of 'next generation' VATS techniques that promise further improvements in terms of post-operative results [1, 2].

Studying the process of this evolution is not simply a matter of re-reading history. Instead, by understanding what drove evolution, and appreciating why particular advances succeeded (or failed), surgeons may gain insight into what really matters for patients. This will help refine their techniques and inspire the next step in the perpetual evolution towards better surgery.

This chapter aims to summarize the evolutionary history of Minimally Invasive Thoracic Surgery culminating in Uniportal VATS, and to demonstrate how the lessons from that evolution may guide surgeons learning this technique. VATS being such a broad topic today, this chapter will focus mainly on VATS lobectomy—which is both the main thread of the evolutionary storyline and also the focus of the most significant developments in VATS.

The Early History of VATS

Performing any surgery within the chest requires the surgeon to put a right hand, a left hand, and a pair of eyes to look inside [1]. Because the space between the ribs cannot naturally admit these three things, it follows that to perform the operation the ribs must be spread apart with force for the duration of the operation—often up to several hours. It is this rib-spreading that is now recognized to contribute most to the pain and morbidity associated with an open thoracotomy [5–7].

Conventional VATS actually maintains the same principle, but uses surgical instruments to replace the right and left hands, and a video-thoracoscope is to replace direct vision through the wound. This allows the same thoracic surgery to be done using three small ports without forcible rib-spreading [1, 3, 4].

When applied to lobectomy, one of the earliest described techniques involved the simultaneous stapling of the skeletonized pulmonary artery, pulmonary vein and lobar bronchus [8, 9]. Though good safety was reported and no evidence was produced to repudiate its usage [8, 10], the approach came under philosophical criticism from conservative opinion leaders at the time [11]. As a result, the principle of individual dissection and division of the hilar structures became the mainstream approach for VATS lobectomy ever since [12–15].

Early evidence suggested that the VATS approach gave less immediate post-operative pain than thoracotomy in terms of reduced analgesic requirements [15–17], or lower

Electronic Supplementary Material The online version of this chapter (https://doi.org/10.1007/978-981-13-2604-2_1) contains supplementary material, which is available to authorized users.

A. D. L. Sihoe (✉)
International Medical Centre Hong Kong,
Hong Kong SAR, China

D. Gonzalez-Rivas et al. (eds.), *Atlas of Uniportal Video Assisted Thoracic Surgery*,
https://doi.org/10.1007/978-981-13-2604-2_1

subjective pain scores [15, 18, 19]. The reduced pain translated into faster recovery, resulting in significantly shorter hospital stays and earlier return to pre-operative work or activities [16, 18].

However, despite the early promise, other studies began to emerge casting doubt on the desirability of the VATS approach. In 1995, a randomized, prospective study failed to demonstrate any advantage of VATS over open lobectomy in reducing post-operative pain [20]. In another questionnaire-based study, the incidence of chronic post-operative pain at 1 year was no better after VATS than after thoracotomy [21]. A study from Japan then compared pain, respiratory muscle strength and 6-min walking distance at 1 week after surgery between VATS and open surgery, and again no difference was found [22]. Such studies cast doubt over the purported advantages of VATS. It therefore came as little surprise that a survey of the General Thoracic Surgery Club members in 1997 showed that most remained skeptical about the VATS approach [23].

The Evolution of VATS Outcomes Assessment

From such inauspicious beginnings, a great change must have occurred to allow VATS to reach its universally accepted status today as the preferred surgical approach for thoracic surgery [24]. That change came not in the operating room, but on the pages of surgical journals. It was the result of pioneer VATS surgeons realizing that in order to establish this new approach to surgery, it was necessary to build up a convincing body of evidence. It was not enough to make loud claims of 'less pain, faster recovery'. Instead, a systematic accumulation of clinical data was called for. This occurred in a number of very distinct stages [25].

Birth: Defining the Technique

It soon became clear to the early VATS pioneers that 'VATS' was not a unified technique [3, 26]. Considerable variations existed in terms of number of ports, size of incisions, and even use of rib-spreading [22, 26]. However, in a couple of landmark papers, Shigemura and colleagues elegantly demonstrated that maintaining a 'complete' VATS approach (with purely endoscopic techniques, 100% monitor vision, and no rib-spreading) resulted in significantly better patient mobilization and shorter hospital stays [27, 28]. Clearly, not all iterations of 'VATS' gave good outcomes. As a consequence of this realization, the Cancer and Leukemia Group B (CALGB) 39,802 trial of the American Society of Clinical Oncology has now clearly defined a VATS lobectomy by the following criteria: no rib spreading; a maximum length of 8 cm of the access incision for removal of the lobectomy specimen; individual dissection of the vein, arteries, and airway for the lobe in question; and standard node sampling or dissection identical to an open thoracotomy [29].

Adherence to a strict definition of VATS allowed the real advantages of VATS to emerge—free from confounding by the worse results of 'pseudo-VATS'. It also allowed surgeons to contemplate *why* elements of the definition gave better results. In particular, the avoidance of rib-spreading is now appreciated as critical and has highlighted the central role of the intercostal nerves in thoracic surgical morbidity.

The characteristics of post-thoracotomy pain were observed to be the same as those of recognized neuropathic pain syndromes, such as post-herpetic neuralgia and diabetic peripheral neuropathy [6, 7, 30, 31]. Physiological studies then confirmed that rib-spreading during thoracotomy could indeed cause neuropraxic damage to the intercostals nerves [32–35]. Evidently, by avoiding rib-spreading, VATS reduced this key element of post-thoracotomy discomfort.

Infancy: Safety and Feasibility

The next step is to demonstrate that VATS is a safe and feasible technique, and for this purpose simple case reports, followed by larger case series, can suffice. Before long, a number of landmark case series were published—each recognized today as having been pivotal in establishing the basic practicality of VATS lobectomy [12–15].

Childhood: Crude Benefit

VATS surgeons then had to show that the new approach held advantages over the old approach (open thoracotomy). The obvious plan was to compare the approaches in terms of post-operative pain, morbidity rates, and lengths of stay. Early studies were relatively simplistic: data for VATS patients were compared with those of historical cohorts who had open thoracotomy [19]. Later, the studies progressed to more elegant comparisons using case-matching of patients in the study arms to reduce bias [18]. There was even a randomized trial as early as 1995 [20]. Oddly, although the authors noted "significantly more postoperative complications occurred in the thoracotomy group", their conclusion was somehow that VATS "continues to expose the patient to the risk of major pulmonary resection being done in an essentially closed chest". This serves as a reminder that perhaps randomization is no guarantee of reasonable conclusions. Thankfully, accumulated clinical experience in the years since then have consistently shown benefits for VATS, and gradually established the consensus that VATS gives less pain, fewer complications and shorter hospital stays [1, 3, 25]. Today, the advantages of VATS in terms of these outcome measures is so well accepted that one can argue that randomized trials comparing VATS and thoracotomy for these are probably no longer necessary [36].

Adolescence: Objective, Quantifiable Benefit

The problem with relying on pain scores, chest drain durations and lengths of stay as outcome measures was that these were subjective measurements. Many confounding variables could affect these, including differences in patient pain thresholds, the use of different analgesic regimens after surgery, variations in chest drain management and removal protocols, socio-cultural factors affecting when patients felt ready to go home, and so on [1, 37]. Hence, VATS surgeons increasingly turned to using more sophisticated, objective outcome measurements. These included, validated quality-of-life questionnaire assessments; landmarks of patient mobilization; testing of shoulder function; and so on [27, 38, 39]. Most objective of all, inflammatory cytokines and indicators of humoral and cellular immune activation were measured after surgery. A number of such studies around the turn of the century elegantly demonstrated that the systemic and physiological disruption after VATS was measurably less than after open thoracotomy [40–42]. The objectivity of these new outcome measures provided conclusive evidence for the advantages of VATS that could not be denied by the remaining sceptics.

Adulthood: Treatment Efficacy

The last hurdle for VATS was to prove the most important: it doesn't matter that VATS caused less surgical trauma than open surgery if it could not deliver equally effective treatment of the disease. It was therefore essential to show that VATS could offer equivalent completeness of resection and survival as open surgery. Yields from mediastinal lymph node dissection was the chosen parameter for comparing completeness of resection, and in this contest a series of studies pointed to equivalency for VATS and open surgery [43–45]. More importantly, a number of systematic reviews and meta-analyses in recent years have now concluded that the survival rates for early-stage lung cancer after VATS were as good as those after open thoracotomy—perhaps even slightly better [46–48]. As a results of these crucial findings, international guidelines today no longer see VATS as an 'alternative' to open surgery, but as "preferred over a thoracotomy for anatomic pulmonary resection" for stage I lung cancer [24].

The Evolution of VATS Technique

The establishment of VATS through scientific evidence is not the end of its evolution. Conventional VATS *reduced* pain but it did not *eliminate* it. Pain and chest wall paresthesia continued to afflict a significant proportion of patients after VATS [49–51]. This was most likely caused by the torquing of the video-thoracoscope and instruments at the ports during surgery, and by the placement of a chest tube that is kept for a few days after surgery [1]. To combat residual pain after VATS, the use of Gabapentin—a drug previously used to treat trigeminal and post-herpetic neuralgia—was shown to be effective in alleviating post-operative discomforts after thoracic surgery [52]. Furthermore, a randomized trial has shown that pre-incisional blockade to pre-empt nerve-mediated pain also significantly reduce post-operative pain for up to a week after VATS [53].

Nonetheless, to the VATS surgeon, it is more interesting to seek surgical solutions to reduce surgical morbidity, instead of relying on pharmaceutical 'bail outs'.

Early Three-Port VATS

The earliest descriptions of VATS lobectomy describe a 'baseball diamond' (Fig. 1). This has been previously described [1, 3]. The 10 mm camera port is at the 'home base' (typically in about the seventh or eighth intercostal space in the mid-axillary line), and the other two ports are placed at 'first base' and 'third base' positions to allow the right and left hand instruments to be placed and triangulated forwards towards the target at 'second base'. The latter two are typically an anterior 3–6 cm 'utility' incision in the fourth

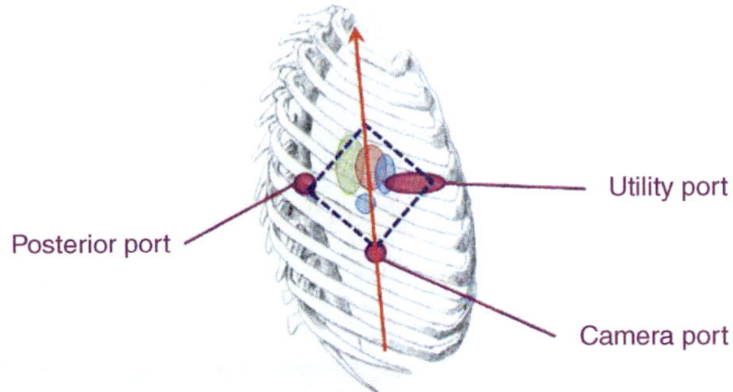

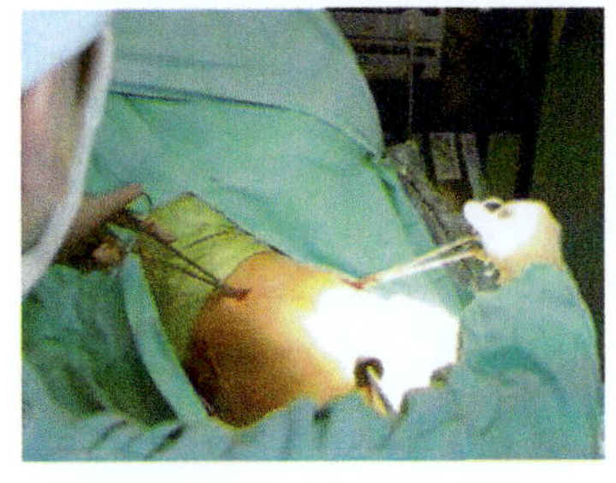

Fig. 1 The 'classic' three-port VATS lobectomy. In a right-side operation, the 'baseball diamond' (dotted blue line) has a 10 mm camera port at 'home base', a 3–5 cm utility port at 'first base', and a 10 mm posterior port at 'third base'. The axis of the operation (red arrow) is a straight line from 'home base' through the 'second base'—and in this classic early VATS approach the axis is essentially in a hip-to-head direction along the patient's body's longitudinal axis. (Reproduced with permission from [2])

or fifth intercostal space for delivery of the resected lobe, and a posterior 10 mm port just anterior the tip of the scapula for retraction or insertion of a stapler.

The imaginary straight line from the 'home base' through the 'second base' approximates the natural axis from the patient's feet towards the head. By placing the instrument ports at the 'first and third bases', the surgeon's right and left hands comfortably straddle this axis on either sides and this will minimize 'sword-fighting' between the instruments and camera.

With the classic three-port approach, the often stands on the opposite side of the operating table from the surgeon. However, this placement means that the assistant's visual axis would be completely different to the surgeon's—a key reason for 'mirror imaging' and fencing between camera and the surgeon's instruments commonly noted in the early experience with VATS.

Modified Three-Port VATS

The conventional three-port VATS approach above imagines the axis of the operation running longitudinally from the patient's feet to the head, but during an operation the surgeon actually stands anterior to the lateral-lying patient [2, 4]. Hence, the actual axis of the operation actually runs slightly diagonally in an anterior-to-posterior as well as an inferior-to-superior direction. In view of this, this author and many others actually adopt a 'modification' of the three-port strategy and place the 'home base' at the anterior rather than the mid-axillary line (Fig. 2). The posterior port was lowered from anterior to the scapula tip to a lower intercostal level. The utility port position is unchanged. The end result of this modification was a posterior rotation of the 'baseball diamond' with the axis of operation running roughly in an umbilicus-towards-shoulder direction [1, 2]. Because the posterior port is lower to properly straddle the new axis, the surgeon's arm does not have to reach as far to the posterior port, making the ergonomics of the operation more comfortable.

An upshot of this modification is that the camera-holding assistant now stands on the same side of the operating table as the surgeon and slightly behind. The assistant thus shares the same axis as the surgeon, improving surgeon-assistant co-ordination and essentially eliminating 'mirror imaging'.

Robot-Assisted Thoracic Surgery

In the early years of the Twenty-first Century, master-slave robotic surgical systems entered the surgical market in earnest, and some pioneering thoracic surgeons quickly adapted it for simple mediastinal operations, and eventually even for major lung cancer resections [54, 55]. However, early enthusiasm was later tempered by concerns over the costs of buying and maintaining the systems, purchase of expensive consumables, and use of longer operating room. The potential advantages of the robotic system in terms of 3D vision, greater intra-thoracic dexterity and steadier instrumentation were also thought by some to be negated by the loss of tactile feedback [56]. Established VATS surgeons also pointed out that the robot did not reduce the number and

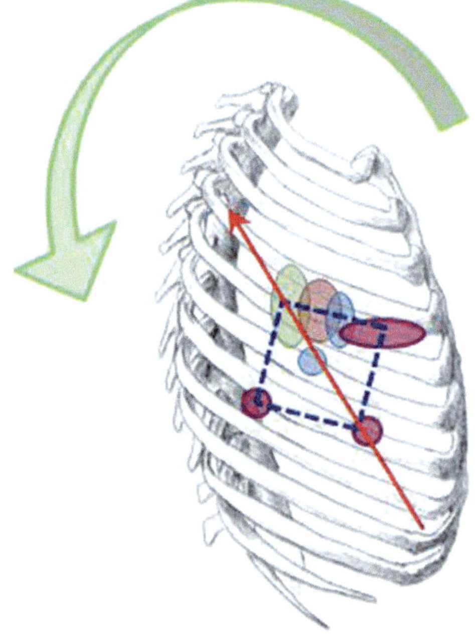

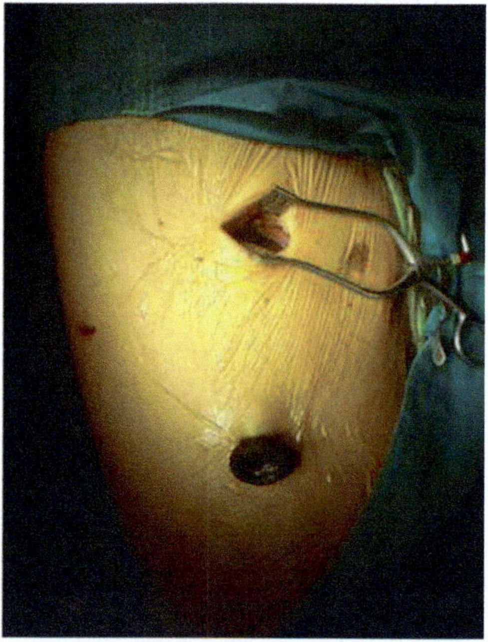

Fig. 2 The 'modified' three-port VATS lobectomy. The 'baseball diamond' (dotted blue line) and axis of the operation (red arrow) have essentially been rotated in a posterior direction—and the axis direction is now umbilicus-to-shoulder. (Reproduced with permission from [2])

sizes of the wounds as classic three-port VATS, and indeed sometimes necessitated the addition of a fourth port.

Many Thoracic Surgeons today would accept that robotics have a potentially important role to play in the future of Minimally Invasive Thoracic Surgery. However, for the present, the greatest strides seem to be made not in the import of such advanced technology, but in the refinement of technique to create the 'next generation' of VATS.

Needlescopic VATS

Thoracoscopes and instruments of only 2–5 mm diameter were first used to perform VATS sympathectomy to treat palmar hyperhidrosis and facial blushing, Raynaud's disease and reflex sympathetic dystrophy [51, 57]. This needlescopic promised even less pain and better cosmesis than conventional VATS, and was later used to treat pneumothorax [58].

In recent years, Needlescopic VATS approach has been used even for lung cancer surgery [1, 2]. The same ports placement strategy as the modified three-port strategy is used, with the posterior port reduced from 10 mm to 3 mm (Fig. 3, Video 1). The camera port begins with a 3 mm skin puncture using a no. 11 scalpel blade, and a 3 mm trocar is pushed through the puncture to admit a 3 mm 30° video-thoracoscope into the chest. Alternatively, a 5 mm 30° video-thoracoscope can be pushed directly through the skin stab without a trocar, and the lens tip cleaned inside the chest using a forceps-mounted pledget held on a curved forceps inserted via the utility port. The utility port has to remain at 3–4 cm simply because this is the minimum required to deliver the resected lobe of lung at the end of the operation. This Needlescopic VATS approach with a very thin scope means there is less torqueing by the camera in the intercostal space during the surgery and there is significantly better cosmesis compared to conventional VATS. At the same time, use of the same port sites means that the axis of operation is the same as for conventional/modified VATS, making it relatively simple for the conventional VATS surgeon to adopt.

Two-Port VATS

After gaining experience with a three-port Needlescopic VATS approach, it was soon realized that the posterior 3 mm port was not really essential useful since it only allowed a 3 mm grasper to be placed [2]. The natural progression was therefore to omit that posterior port altogether—resulting in a two-port VATS technique (Fig. 4, Video 2). The use of only one utility port for all the instrumentation requires that both instruments for the right and left hand are used coaxially via the utility incisions. However, the axis of the operation and the camera-handling by the assistant are unchanged from the conventional three-port approach, making this a simple approach to adapt for those with prior VATS experience.

Early experience confirmed that the technique was compatible with prompt recovery and short hospital stays [2]. Compared to robot-assisted surgery, Needlescopic and two-port VATS evolutions require no expensive equipment (most hospitals already have Needlescopic instruments), take no longer than conventional VATS, and can be quickly learned by experienced VATS surgeons by further honing their skills.

Uniportal VATS

Progressing from conventional three-port VATS to two-port VATS, the surgeon becomes accustomed to working with both hands' instruments via the same utility port. From there, it was merely a matter of also bringing the video-thoracoscope placed through the utility port to evolve into a Uniportal technique [2, 59]. The concept of Uniportal VATS was actually first pioneered by Dr. Gaetano Rocco for simpler intrathoracic procedures [60, 61]. It was eventually developed in

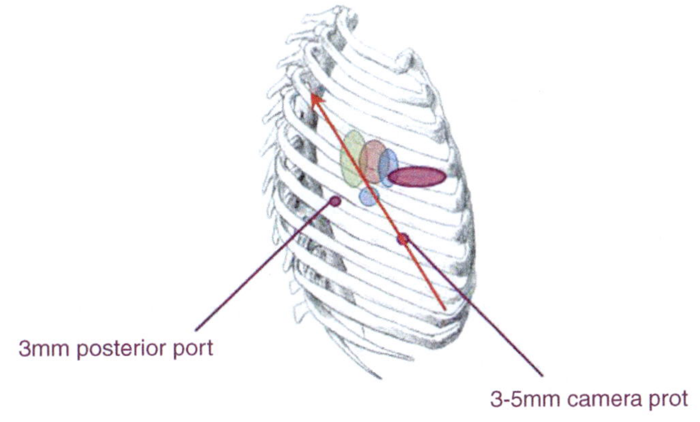

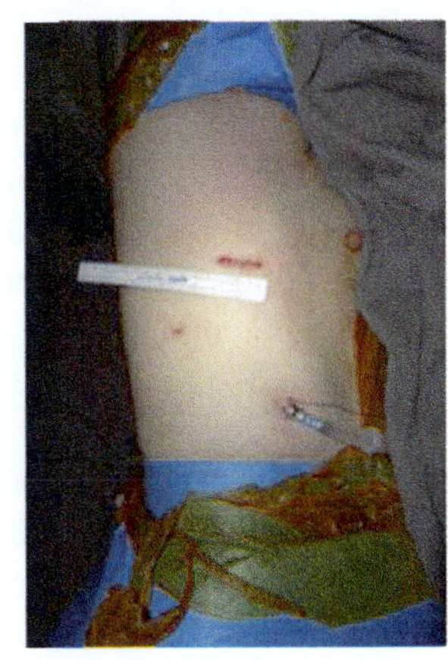

Fig. 3 The Needlescopic VATS lobectomy. The ports positions (purple) and axis of the operation (red arrow) are the same as for the 'modified' three-port VATS approach. However the posterior and camera ports have been reduced in size to 3 mm in diameter only. (Reproduced with permission from [2])

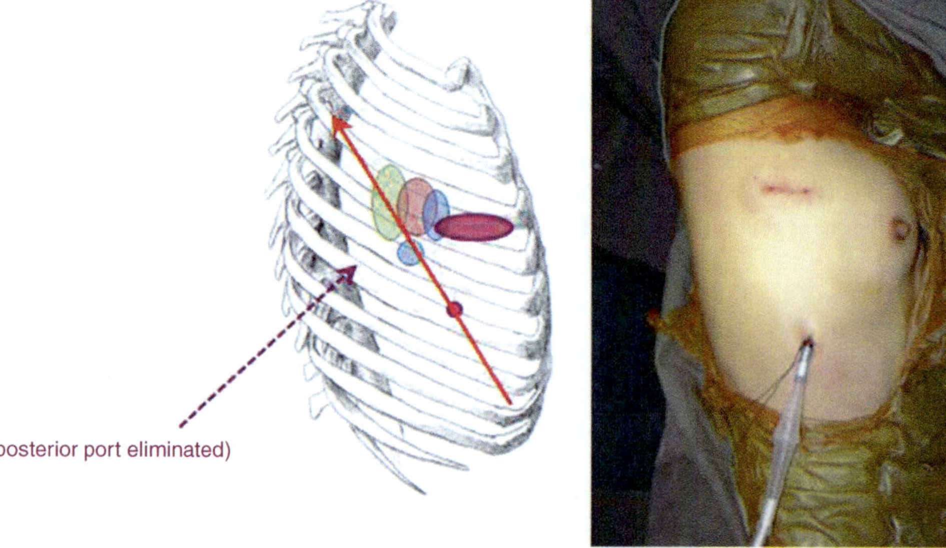

Fig. 4 The two-port VATS lobectomy. The utility and camera ports are identical to the Needlescopic approach, but the posterior port has been eliminated. (Reproduced with permission from [2])

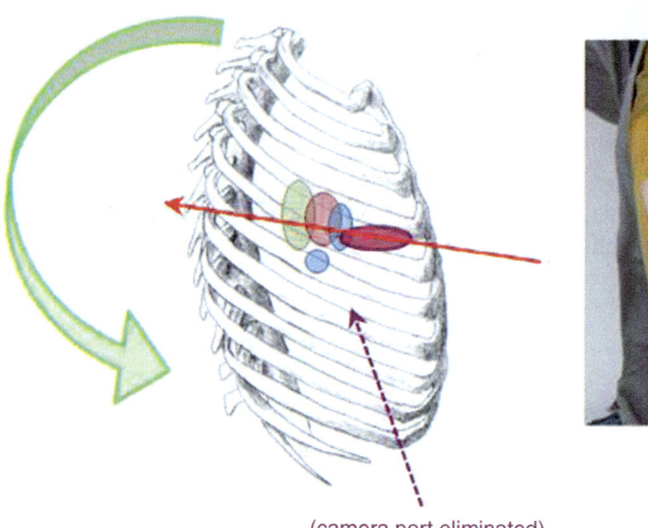

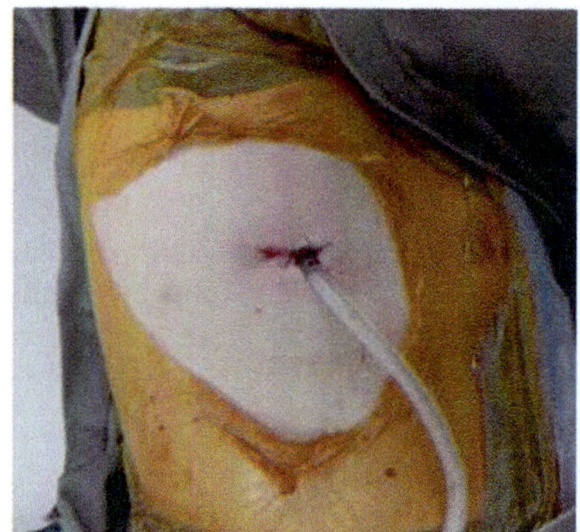

Fig. 5 The Uniportal VATS lobectomy. Compared to the two-port approach, the camera port has been eliminated. The Uniport is in the fifth intercostal space and is largely unchanged from the utility port of all previous iterations of VATS lobectomies. (Reproduced with permission from [2])

more recent years to allow major lung resections by Dr. Diego Gonzalez-Rivas of A Coruna, Spain [62, 63].

The author's technique for Uniportal VATS major lung resections has been described previously [59]. Typically, a 3–4 cm incision in the anterior axillary line in the fifth intercostal space is used (Fig. 5, Video 3). A 5 mm diameter 30° video-thoracoscope is placed coaxially with the instruments used by the surgeon's right and left hands in a 'traffic light' configuration (Fig. 6). The video-thoracoscope is kept in the uppermost 'red light' position, and the surgeon's left and right hand instruments are inserted underneath in the 'yellow' and 'green light' positions. This is the ideal configuration because a human's eyes are always above his/her hands. Compared with the three-port approach, the axis of operation during a Uniportal lobectomy is changed from an umbilicus-to-shoulder direction to a nipple-to-scapula tip direction. Consequently, the surgeon and the assistant must to some extent re-learn the hand-eye co-ordination.

Implications of Evolution on Technique

The above sequence illustrates that Uniportal VATS is a product of a gradual evolution of Minimally Invasive Thoracic Surgery: from classical three-port VATS, through Needlescopic and two-port VATS, to eventually Uniportal VATS. That this is an evolutionary—not revolutionary—process has several important implications for any surgeon learning the technique(s).

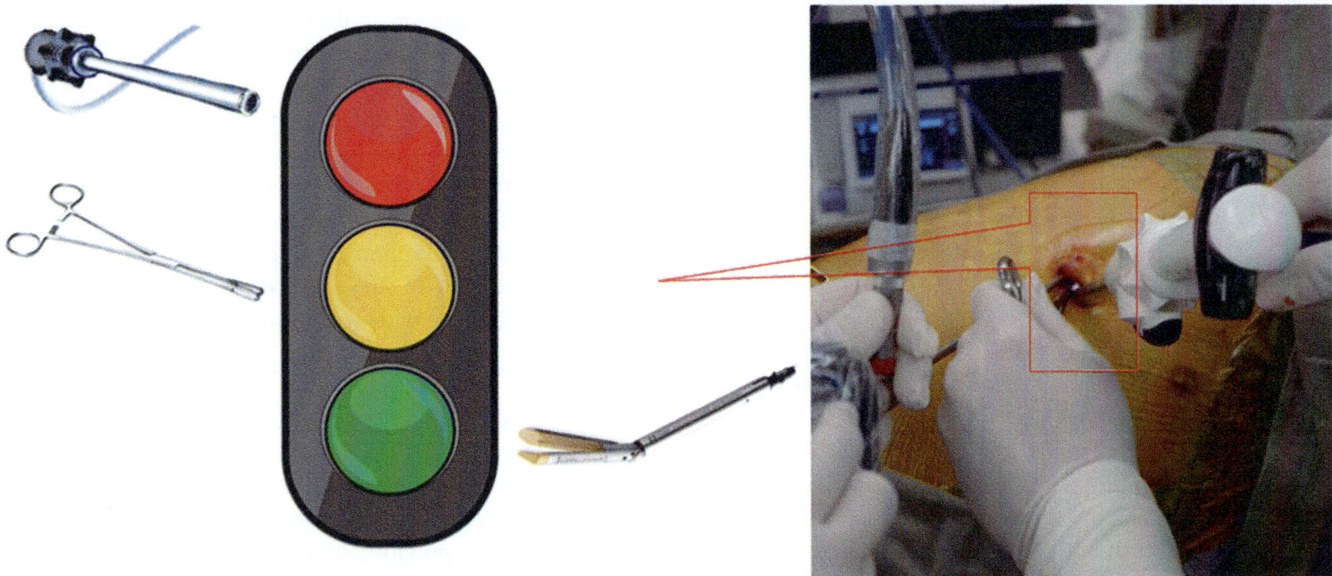

Fig. 6 Standing in front of the patient, the surgeon and assistant's view of the Uniport before them resembles a vertical slit with just enough room for the video-thoracoscope and two instruments to be inserted, one above the other. In this 'traffic light' configuration, the video-thoracoscope should be kept at the top 'red light' position, and the left and right hand instruments are inserted at the 'yellow light' and 'green light' positions. This view keeps the visualization above the level of the instruments on the monitor, just like humans have eyes above the level of the hands. Occasionally, the scope may be relocated to the 'yellow' or 'green light' positions for specific views. Using this traffic light imagery, the surgeon can verbally communicate exactly where the assistant should be placing the scope in the uniport

Step-wise Learning: Manual Skills, Then Visual

Transitioning from a conventional three-port VATS technique directly to Uniportal VATS can be challenging because the surgeon must adapt two new things: shared instrumentation through a single port *and* a new camera viewing perspective. In this author's experience, it may be easier and safer for an experienced three-port VATS surgeon to progress step-by-step through the next generation VATS approaches. First, when changing from a conventional three-port to a Needlescopic approach, the surgeon can no longer use the posterior or camera ports to admit a stapler and must learn how to apply the stapler via the utility incision only and yet access all the hilar structures for stapling. Second, on changing from a Needlescopic to a two-port approach, the surgeon must learn how to use both right and left hand instruments coaxially via the same utility incision to allow adequate retraction and safe dissection. In these first two steps, the axis of the operation and the camera port position are unchanged, so the surgeon retains the same view as with three-port VATS, eliminating visualization difficulties for both surgeon and camera assistant. Thirdly, by the time the surgeon is familiar with the two-port approach and switches to a Uniportal approach, the surgeon only needs to become accustomed to viewing the operation from a different perspective—having already acquired the manual skills for bimanual instrumentation through the same incision. Breaking the transition down into three steps means learning stapling from a single port access, coaxial instrumentation, and Uniportal visualization can be learned individually, and this potentially facilitates the adoption of Uniportal VATS for conventional VATS surgeons. This author suggests that for experienced VATS surgeons, 10–20 cases at each step may be adequate at each before moving on.

Instruments: Try Before You Buy

Because each step along the evolution is small, there is no need to radically change the instruments used along the way. Almost all the same instruments used for conventional three-port VATS—including standard Metzenbaum scissors, Debakey forceps, hand-control diathermy devices with long-tip extensions, and so on—can be used for Needlescopic VATS. Similarly, the gap between Needlescopic to two-port VATS is also so small that the transition does not necessitate a change in inventory. This proved invaluable by allowing a familiar set of instruments to be maintained without the surgeon having to learn to use new ones alongside learning a new technique. It is daunting enough to attempt a new surgical approach, and the need to simultaneously try completely new instruments at the same time can only make that more difficult (and risky). That is not to say that expensive new

'VATS' or 'Uniportal' instruments are not useful. They often do facilitate surgery considerably. However, it is perhaps easier for surgeons to learn the next step along the evolution using trusted, familiar instruments first—and then consider what new instruments to buy after initial experience reveals which specific ones may be helpful to him/her.

Coping Without the Posterior Port

With conventional three-port VATS, the posterior port allows retraction of the lung or introduction of a stapler from an alternative direction other than the utility incision. Without that posterior port in two-port and Uniportal VATS, retraction calls for more flexibility in thinking about how to retract the lung. Simply 'pulling up' the lung (as one would do in three-port VATS) can result in the wrong angle of approach for the stapler, with medial or posterior structures impeding the passage of the anvil (Fig. 7). Instead, the retraction should often be in a counter-intuitive direction away from the utility incision aim to present vessel in a direction perpendicular to stapler approach for easier stapling. Use of long curved ring forceps facilitates the maneuvering of the lung inside the chest.

When inserting a stapler straight in via the utility incision only, the anvil may impact on the structures behind and prevent satisfactory closing and firing. This is most evident when stapling upper lobe pulmonary veins. The author has described the 'Rotation Trick' to overcome this [59]. The anvil is 'engaged' at one side of the vein, and the lung is then rotated forwards and in a cephalad direction (Fig. 8). This movement opens up space behind the vein, between it and the artery behind it. At the same time, the stapler is also gently rotated clockwise so that the reticulated head is not pointing straight into the hilum, but instead towards a more cephalad direction. In this direction, the anvil can be advanced through the widened-up space behind the vein.

Troubleshooting

Because this is an evolution, if any difficulties are encountered at each step, the same solutions that the surgeon is familiar with from previous steps can still be applied just as effectively [2–4]. Some examples include:

- Bleeding: compression, topical hemostats, endoscopic suturing.
- Fused interlobar fissure: 'fissure-less' (or 'fissure *last*') approach.
- Air leaks detected on-table: endoscopic suturing, topical sealants, pleural tent, etc.
- Large tumors: anterior rib-cutting technique [64].

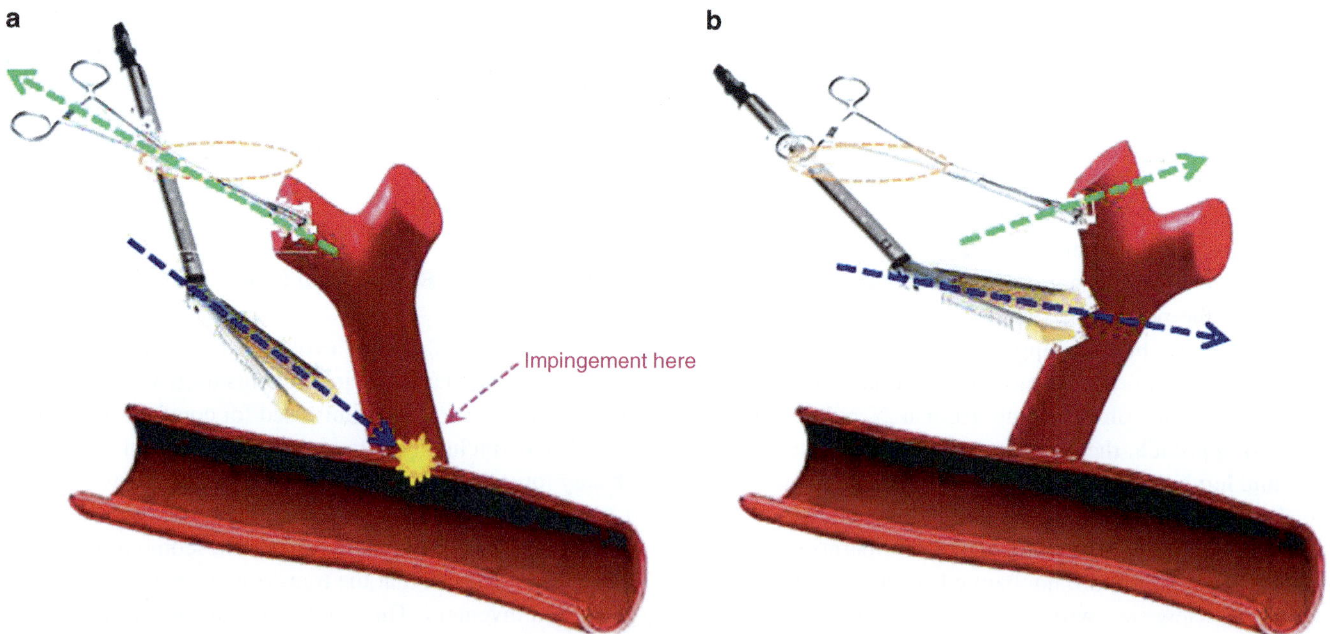

Fig. 7 Example of manoeuvring the lung to enable the correct angulation for stapling. (**a**) If the lung is simply retracted upwards (green arrow) or towards the Uniport (yellow ring), the stapler is inserted downwards near-vertically (blue arrow) and even with reticulation of the stapler head the stapler tip will impinge against the mediastinal or hilar structures, impeding passage of the stapler around the vessel branch. (**b**) If the lung is instead distracted away (green arrow) from the Uniport (yellow ring), the target vessel branch is better displayed, allowing the reticulated stapler to approach perpendicularly at a 'flatter' angle (blue arrow) and avoid impingement against any structures on the far side. (Reproduced with permission from [2])

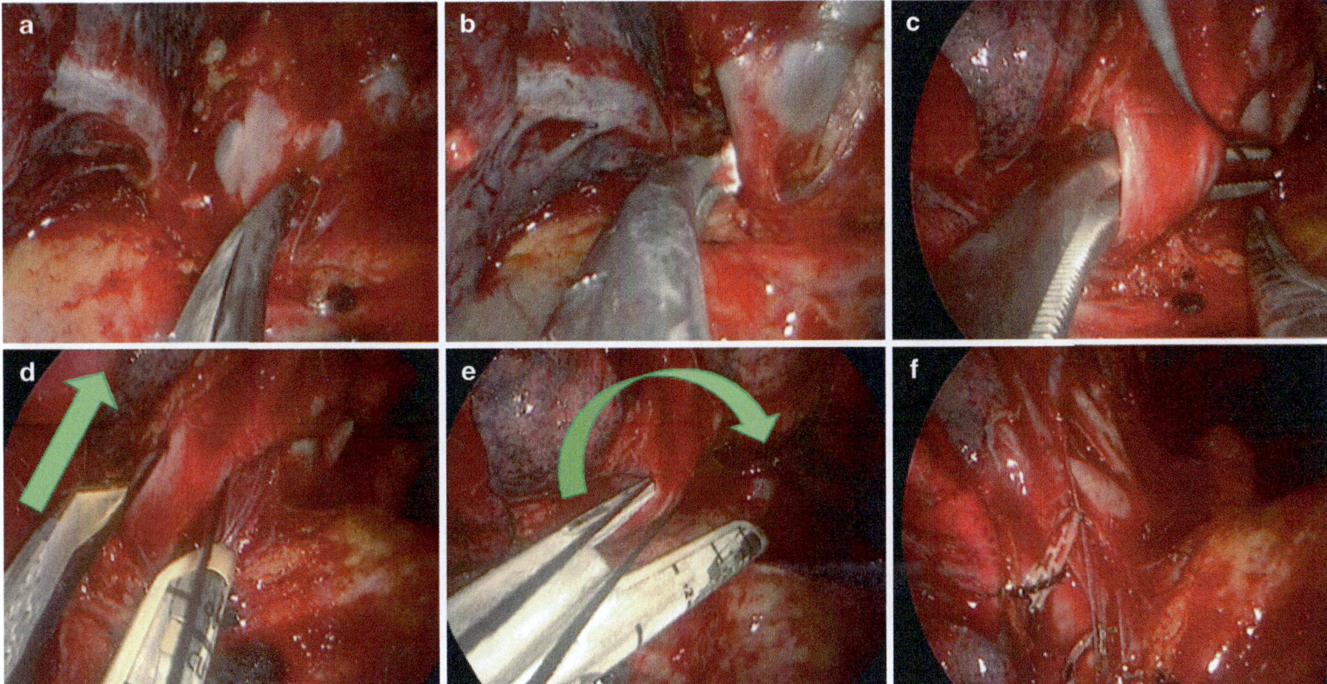

Fig. 8 Dissection of the RUL pulmonary artery truncus, illustrating the 'Rotation Trick': (**a**) The lung is retracted laterally, displaying the RUL pulmonary artery truncus running vertically up to the RUL on the monitor. Long Metzenbaum scissors are used to dissect around the truncus onto the subadventitial layer. (**b**) Blunt dissection using a Yankauer sucker allows further gentle dissection around and behind the artery. (**c**) A curved Rumel forceps is used to get around the back of the artery. It is then used to open up the space behind by gentle opening and closing, facilitating subsequent passage of the stapler. (**d**) The stapler is inserted directly towards the artery, with the thinner anvil engaging the caudal side of the vessel. Notice that if the stapler were advanced further in this direction it would be forced to stop as it impinges on the RUL bronchus behind the artery. (**e**) With the anvil engaged on the left of the artery, the lung is retracted slightly cepahald and forwards. This widens up the space behind the artery. Simultaneously, the reticulated stapler is also rotated clockwise very subtly. In this angulation, the anvil can be advanced in an anterior-to-posterior and slight caudal-to-cranial direction, and it will emerge from behind the right side of the artery no longer impinging on anything. (**f**) After the artery is divided, using the original lateral retraction of the RUL, the RUL bronchus can now be seen clearly behind where the artery once ran

Peri-operative Care

If a patient receiving a VATS procedure was nursed and rehabilitated in exactly the same way as a patient who received an open thoracotomy, the potential benefits of Minimally Invasive Surgery cannot be realized. Patients receiving any form of VATS must be managed according a bespoke Clinical Pathway if they are to fully take advantage of the reduction in surgical trauma [65, 66]. The Pathway (equivalents are also referred to as 'fast track' or 'expedited recovery' in other centers) covers every aspect of nursing, physiotherapy, mobilization schedules, peri-operative investigations, pain management, chest drain management, nutrition, communication with the family, and so on. Goals for each day are set and monitored. Using a Clinical Pathway ensures the significant benefits or VATS are realized in terms of: pre- and post-operation lengths of stay; morbidity; readmission rates; and so on [65, 66]. The implications of evolution in VATS here is that with each step of the technique evolution, the Pathway should also be updated to best complement the potential advantages.

Implications of Evolution on the Future of VATS

Trial by Evidence

It can be seen from the above that there are two processes of evolution in VATS: one is of the technique, and the other is in the assessment of the technique. For a new approach to succeed, it must undergo scrutiny by peer surgeons and the trial will be whether convincing clinical evidence can be produced to validate its use.

Previously, three-port VATS underwent such trial by evidence. Currently, the latest VATS development is Uniportal VATS, and this too must pass the trial if it is to be widely accepted. Following the stages from infancy to adulthood described above, how does the Uniportal approach fare?

A rudimentary literature search in 2015 revealed that the vast majority of publications on the Uniportal approach were still case reports and case series [25]. These have validate the feasibility and safety of the Uniportal approach for a wide range of major pulmonary resections, including complex reconstructions and in high-risk patients [63, 67, 68]. At the same time, no consistent data has emerged suggesting any compromise of patient safety when using the Uniportal approach. It is safe to say that clinical evidence for Uniportal VATS has passed the infancy stage or proving safety and feasibility.

However, when looking at the next stages of evidence—the comparative studies to show benefit—there were only a handful of limited, small studies [25]. In terms of post-operative pain, the Uniportal approach for lobectomy gave better or at least no worse outcomes than three-port VATS [69, 70]. However, studies have reported conflicting results in terms of intra-operative (operation times, nodal clearance) and post-operative outcomes (lengths of stay)—with data showing both favorable and unfavorable comparisons for Uniportal versus three-port VATS [70–73]. Clearly, evidence for Uniportal VATS has not emerged from the childhood stage of trying to demonstrate comparative benefits in the crudest outcome measures. No good evidence has yet emerged for Uniportal VATS in the adolescent and adult stages. From this, one can conclude that at the time of this writing, there is enough evidence to say that Uniportal VATS *can* be performed, but not enough to say that it *should* be performed in every patient.

Given that the evolution of VATS is an ongoing process, it is inevitable that each next step 'forwards' in technique must undergo the same trial by evidence. Those steps that pass may be accepted in the way three-port VATS is today. Those that fail may become discarded.

Training in VATS

Because VATS is constantly evolving, there is strictly speaking no one single technique of VATS [1]. Considerable variations exist within the practice of conventional three-port VATS, and the 'next generation' VATS approaches above represent even greater variability. For the thoracic surgeon, VATS is such a moving target that it is hard to say where he/she should aim for in terms of training.

There are proponents of 'jumping in at the deep end' and proceeding immediately from open surgery to Uniportal VATS [74, 75]. There is no reason to argue against this when training takes place at expert centers under the tutelage of highly experienced Uniportal surgeons [75].

As noted above, this author suggests that for surgeons familiar with conventional three-port VATS, it may be easier (though not essential) for take a step-wise approach when learning to perform Uniportal VATS. The first step is to familiarize oneself with applying the stapler only via the utility port (as occurs with Needlescopic VATS). The second is to acquire the skill of coaxial instrumentation via the single utility port only (as in two-port VATS). The third step is to then learn the new views when the camera is brought up and inserted via the single port in Uniportal VATS. There are a few good reasons to consider this step-wise approach. First, as said above, It is easier for the conventional VATS surgeon—and safer for the patient—to learn one skill at a time. Second, it allows the entire surgical team (including assistants, anesthetists and nurses) to also learn one step at a time, minimizing anxiety and possible error. Thirdly, during the transition, the surgeon may feel comfortable enough with the Needlescopic or two-port VATS technique that it is felt the final transition to Uniportal VATS is unnecessary. Surgeons should be reminded that there is as yet insufficient evidence to conclude that Uniportal VATS is necessarily 'superior' to the other VATS approaches [25]. Surgeons should therefore not feel pressured now to adopt Uniportal VATS, and rest assured that settling with Needlescopic or two-port VATS will not give inferior outcomes.

Technology and Technique

With each step in the evolution of the VATS technique, there is an expectation of potentially improved outcomes for the patients. This is counter-balanced by the reality of increased demand on the surgeon because of greater technical difficulty. As one evolves further, the law of diminishing returns applies: the increased difficulty is not reciprocated by a proportionate increase in patient benefit [25]. When going from open thoracotomy to conventional three-port VATS, the benefit was large because of the morbidity posed by open surgery [1]. However, when evolving from three-ports to two-ports to Uniportal, it becomes hard to demonstrate substantially more improvement because the morbidity from three-ports is already so low.

On this basis, it is easy for a surgeon to declare that he/she has no interest to evolve his/her technique further. However, this complacency is short-sighted and underestimates the power of human innovation. Every so often, a new disruptive technology emerges that resets the diminishing returns curve, allowing more benefits to be realized from greater investment of surgeon effort. In the past, just when thoracotomy reached its peak, the introduction of surgical video systems allowed the birth of VATS. When early VATS surgeons were preparing to accept that VATS was only useful for simple biopsy procedures, the arrival of endoscopic staplers allowed the progression into the realms of major, complex lung resections by VATS. Today, the emergence of Uniportal VATS appears to be the pinnacle of minimally invasive surgery in the chest—and may not even seem to be worth the extra effort over three-port VATS. However, that is merely turning a blind eye to exciting new technology advances that may be only months to a few years again, and which could radically realize the full potential of Uniportal VATS. These could include: wireless steerable endoscopy devices; natural orifice transluminal endoscopic surgery (NOTES) platforms for the chest; and new robotic surgery systems designed for Uniportal access [76].

The modern surgeon should anticipate the emergence of such new disruptive technologies, and prepare for them rather than belatedly react to them. One reason to stay ahead of the VATS evolution is to master the newer techniques so that when the technology arrives, one is already in a position to safely incorporate into surgical practice it to benefit patients. In the fable of the ant and the grasshopper, it is the ant who anticipates and prepares for the future that ultimately fares best when the future (winter) arrives. Similarly, surgery requires pioneers willing to seek out the next step of the evolution to guarantee its future relevance to patients. Today, one has Uniportal VATS—but who will look for the next breakthrough to take advantage of future technologies as they emerge?

Conclusion

Although this book celebrates the Uniportal VATS approach, it is important to appreciate it in the context of the evolution of VATS. Evolution teaches us that past lessons from the rise of conventional three-port VATS will dictate how best to develop clinical evidence to establish the Uniportal approach today. Evolution shows how best to learn, perform and teach 'next generation' VATS techniques safely and effectively. Evolution reminds us that Uniportal VATS is not a destination, but merely a step along the never-ending journey in search of better patient outcomes.

Acknowledgements The author wishes to thank Dr. Stephen Wang and the AME Publishing Company for technical support and permission to reproduce Figs. 1, 2, 3, 4, 5 and 7 from the *Journal of Thoracic Disease*.

References

1. Sihoe ADL. The evolution of VATS lobectomy. In: Cardoso P, editor. Topics in thoracic surgery. Rijeka: Intech; 2011. p. 181–210.
2. Sihoe ADL. The evolution of minimally invasive thoracic surgery: implications for the practice of uniportal thoracoscopic surgery. J Thorac Dis. 2014;6(Suppl 6):S604–17. https://doi.org/10.3978/j.issn.2072-1439.2014.08.52.
3. Sihoe ADL, Yim APC. Video-assisted pulmonary resections. In: Patterson GA, Cooper JD, Deslauriers J, Lerut AEMR, Luketich JD, Rice TW, Pearson FG, editors. Thoracic surgery. 3rd ed. Philadelphia: Elsevier; 2008. p. 970–88.
4. Sihoe ADL, Yim APC. VATS as a diagnostic tool. In: Shields TW, Locicero J, Ponn RB, Rusch VW, editors. General thoracic surgery. 7th ed. Philadelphia: Lippincott Williams & Wilkins; 2009. p. 313–32.
5. Braimbridge MV. Thoracoscopy: a historical perspective. In: Yim APC, Hazelrigg SR, Izzat MB, et al., editors. Minimal access cardiothoracic surgery. Philadelphia: WB Saunders; 2000. p. 1–10.
6. Karmakar MK, Ho AMH. Postthoracotomy pain syndrome. Thorac Surg Clin. 2004;14:345–52.
7. Rogers ML, Duffy JP. Surgical aspects of chronic post-thoracotomy pain. Eur J Cardiothorac Surg. 2000;18:711–6.
8. Lewis RJ. Simultaneously stapled lobectomy: a safe technique for video-assisted thoracic surgery. J Thorac Cardiovasc Surg. 1995;109:619–25.
9. Lewis RJ, Caccavale RJ, Sisler GE, et al. One hundred consecutive patients undergoing video-assisted thoracic operations. Ann Thorac Surg. 1992;54:421–6.
10. Lewis RJ, Caccavale RJ. Video-assisted thoracic surgical non-rib-spreading simultaneously stapled lobectomy. In: Yim APC, Hazelrigg SR, Izzat MB, et al., editors. Minimal access cardiothoracic surgery. Philadelphia: WB Saunders; 2000. p. 135–49.
11. Pearson FG. Commentary. In: Yim APC, Hazelrigg SR, Izzat MB, et al., editors. Minimal access cardiothoracic surgery. Philadelphia: WB Saunders; 2000. p. 151.
12. Kirby TJ, Mack MJ, Landreneau RJ, et al. Initial experience with video-assisted thoracoscopic lobectomy. Ann Thorac Surg. 1993;56:1248–53.
13. McKenna RJ. Lobectomy by video-assisted thoracic surgery with mediastinal node sampling for lung cancer. J Thorac Cardiovasc Surg. 1994;107:879–82.
14. Roviaro CG, Varoli F, Rebuffat C, et al. Videothoracoscopic major pulmonary resections. Ann Thorac Surg. 1993;56:779–83.
15. Yim APC, Ko KM, Chau WS, et al. Video-assisted thoracoscopic anatomic lung resections: the initial Hong Kong experience. Chest. 1996;109:13–7.
16. Sugiura H, Morikawa T, Kaji M, et al. Long-term benefits for the quality of life after video-assisted thoracoscopic lobectomy in patients with lung cancer. Surg Laparosc Endosc. 1999;9:403–8.
17. Walker WS, Pugh GC, Craig SR, Carnochan FM. Continued experience with thoracoscopic major pulmonary resection. Int Surg. 1996;81:255–8.
18. Demmy TL, Curtis JJ. Minimally invasion lobectomy directed toward frail and high-risk patients: a case control study. Ann Thorac Surg. 1999;68:194–200.
19. Giudicelli R, Thomas P, Lonjon T, et al. Video-assisted minithoracotomy versus muscle sparing thoracotomy for performing lobectomy. Ann Thorac Surg. 1994;58:712–8.
20. Kirby TJ, Mack MJ, Landreneau RJ, Rice TW. Lobectomy video-assisted thoracic surgery versus muscle-sparing thoracotomy: a randomized trial. J Thorac Cardiovasc Surg. 1995;109:997–1002.
21. Landreneau RJ, Mack MJ, Hazelrigg SR, et al. Prevalence of chronic pain after pulmonary resection by thoracotomy or video-assisted thoracic surgery. J Thorac Cardiovasc Surg. 1994;107:1079–86.
22. Nomori H, Horio H, Naruke T, Suemasu K. What is the advantage of a thoracoscopic lobectomy over a limited thoracotomy procedure for lung cancer surgery? Ann Thorac Surg. 2001;72:879–84.
23. Mack MJ, Scruggs GR, Kelly KM, et al. Video-assisted thoracic surgery: has technology found its place? Ann Thorac Surg. 1997;64:211–5.
24. Howington JA, Blum MG, Chang AC, Balekian AA, Murthy SC. Treatment of stage I and II non-small cell lung cancer: diagnosis and management of lung cancer, 3rd ed: American College of Chest Physicians evidence-based clinical practice guidelines. Chest. 2013;143:e278S–313S.
25. Sihoe DLA. Reasons not to perform uniportal VATS lobectomy. J Thorac Dis. 2016a;8:S333–43.
26. Yim APC, Landreneau RJ, Izzat MB, Fung ALK. Is video assisted thoracoscopic lobectomy a unified approach? Ann Thorac Surg. 1998;66:1155–8.
27. Shigemura N, Akashi A, Nakagiri T, Ohta M, Matsuda H. Complete vs assisted thoracoscopic approach. A prospective randomized trial comparing a variety of video-assisted thoracoscopic lobectomy techniques. Surg Endosc. 2004;18:1492–7.

28. Shigemura N, Akashi A, Funaki S, Nakagiri T, Inoue M, Sawabata N, Shiono H, Minami M, Takeuchi Y, Okumura M, Sawa Y. Long-term outcomes after a variety of video-assisted thoracoscopic lobectomy approaches for clinical stage IA lung cancer: a multi-institutional study. J Thorac Cardiovasc Surg. 2006;132:507–12.
29. Swanson SJ, Herndon JE 2nd, D'Amico TA, et al. Videoassisted thoracic surgery lobectomy: report of CALGB 39802-a prospective, multi-institution feasibility study. J Clin Oncol. 2007;25:4993–7.
30. Laird MA, Gidal BE. Use of gabapentin in the treatment of neuropathic pain. Ann Pharmacother. 2000;34:802–7.
31. Nicholson B. Gabapentin use in neuropathic pain syndromes. Acta Neurol Scand. 2000;101:359–71.
32. Benedetti F, Vighetti S, Ricco C, Amanzio M, Bergamasco L, Casadio C, Cianci R, Giobbe R, Oliaro A, Bergamasco B, Maggi G. Neuorphysiologic assessment of nerve impairment in posterolateral and muscle-sparing thoracotomy. J Thorac Cardiovasc Surg. 1998;115:841–7.
33. Bolotin G, Buckner GD, Jardine NJ, Kiefer AJ, Campbell NB, Kocherginsky M, Raman J, Jeevanandam V. A novel instrumented retractor to monitor tissue-disruptive forces during lateral thoracotomy. J Thorac Cardiovasc Surg. 2007;133:949–54.
34. Maguire MF, Latter JA, Mahajan R, David Beggs F, Duffy JP. A study exploring the role of intercostal nerve damage in chronic pain after thoracic surgery. Eur J Cardiothorac Surg. 2006;29:873–9.
35. Rogers ML, Henderson L, Duffy JP. Preliminary findings of a neurophysiological assessment of intercostal nerve injury during thoracotomy. Eur J Cardiothorac Surg. 2002;21:298–301.
36. D'Amico TA. Thoracoscopic lobectomy: evolving and improving. J Thorac Cardiovasc Surg. 2006a;132:464–5.
37. Bachiocco V, Morselli-Labate AM, Rusticali AG, Bragaglia R, Mastrorilli M, Carli G. Intensity, latency and duration of post-thoracotomy pain: relationship to personality trials. Funct Neurol. 1990;5:321–32.
38. Li WWL, Lee TW, Lam SSY, Ng CSH, Sihoe ADL, Wan IYP, Yim APC. Quality of life following lung cancer resection: video-assisted thoracic surgery versus thoracotomy. Chest. 2002;122:584–9.
39. Li WW, Lee RL, Lee TW, Ng CS, Sihoe AD, Wan IY, Arifi AA, Yim AP. The impact of thoracic surgical access on early shoulder function: video-assisted thoracic surgery versus posterolateral thoracotomy. Eur J Cardiothorac Surg. 2003;23:390–6.
40. Craig SR, Leaver HA, Yap PL, et al. Acute phase responses following minimal access and conventional thoracic surgery. Eur J Cardiothorac Surg. 2001;20:455–63.
41. Ng CS, Lee TW, Wan S, Wan IY, Sihoe ADL, Arifi AA, Yim AP. Thoracotomy is associated with significantly more profound suppression in lymphocytes and natural killer cells than video-assisted thoracic surgery following major lung resections for cancer. J Investig Surg. 2005;18:81–8.
42. Yim APC, Wan S, Lee TW, Arifi AA. VATS lobectomy reduces cytokine responses compared with conventional surgery. Ann Thorac Surg. 2000;70:243–7.
43. Denlinger CE, Fernandez F, Meyers BF, et al. Lymph node evaluation in video-assisted thoracoscopic lobectomy versus lobectomy by thoracotomy. Ann Thorac Surg. 2010;89:1730–6.
44. Sagawa M, Sato M, Sakurada A, et al. A prospective trial of systematic nodal dissection for lung cancer by video-assisted thoracic surgery: can it be perfect? Ann Thorac Surg. 2002;73:900–4.
45. Watanabe A, Koyanagi T, Ohsawa H, et al. Systematic node dissection by VATS is not inferior to that through an open thoracotomy: a comparative clinicopathologic retrospective study. Surgery. 2005;138:510–7.
46. Rueth NM, Andrade RS. Is VATS lobectomy better: perioperatively, biologically and oncologically? Ann Thorac Surg. 2010;89:S2107–11.
47. Whitson BA, Groth SS, Duval SJ, Swanson SJ, Maddaus MA. Surgery for early-stage non-small cell lung cancer: a systematic review of the video-assisted thoracoscopic surgery versus thoracotomy approaches to lobectomy. Ann Thorac Surg. 2008;86:2008–18.
48. Yan TD, Black D, Bannon PG, McCaughan BC. Systematic review and meta-analysis of randomized and nonrandomized trials on safety and efficacy of video-assisted thoracic surgery lobectomy for early-stage non-small-cell lung cancer. J Clin Oncol. 2009;27:2553–62.
49. Passlick B, Born C, Sienel W, Thetter O. Incidence of chronic pain after minimal invasive surgery for spontaneous pneumothorax. Eur J Cardiothorac Surg. 2001;19:355–9.
50. Sihoe ADL, Au SS, Cheung ML, Chow IK, Chu KM, Law CY, Wan M, Yim APC. Incidence of chest wall paresthesia after video-assisted thoracic surgery for primary spontaneous pneumothorax. Eur J Cardiothorac Surg. 2004;25:1054–8.
51. Sihoe ADL, Cheung CS, Lai HK, Lee TW, Thung KH, Yim APC. Incidence of chest wall paresthesia after needlescopic video-assisted thoracic surgery for palmar hyperhidrosis. Eur J Cardiothorac Surg. 2005;27:313–9.
52. Sihoe AD, Lee TW, Wan IY, Thung KH, Yim AP. The use of gabapentin for post-operative and post-traumatic pain in thoracic surgery patients. Eur J Cardiothorac Surg. 2006;29:795–9.
53. Sihoe AD, Manlulu AV, Lee TW, Thung KH, Yim AP. Pre-emptive local anesthesia for needlescopic video-assisted thoracic surgery: a randomised controlled trial. Eur J Cardiothorac Surg. 2007;31:103–8.
54. Melfi FM, Menconi GF, Mariani AM, et al. Early experience with robotic technology for thoracoscopic surgery. Eur J Cardiothorac Surg. 2002;21:864–8.
55. Veronesi G, Galetta D, Maisonneuve P, Melfi F, Schmid RA, Borri A, et al. Four-arm robotic lobectomy for the treatment of early-stage lung cancer. J Thorac Cardiovasc Surg. 2010;140:19–25.
56. D'Amico TA. Robotics in thoracic surgery: applications and outcomes. J Thorac Cardiovasc Surg. 2006b;131:19–20.
57. Yim APC, Sihoe ADL, Lee TW, Arifi AA. A simple maneuver to detect airleak on-table following 'needlescopic' VATS. J Thorac Cardiovasc Surg. 2002;124:1029–30.
58. Sihoe ADL, Yu PA, Wong JCC, Lee KM, Heung TCY, Ho TSY. Needlescopic video-assisted thoracic surgery for primary spontaneous pneumothorax. Respirology. 2012;17(Suppl 2):17–24.
59. Sihoe DLA. Uniportal videoassisted thoracic surgery (VATS) lobectomy. Ann Cardiothorac Surg. 2016b;5:133–44.
60. Jutley RS, Khalil MW, Rocco G. Uniportal vs standard three-port VATS technique for spontaneous pneumothorax: comparison of post-operative pain and residual paraesthesia. Eur J Cardiothorac Surg. 2005;28:43–6.
61. Rocco G, Khalil M, Jutley R. Uniportal video-assisted thoracoscopic surgery wedge lung biopsy in the diagnosis of interstitial lung diseases. J Thorac Cardiovasc Surg. 2005;129:947–8.
62. Gonzalez D, Paradela M, Garcia J, de la Torre M. Single-port video-assisted thoracoscopic lobectomy. Interact Cardiovasc Thorac Surg. 2011;12:514–5.
63. Gonzalez-Rivas D, Delgado M, Fieira E, Mendez L. Single-port video-assisted thoracoscopic lobectomy with pulmonary artery reconstruction. Interact Cardiovasc Thorac Surg. 2013a;17:889–91.
64. Sihoe AD, Chawla S, Paul S, Nair A, Lee J, Yin K. Technique for delivering large tumors in video-assisted thoracoscopic lobectomy. Asian Cardiovasc Thorac Ann. 2014;22:319–28.
65. Sihoe DLA. Clinical pathway for videoassisted thoracic surgery: the Hong Kong story. J Thorac Dis. 2016c;8:S1222.
66. Sihoe DLA, Yu SYP, Kam TH, Lee SY, Liu X. Adherence to a clinical pathway for videoassisted thoracic surgery: predictors and clinical importance. Innovations. 2016;11:179–86.
67. Gonzalez-Rivas D, Paradela M, Fernandez R, Delgado M, Fieira E, Mendez L, et al. Uniportal video-assisted thoracoscopic lobectomy: two years of experience. Ann Thorac Surg. 2013b;95:426–32.

68. Gonzalez-Rivas D, Fieira E, Delgado M, Mendez L, Fernandez R, de la Torre M. Is uniportal thoracoscopic surgery a feasible approach for advanced stages of non-small cell lung cancer? J Thorac Dis. 2014;6:641–8.
69. Hirai K, Takeuchi S, Usuda J. Single-incision thoracoscopic surgery and conventional video-assisted thoracoscopic surgery: a retrospective comparative study of perioperative clinical outcomes. Eur J Cardiothorac Surg. 2016;49:i37–41.
70. Zhu Y, Liang M, Wu W, Zheng J, Zheng W, Guo Z, Zheng B, Xu G, Chen C. Preliminary results of single-port versus triple-port complete thoracoscopic lobectomy for non-small cell lung cancer. Ann Translat Med. 2015;3(7):92. https://doi.org/10.3978/j.issn.2305-5839.2015.03.47.
71. Liu CC, Shih CS, Pennarun N, Cheng CT. Transition from a multiport technique to a single-port technique for lung cancer surgery: is lymph node dissection inferior using the single-port technique? Eur J Cardiothorac Surg. 2016;49:i64–72.
72. Mu JW, Gao SG, Xue Q, Zhao J, Li N, Yang K, Su K, Yuan ZY, He J. A matched comparison study of uniportal versus triportal thoracoscopic lobectomy and sublobectomy for early-stage nonsmall cell lung cancer. Chin Med J. 2015;128:2731–5.
73. Wang BY, Liu CY, Hsu PK, Shih CS, Liu CC. Single-incision versus multiple-incision thoracoscopic lobectomy and segmentectomy: a propensity-matched analysis. Ann Surg. 2015;261:793–9.
74. Guido Guerrero W, Gonzalez-Rivas D, Hernandez Arenas LA, et al. Techniques and difficulties dealing with hilar and interlobar benign lymphadenopathy in uniportal VATS. J Visc Surg. 2016;2:23.
75. Sihoe DLA. Opportunities and challenges for thoracic surgery collaborations in China: a commentary. J Thorac Dis. 2016d;8:S414–26.
76. Li Z, Ng CS. Future of uniportal video-assisted thoracoscopic surgery—emerging technology. Ann Cardiothorac Surg. 2016;5(2):127–32. https://doi.org/10.21037/acs.2016.02.02.

The New Era of Uniportal VATS

Peter Sze Yuen Yu and Calvin S. H. Ng

Introduction

Since its advent in the early twenty-first century, uniportal VATS has expanded its utility from simple procedures (such as thoracic sympathectomy, pleural deloculations, mediastinal biopsies, pneumothorax, and wedge resections) [1–4] to major lung resections [5, 6]. For over a decade, this technique has become in vogue as surgeons gradually overcome the technical challenges, and perceived its potential benefits for patients in terms of reduced access trauma and postoperative discomfort, reduced chest wall pain and paresthesia, and quicker recovery [7].

The extension of application of uniportal VATS to major lung resection does not mark the end of its growth. In fact, it is the beginning of all the continuous development of various technologies which make uniportal VATS easier (e.g. scope technologies, instrument design). The single incision also fostered the application and evolution of novel surgical approaches (e.g. subxiphoid approach, image-guided VATS, natural orifice transluminal endoscopic surgery) in a pace more rapid than ever before (Fig. 1).

What Made Uniportal VATS Easier

Scope Technologies

Quality of image by the thoracoscope is important as in every endoscopic surgery. Quality of visualization is further improved with the 3-dimensional imaging of intrathoracic structures using a double lens binocular system. It allows natural 3D vision and better depth perception, facilitating faster and more accurate grasping, suturing, and dissection during surgery [8].

The classical thoracoscope used in VATS has the rigid rod lens design with a beveled tip which defines the viewing angle. The field of view can only be modified by steering the endoscope shaft, and this is an important cause of instrumental fencing in the single narrow working channel where all instruments pass through in nearly the same direction. It is important to visualize the whole pleural cavity with unparalleled vision, and avoid torqueing scope at the incision site. One of the way is to use the wide-angled rigid thoracoscope (Endocameleon, Karl Storz, Germany), which allows vision between 0° and 120° through a rotating prism mechanism at the tip. Alternatively, the distal tip of the scope can be made flexible to change the field of view without moving the shaft of the scope [9]. An early example brought into use is the EndoEye [Olympus, Tokyo, Japan] which has a flexible tip able to angulate to over 100°. Furthermore, the developing Cardioscope [10] added in an adjustable length to its flexible tip section, providing even a higher flexibility of the field of vision.

But ideally, the instrumental fencing of the working space should be minimized if the scope does not occupy the space. The currently-developing remote wireless steerable endoscope is a potential solution. It is placed into the thorax via the single port and magnetically anchored to the internal thoracic wall at the beginning of operation. The image signal is transmitted to the monitor, and the field of vision is modified by remotely controlling the scope. This technology can reduce the occupancy of the thoracic cavity by the scope, and reduce the uniportal incision size [11].

Instrumental Design

Manipulation via a small single incision is greatly facilitated by the evolutionary modifications of the thoracoscopic instruments [4]. As the angle for passage of endostapler is

P. S. Y. Yu · C. S. H. Ng (✉)
Division of Cardiothoracic Surgery, Department of Surgery, Prince of Wales Hospital, The Chinese University of Hong Kong, Hong Kong SAR, China
e-mail: calvinng@surgery.cuhk.edu.hk

D. Gonzalez-Rivas et al. (eds.), *Atlas of Uniportal Video Assisted Thoracic Surgery*,
https://doi.org/10.1007/978-981-13-2604-2_2

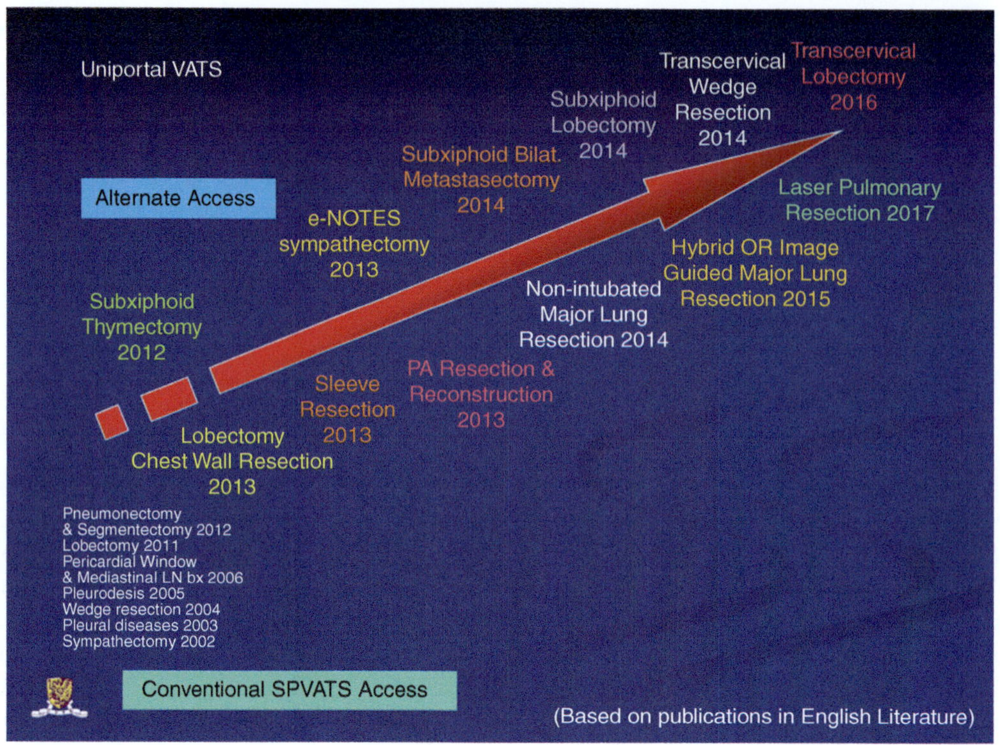

Fig. 1 A chronological chart illustrating some of the developments in Uniportal VATS over the past decade and a half. (Modified from Ng CSH. Uniportal video assisted thoracic surgery—a look into the future. *Eur J Cardiothorac Surg*. 2016 Jan;48(S1):i1–i2)

often more acute than the conventional VATS, stapling of hilar structures via single incision is more challenging. Endostapler modifications have at least in part addressed these difficulties, by having 'curved tip' staple end which allows the staple to pass through narrow gaps and at more acute angles. The electrically driven endostaplers (Powered Echelon Flex [Ethicon, Johnson & Johnson, New Brunswick, NJ, USA]; and Signia Tri-staple [Covidien, Mansfield, MA, USA]) add stability to stapling and hence more secure stapling line, as stapler movement during firing can be reduced, to decrease movement disturbance of the stapler to the other instruments which are often in very close proximity. Designing narrower staplers by reducing the number of rows for metallic staples [ECHELON FLEX™ PVS, Ethicon, Johnson & Johnson, New Brunswick, NJ, USA] further pushes the balance between haemostasis and surgeons' comfort and control [12]. Allowing a stapler to have larger range of angulation [MicroCutter XCHANGE 30, Cardica Inc., Redwood City, CA, USA] can potentially allow surgery through a smaller incision with larger degrees of freedom for stapling.

The VATS-specific instruments accommodating the small incision of uniportal VATS have also expanded rapidly. In one example, the Scanlan instruments [Scanlan, Minnesota, MN, USA] redeveloped their double-hinged VATS instruments into more narrow-shafted designs, which are particularly useful for patients with small stature and narrower rib space, as well as during uniportal VATS when instrument crowding can occur. Instruments with curved or mobile shaft [Karl Storz, Tuttlingen, Germany] also facilitate the reach within the thorax particularly for anterior chest wall adhesiolysis, and reduce instrument fencing.

To further reduce access incision size, other forms of energy for lung resection with haemo- and pneumostatic properties are under investigation. Laser resection of small peripheral lung nodules has recently been reported to be safe and feasible method to replace the space-occupying endostapler, achieving satisfactory haemostasis and pneumostasis [13]. Replacement of the endostapler with a finer instrument may potentially reduce instrumental fencing at the single port wound.

Image-Guided VATS for Tiny Pulmonary Nodules

Diagnostic challenge for subcentimeter, soft and deep pulmonary nodules is greater with uniportal VATS due to limited access and increased instrumental fencing with the palpating finger for localization of the lung nodule. Various adjuncts, such as hookwire, dye marking, microcoil implantation etc., were described to aid the intraoperative localization [9]. However, the interdepartmental transfer time between the localization procedure and the VATS operation may increase the risk of hookwire dislodgement, dye dispersing, or progression of pneumothorax or haemothorax that may endanger the patient. Nowadays all these diagnostic adjuncts can be immediately followed by uniportal VATS lung resection in the same operation setting if they are performed in the hybrid operating theatre [14], which comprises an imaging C-arm for real-time cone beam CT scanning, a conventional operating table, and a radiology control room for real-time image reconstruction to guide the placement of hookwire [15, 16] or microcoils, and entry of navigational bronchoscope [17]. Should the lesion be found to be suboptimally localized, the real-time imaging can be implemented on the table to relocalize the lesion. With the future development of radiolucent instruments, thoracic imaging and image-guided uniportal VATS may be performed simultaneously in the hybrid theatre, further improving resection accuracy and safety.

What Has Been Made Possible by Uniportal VATS?

Non-intubated VATS Lung Resection

Uniportal VATS involves only one intercostal space, therefore is less demanding on local or regional anaesthetic techniques. Nonintubated uniportal VATS, first described for major lung resection in 2014 [18], is a further less invasive version of uniportal VATS [19]. It can avoid the perioperative morbidity from the effect of general anesthesia and one-lung mechanical ventilation, while having safety similar to conventional VATS lung resection under general anaesthesia [20]. Also, it allowed a fast-track postoperative recovery. During the procedure, patient was sedated with oxygenation via nasal cannulae or face mask. Paravertebral blockade or intercostal infiltration under thoracoscopic view were performed as regional pain control. Intraoperative vagus blockade is needed to suppress coughing when performing lung traction and manipulation of hilar structures. As intraoperative conversion may be necessary, non-intubated VATS must be performed by experienced thoracic surgeons (with experience in complex cases and complication management) and anaesthesiologist (with ability to perform bronchoscopic intubation, placing a double-lumen tube or an endobronchial blocker in a lateral decubitus position).

Alternative Surgical Access

Intercostal incision inadvertently causes nerve injury causing postoperative chronic chest wall pain and neuralgia. Creating an alternative incision site can avoid intercostal nerve damage, and may potentially avoid the limitation imposed by narrow rib spaces. Subcostal incision is one of the approach first successfully performed for uniportal VATS major lung resection [21]. The subxiphoid approach also allows simultaneous access to bilateral thoracic space via a single incision [22], making bilateral pulmonary wedge resection less invasive. There remains a number of limitations awaiting further technical refinement. First, extension of subxiphoid incision is unlikely to be useful, and an addition thoracotomy would be necessary for open conversion for major operative complications. Second, complete lymph node dissection is difficult due to angulation and distance from the subxiphoid to the hilum which makes instrumental fencing more severe. Third, transmitted pulsation from the heart to the VATS instruments, especially during left-side surgery, may be cumbersome. Approaching from the other side of the sternum is the trans-cervical approach. It is an expanded application of the suprasternal incision of mediastinoscopy, allowing simultaneous lung resection and mediastinal lymph node dissection [23]. Same as the subxiphoid approach, it allows access to bilateral thoracic cavity with a single incision [24]. Recently its application was further extended to major lung resections [25].

Natural orifice transluminal endoscopic surgery (NOTES) is another form of single-access platform. It was first reported in 2013 for thoracic sympathectomy for palmar hyperhidrosis [26]. Their transumbilical embryonal-NOTES approach used a 5-mm flexible gastroscope, and used a needle knife to cut open the diaphragm to reach the pleural space. Less pain and higher cosmetic satisfaction compared with needlescopic VATS sympathectomy were reported [27]. Since the success of sympathectomy, other procedures, such as pericardial window and wedge lung resection, via the e-NOTES approach have been reported [28]. Endoscopic platforms catering for NOTES are required for its application. Passage of natural orifices or lumens required the instruments having flexible shafts. The better-known examples include Cobra [USGI], Anubiscope [Karl Storz, Tuttlingen, Germany], EndoSamurai [Olympus, Tokyo, Japan], MASTER system [EndoMaster], and the Flex System [Medrobotic]. Further development of these platforms should address stable positioning of the flexible instruments, easy exchange of instruments, and improved triangulation between the scope and instrument arms [11].

Robotic Uniportal VATS

Robotic platform facilitates VATS by providing 3D visual feedback coupled with dexterity and precision from the robotic arm. Uniportal VATS joined the trend of development of single-access robotic platforms, such as the da Vinci single site robot [Intuitive Surgical Inc.], the SPORT surgical system [Titan Medical Inc.], the SPIDER surgical system [TransEnterix], and the SJTU unfoldable robotic system (SURS). The surgical arms for robotic uniportal VATS mostly have a rigid shaft with a distal flexible section. The rigid shaft stabilizes and positions the surgical arms, whose movement is controlled by wires or cables. The distal flexible section usually contains multiple bending segments, providing much improved dexterity and triangulation. However, a more flexible arm results in a more complex actuation unit, limited payload ability, and difficult sterilization. The application and results of robotic uniportal VATS remain to be seen.

Summary

Uniportal VATS is a concept and approach to minimally invasive thoracic surgery that has stood the test of time from its application in relatively minor thoracic procedures to ultra-major lung resections in recent few years. Furthermore, the ethos of uniportal VATS of fewer and ultimately smaller access incision has encouraged creativity from surgeons and industry through improved techniques and instruments to attain a higher level of surgical refinement. Together with these new developments, another future challenge would be to acquire quality evidence to demonstrate the potential benefits of uniportal VATS, requiring the continuous efforts of all thoracic surgeons.

References

1. Rocco G, Martin-Ucar A, Passera E. Uniportal VATS wedge pulmonary resections. Ann Thorac Surg. 2004;77(2):726–8. https://doi.org/10.1016/S0003-4975(03)01219-0.
2. Rocco G, Brunelli A, Jutley R, Salati M, Scognamiglio F, La Manna C, La Rocca A, Martucci N. Uniportal VATS for mediastinal nodal diagnosis and staging. Interact Cardiovasc Thorac Surg. 2006;5(4):430–2. https://doi.org/10.1510/icvts.2006.128603.
3. Jutley RS, Khalil MW, Rocco G. Uniportal vs standard three-port VATS technique for spontaneous pneumothorax: comparison of post-operative pain and residual paraesthesia. Eur J Cardiothorac Surg. 2005;28(1):43–6. https://doi.org/10.1016/j.ejcts.2005.02.039.
4. Ng CS, Rocco G, Wong RH, Lau RW, Yu SC, Yim AP. Uniportal and single-incision video-assisted thoracic surgery: the state of the art. Interact Cardiovasc Thorac Surg. 2014;19(4):661–6. https://doi.org/10.1093/icvts/ivu200.
5. Gonzalez D, Paradela M, Garcia J, Dela Torre M. Single-port video-assisted thoracoscopic lobectomy. Interact Cardiovasc Thorac Surg. 2011;12(3):514–5. https://doi.org/10.1510/icvts.2010.256222.
6. Ng CS, Kim HK, Wong RH, Yim AP, Mok TS, Choi YH. Single-port video-assisted thoracoscopic major lung resections: experience with 150 consecutive cases. Thorac Cardiovasc Surg. 2016;64(4):348–53. https://doi.org/10.1055/s-0034-1396789.
7. Ng CS, Lau KK, Gonzalez-Rivas D, Rocco G. Evolution in surgical approach and techniques for lung cancer. Thorax. 2013;68(7):681. https://doi.org/10.1136/thoraxjnl-2012-203157.
8. Bagan P, De Dominicis F, Hernigou J, Dakhil B, Zaimi R, Pricopi C, Le Pimpec Barthes F, Berna P. Complete thoracoscopic lobectomy for cancer: comparative study of three-dimensional high-definition with two-dimensional high-definition video systems dagger. Interact Cardiovasc Thorac Surg. 2015;20(6):820–3. https://doi.org/10.1093/icvts/ivv031.
9. Ng CS, Wong RH, Lau RW, Yim AP. Minimizing chest wall trauma in single-port video-assisted thoracic surgery. J Thorac Cardiovasc Surg. 2014;147(3):1095–6. https://doi.org/10.1016/j.jtcvs.2013.10.043.
10. Li Z, Oo M, Nalam V, et al. Design of a novel flexible endoscope-cardioscope. ASME. International design engineering technical conferences and computers and information in engineering conference, Vol. 5B: 39th mechanisms and robotics conference.
11. Li Z, Ng CS. Future of uniportal video-assisted thoracoscopic surgery-emerging technology. Ann Cardiothorac Surg. 2016;5(2):127–32. https://doi.org/10.21037/acs.2016.02.02.
12. Ng CS, Pickens A, Siegel JM, Clymer JW, Cummings JF. A novel narrow profile articulating powered vascular stapler provides superior access and haemostasis equivalent to conventional devicesdagger. Eur J Cardiothorac Surg. 2016;49(Suppl 1):i73–8. https://doi.org/10.1093/ejcts/ezv352.
13. Ng CSH, Capili F, Zhao ZR, Yu PSY, Ho JYK, Lau RWH. Laser resection of pulmonary nodule via uniportal thoracoscopic surgery. J Thorac Dis. 2017;9(3):846–8. https://doi.org/10.21037/jtd.2017.02.100.
14. Zhao ZR, Lau RW, Yu PS, Wong RH, Ng CS. Image-guided localization of small lung nodules in video-assisted thoracic surgery. J Thorac Dis. 2016;8(Suppl 9):S731–7. https://doi.org/10.21037/jtd.2016.09.47.
15. Ng CS, Man Chu C, Kwok MW, Yim AP, Wong RH. Hybrid DynaCT scan-guided localization single-port lobectomy. [corrected]. Chest. 2015;147(3):e76–8. https://doi.org/10.1378/chest.14-1503.
16. Yu PSLR, Capili GF, Wan IYP, Underwood MJ, Chu CM, Yu SCH, Ng CSH. Minimally-invasive sublobar resection of tiny pulmonary nodules with real-time image guidance in the hybrid theatre. Innovations (Phila). 2016;11:S98–9.
17. Ng CS, Yu SC, Lau RW, Yim AP. Hybrid DynaCT-guided electromagnetic navigational bronchoscopic biopsy†. Eur J Cardiothorac Surg. 2016;49(Suppl 1):i87–8. https://doi.org/10.1093/ejcts/ezv405.
18. Gonzalez-Rivas D, Fernandez R, de la Torre M, Rodriguez JL, Fontan L, Molina F. Single-port thoracoscopic lobectomy in a non-intubated patient: the least invasive procedure for major lung resection? Interact Cardiovasc Thorac Surg. 2014;19(4):552–5. https://doi.org/10.1093/icvts/ivu209.
19. Zhao ZR, Lau RW, Ng CS. Non-intubated video-assisted thoracic surgery: the final frontier? Eur J Cardiothorac Surg. 2016;50(5):925–6. https://doi.org/10.1093/ejcts/ezw183.
20. Liu J, Cui F, Pompeo E, Gonzalez-Rivas D, Chen H, Yin W, Shao W, Li S, Pan H, Shen J, Hamblin L, He J. The impact of non-intubated versus intubated anaesthesia on early outcomes of video-assisted thoracoscopic anatomical resection in non-small-cell lung cancer: a propensity score matching analysis. Eur J Cardiothorac Surg. 2016;50(5):920–5. https://doi.org/10.1093/ejcts/ezw160.
21. Liu CC, Wang BY, Shih CS, Liu YH. Subxiphoid single-incision thoracoscopic left upper lobectomy. J Thorac Cardiovasc Surg. 2014;148(6):3250–1. https://doi.org/10.1016/j.jtcvs.2014.08.033.
22. Suda T, Ashikari S, Tochii S, Sugimura H, Hattori Y. Single-incision subxiphoid approach for bilateral metastasectomy. Ann Thorac Surg. 2014;97(2):718–9. https://doi.org/10.1016/j.athoracsur.2013.06.123.
23. Kim AW, Kull DR, Zielinski M, Boffa DJ, Detterbeck FC. Transcervical wedge resection after transcervical extended mediastinal lymphadenectomy. Innovations (Phila). 2014;9(4):327–9. https://doi.org/10.1097/IMI.0000000000000079.
24. Obiols C, Call S, Rami-Porta R, Trujillo-Reyes JC. Utility of the transcervical approach in bilateral synchronous lung cancer. Asian Cardiovasc Thorac Ann. 2015;23(8):991–4. https://doi.org/10.1177/0218492315579554.

25. Tezel C, Dogruyol T, Baysungur V, Yalcinkaya I. The most minimally invasive lobectomy: videomediastinoscopic lobectomy. Surg Laparosc Endosc Percutan Tech. 2016;26(4):e73–4. https://doi.org/10.1097/SLE.0000000000000292.
26. Zhu LH, Chen L, Yang S, Liu D, Zhang J, Cheng X, Chen W. Embryonic NOTES thoracic sympathectomy for palmar hyperhidrosis: results of a novel technique and comparison with the conventional VATS procedure. Surg Endosc. 2013;27(11):4124–9. https://doi.org/10.1007/s00464-013-3079-0.
27. Zhu LH, Du Q, Chen L, Yang S, Tu Y, Chen S, Chen W. One-year follow-up period after transumbilical thoracic sympathectomy for hyperhidrosis: outcomes and consequences. J Thorac Cardiovasc Surg. 2014;147(1):25–8. https://doi.org/10.1016/j.jtcvs.2013.08.062.
28. Wu YC, Yen C, Yeh CJ, Hsieh MJ, Chen TP, Chao YK, Wu CY, Yuan HC, Ko PJ, Liu YH, Liu HP. Feasibility of transumbilical surgical lung biopsy and pericardial window creation. Surg Innov. 2014;21(1):15–21. https://doi.org/10.1177/1553350613484825.

Room Set Up and Instrumentation

Mahmoud Ismail

Abstract

Uniportal VATS is becoming nowadays a more common procedure in several thoracic units worldwide. With this technique, all advantages of minimally invasive surgery are applied and the oncological principles of open surgery are respected. The use of this approach is described not only for minor lung resections but also for major lung resections (Gonzalez D, Paradela M, Garcia J, et al. Interact Cardiovasc Thorac Surg 2011;12:514–5) Various standardized steps, starting with the preoperative setting and ending with the immediate postoperative care, can help establish development of this procedure. As the surgeon gains more experience with setting up of this procedures, this could enable to manage even complex cases. The objectives of this chapter are to set the basic steps for room set-up and instrumentation for starting or improving a uniportal program in thoracic surgery units.

Introduction

In 1924 *Singer & Graham* published the first article dealing with the technical difficulties of minimally invasive thoracic surgery [1]. One of their concerns was the necessity of new instrumentations and set-up. Since that, several innovations in surgery have been introduced which led in the 1990s to a revolution in minimally invasive surgery [2, 3]. The principles of minimally invasive abdominal surgery were transferred and applied in thoracic surgery. Nowadays, international guidelines consider multiportal VATS techniques to be the preferred procedure for early stage lung cancer [4]. Similar to other surgical fields, thoracic surgeons aimed to reduce the number and length of their incisions. The one incision technique is called the "uniportal VATS" technique; it has been used for minor lung resections and has been described since 1998 [5, 6]. Since that only limited number of thoracic surgeons has started to use this technique for minor lung procedures. In 2010, and after the publication of Gonzalez Rivas describing a successful major lung resection through a single thoracic incision, a rapid growth of this technique was recognised [7]. Standardisation of perioperative management is a key point in development of such new promising techniques. Lessons learned and developed in big centres performing this procedure are essential.

Perioperative Preparation

The first steps of preparation start before entering the operating room. Optimally it is the application of the fast-track thoracic surgery that defines these steps and optimises the patient for this surgery [8]. The operation side is controlled and marked before the operation. The procedure is performed under general anaesthesia, in specialised thoracic centres it could be even performed as a non-intubated procedure. There is no need for a peridural catheter and neither for a central venous catheter.

Patient Positioning and Incision Marking

There are different types of operating tables which facilitate positioning the patients in thoracic surgery. In general the aim is to have the patient placed in a comfortable lateral decubitus position. This can be achieved be flexing the table in a wedge–shape or placement of a rolled blanket under the patient (Fig. 1). This is crucial in allowing better spreading of the intercostal spaces. The arms of the patient are flexed and stretched towards the head in order to give the space and

M. Ismail (✉)
Department of Thoracic Surgery, Klinikum Ernst von Bergmann, Academic Hospital of the Charité—Universitätsmedizin Humboldt University Berlin, Potsdam, Germany

D. Gonzalez-Rivas et al. (eds.), *Atlas of Uniportal Video Assisted Thoracic Surgery*,
https://doi.org/10.1007/978-981-13-2604-2_3

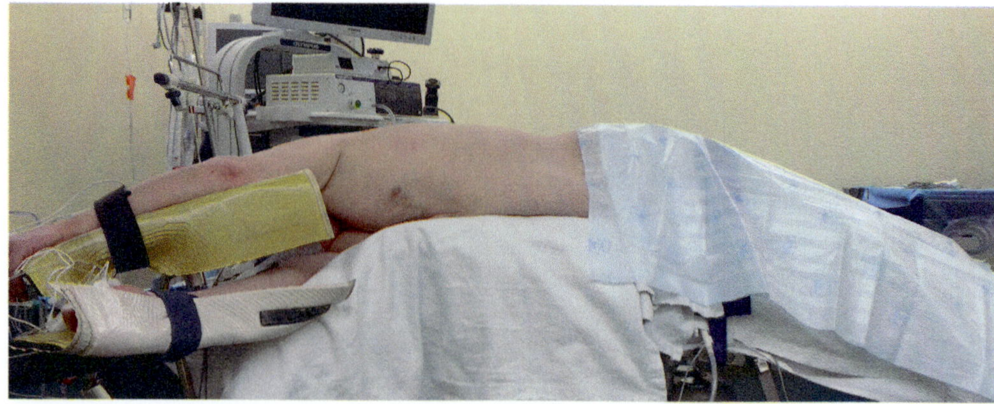

Fig. 1 Patient's position with his arms flexed and stretched upwards, giving more space to the surgeon and his assistant

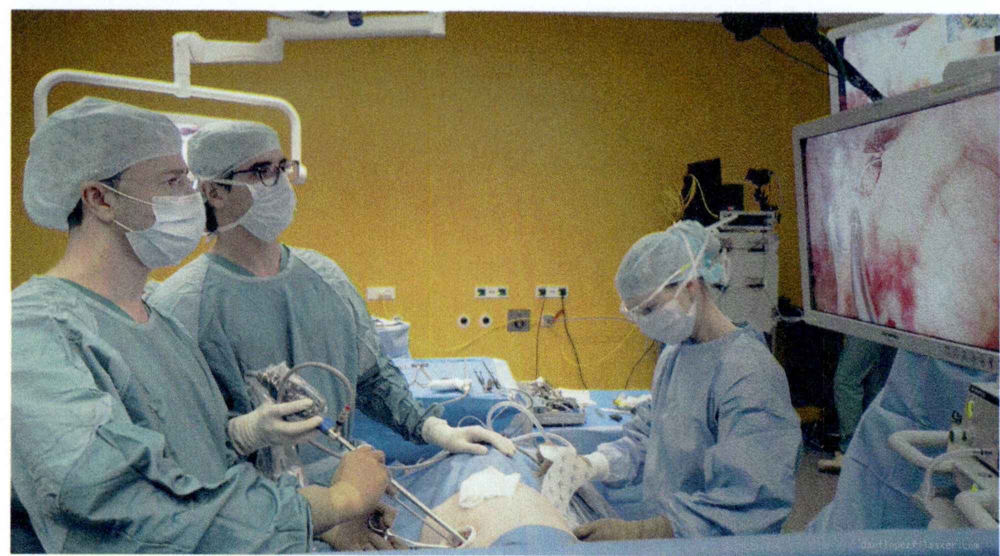

Fig. 2 Room set-up: the scrubbed nurse is opposite to the surgeons. The camera is inserted in the upper part of the incision and the working instruments in the lower part of the incisions

possibility for the surgeon and his assistance to stand in front of the patient. For better stabilization and preventing an incorrect decubitus, vacuum mattress can be used. For achieving an optimal early extubation, the use of thermal blankets is necessary. After positioning the patient, the 2–4 cm single incision is marked usually in the fifth intercostal space between the anterior and middle axillary line. But sometimes variations are necessary according to the lesion and procedure. For lower lobe it could be necessary to perform the incision in the sixth intercostal space. For central tumors or sleeve resections an incision in the fourth intercostal space can offer better exposure and management.

Staff Positioning

The place of both surgeons is mainly depending on which lobe to be operated on. Usually both surgeons are standing in front of the patient watching the same monitor where as the scrub nurse opposite to them (Fig. 2). When the surgeon is operating on the upper and middle part of the thoracic cavity, the assistance must stand caudally. On the other hand when the surgeon is operating in the lower chest cavity the assistance is standing in the cranial side. This allows more room for the surgeon and prevents surgeon and assistance discomfort. In operating theaters where only one monitor is available an optimal organization will be if the monitor is placed cranially with the assistance and scrub nurse on the opposite side of the surgeon who is standing in front of the patient. For the uniportal VATS technique, the availability of two monitors is optimal.

Instrumentation

For uniportal VATS procedures, special instruments are necessary. Instruments with a dual pivot point design enables the full functional when placed through this small thoracic incision. The shaft of these instruments must be as thin as possible in order to allow the introduction of more than one instrument in the uniportal incision when necessary. These

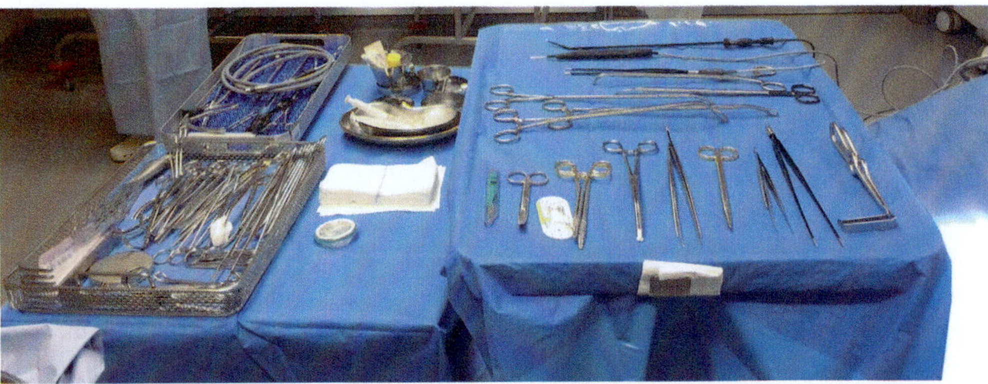

Fig. 3 Tables of instruments: frequent instruments are put on above table, complementary instruments are in the lower one

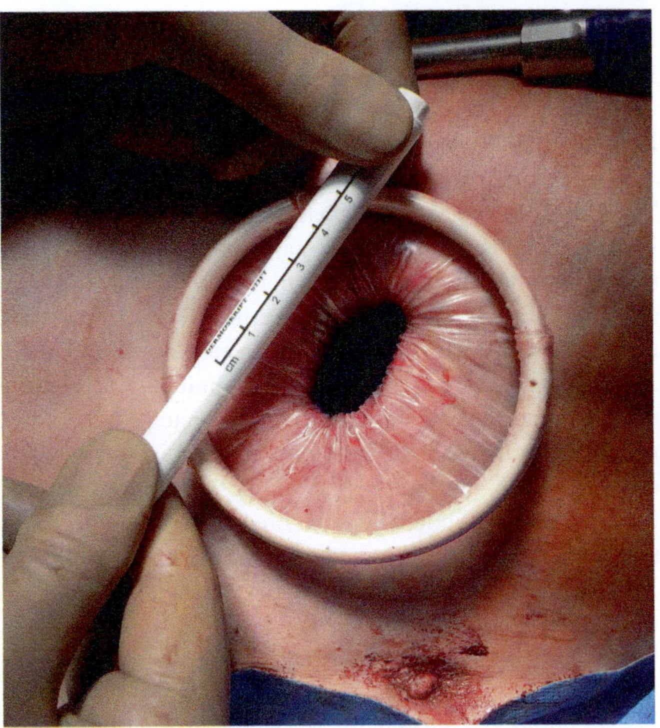
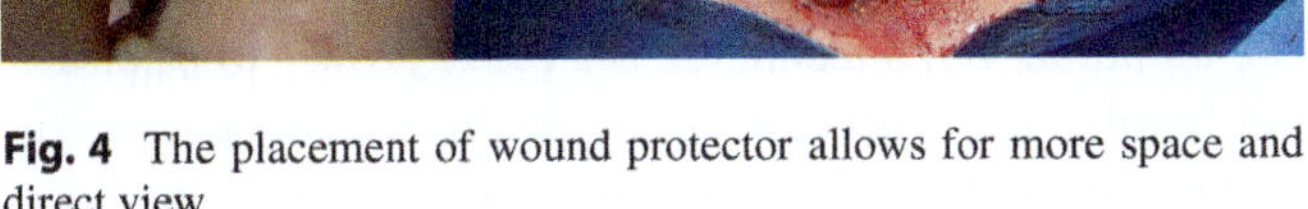

Fig. 4 The placement of wound protector allows for more space and direct view

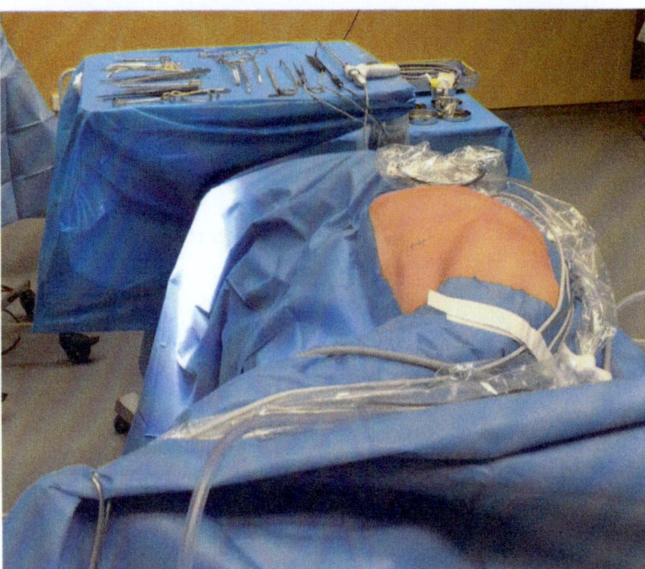

Fig. 5 All cables are fixed on the backside of the patient

instruments can be even used for conventional surgery, making it easier when a conversion is required. It is suggested to have a complete set of instruments in order to be prepared as in conventional surgery to any surprising events like intrathoracic suturing or sleeve resections (Fig. 3). For this aim, some companies designed special sets for the uniportal surgery [9]. A 10 mm 30° thoracoscpe is used. A 5 or 10 mm 30° thoracoscope is used. The optimal one is the one requiring only one hand for handling. This gives the assistance surgeon the possibility to help easily with the second hand. After performing the incision in an anatomical way [10], a wound protector is used without any rib spreading (Fig. 4). In anyway, a rib spreader must be prepared on the table in case of conversion.

Intraoperative Tips and Tricks

- All cables from energy devices and camera should be placed on the backside of the patient. This prevents instrument crowding (Fig. 5).
- The uniportal VATS incision is a muscle-sparing one; the muscles of the serratus anterior are opened without cutting their fibers.
- Cutting the intercostal muscle along the upper edge of the lower rib; this muscle may be used for plastic patch of the bronchus.
- Trying not to enlarge the intercostal incision more than necessary; this can prevent postoperative skin emphysema.
- The use of wound protector could prevent soiling of the camera as well as decreasing the risk of wound infection.

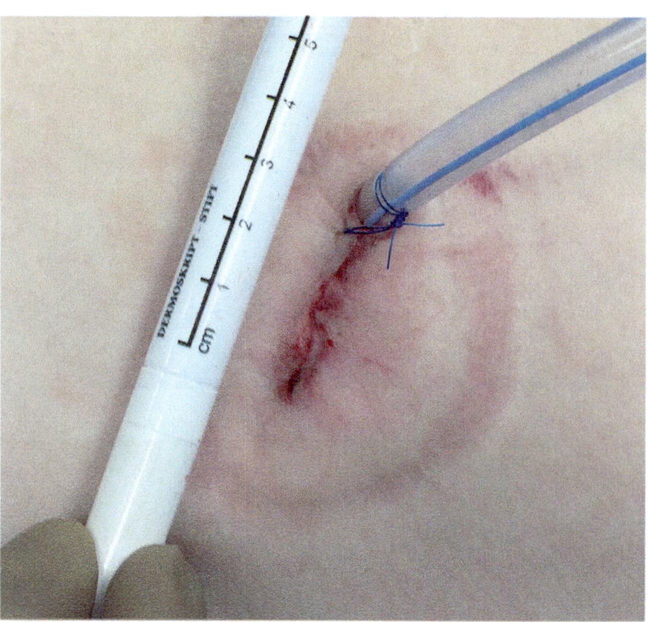

Fig. 6 The 24 Fr chest tube is fixed in the upper part of the incision

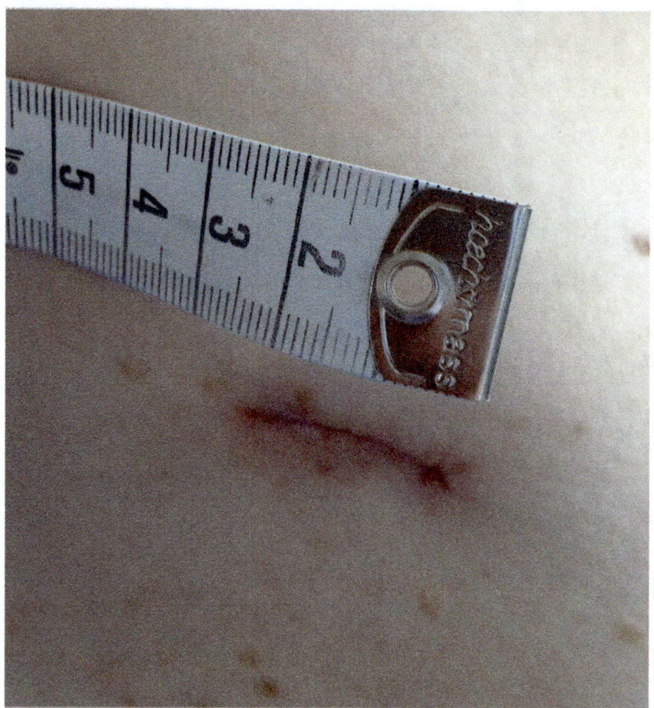

Fig. 7 Postoperative cosmetic results

- In case of adhesions sometimes it is more convenient to dissect them without the use of a wound protector.
- The camera is placed all the time in the upper part of the incision (Fig. 2).
- The assistance surgeon holds the thoracoscope either with right or left hand to allow more space for the surgeon.
- The working instrument is usually coming from the lower part of the incision.
- Usually a lung grasper and two working instruments are necessary, one of them is either energy devise or the stapler.
- For each step in dissection you have to expose the lung in a special way [10].
- No epidural catheter is necessary; the use of intraoperative intercostal/paravertebral block is enough [10].
- The chest tube is inserted and fixed in the upper part of the incision (Fig. 6); in some cases like empyema two tubes can be inserted in the incision.
- The incision is closed without using intercostal sutures. For better cosmetic results skin is closed by resorbable intradermal suture (Fig. 7).
- The use of digital thoracic drain systems is recommended.

Immediate Postoperative Care

The patient is optimally extubated while still lying on the lateral decubitus position. After major lung resections patient should be admitted to an intermediate care unit. If they are cardiopulmonary stable, they can be transferred to the normal ward after 2–6 h. Otherwise, or in case of patients with ASA III or higher, patients have to be admitted to the intensive care unit for one night. In the immediate postoperative phase the patients should be monitored and undergo blood analysis. No X-ray is necessary in the operation day. The thoracic drainage should be monitored and set on a negative pressure of −7 cm H_2O immediately from the beginning.

Conclusion

The uniportal VATS technique is already proven to be a safe and feasible technique for even complicated thoracic surgical procedures [11]. Special instruments with proximal and distal articulation are recommended. This allows the simultaneous use of multiple instruments when necessary. The use of modern thoracoscopes is of advantage. The standardisation of room set-up and instrumentation helps to prevent difficulties during the start and also optimizing the existing experience. Visiting experienced uniportal VATS centres and attending wetlabs and hands-on courses could facilitate the learning curve of this procedure.

References

1. Moisiuc FV, Colt HG. Thoracoscopy: origins revisited. Respiration. 2007;74(3):344–55. Epub 2006 Dec 21.
2. Landreneau RJ, Mack MJ, Hazelrigg SR, Dowling RD, Acuff TE, Magee MJ, Ferson PF. Video-assisted thoracic surgery: basic technical concepts and intercostal approach strategies. Ann Thorac Surg. 1992;54(4):800–7.

3. Rocco G. One-port (uniportal) video-assisted thoracic surgical resections—a clear advance. J Thorac Cardiovasc Surg. 2012; 144:S27–31.
4. Howington JA, et al. Treatment of stage I and II non-small cell lung cancer: diagnosis and management of lung cancer, 3rd ed: American College of Chest Physicians evidence-based clinical practice guidelines. Chest. 2013;143(Suppl 5): e278S–313S.
5. Rocco G, Martin-Ucar A, Passera E. Uniportal VATS wedge pulmonary resections. Ann Thorac Surg. 2004;77(2):726–8.
6. Yamamoto H, et al. Video-assisted thoracic surgery through a single skin incision. Arch Surg. 1998;133(2):145–7.
7. Ismail M, Swierzy M, Nachira D, Rückert JC. Fast-tracking patients through the diagnostic and therapeutic pathways of intrathoracic conditions: the role of uniportal vats. Thorac Surg Clin. 2017;27(4):425–30. https://doi.org/10.1016/j.thorsurg.2017.06.011.
8. Gonzalez-Rivas D. Recent advances in uniportal video-assisted thoracoscopic surgery. Chin J Cancer Res. 2015;27(1):90–3. https://doi.org/10.3978/j.issn.1000-9604.2015.02.03.
9. Ismail M, Swierzy M, Nachira D, Rückert JC, Gonzalez-Rivas D. Uniportal video-assisted thoracic surgery for major lung resections: pitfalls, tips and tricks. J Thorac Dis. 2017;9(4):885–97. https://doi.org/10.21037/jtd.2017.02.04.
10. Wang L, Liu D, Lu J, Zhang S, Yang X. The feasibility and advantage of uniportal video-assisted thoracoscopic surgery (VATS) in pulmonary lobectomy. BMC Cancer. 2017;17(1):75. https://doi.org/10.1186/s12885-017-3069-z.
11. Gonzalez D, Paradela M, Garcia J, et al. Single-port video-assisted thoracoscopic lobectomy. Interact Cardiovasc Thorac Surg. 2011;12: 514–5.

Anaesthesia for Uniportal VATS

Sonia Alvarado, César Bonome, and Diego Gonzalez-Rivas

Abstract

With the emergence of video-assisted thoracic surgery and more recently, thoracic surgery performed through a single incision (uniportal video-assisted thoracoscopic surgery) we have witnessed a move towards less aggressive thoracic procedures which lead us to search for minimally invasive surgical approaches and more secure anaesthesic strategies, always trying to decrease secondary injuries. However, anaesthesiologists should not believe that this necessarily implies safer or more simple procedures. In fact, anaesthesia for video-assisted thoracic surgery, requires the same level of monitoring and security than conventional open surgeries.

Success resides not only in a sophisticated surgical technique but also in an adequate anaesthetic management which includes a correct selection of the patients, a suitable and personalized patient monitoring, a safe airway management, and an efficient postoperative analgesia strategy.

Introduction

VATS (video-assisted thoracic surgery) and more recently, thoracic-surgery performed through a single incision (uniportal VATS) represents an excellent minimally invasive strategy for major procedures [1, 2]. Benefits such as less pain, better pulmonary function or shorter period of hospitalization are being achieved with the expansion of this novel surgical approach. Therefore, it is not surprising that uniportal VATS is becoming increasingly popular and requested by the patient. We can proudly state that nowadays VATS can be virtually used in almost every thoracic surgery procedure. However, in order to obtain all the benefits that VATS and specifically uniportal VATS can offer, both thoracic surgeons and anaesthesiologists must work effortlessly together in the operating room. Anaesthesiologists must keep in mind that in spite of VATSs being an apparently minimally invasive approach (compared to a classical thoracotomy), anaesthesia for VATS require the same level of safety and monitoring as conventional surgery.

Preoperative Evaluation

Preoperative evaluation for VATS should be the same as for open surgery. This is necessary not only because operability criteria remain the same, but also because until now, studies have shown that 1–8% of VATS procedements are converted to open surgery. Therefore, patients undergoing VATS or uniportal VATS must be well investigated prior to surgery, including respiratory function tests and in numerous cases cardiac function tests [3].

Monitoring

Monitoring for VATS/uniportal VATS has been a matter of much controversy; the general opinion is that the level of monitoring should be the same as for open surgery and its complexity will depends greatly on patients comorbidities as well as the extension of the surgical interventions.

Aside from conventional anaesthesia monitoring, it is strongly recommended to have arterial cannulation for invasive arterial blood pressure measurement as well as for the extraction of blood samples.

S. Alvarado · C. Bonome (✉)
Anesthesiology Department, University Hospital La Coruña, La Coruña, Spain
e-mail: cesar@bonome.es

D. Gonzalez-Rivas
Department of Thoracic Surgery, Shanghai Pulmonary Hospital, Tongji University School of Medicine, Shanghai, China

Department of Thoracic Surgery and Minimally Invasive Thoracic Surgery Unit (UCTMI), Coruña University Hospital, Coruña, Spain
e-mail: diego@uniportal.es

D. Gonzalez-Rivas et al. (eds.), *Atlas of Uniportal Video Assisted Thoracic Surgery*,
https://doi.org/10.1007/978-981-13-2604-2_4

We should not forget that intrathoracic vascular structures can be damaged during surgery; in case of massive intraoperative hemorrhage, it can become necessary to convert immediately to an open thoracotomy, which can take at least five minutes. In this situation, to maintain hemodynamic stability large caliber venous lines are indispensable; and so it is essential to have established good venous access from the beginning of the surgery, being necessary in some cases to have central venous lines.

Airway Management

During uniportal VATS the goal is to achieve lung isolation, providing proper ventilation to the non-operated lung (dependent) and obtaining a complete collapse of the operating lung (non-dependent), allowing an appropriate visualization of the surgical field thus facilitating the work of the surgeon.

Furthermore this would prevent future air leaks which can be generated with the use of surgical staplers on the surface of an inflated lung, increasing the risk of postoperative complications.

An early and adequate lung collapse will promote faster and safer surgeries together with shorter times of one-lung ventilation (OLV), reducing complications and the possibility of an emergency thoracotomy.

The left double-lumen endotracheal tube is the "gold standard" for lung isolation. Other options include the use of endobronchial blockers (Arndt, Cohen, Fuji Uniblocker®), and there are well-designed studies that have demonstrated good results, positioning these devices as valid alternatives, being particularly useful in cases where double-lumen endotracheal tubes (DLET) are contraindicated or their placement is difficult. However, studies also have shown that DLET provide a quicker deflation of the lungs as well as less need for repositionings (Figs. 1 and 2).

Unlike thoracotomies, with VATS we need to achieve a complete lung collapse before the surgical incision is executed to avoid parenchymal damage, because the operation starts with the introduction of a trocar into the hemithorax [4].

We can deduce, that concerning airway management for VATS, the main challenge for the anaesthesiologist is to achieve and to keep a complete lung collapse throughout the surgery.

The possibility of hypoxemia during OLV is independent of the surgical approach, but its management may be more challenging during VATS, as some of the rescue maneuvers could be inappropriate as they can interfere with our surgeons work, such as the use of continuous airway pressure (CPAP). Taking this into consideration, the importance of hypoxemia prevention is capital [5, 6].

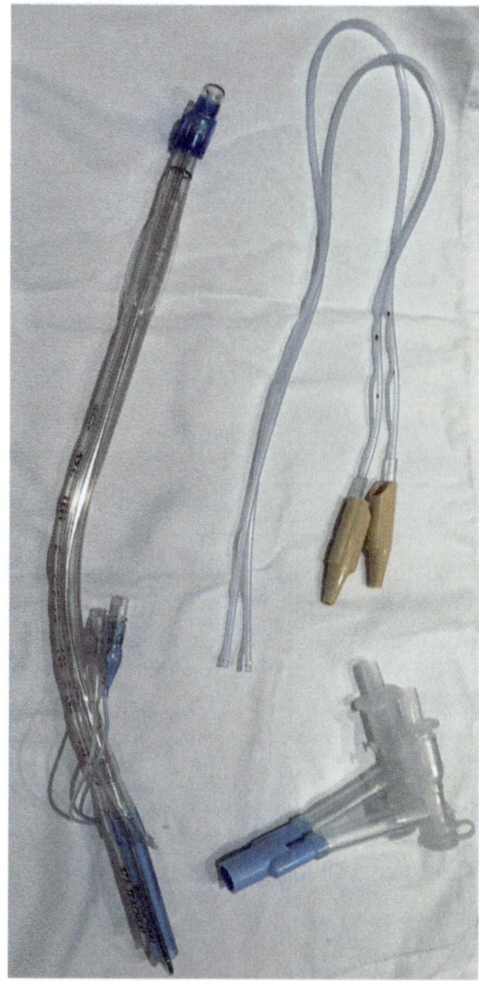

Fig. 1 DLET remains the gold standard for airway management during VATS

These Include

- Ventilate with Fi02 1 during 3–5 min previous to OLV, once it is initiated we should ventilate with a mixture of oxygen plus medical air, to avoid reabsorption atelectasis.
- Pulmonary recruitment maneuvers and implementation of an optimal PEEP level, according to the best pulmonary compliance, as part of the overall strategy of protective lung ventilation.
- Optimize tissue oxygenation: adequate haemoglobin levels, appropriated cardiac output, avoid hypovolemia, use inotropic drugs or prevent anaesthetic overdosing may be useful.

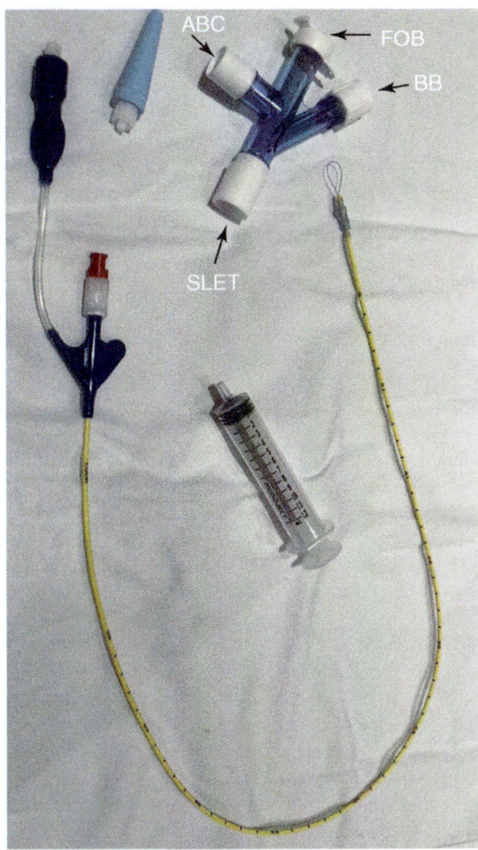

Fig. 2 Arndt endobronchial blocker. *FOB* fiberoptic bronchoscopy port, *BB* bronchial blocker port, *ABC* anaesthesia breathing circuit, *SLET* single-lumen endotracheal tube connection

Table 1 Strategies to manage hypoxemia during VATS

When hypoxemia appears	The first thing to do is to ensure the correct position of our DLET. Its malposition is the first cause of intraoperative hypoxemia
If hypoxemia persists	Increase Fi02 Recruitment maneuvers/use of PEEP Optimize tissue oxygenation
Exceptional measures	High frequency jet ventilation Low levels of CPAP (<5 cmH_2O) Direct insufflation of oxygen guided by fibre-optic bronchoscopy

- Encourage mechanisms that facilitate the phenomenom of hypoxic pulmonary vasoconstriction.
- Use of CPAP considering that its implementation can reduce the surgical field and operating space. And preferably low CPAP levels (<5 cmH_2O).
- Others: high frequency jet ventilation, direct insufflation of oxygen guided by fibre-optic bronchoscopy, oxygen flow of 5 L per minute through the suction channel of the fibre-optic bronchoscopy to collapse areas (Table 1).

Pain Management

According to most recent studies, VATS is associated with less postoperative pain; however some patients still suffer from severe postoperative pain, and even in a high percentage of cases (47% in some studies) patients develop chronic pain. This is mainly due to the damage of intercostal nerves with the introduction and manipulation of the trocars.

Epidural analgesia is considered the "gold standard" for analgesia after thoracotomies and it also seems useful for VATS. However an increasingly popular alternative is paravertebral analgesia, obtained through a paravertebral blockade (with or without the placement of a catheter). When performed at T_4 level we can achieve ipsilateral analgesia from T_2 to T_6 approximately, also it provides a lower rate of complications and adverse side effects, comparing to epidural analgesia.

More recently the widespread use of ultrasounds has contributed to the expand use of this type of blockade, allowing higher success rates, and decreasing its complications: pneumothorax or intravascular punctures… (Fig. 3) [7].

Other alternatives, indicated specifically for uniportal VATS thanks to its minimal aggressiveness, include intercostal blockades or even wound infiltration with local anaesthesia, with an increasing number of recent studies showing good results, with patients experiencing a high degree of satisfaction. It is recommended to start using these alternatives after shorter and less invasive surgical procedures, specially in groups not experienced in uniportal VATS (Fig. 4) [8].

Nevertheless, we must remember that as in any other surgical interventions, the most appropriate strategy is that based on the application of multimodal analgesia principles, which combine the use of regional techniques with non-opioid and opioid analgesics.

Certainly, we have to consider always our patients comorbidities and therefore individualize each case in search of optimisation.

Conclusion

Video-assisted thoracic surgery, initially developed and used only in minor procedures like biopsies or athipical resections, has been extended swiftly; and nowadays it is positioned as the first option for almost all thoracic procedures, so anaesthesiologists should be familiar to its peculiarities and how they can modify their clinical practice. An efficient communication and cooperation between surgeons and anaesthesiologist is an essential point for achieving the best possible results.

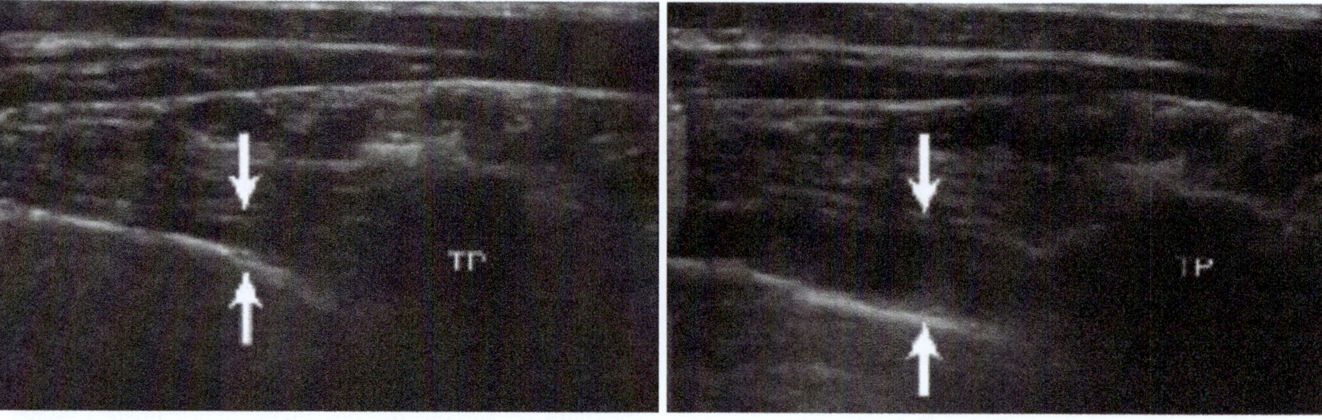

Fig. 3 Paravertebral blockade, ultrasound image, the white arrows are pointing at the paravertebral space. Left image is before anaesthetic infiltration, right image after anaesthetic infiltration. TP: Transverse process

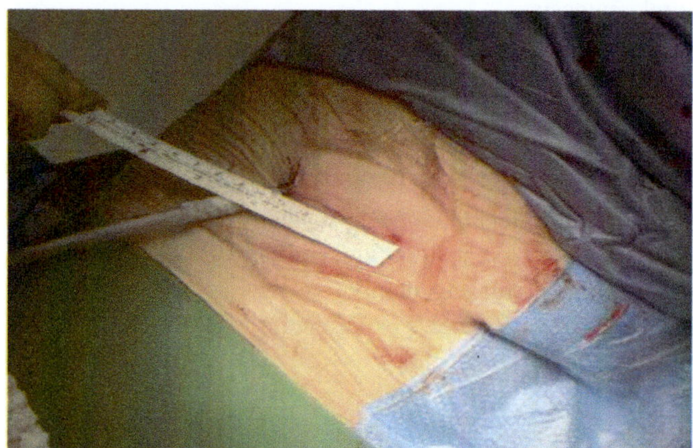

Fig. 4 Uniportal VATS, standard incision size. Wound infiltration with local anaesthesia can be a valid option for this minimal incisions

References

1. Shaw JP, Dembitzer FR, Wisnivesky JP, Litle VR, Weiser TS, Yun J, et al. Video-assisted thoracoscopic lobectomy: state of the art and future directions. Ann Thorac Surg. 2008;85(2):S705–9.
2. Gónzalez-Rivas D, Aymerich H, Bonome C, Fieira E. From open operations to nonintubated video-assisted thoracoscopic lobectomy: minimizing the trauma to the patient. Ann Thorac Surg. 2015;100(6):2003–5.
3. Matsuguma H, Nakahara R, Anraku M, Kondo T, Tsuura Y, Kamiyama Y, et al. Objective definition and measurement method of ground-glass opacity for planning limited resection in patients with clinical stage IA adenocarcinoma of the lung. Eur J Cardiothorac Surg. 2004;25:1102–6.
4. Gothard J. Lung injury after thoracic surgery and one-lung ventilation. Curr Opin Anaesthesiol. 2006;19(1):5–10.
5. Brassard C, Lohser J, Donati F, Bussières J. Step-by-step clinical management of one-lung ventilation: continuing professional development. Can J Anesth. 2014;61:1103–21.
6. Nagendran J, Stewart K, Hoskinson M, Archer SL. An anesthesiologist's guide to hypoxic pulmonary vasoconstriction: implications for managing single-lung anesthesia and atelectasis. Curr Opin Anaesthesiol. 2006;19(1):34–43.
7. Hausman MS Jr, Jewell ES, Engoren M. Regional versus general anesthesia in surgical patients with chronic obstructive pulmonary disease: does avoiding general anesthesia reduce the risk of postoperative complications? Anesth Analg. 2014;120(6): 1405–12.
8. Katlic MR, Facktor MA. Video-assisted thoracic surgery utilizing local anesthesia and sedation: 384 consecutive cases. Ann Thorac Surg. 2010;90(1):240–5.

Geometric Considerations in Uniportal VATS

Luca Bertolaccini

Abstract

As laparoscopy in the abdomen, Video-Assisted Thoracic Surgery (VATS) has represented the revolution of the surgical approach to the lungs. Compared to open thoracotomy, VATS has demonstrated a significant reduction in pain, time for recovery, complications, and, not least, an improvement in the daily quality of life. Uniportal VATS (UniVATS) may be seen as a further step of minimally invasive thoracic surgery, consisting in only one small incision allowing simultaneous introduction of instruments parallel to the thoracoscope through an ideal cylindrical space as vast as a surgeon's finger-breadth without further dissection of the intercostal space. An enhanced hand-eye coordination to visualise and operate the thoracoscope-surgical instruments ensemble is required. In particular, the thoracoscope is handled to view the position of the instruments at any time during the procedure with simple zooming in or out. UniVATS geometric configuration of the approach is entirely different from the standard three-port VATS settings. The use of a single port favours a translational approach of VATS instruments along with a sagittal plane. The single port configuration enables the devices to move along two parallel lines on a plane approaching the target lesion from a craniocaudal perspective, and this allows to bring the effective fulcrum inside the chest in a way comparable to open surgery.

Introduction

During the last three decades, Video-Assisted Thoracic Surgery (VATS) was a revolution in the surgical approach to the lungs [1]. Compared to open thoracotomy, VATS, as previously demonstrated in several papers, entails a significant reduction in pain, time for recovery, complications, and, not least, an improvement in the daily quality of life [2]. In 2004, Gaetano Rocco first described the technique of uniportal VATS (UniVATS) for pulmonary wedge resection [3]. From this early report, the progressive refinements of UniVATS have broadened its use, in particular in major anatomic pulmonary resections for lung cancers. More papers have already demonstrated the advantage of the UniVATS approach in comparison to standard techniques with three-port in the reduction of postoperative pain, postoperative hospital stay, and in a faster recovery of daily life activities. The main characteristic of UniVATS is only one small incision with the simultaneous introduction of instruments parallel to the thoracoscope through an ideal cylindrical shape as full as a surgeon's finger-breadth without further dissection of the intercostal space. An enhanced hand-eye coordination to visualise and operate the thoracoscope-instruments ensemble is required [4]. In particular, the thoracoscope is handled to visualise the position of the instruments at any time during the procedure with simple zooming in or out of the operative field [5]. UniVATS approach was initially described in the management of pneumothorax, wedge resection and other minor procedures.

Nevertheless, one of the most challenging tasks in the uniportal VATS had been the anatomic major lung resections. Diego Gonzalez-Rivas described a comprehensive array of techniques for anatomic lung resection, covering every important aspect encountered in lung cancer surgery, including lobectomy, segmentectomy, pneumonectomy, including complex broncho-vascular reconstructions [6–10]. In this chapter, we reviewed the geometric approach of UniVATS.

A Bird Fly on Plane Geometry Concepts

Geometry is the mathematical discipline used to describe the space and those elements that compose it. For 2500 years, the natural geometry was the Euclidean plane: a formal

L. Bertolaccini (✉)
Department of Thoracic Surgery, Maggiore Teaching Hospital, Bologna, Italy

D. Gonzalez-Rivas et al. (eds.), *Atlas of Uniportal Video Assisted Thoracic Surgery*, https://doi.org/10.1007/978-981-13-2604-2_5

system to characterise two-dimensional plane according to distance, angle, and the relationships among them. The geometrical equivalence of two forms with the same length, angle, and relations is rather evident to the human mind. So, mathematicians and philosophers have believed for millennia that Euclidean geometry constituted the only logically possible geometric system. Although this view was changed more than two centuries ago with Nikolaj Ivanovič Lobačevskij ad his non-Euclidean geometry, Euclidean remains the first formal geometry students learn.

Αγεωμετρετος μεδεις εισιτω (let no one ignorant of geometry enters): tradition tells that this phrase was engraved on the door of Plato's Academy in Athens. For Plato, geometry and mathematics was a prerequisite for testing and developing the power of abstraction. All of us could remember this famous dialogue of Meno.

> Socrates: I cause doubt in others. So now, for my part, I have no idea what virtue is, while you, though perhaps you may have known before you came in touch with me, are now as good as ignorant of it also. However, none the less I am willing to join you in examining it and inquiring into its nature.
>
> Meno: Why, on what lines will you look, Socrates, for a thing of whose nature you know nothing at all? Pray, what sort of thing, amongst those that you know not, will you treat us to as the object of your search? Alternatively, even supposing, at best, that you hit upon it, how will you know it is the thing you did not know?
>
> Socrates: I understand the point you would make, Meno [6].

Processes of association learn geometry, adaptive learning, applied to the spatially structured world projected to our senses. Like natural numbers, physical geometry is founded on two evolutionarily ancient and universal cognitive systems that capture pieces of information from the surrounding world and translating them into abstract ideas [11]. The abundance of morphological diversity of the anatomical structures is often simplified because they are both conceptually and empirically approximated to ideally regular Euclidean shapes, such as spheres, ellipses, triangles, etc. [12]. In geometrical terms, Human bodies become objects featuring angles and relative lengths, thus defining three-dimensional (3D) structures or two dimensions (2D) shapes. In perception, the spatial relationships of objects are more important than their absolute sizes [13].

What is more, under natural circumstances the human brain tends to perceive 3D scenes as plausible. This strategy encourages our mind to elaborate images in geometrical terms. Perceptual effects are useful, such as the effect of depth cues on judging the aspect ratio of an ellipse, or the joint effect of texture. Human 3D perception is based on the direction of gravity, a horizontal plane upon which all objects reside, and the inherent symmetry of 3D objects [14]. Objects seem slighter when they are far away from us than when they are near, and this explains that the perceived size of things does not equal their physical size. The perceived size depends on the physical size and the stimuli that carry information about space. The retinal image decreases in size in proportion to the object distance, and this explains the perceptual shrinking as distance increases. Euclid's Optics described that perceived size does not decrease in proportion to distance. Indeed, in many well-lighted situations perceived size changes little with distance when distances are short, and the perceived size depends on the perceived distance. The visual angle α is proportional to retinal image size, and both is inversely proportional to distance and implies that perceived size will fill the visual angle at the perceived distance (Fig. 1) [15].

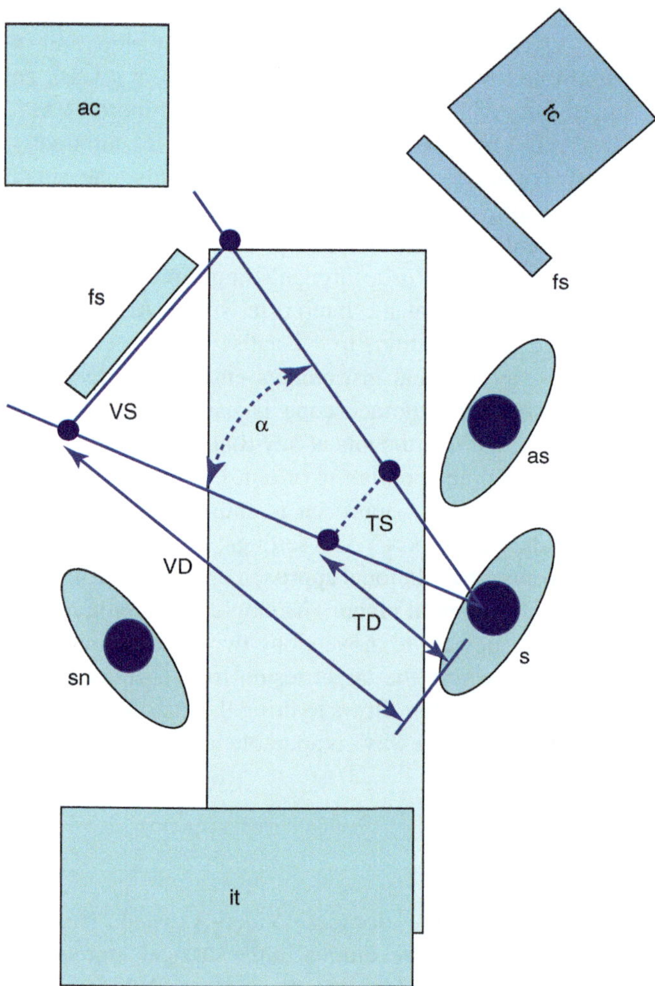

Fig. 1 Size perception in the operative setup of the uniportal VATS approach. Perceived size fills the visual angle at the perceived distance. The dashed line indicates the perceived extent. α = visual angle; VD = view distance; VS = visual size; TD = target distance; PS = physical size; ac = anaesthesia console; tc = thoracoscopic console; fs = flat screen; s = surgeon; as = assisting surgeon; sn = scrub nurse; it = instrument table. Elaborated from [4, 15]

Geometrical Characteristics of Uniportal VATS

The UniVATS approach has a geometric configuration entirely different from the standard three-port VATS setting. The use of a single port favours a translational approach of VATS instruments along with a sagittal plane. The single port configuration enables the devices to move in the direction of two parallel lines on that plane approaching the target lesion from a craniocaudal perspective. This allows bringing the effective fulcrum inside the chest in a fashion similar to open surgery. The three-port VATS lobectomy approach typically employs small ports without rib spreading. The strategy for ports placement was described in the literature as the baseball diamond and corresponds in plane geometry to a trapezoid (Fig. 2). The surgeon's eyes (the thoracoscope) are in point A; the target lesion lays in front of surgeon's eyes in point B; the other two ports are placed at points C and D to allow the left and right-hand instruments to be placed and triangulated forwards towards the target in point B along two vectorial planes $\overrightarrow{CB}$ and $\overrightarrow{DB}$. The viewing axis, the vector $\overrightarrow{AB}$, is perpendicular to the operation port axis CD and follows the natural longitudinal axis of the patient from feet towards the head. Nevertheless, this setting fails to reproduce the real-life setting, where the surgeons and assistants place themselves around the operating table. In real settings, many surgeons stand anteriorly to the patient in lateral decubitus. Consequently, the real axis of the operation is translated posteriorly (Fig. 3). The posterior port (D) is translated along the viewing axis and the surgeon is too far to comfortably effect the instrumentation there. In addition, if the assistant stands on the opposite side of the operating table, the visual axis would be completely different. In order to cope with these technical and ergonomic blemishes, the three-port VATS port placement strategy has been modified, as proposed by Hansen and co-workers, with the translation of the trapezoid (Fig. 4). The camera port (A) was brought more anterior to the anterior axillary line (A'). The posterior port

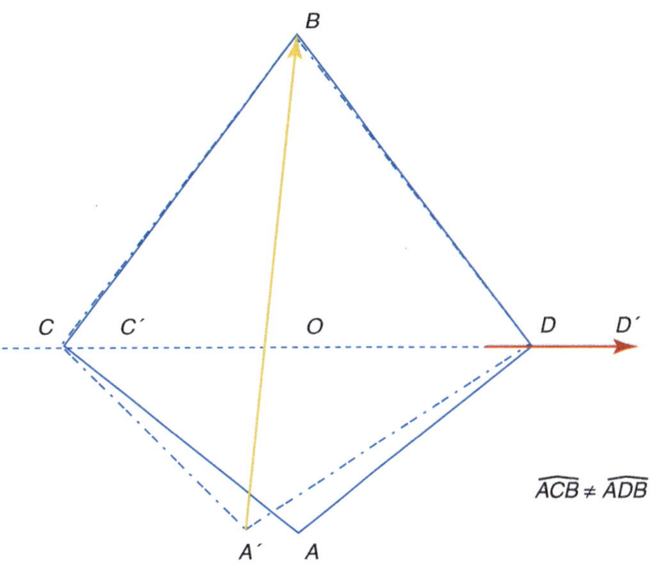

Fig. 3 Real three-port VATS lobectomy settings. The real axis ($\overrightarrow{A'B}$) of the operation is translated posteriorly. A = thoracoscope port; B = target lesion; C and D = operative ports. $\overrightarrow{A'B}$ = axis of vision. Elaborated from [18]

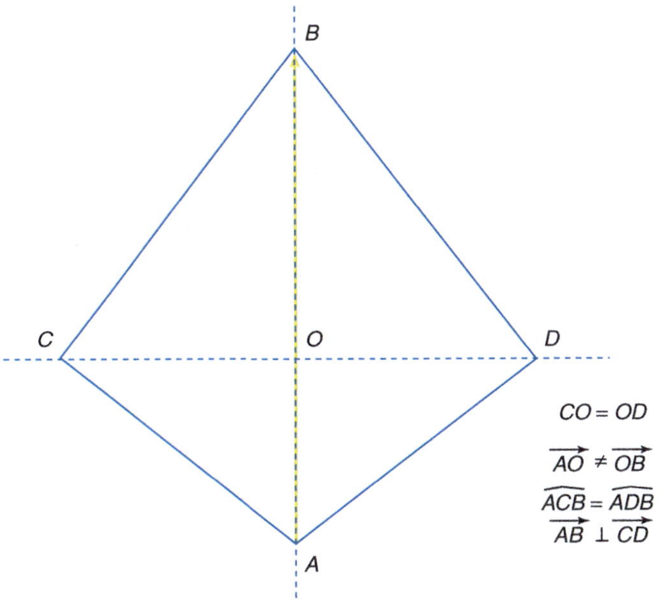

Fig. 2 Ideal three-port VATS lobectomy settings. A = thoracoscope port; B = target lesion; C and D = operative ports. $\overrightarrow{AB}$ = axis of vision. Elaborated from [18]

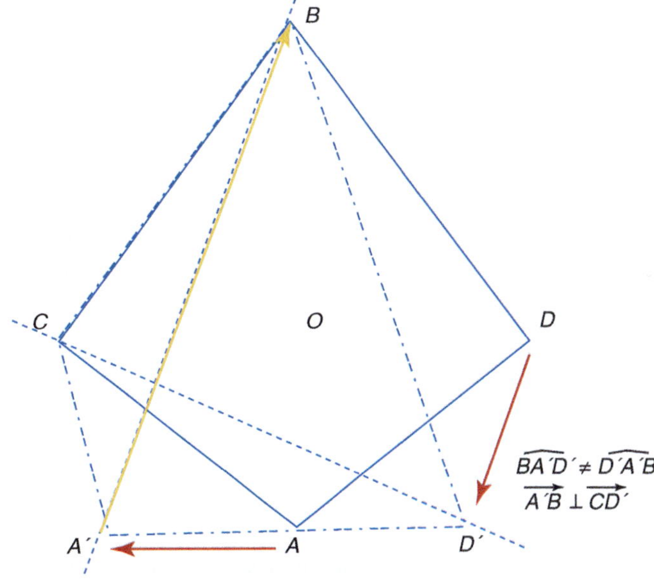

Fig. 4 Anterior three-port VATS lobectomy settings. A' = thoracoscope port; B = target lesion; C and D' = operative ports. $\overrightarrow{A'B}$ = axis of vision. Elaborated from [18]

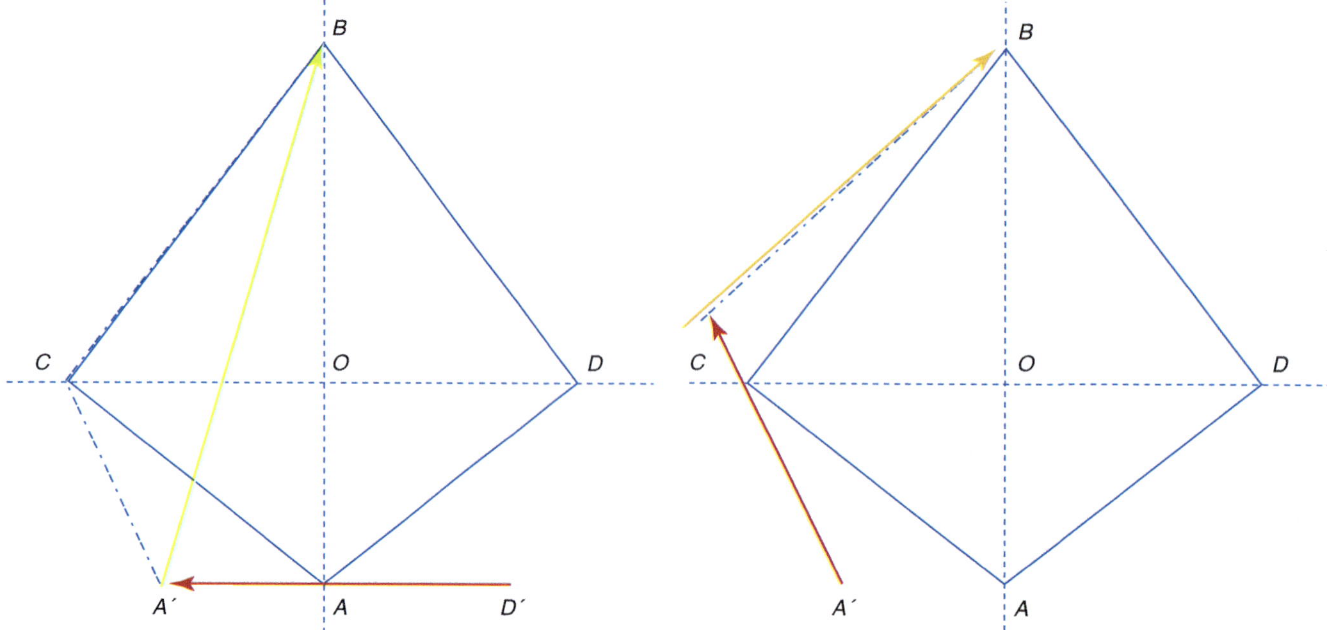

Fig. 5 Two-port VATS lobectomy settings. A' = thoracoscope port; B = target lesion; C = operative ports. $\overrightarrow{A'B}$ = axis of vision. Elaborated from [18]

Fig. 6 Uniportal VATS settings. The thoracoscope instruments are translated of 90° along a sagittal plane passing through the point C, bringing the operative tools to address the target lesion from a vertical, caudocranial perspective. Elaborated from [18]

(D) was placed further caudally (D'). The utility port position (C) remains unchanged. Although the trapezoid was preserved, the axis $A'B$ was more comfortable for the operating surgeon. The assistant stands on the same side of the operating table improving the coordination. After gaining experience with the three port VATS approach, it was realized that the posterior 3 mm (D') port was not always essential, resulting in a two port VATS technique (Fig. 5). Therefore, the three-port approach, in which the trapezoid configuration allows maximal convergence of operative instruments from each side of target lesion, thus meddling with the optical source [2]. The UniVATS approach requires the translation of the thoracoscope instruments 90° along a sagittal plane passing from point C, placing the operative instruments so to address the target lesion from a vertical, caudo-cranial perspective (Fig. 6). To avoid mutual interference, the use of articulating instruments is of paramount importance, owing the possibility to rotate their tip independently on different planes and with multiple angles. In fact, the approach to the target lesion in the lung is substantially similar to the approach that the surgeon would use in open surgery [9]. In the UniVATS approach, the target lesion is located in a projective plane with homogeneous coordinates and represents the point at infinity and it is elevated with forceps perpendicularly from the parenchymal profile and resected by applying a stapler (or a curved clamp and overseen) at the base of this newly created, cone-shaped parenchymal area. The approach for a target lung lesion is then similar to a coaxial approach: surgeons work with their eyes and hands in the same plane (coaxial path), much like open surgery and in contrast to three-port VATS (para-axial approach) [16, 17]. UniVATS implemented through a tailored minimal single incision through which some thoracoscopic instruments access [17]. This single incision site usually functions as an access port entering into the chest cavity, a specimen-extracting orifice, and a pathway for the drain. The preferred single incision site is the fourth or fifth intercostal space. Furthermore, UniVATS can provide a shortcut to various lobes. Thoracic surgeons could perform traction and dissection thanks to the triangulation (Fig. 7a, b). UniVATS, however, could provide the unfavourable surroundings for triangulation, often resulting in the chopsticks or sword fighting effect due to parallel alignment of instruments. Inverse triangulation refers to the formation of an inverted triangle viewed from the operator; one single-incision port site and two instrumental ends, which are positioned in a crossing-over pattern, comprise three triangles. The two instrumental terms do not encounter but assist each other by creating tension. The operation is carried out with the two instruments crossed-over (Fig. 7c). The surgeon's right-hand holds the left-sided instrument and vice versa. Moreover, inverse triangulation does not increase the chest wall pain because the range of motion of the instruments is restricted within the port [18].

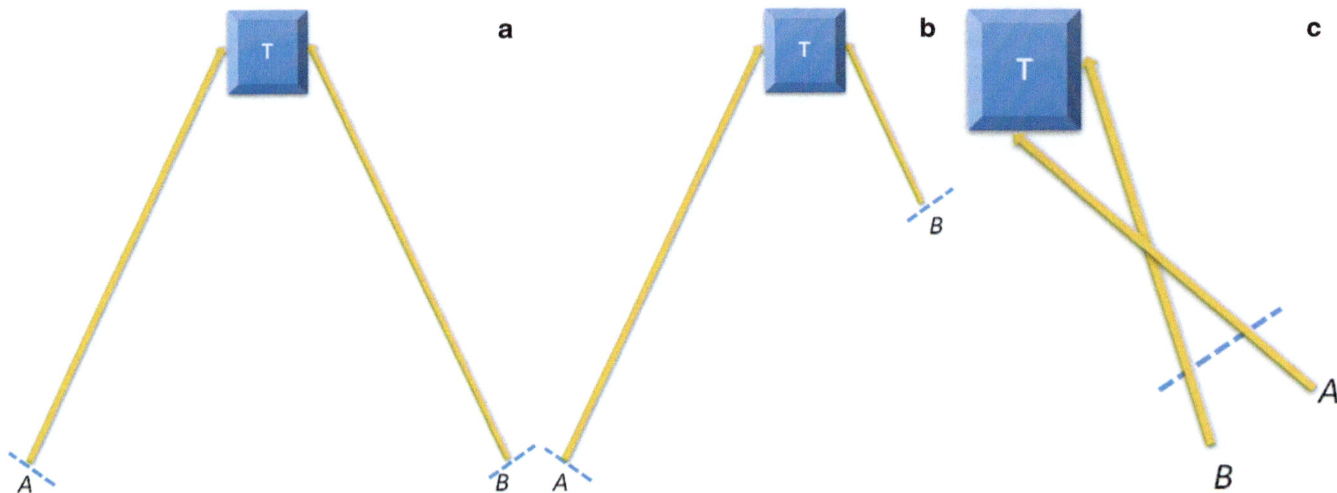

Fig. 7 (**a**) The direct triangulation in the standard three-port VATS access allows traction on tissues and improve the dissection along the anatomical planes. (**b**) The direct triangulation in three port anterior VATS access allows better traction helping the dissection along the anatomical planes. (**c**) In uniportal VATS, the inverse triangulation of the two instruments ends do not encounter themselves but assist each other creating tension. Therefore, the manoeuvres are carried out with the two instruments crossed-over. A and B = thoracoscopic instruments; T = target lesion. Elaborated from [18]

Conclusions

UniVATS represents an advantage and valuable addition to the surgical *armamentarium.* Further developments in UniVATS will be its use as a technique of choice for pulmonary tissue procurement aimed at biomolecular investigations, as the geometric approach to the chest cavity is used to minimise surgical trauma [19]. UniVATS approach the lesion along a sagittal plane. The target lesion is reached for caudocranial perspectives that realise a projective plane that preserves the depth of intraoperative visualisation. The instruments are parallel lines drawn on the plane that enables the surgeon to bring the effective fulcrum inside the chest [20].

References

1. Anile M, Diso D, Mantovani S, Patella M, Russo E, Carillo C, et al. Uniportal video assisted thoracoscopic lobectomy: going directly from open surgery to a single port approach. J Thorac Dis. 2014;6:S641–3.
2. Sihoe AD. The evolution of minimally invasive thoracic surgery: implications for the practice of uniportal thoracoscopic surgery. J Thorac Dis. 2014;6:S604–17.
3. Rocco G, Martucci N, La Manna C, Jones DR, De Luca G, La Rocca A, et al. Ten-year experience on 644 patients undergoing single-port (Uniportal) video-assisted thoracoscopic surgery. Ann Thorac Surg. 2013;96:434–8.
4. Bertolaccini L, Viti A, Terzi A. Ergon-trial: ergonomic evaluation of single-port access versus three-port access video-assisted thoracic surgery. Surg Endosc. 2015;29:2934–40.
5. Tu CC, Hsu PK. Global development and current evidence of uniportal thoracoscopic surgery. J Thorac Dis. 2016;8:S308–18.
6. Gonzalez-Rivas D, Yang Y, Sekhniaidze D, Stupnik T, Fernandez R, Lei J, et al. Uniportal video-assisted thoracoscopic bronchoplastic and carinal sleeve procedures. J Thorac Dis. 2016;8:S210–22.
7. Fieira Costa E, Delgado Roel M, Paradela de la Morena M, Gonzalez-Rivas D, Fernandez-Prado R, de la Torre M. Technique of Uniportal VATS major pulmonary resections. J Thorac Dis. 2014;6:S660–4.
8. Gonzalez-Rivas D, Fieira E, Delgado M, de la Torre M, Mendez L, Fernandez R. Uniportal video-assisted thoracoscopic sleeve lobectomy and other complex resections. J Thorac Dis. 2014;6: S674–81.
9. Gonzalez-Rivas D, Fieira E, Delgado M, Mendez L, Fernandez R, de la Torre M. Is Uniportal thoracoscopic surgery a feasible approach for advanced stages of non-small cell lung cancer? J Thorac Dis. 2014;6:641–8.
10. Lyscov A, Obukhova T, Ryabova V, Sekhniaidze D, Zuiev V, Gonzalez-Rivas D. Double-sleeve and carinal resections using the Uniportal VATS technique: a single centre experience. J Thorac Dis. 2016;8:S235–41.
11. Plato, Meno, section 80d. Available: http://www.perseus.tufts.edu/hopper/text?doc=Perseus%3Atext%3A1999.01.0178%3Atext%3DMeno%3Asection%3D80d
12. Elizabeth S, Sang AL, Véronique I. Beyond core knowledge: natural geometry. Cogn Sci. 2010;34:863–84.
13. Maina JN. Is the sheet-flow design a 'frozen core' (a Bauplan) of the gas exchangers? Comparative functional morphology of the respiratory microvascular systems: illustration of the geometry and rationalization of the fractal properties. Comp Biochem Physiol A Mol Integr Physiol. 2000;126:491–515.
14. Moira RD, Yi H, Elizabeth SS. Core foundations of abstract geometry. Proc Natl Acad Sci U S A. 2013;110:14191–5.
15. TaeKyu K, Yunfeng L, Tadamasa S, Zygmunt P. Gestalt-like constraints produce veridical (Euclidean) percepts of 3D indoor scenes. Vis Res. 2015;126:264–77.

16. John MF, Nilton PRF, José ADS. Visual perception of extent and the geometry of visual space. Vis Res. 2004;44:147–56.
17. Kamiyoshihara M, Igai H, Ibe T, Kawatani N, Shimizu K, Takeyoshi I. A 3.5-cm single-incision VATS anatomical segmentectomy for lung cancer. Ann Thorac Cardiovasc Surg. 2015;21:178–82.
18. Bertolaccini L, Viti A, Terzi A, Rocco G. Geometric and ergonomic characteristics of the Uniportal video-assisted thoracoscopic surgery (VATS) approach. Ann Cardiothorac Surg. 2016;5:118–22.
19. Rocco G. One-port (Uniportal) video-assisted thoracic surgical resections—a clear advance. J Thorac Cardiovasc Surg. 2012;144: S27–31.
20. Bertolaccini L, Rocco G, Viti A, Terzi A. Geometrical characteristics of Uniportal VATS. J Thorac Dis. 2013;5:S214–6.

Modified Uniportal Approach

H. Volkan Kara, Stafford S. Balderson, and Thomas A. D'Amico

Abstract

Video Assisted Thoracoscopic Surgery (VATS) for anatomical lung resection has been performed utilizing 2–4 ports in experienced thoracic surgery centers. The efforts to reduce the number of ports and incision length led to innovations in a uniportal VATS approach. These innovations have gained much popularity over the last decade. The described uniportal technique has disadvantages with regards to surgical instrumentation, ergonomic distribution of the surgical team and how a surgical trainee can be taught. Inspired by our dual port VATS approach and calling upon our experience, we have described a modified uniportal VATS technique. Our new technique also uses a single intercostal space and has potential advantages over the classical uniportal approach with a more stable camera platform, better ergonomics for the surgical team and a more productive experience for the surgeon trainee and surgeon instructor.

Introduction

Video Assisted Thoracoscopic Surgery (VATS) has been utilized in thoracic surgery beginning in the 1990s. Compared with traditional open thoracotomy, minimally invasive surgery in the form of VATS offers the surgeon the opportunity to perform all dissection of pulmonary structures (pulmonary veins, arteries and bronchi) under visualization via high definition videothoracoscopic camera systems and ergonomically oriented video monitors in the operating room (OR). The surgeon performs every surgical maneuver within the thoracic cavity without rib spreading. The surgical team uses thoracoscopic surgical instruments specifically designed to operate through small incisions (port sites) varying from 2 to 4 in number [1–3]. The procedure has been proven to be safe, with low morbidity and mortality in large patient groups [3–5]. Patients who have undergone VATS pulmonary resections have had fewer respiratory complications, fewer cardiac arrhythmias, and better pain management post operatively. They have had shorter hospital stays, less need for blood transfusion [6, 7] and better cost effectiveness [8, 9]. The Duke University Division of Thoracic Surgery has been performing VATS lobectomy for lung cancer surgery since 1999. Duke's classical VATS approach is via two incisions (dual port); a 3–4 cm utility incision in the fifth intercostal space, anterior axillary line and a 10 mm camera port in the seventh or eighth intercostal space, posterior axillary line [4]. We have been using this approach for resection of complex cases, some of which require chest wall and bronchoplastic sleeve resections [10, 11].

The movement towards decreasing the port sites and the incision length began in the 2000s with authors subsequently publishing their experience with uniportal VATS [12, 13]. The initial cases were for minor indications such as pleural biopsy and pulmonary wedge resection. As the experience progressed the first anatomic lobectomy was performed in 2010 [14] and subsequently gained increasing popularity with all pulmonary resections and intrathoracic interventions [15, 16].

Our impression is that the defined classical uniportal VATS approach using a single incision and placing the videothoracoscope within the incision has an unstable camera platform due to competition with instruments for space as well as no defined pivot point with which the thoracoscope can be balanced. Additionally, the camera holder stands on the patient's anterior and the surgeon has to share the space.

Electronic Supplementary Material The online version of this chapter (https://doi.org/10.1007/978-981-13-2604-2_6) contains supplementary material, which is available to authorized users.

H. V. Kara (✉)
Cerrahpasa Medical Faculty, Department of Thoracic Surgery, Istanbul University-Cerrahpasa, Istanbul, Turkey

S. S. Balderson · T. A. D'Amico
Division of Thoracic Surgery, Department of Surgery, Duke University Medical Center, Durham, NC, USA

D. Gonzalez-Rivas et al. (eds.), *Atlas of Uniportal Video Assisted Thoracic Surgery*,
https://doi.org/10.1007/978-981-13-2604-2_6

If a surgical trainee is present the position of the surgical team makes it difficult for the trainee to perform the surgical maneuvers with limited space and access, thus marginalizing the ability for the trainee to engage and unsafe for the surgeon instructor to manage any intraoperative complications. This suboptimal ergonomic distribution may also negatively impact the ability to teach VATS to new generations. As an alternative to this existing uniportal VATS approach we have designed a new modified technique by utilizing our existing dual port VATS experience with further innovation. This new technique is based on our existing OR facilities and thoracoscopic surgery instruments [17].

Surgical Technique

The surgical table set up is the same as our classical dual port VATS approach. The patient is intubated selectively with a dual lumen endotracheal tube (less frequently an endobronchial blocker may be used) for single lung ventilation, which is essential during surgery. The patient is placed lateral decubitus position; the non-operative side down, with slight flexion of the table at the hips which helps splaying of the ribs. This creates an easier and better exposure of the intercostal space for surgical instruments' movements and removal of the surgical specimen. The patient is secured with a belt, prepped and draped. The instrument table extends over the patient's feet. The camera equipment (light cord and camera cable) are attached to the drape at the level of the up-side axilla with available length of cable to reach the instrument table. Dual monitors are positioned at the patient's head on both sides (anteriorly and posteriorly) facilitating each member of the surgical team to have an unobstructed view of a monitor from either side of the OR table [4, 18].

At the level of fifth intercostal space over the anterior axillary line we make the approximately 4–5 cm utility incision (Fig. 1). In the deeper intercostal muscle layer in the fifth intercostal space we extend the most inner layer of the incision 1 cm on either anterior or posterior directions of the skin incision. This inner extension helps for better instrument working area thus better retrieval of the resected specimen. Adjacent to the utility incision positioned postero-inferiorly we add a 5 mm camera port incision, which enters the hemithorax within the same fifth intercostal space that had been extended previously. Through a trocar a 5 mm 30-degree angled video camera is placed for the visualization of the surgical field (Fig. 2). We position an experienced camera holder on the posterior side of the patient. The surgeon instructor and the surgical trainee are positioned on the anterior side of the patient in the working area (Fig. 3). This distribution facilitates the surgeon instructor to have his–her attention on teaching the procedure and also provides more opportunity for the surgeon trainee to participate in the steps of the procedure (Fig. 4). As the visualization from the hemithorax is achieved, the lung and the pleural space should be inspected carefully to confirm the operative plan. The procedure is conducted according to the defined steps with specific anatomic considerations. The initial goal is to lengthen the hilum with dissection. The dissection is carried out via the uniportal incision. The surgeon instructor may guide the surgeon trainee through suitable steps of the procedure according level of experience with a graduating level of responsibility while the surgeon instructor may

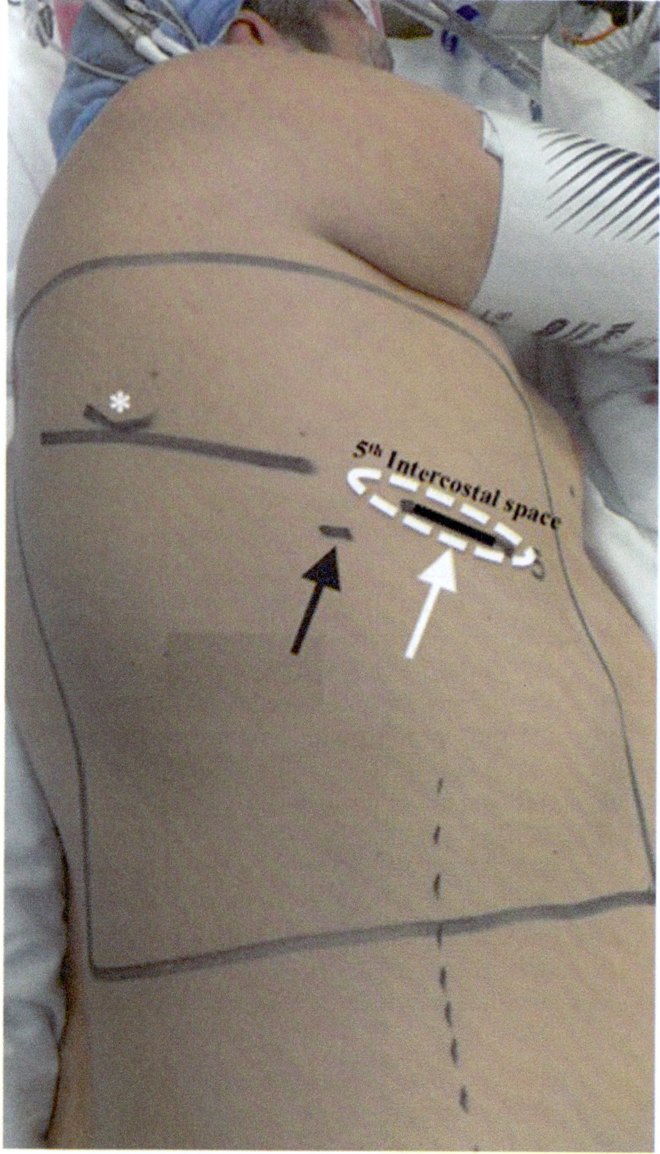

Fig. 1 Distribution of the surgical area for a right-sided modified uniportal VATS: Iliac crest and tip of the scapula (asterisk) is marked as landmarks. The utility incision (black line) is placed on the fifth intercostal space (white arrow), in the most inner layer of the incision is extended 1 cm on either anterior or posterior directions. The 5 mm camera incision (Black arrow) is placed on the posteroinferior of the utility incision using the same (5th) intercostal space with the utility incision

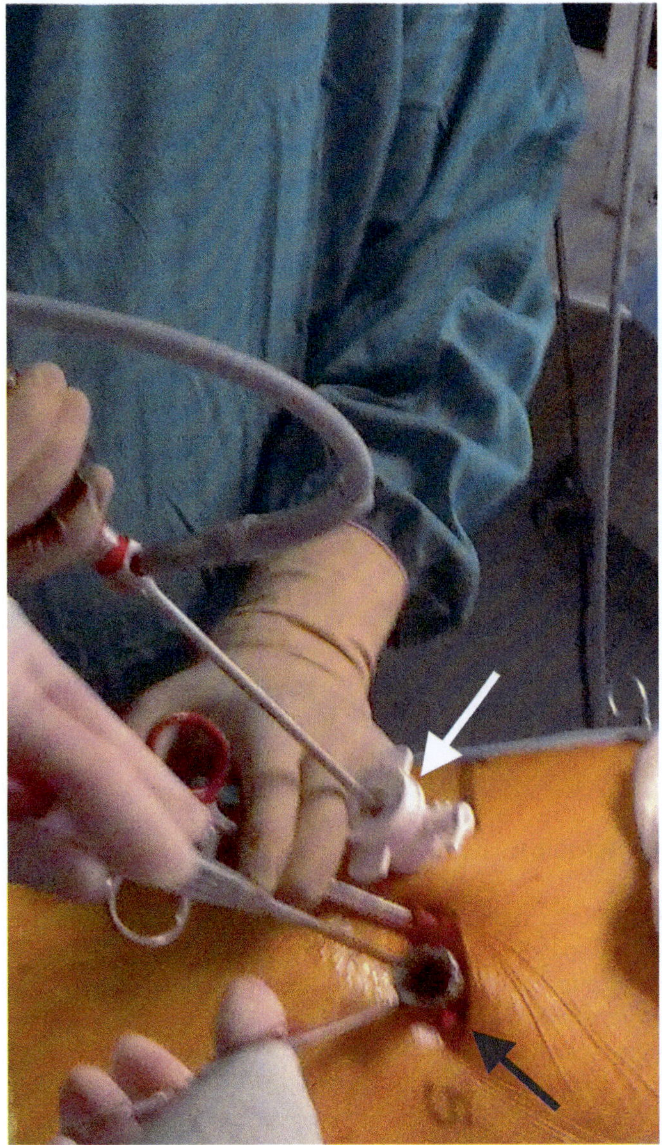

Fig. 2 The 5 mm camera uses the separate incision (White arrow), the surgical instrumentation including staping devices are placed through the utility incision (Black arrow)

provide retraction of the lung in order to optimize exposure of the hilar structures. Standardized (angulated or non angulated) endoscopic linear and vascular stapling devices are used for each vascular, bronchial and parenchymal ligation. A specimen bag is a must for the retrieval of the resected pulmonary tissue for avoiding potential seeding of the tumour cells in pleural cavity and utility incision. The extension on the intercostal muscle facilitates removal of the specimen from the hemithorax. Hilar lymph nodes should be dissected and removed as they are encountered in transit which also frequently clarifies the hilar anatomy for resection. We perform a systematic mediastinal lymph node dissection in all lung cancer cases. After the specimen has been removed, we perform five levels of intercostal blockage with a long acting local anesthetic (bupivacaine) under thoracoscopic vision. We then place a 24 F chest tube apically from the camera incision and using the camera from the utility incision to verify the positioning of the chest tube. The chest tube is secured with a single suture to be tied when the tube is removed. The utility incision is then closed with absorbable suture in the inner layers as well as subcutaneously [17, 19].

Discussion

Utilization of a single intercostal incision and adding a skin incision for a 5 mm thoracoscope has advantages. The extension of the intercostal tissue beneath the incision decreases the tension and avoids uncontrolled pressure during surgery and removal of the specimen. Each layer of the utility incision is sutured without the need for sparing a space for the chest tube. The camera port incision is used to place a 24 F chest tube into the thoracic cavity. Having the camera in a separate skin incision decreases competition with the surgical instruments, surgical maneuvers, and the thoracoscope is better stabilized by the pivot point provided by the trocar within the incision. Positioning the camera holder at the patient's posterior creates an ergonomically free space for the surgeon instructor and the surgeon trainee. The combination of the separate skin incision over the same interspace for the thoracoscope and the judicious positioning of the operative team maximizes the opportunity for the surgeon instructor to incorporate and guide the surgeon trainee facilitating a better teaching experience. Of note, this modified approach is less complicated in the resection of lower lobes as there is no need to pass the stapler from a medial port.

The use of a 5 mm thoracoscope should be gentle. The instrument is thin and fragile therefore maneuvers of the camera navigator and the surgeon must be synchronized for avoiding uncontrolled manipulation, which may easily damage the instrument.

The safety and the beneficial advantages of VATS over conventional open thoracotomy have been proven over the last decades. Aiming to decrease the number of incisions and shortening the length of the incisions has caused a recent gain in popularity for uniportal VATS. The published data comparing uniportal to multiportal demonstrates similar results for operating time, patient controlled analgesia (PCA) duration, chest tube duration, and length of hospital stay [20]. Pain scores appear to be better in uniportal VATS series [16] therefore the use of a single intercostal space appears to be more reasonable.

According to recent data from the Society of Thoracic Surgeons (STS) nearly 60% of lobectomies for lung cancer have been performed by VATS [18, 21] demonstrating significant increase since 2010 when VATS resections accounted

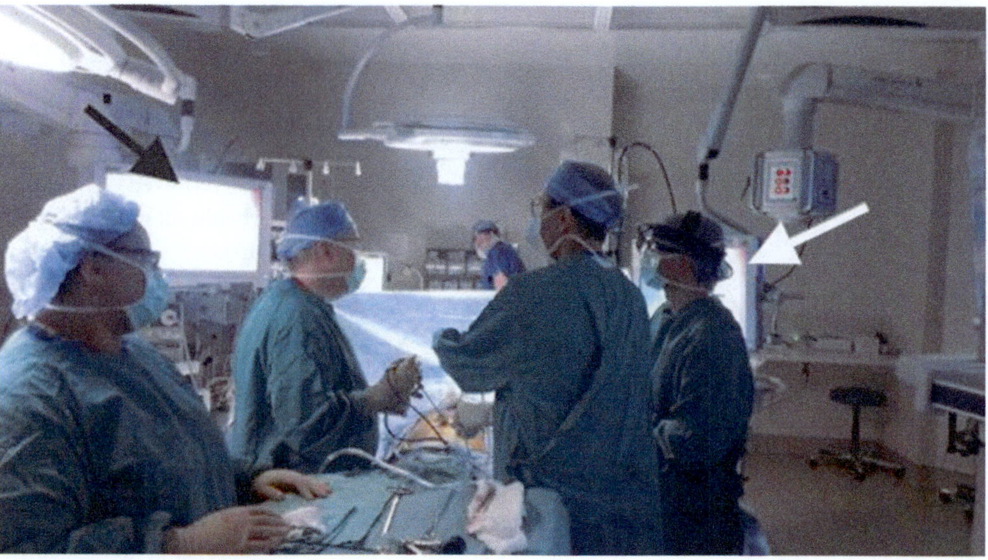

Fig 3 The surgeon and the trainee stands anterior of the patient (White arrow). The camera holder and the OR nurse stands posteriorly (Black arrow)

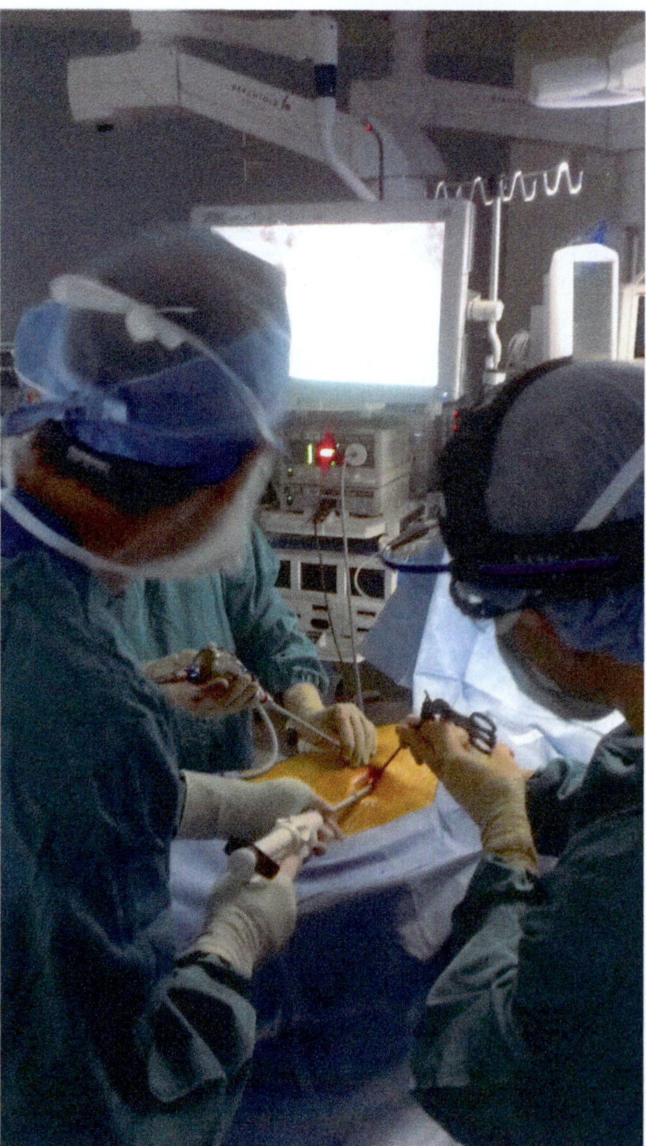

Fig. 4 Anteriorly positioning helps instructor and the surgical trainee to move more comfortably

for less than 45% [22]. This underscores the importance of teaching VATS techniques and the effect of increased numbers of new surgeon trainees whom had the opportunity to practice VATS [18].

Conclusion

Our modified uniportal VATS technique uses a single intercostal space with a more stable camera platform. We are advocating better ergonomics for surgical team members, easier surgical instrumentation, and better teaching-learning opportunities. Our routine approach for VATS resections is via our classical dual port approach. We are using this modified uniportal technique for selected patients. There is still need for evidence to prove the hypothetical advantages of uniportal VATS to multiportal VATS. Either way, the current rate of adoption indicates that there is still improvement to be made in order to make VATS the standard approach worldwide, thus training the next generation is important.

References

1. Burfeind WR, D'Amico TA. Thoracoscopic lobectomy. Oper Tech Thorac Cardiovasc Surg. 2004;9:98–114.
2. Onaitis M, D'Amico TA. Minimally invasive management of lung cancer. In: Sellke F, Swanson S, del Nido PJ, Swanson S, editors. Sabiston and Spencer's surgery of the chest. Philadelphia: Elsevier; 2004. p. 277–84.
3. Shaw JP, Dembitzer FR, Wisnivesky JP, et al. Video-assisted thoracoscopic lobectomy: state of the art and future directions. Ann Thorac Surg. 2008;85(2):S705–9.
4. Onaitis MW, Petersen RP, Balderson SS, et al. Thoracoscopic lobectomy is a safe and versatile procedure: experience with 500 consecutive patients. Ann Surg. 2006;244:420–5.
5. McKenna RJ Jr, Houck W, Fuller CB. Video-assisted thoracic surgery lobectomy: experience with 1,100 cases. Ann Thorac Surg. 2006;81:421–5;discussion 425–6.

6. Paul S, Altorki NK, Sheng S, et al. Thoracoscopic lobectomy is associated with lower morbidity than open lobectomy: a propensity-matched analysis from the STS database. J Thorac Cardiovasc Surg. 2010;139:366–78.
7. Villamizar NR, Darrabie MD, Burfeind WR, et al. Thoracoscopic lobectomy is associated with lower morbidity compared with thoracotomy. J Thorac Cardiovasc Surg. 2009;138:419–25.
8. Swanson SJ, Meyers BF, Gunnarsson CL, Moore M, et al. Video-assisted thoracoscopic lobectomy is less costly and morbid than open lobectomy: a retrospective multiinstitutional database analysis. Ann Thorac Surg. 2012;93(4):1027–32.
9. Burfeind WR, Jaik N, Villamizar N, et al. A cost-minimisation analysis of lobectomy: thoracoscopic versus posterolateral thoracotomy. Eur J Cardiothorac Surg. 2010;37:827–32.
10. Berry MF, Onaitis MW, Tong BC, et al. Feasibility of hybrid thoracoscopic lobectomy and en-bloc chest wall resection. Eur J Cardiothorac Surg. 2012;41:888–92.
11. Kara HV, Balderson SS, D'Amico TA. Challenging cases: thoracoscopic lobectomy with chest wall resection and sleeve lobectomy-Duke experience. J Thorac Dis. 2014;6(Suppl 6):S637–40.
12. Nesher N, Galili R, Sharony R, Uretzky G, Saute M. Videothorascopic sympathectomy (VATS) for palmar hyperhidriosis: summary of a clinical trial and surgical results. Harefuah. 2000;138:913–6.
13. Rocco G, Martucci N, La Manna C, et al. Ten-year experience on 644 patients undergoing single-port (uniportal) video-assisted thoracoscopic surgery. Ann Thorac Surg. 2013;96(2):434–8.
14. Gonzalez D, Paradela M, Garcia J, Dela Torre M. Single-port video-assisted thoracoscopic lobectomy. Interact Cardiovasc Thorac Surg. 2011;12:514–5.
15. Ng CS, Gonzalez-Rivas D, D'Amico TA, Rocco G. Uniportal VATS-a new era in lung cancer surgery. J Thorac Dis. 2015;7(8): 1489–91.
16. Chung JH, Choi YS, Cho JH, Kim HK, Kim J, Zo JI, Shim YM. Uniportal video-assisted thoracoscopic lobectomy: an alternative to conventional thoracoscopic lobectomy in lung cancer surgery? Interact Cardiovasc Thorac Surg. 2015;20(6):813–9.
17. Kara HV, Balderson SS, D'Amico TA. Modified uniportal video-assisted thoracoscopic lobectomy: Duke approach. Ann Thorac Surg. 2014;98:2239–41.
18. Zwischenberger BA, D'Amico TA, Tong BC. How I teach a thoracoscopic lobectomy. Ann Thorac Surg. 2016;101(3):846–9.
19. Kara HV, Balderson SS, D'Amico TA. Modified uniportal video-assisted thoracoscopic surgery (VATS). Ann Cardiothorac Surg. 2016;5(2):123–6.
20. McElnay PJ, Molyneux M, Krishnadas R, Batchelor TJ, West D, Casali G. Pain and recovery are comparable after either uniportal or multiport video-assisted thoracoscopic lobectomy: an observation study. Eur J Cardiothorac Surg. 2015;47(5):912–5.
21. Fernandez FG, Kosinski A, Burfeind W, et al. The Society of Thoracic Surgeons lung cancer resection risk model: higher quality data and superior outcomes. Presented at the 62nd annual meeting of the southern thoracic surgical association, November 5, 2015, Orlando, FL.
22. Ceppa DP, Kosinski AS, Berry MF, et al. Thoracoscopic lobectomy has increasing benefit in patients with poor pulmonary function: a Society of Thoracic Surgeons database analysis. Ann Surg. 2012;256:487–93.

Part II

Uniportal VATS in Pleural and Mediastinal Diseases

Uniportal Video-Assisted Thoracoscopic Surgery for the Management of Pleural Effusions, Empyema and Pleural Biopsy

Marco Scarci, Fabrizio Minervini, and Gaetano Rocco

Uniportal Video-Assisted Thoracoscopic Surgery (Vats) for Pleural Effusions and Pleural Biopsy

Uniportal VATS represents an excellent compromise to medical thoracoscopy and three ports VATS and we believe it brings the best of both worlds. It can be easily performed under spontaneous ventilation, much like medical thoracoscopy, but offers the same wide range of therapeutic possibilities as three ports VATS. In fact, in our experience, uniportal VATS is ideal in debriding complex pleural spaces due to the increased visibility afforded by the direct view; the thoracoscope and the instruments are in the same viewing plane allowing easier division of complex adhesions.

We perform a 3 cm incision in the fifth intercostal space, anterior axillary line. If the space is complex and the ribs are crowded a soft tissue retractor facilitates the initial dissection and introduction of instruments. The chest is then thoroughly freed up from adhesions and inspected for abnormal findings. Any fluid is collected for cytological examination and/or tissue banking.

Multiple biopsies are then taken from several areas (most suspicious and relatively normal looking for histological comparison). If there is a clear evidence of a malignant process, then we ventilate the lung to check whether the lung fully expand. In that case 8 g of talcum powder is insufflated to achieve full coverage. Using the European French talc we never experienced any issue with ARDS as described by several American articles. We believe that a good amount of talc will reduce the incidence of recurrence. If the lung is clearly trapped, then we then consider the overall fitness of the patient and the potential life expectancy. In fit patients the recent MESOVATS trial confirmed that there is no survival advantage in performing a limited vats pleurectomy decortication, but there is a symptomatic advantage. If the patient is frail, then we insert an indwelled pleural catheter. Limited VATS pleurectomy decortication is achieved by freeing up the most trapped part of the lung. The idea is not to achieve an R0 resection, but simply to obtain lung re-expansion. When the procedure is carried out there is still macroscopic tumor visible.

Once the initial incision in the fifth intercostal space is made, we proceed to the exploration of the pleural space. In determining the likely success of the procedure versus unacceptable morbidity (excessive blood loss or prolonged airleak) we consider the amount of lung trapped and the thickness of the malignant rind. If most of the lung is affected then we would not proceed with a decortication, on the other hand, if up to 50% of the lung is trapped (mostly lower lobe) then the procedure has a good chance of success. Usually we start incising the cortex on the lung and then proceeding to decorticating the lung with a mix of sharp and blunt dissection. It is easier to perform the incision of the rind with the lung inflated, visibility is usually not compromised as the lung is trapped anyhow. If there are area that are excessively expanded, then reducing the peep is advantageous. In any case warn the anesthetist not to reinflate the lung using excessive pressure in the attempt to facilitate dissection and free up the lung. Such maneuver usually determines a tear of the parenchyma at the interface between the islets of trapped lung and the relatively spared lung, as different areas react to the tangential stress differently. Those tears create a bothersome oozing that makes further decortication quite tedious. Although tempting to start the dissection of the visceral pleura near the incision site, relaying on the apparent convenience of doing under direct vision through the incision,

M. Scarci (✉)
Thoracic Surgery Unit, S. Gerardo Hospital, Monza, Italy
e-mail: m.scarci@asst-monza.it

F. Minervini
Department of Thoracic Surgery, McMaster University, Hamilton, ON, Canada

G. Rocco (✉)
Service of Thoracic Surgery, Department of Surgery Memorial Sloan Kettering Cancer Center, New York, NY, USA
e-mail: roccog@mskcc.org

D. Gonzalez-Rivas et al. (eds.), *Atlas of Uniportal Video Assisted Thoracic Surgery*,
https://doi.org/10.1007/978-981-13-2604-2_7

we would recommend otherwise. The initial dissection might be easier, but further mobilization of the visceral pleura is made really difficult by the forced acute angle of the instruments in relationship to the rest of the lung parenchyma. Our suggestion is to start away from the fissure, in a relatively flat area of the lung. Doing the dissection under ventilation allows to clearly visualize the lung underneath as the incision start to spread gently on its own. Once the correct plane is entered, we proceed in cephalad and caudal direction with a combination of blunt and diathermy dissection. Particular care is taken not to push downward toward the lung. Such maneuver comes naturally, but will result in a tear of the lung. We suggest to dissect parallel to the surface of the lung. The key point is to get into the right plane, this is identified by the shiny appearance of the lung underneath. Sometime the tumor grows in sheets and particular care must be taken to get to the bottom of them, like peeling an onion. During the dissection traction on the lung and counter traction onto the dissected pleura is essential and it is best achieved using curved instruments. Once an appropriate amount of lung is freed up and the lung fills the chest cavity, the removal of the visceral pleura is deemed complete. The last step in the procedure is the partial parietal pleurectomy. We believe that patients with advanced pleural malignancy have a restrictive chest wall movement and the ribs are crowded. To facilitate chest re-expansion we perform a bottom half parietal pleurectomy. The purpose of this procedure is three-fold:

1. Facilitate chest wall expansion as already mentioned
2. Create diffuse oozing that seals most of the ongoing air-leak. We keep the patients on suction of 2 kPa for 24–48 h. Although intuitively this is thought to prolonge the air-leak, the presence of the film of blood that results from the pleurectomy seal them, very much like the blood pleurodesis described for emphysematous patients
3. Allows effective pleurodesis to manage fluid accumulation.

Uniportal Video-Assisted Thoracoscopic Surgery (Vats) for Empyema

The use of video-assisted thoracoscopic surgery (VATS) in the treatment of pleural empyema has evolved over the last years. The role of the VATS was initially limited to confirm the diagnosis presence of empyema [1]. Only afterwards, VATS was considered as a successful approach in order to treat early fibrinopurulent empyema [2, 3]. The low morbidity and mortality in addition to better cosmetic results associated with Uniportal VATS produced a great deal of enthusiasm for the procedure.

Many retrospective analysis have shown lower morbidity and higher success rates with early surgical approach rather than delayed surgery [4] and therefore VATS played an important role in the management of empyema [5, 6]. VATS for empyema produced a shorter length of stay as well as better outcomes when compared to chest tube drainage [7–12]. In support of this conclusion, two prospective randomized studies comparing primary VATS treatment to non-image guided chest tube drainage were published demonstrating lower treatment failures and reduced need for conversion to an open approach with primary VATS [13, 14]. On the contrary similar studies in children showed no advantages of a VATS approach [15, 16]. No significant variation in cost between primary VATS and chest tube drainage was observed [17, 18].

Use of fibrinolytic agents like streptokinase/urokinase has spread recently but a large randomized double-blind trial showed that intrapleural streptokinase did not reduce the need for surgery and had a small impact on mortality [19]. Fibrinolysis provides also a viable option for chronic empyema [20] even if VATS has been shown to produce similar mortality rates, lower length of stay and greater success rates than fibrinolysis [21].

Initial trials limited the use of VATS decortication only to uncomplicated, Stage I empyema [2]. More recently, surgical decortication was performed in order to treat stage I/II empyema after failure of a trial of chest drainage. Further studies have also highlighted its effectiveness in treating multiloculated and chronic empyemas but these are associated with lower success rates than those for lower stage empyemas [14, 22, 23]. VATS surgery for empyema is usually carried out after a trial of chest tube drainage with antibiotic irrigation [24] due to the high success rates and low morbidity with tube thoracostomy [20]. Some recent studies suggest that VATS decortication could represent the first line treatment for fibrinopurulent empyema [6, 14].

VATS decortication has been shown to be effective in treating empyemas of various aetiology. Many studies have shown its efficacy at managing empyema secondary to parapneumonic effusions, to tuberculosis [25, 26] or post-pneumonectomy empyemas [7, 27].

One particular advantage of a Uniportal VATS could be potentially represented by the possibility of performing surgery without general anaesthetic. This is of particular relevance in patients with several co-morbidities not suitable for general anaesthesia. Uniportal VATS decortication could effectively manage empyema in awake patients using epidural or paravertebral nerve block [28, 29] without increasing the mortality but delivering an easier dissection during the surgery and thus lower post-operative complication rate.

The above findings indicate Uniportal that VATS holds a bright future in the treatment of empyema. Its increasing use as first-line treatment in the management of early and chronic empyema could mark a turning point in the empirical practice.

References

1. Medford AR, Awan YM, Marchbank A, Rahamim J, Unsworth-White J, Pearson PJ. Diagnostic and therapeutic performance of video-assisted thoracoscopic surgery (VATS) in investigation and management of pleural exudates. Ann R Coll Surg Engl. 2008;90(7):597–600.
2. Yamaguchi M, Takeo S, Suemitsu R, Matsuzawa H, Okazaki H. Video-assisted thoracic surgery for fibropurulent thoracic empyema: a bridge to open thoracic surgery. Ann Thorac Cardiovasc Surg. 2009;15(6):368–72.
3. Potaris K, Mihos P, Gakidis I, Chatziantoniou C. Video-thoracoscopic and open surgical management of thoracic empyema. Surg Infect. 2007;8(5):511–7.
4. Chen LE, Langer JC, Dillon PA, et al. Management of late-stage parapnuemonic empyema. J Pediatr Surg. 2002;37:371–4.
5. Wozniak CJ, Paull DE, Moezzi JE, Scott RP, Anstadt MP, York VV, Little AG. Choice of first intervention is related to outcomes in the management of empyema. Ann Thorac Surg. 2009;87(5):1525–30;discussion 1530–1;15(6):368–72.
6. Petrakis IE, Heffner JE, Klein JS. Surgery should be the first line of treatment for empyema. Respirology. 2010;15(2):202–7.
7. Gossot D, Stern JB, Galetta D, Debrosse D, Girard P, Caliandro R, et al. Thoracoscopic management of postpneumonectomy empyema. Ann Thorac Surg. 2004;78(1):273–6.
8. Cremonesini D, Thomson AH. How should we manage empyema: antibiotics alone, fibrinolytics, or primary video-assisted thoracoscopic surgery (VATS)? Semin Respir Crit Care Med. 2007;28:322–32.
9. Cassina PC, Hauser M, Hillejan L, et al. Video-assisted thoracoscopy in the treatment of pleural empyema: stage-based management and outcome. J Thorac Cardiovasc Surg. 1999;117:234–8.
10. Striffeler H, Gugger M, Im Hof V, et al. Video-assisted thoracoscopic surgery for fibrinopurulent pleural empyema in 67 patients. Ann Thorac Surg. 1998;65:319–23.
11. Waller DA, Rengarajan A. Thoracoscopic decortication: a role for video-assisted surgery in chronic postpneumonic pleural empyema. Ann Thorac Surg. 2001;71:1813–6.
12. Aziz A, Healey JM, Qureshi F, Kane TD, Kurland G, Green M, Hackam DJ. Comparative analysis of chest tube thoracostomy and video-assisted thoracoscopic surgery in empyema and parapneumonic effusion associated with pneumonia in children. Surg Infect. 2008;9(3):317–23.
13. Bilgin M, Akcali Y, Oguzkaya F. Benefits of early aggressive management of empyema thoracis. ANZ J Surg. 2006;76(3):120–2.
14. Wait MA, Sharma S, Hohn J, Nogare AD. A randomised trial of empyema therapy. Chest. 1997;111:1548–51.
15. St Peter SD, Tsao K, Harrison C, et al. Thoracoscopic decortication vs tube thoracostomy with fibrinolysis for empyema in children: a prospective, randomised trial. J Pediatr Surg. 2009;44:106–11.
16. Sonanappa S, Cohen G, Owens CM, et al. Comparison of urokinase and video-assisted thoracoscopic surgery for treatment of childhood empyema. Am J Respir Crit Care Med. 2006;174:221–7.
17. Shah SS, Ten Have TR, Metlay JP. Costs of treating children with complicated pneumonia: a comparison of primary video-assisted thoracoscopic surgery and chest tube placement. Pediatr Pulmonol. 2010;45:71–7.
18. Cohen E, Weinstein M, Fisman DN. Cost-effectiveness of competing strategies for the treatment of pediatric empyema. Pediatrics. 2008;121(5):e1250–7.
19. Maskell NA, Davies CW, Nunn AJ, Hedley EL, Gleeson FV, Miller R, Gabe R, Rees GL, Peto TE, Woodhead MA, Lane DJ, Darbyshire JH, Davies RJ. First multicenter intrapleural sepsis trial (MIST1) group. U.K. Controlled trial of intrapleural streptokinase for pleural infection. N Engl J Med. 2005;352(9):865–74.
20. Demirhan R, Kosar A, Sancakli I, Kiral H, Orki A, Arman B. Management of postpneumonic empyemas in children. Acta Chir Belg. 2008;108(2):208–11.
21. Khan N, Mian I, Javed A, Wazir S, Yousaf M. Efficacy, safety and tolerability of streptokinase in multiloculated empyema. J Ayub Med Coll Abbottabad. 2003;15(4):20–2.
22. Drain AJ, Ferguson JI, Sayeed R, et al. Definitive management of advanced empyema by two-window video-assisted surgery. Asian Cardiovasc Thorac Ann. 2007;15:238–9.
23. Luh SP, Chou MC, Wang LS, Chen JY, Tsai TP. Video-assisted thoracoscopic surgery in the treatment of complicated parapneumonic effusions or empyemas: outcome of 234 patients. Chest. 2005;127(4):1427–32.
24. Shiraishi Y. Surgical treatment of chronic empyema. Gen Thorac Cardiovasc Surg. 2010;58(7):311–6.
25. Barbetakis N, Paliouras D, Asteriou C, Tsilikas C. Ecomment: the role of video-assisted thoracoscopic surgery in the management of tuberculous empyemas. Interact Cardiovasc Thorac Surg. 2009;8(3):337–8.
26. Olgac G, Yilmaz MA, Ortakoylu MG, Kutlu CA. Decision-making for lung resection in patients with empyema and collapsed lung due to tuberculosis. J Thorac Cardiovasc Surg. 2005;130:131–5.
27. Zahid I, Routledge T, Bille A, Scarci M. What is the best treatment of postpneumonectomy empyema? Interact Cardiovasc Thorac Surg. 2010;12(2):260–4.
28. Tacconi F, Pompeo E, Fabbi E, Mineo TC. Awake video-assisted pleural decortication for empyema thoracis. Eur J Cardiothorac Surg. 2010;37(3):594–601.
29. Katlic MR. Video-assisted thoracic surgery utilizing local anaesthesia and sedation. Eur J Cardiothorac Surg. 2006;30:529–32.

Uniportal Approach to Pericardial Window and Sympathectomy

Simon C. Y. Chow and Calvin S. H. Ng

Abstract

Pericardial window creation and thoracic sympathectomy are relatively simple procedures that can be performed by uniportal VATS approach. Successful drainage of pericardial effusion via a pericardial window can improve quality of life of patients and reduce frequency of admissions, while successful elimination of hyperhidrosis can improve patient satisfaction and self esteem. With the evolution of surgical techniques and emergence of uniportal thoracic surgery, excellent procedural outcomes can be achieved while minimizing surgical trauma to patients. In this chapter, we will introduce and describe the latest uniportal approaches to pericardial window and sympathectomy. In addition, technical considerations and select clinical results will also be discussed.

Pericardial Window

Introduction

Pericardial effusion (PE) is a commonly encountered condition in daily clinical practice. Causes can range from thyroid dysfunction, infection, inflammatory disease, uremia to disseminated malignancies. Around half of patients with PE develop cardiac tamponade requiring urgent drainage. Hence PE itself contributes to significant morbidity and carries a risk of mortality. The prognosis of PE depends on the underlying cause, and the ideal intervention for PE should not only achieve palliation of symptoms and prevention of recurrence, but also serves to obtain adequate samples for diagnosis. Options of pericardial drainage vary from non-surgical to surgical means including needle pericardiocentesis, pericardial drains, balloon pericardiotomy, pericardial window and pericardiectomy. Surgical pericardial drainage is preferred for patients with recurrent effusion, while needle pericardiocentesis is a better immediate option for patents with cardiac tamponade and hemodynamic instability. Subxiphoid and open transthoracic pericardial window have been well established as safe and effective options for pericardial drainage, however with the recent surge of interest and advancement in minimal invasive surgery and the rapid development of thoracoscopy, video-assisted thoracoscopic (VATS) pericardial window is increasingly practiced amongst surgeons. Until recently, needlescopic VATS thoracic surgery have been described in the literature [1]. A number of studies have found the VATS approach to be safe and feasible for a wide variety of thoracic and mediastinal conditions and is associated with less wound pain, as well as better and speedier recovery in patients post-operatively [2]. In particular, with the recent rapid expansion and utilization of uniportal surgery, different uniportal approaches to pericardial window have been reported worldwide. In addition, innovative techniques such as natural orifice trans-luminal endoscopic surgery (NOTES) have been explored and are currently under investigation. In this chapter, we will introduce and explore the different methods of pericardial drainage, with particular focus on uniportal VATS pericardial window, patient selection and latest advancements.

Patient Selection and Preoperative Planning

Patients with recurrent PE should be considered for surgery. All patients should have a formal echocardiogram to document the thickness of the pericardium and effusion, as

Electronic Supplementary Material The online version of this chapter (https://doi.org/10.1007/978-981-13-2604-2_8) contains supplementary material, which is available to authorized users.

S. C. Y. Chow · C. S. H. Ng (✉)
Division of Cardiothoracic Surgery, Department of Surgery, Prince of Wales Hospital, The Chinese University of Hong Kong, Hong Kong SAR, China
e-mail: calvinng@surgery.cuhk.edu.hk

D. Gonzalez-Rivas et al. (eds.), *Atlas of Uniportal Video Assisted Thoracic Surgery*,
https://doi.org/10.1007/978-981-13-2604-2_8

well as look for any features of tamponade. Echocardiogram may in some cases provide evidence for an unsuspecting diagnosis for the PE, such as aortic dissection, myocardial infarction or even an infiltrating cardiac tumour. Computed tomography (CT) of the thorax is useful to look for the extent of PE including the presence of loculations and masses both within and surrounding the pericardium, as well as pleural diseases such as pleural effusion that can be managed concomitantly during surgery. Hence, CT scan has an important role in providing information for deciding the type of approach, as well as the laterality of the approach.

Anesthetic concerns also differ for different surgical approaches. Subxiphoid and transthoracic open approach can be performed under local anesthesia with sedation in the supine position. These approaches are recommended in patients who are marginal candidates for surgery or during emergencies as urgent subxiphoid pericardial drainage can be performed if the patient deteriorates on the operating table before the operation. In addition, these approaches do not require one lung ventilation or decubitus positioning. For the VATS approach, patients are often positioned in the lateral decubitus position, or supine with 30 degrees tilt, with double lumen endobronchial tube intubation and one lung ventilation. The VATS approach is not recommended in patients who are hemodynamically unstable or intolerant of one—lung ventilation.

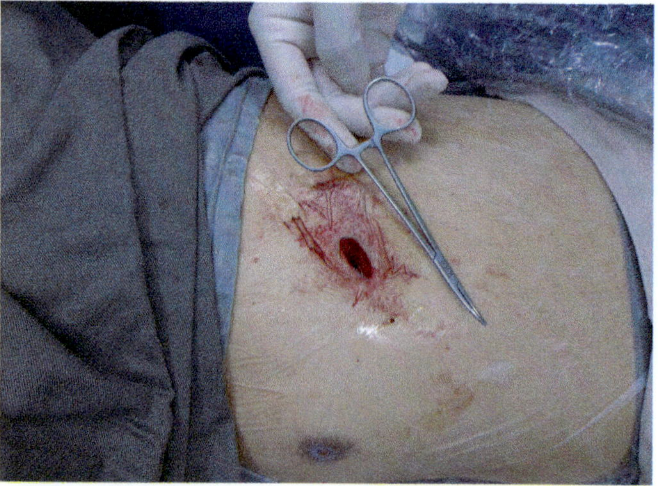

Fig. 1 Two centimetre single incision at fifth intercostal space on the anterior axillary line

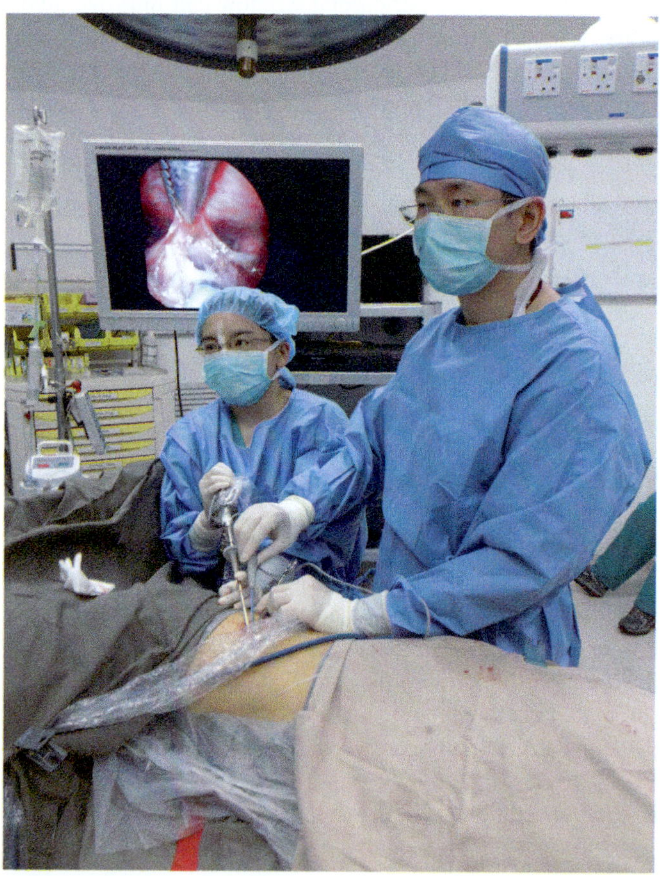

Fig. 2 Cameraman and surgeon on the same side for the uniportal approach to pericardial window

Uniportal VATS Pericardial Window

Uniportal VATS approach has displayed great versatility and is being reported in major lung resections including lobectomies and pneumonectomies, as well as complex bronchoplastic resections. Numerous studies have shown that uniportal VATS is safe and equally effective as conventional three ports VATS for various thoracic conditions [3–5]. Uniportal VATS pericardial window was first described by Rocco and colleagues in 2006 [6]. In that report, four patients with malignant pleuro-pericardial effusions had uniportal pericardial window performed under general anesthesia via single lung ventilation.

In our approach, patients are placed in supine position or with hemithorax elevated 45 degrees with a roll, then a 2.5 cm incision is created in the fifth intercostal space along the mid axillary line (Fig. 1). The assistant cameraman stands on the same side as the surgeon (Fig. 2). The pleural cavity is inspected using a 5 mm 30 degree videothoracoscope. The pericardium is opened under direct vision anterior to the phrenic nerve (Fig. 3). The opening on the pericardium is circumferentially enlarged with endoscissors inserted parallel to the thoracoscope to create the desired window (Video 1). A thoracostomy tube is placed through the same incision and removed post-operatively when drain output decreases (Fig. 4). To date, cases of uniportal VATS pericardial window have been reported as part of larger studies looking into the feasibility and versatility of single port surgery. Song et al. reported their own series of uniportal

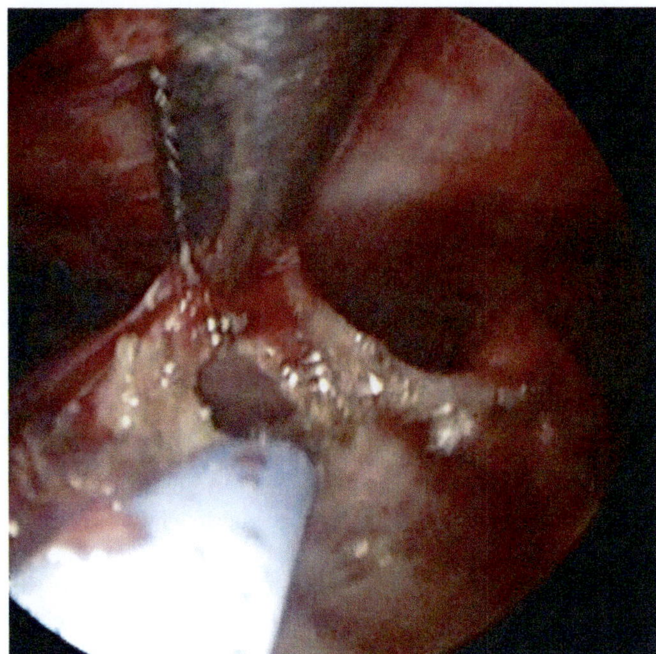

Fig. 3 Creation of pericardial window via uniportal access with diathermy, and variable angulated graspers

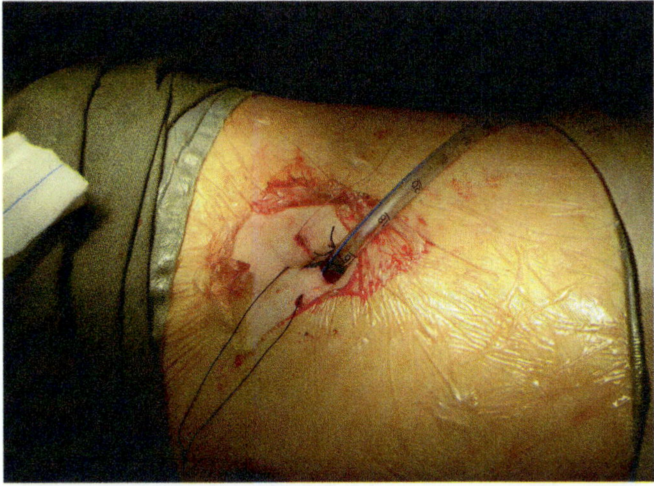

Fig. 4 Post pericardial window chest drain inserted via operative incision

VATS in a heterogeneous group of patients with mediastinal and thoracic pathologies [7]. Of the 264 cases in the series, 3 cases of single port pericardial window were reported. The pleural cavity was accessed via a 2.5–3.0 cm long incision in the sixth to seventh intercostal space. All three cases of pericardial window formation did not require conversion or further incisions, but there was limited data on patients' follow-up. In a recent larger case series of 644 cases of uniportal VATS thoracic surgery spanning 10 years, Rocco et al. further demonstrated the versatility of uniportal VATS. In his cohort, 17.8% of the 644 patients operated

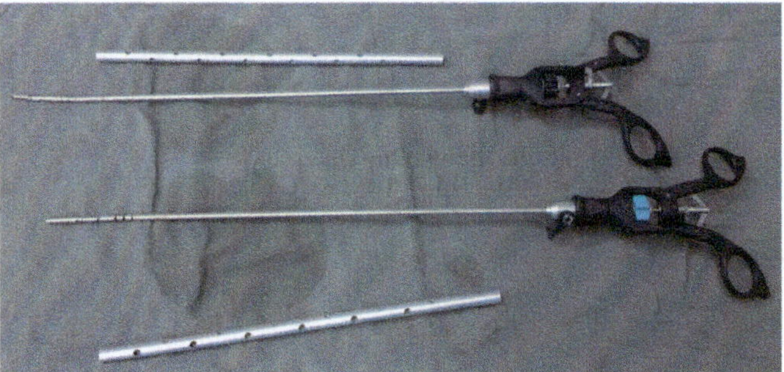

Fig. 5 Endoscopic long graspers (straight and angulated Snowden Pencer endograspers)

under uniportal VATS had pathologies other than lung nodules or pleural effusion. Ninety-five percent of the patients had the surgery done under general anesthesia with reported conversion rates at 3.7% [8]. Although no specific data concerning the number of cases, overall success and complication for uniportal pericardial window is available from the paper; nonetheless this study has further reinforced the increasing consensus that uniportal VATS is feasible and safe in a wide variety of thoracic and mediastinal conditions.

A possible concern regarding uniportal VATS is the limited working space, resulting in instrument fencing and frequent soiling of the videothoracoscope lens. Hence meticulous preoperative planning is important, as application of endoscopic instruments may be hindered by suboptimal positioning of the incision necessitating a second port for better intrathoracic manipulation. As a result, flexible, long curved or variable angled instruments have been developed to facilitate uniportal VATS, and special considerations and techniques are described to minimize fencing [9] (Fig. 5). The proposed advantages of uniportal VATS over three port VATS are less pain and paraesthesia as well as better satisfaction postoperatively, although conclusive large scaled studies are lacking to prove the superiority of uniportal VATS over traditional three port approach. Multiple studies have shown uniportal VATS is an equally effective and safe alternative to 2 or 3 port VATS in a wide variety of thoracic and mediastinal conditions [3–5].

Sympathectomy

Introduction

Primary hyperhidrosis (PH) is a disorder of eccrine glands. Patients experience excessive sweating greater than physiological needs for thermoregulation. PH affects quality of life as well as leads to feelings of shame and low self-esteem. The condition mostly affects young adults with onset during puberty and has no predilection for male or female. Treatment of PH can be categorized into non-surgical and surgical options. Non-surgical treatment includes the use of oral (for example, propantheline and oxybutynin) or topical medications (for example, aluminum chloride and glycopyrrolate), iontophoresis and botulinum toxin. Newer non-surgical options such as ablative ultrasound to destroy cutaneous sweat glands are still under investigation. The efficacy of nonsurgical treatment for PH is unpredictable and modest. Treatments such as iontophoresis and botulinum toxin injections require long term maintenance therapy for sustained effect, and recurrences are common. Lifelong treatment is also less cost effective when compared to surgery, especially in patients with severe hyperhidrosis.

Thoracic sympathectomy was first reported in 1920 by Kotzareff [10]. Sympathectomy was not popularized until Kux reported the thoracoscopic approach for sympathectomy which significantly reduced access trauma, and made sympathectomy more acceptable amongst patients [11]. Formally introduced in the 1980s, endoscopic thoracic sympathectomy (ETS) has become the mainstay treatment for severe cases of PH. Over the past 20 years, there has been substantial improvements in endoscopic techniques and major advances in minimally invasive surgical equipment. Studies have shown that ETS is both a safe and effective treatment for PH with success rates over 90% [12, 13]. The emergence of uniportal surgery and natural orifice transluminal surgery has further reduced surgical access trauma with promising results.

VATS Sympathectomy

Patient Selection

VATS sympathectomy is indicated for patients with severe PH suffering from intolerable sweating that persistently interferes with their daily lives. It is important to rule out secondary causes of hyperhidrosis as sympathectomy is not indicated in patients with secondary hyperhidrosis caused by underlying metabolic, infectious or malignant causes. Generally, VATS sympathectomy is the approach of choice when other non-surgical therapies have failed, and for those sufferers seeking a more permanent solution for PH. Success rates have been quoted from 92 to 100%, with particularly promising results in patients with palmar hyperhidrosis [14].

Extra caution is required in patients with history of chronic lung disease or previous lung surgery as adhesions may be present and make surgical approach to the sympathetic nerve difficult. Chest computed tomography is not necessary in most patients with PH, especially in young adults. Some centres monitor temperature rise via thermometer and sensor probes in bilateral palms or digits to ensure successful sympathectomy, a rise of around 1.5 °C is generally indicative of successful sympathectomy.

Technical Consideration of Sympathectomy

The principle of sympathectomy is to denervate the eccrine glands by interrupting nerve conduction in the sympathetic chain. Techniques and approaches vary. Methods of interruption of sympathetic chain also range from cauterization, cutting, clipping to division. Some centres advocate ganglionectomy and ramicotomy; while others prefer selective sympathicotomy sparing the ganglions. Sympathicotomy as oppose to more radical denervation procedures usually result in less compensatory hyperhidrosis (CH). The level of interruption of the chain is a decision that should be based on the pattern of hyperhidrosis and patient's preference. A set of terminology regarding level of interruption has been proposed for better consistency in research and communication. Level of sympathectomy is presented in relation to the rib number. Hence R2 being above the second rib, R3 above the third rib and so on [15]. R3 and R4 interruption yields the driest hands in patients with palmar hyperhidrosis alone, but entails a higher risk of CH. R3 interruption alone may lead to moister hands but lower incidence of CH. Hence, in general, R3 interruption is recommended for patients with palmar hyperhidrosis alone. For craniofacial hyperhidrosis, Chou and colleagues reported CH rate of 27% following R3 only interruption when compared with CH rate of more than 40% following R2 interruption [16]. In another series, R2 and R3 interruption was found to have higher CH rate than R2 alone [17]. Therefore based on these findings, experts suggest R3 only interruption for craniofacial hyperhidrosis for its lower risk of CH. The debate on whether cauterizing, clipping or ablation of the sympathetic chain achieves better symptom resolution is ongoing, and so far no discernible difference among different techniques has been reported, provided the sympathectomy is done properly with enough separation between ends of chain to prevent regrowth. The proposed extent of lateral cauterization of communicating fibres (Fibres of Kuntz) is around 2–3 cm lateral to the sympathetic ganglion. It is important that regardless of the technique used, we advocate complete cut of the chain down to the rib periosteum and ablation of the nerve of Kuntz to avoid recurrence. Resection of a certain length of the chain is not proven to be superior to cauterization only.

The conventional bilateral ETS is done with 2–3 ports on each side. 10 mm ports and 5 mm ports are created for the insertion of the camera and dissecting instruments respectively. ETS is done under general anaesthesia with double lumen tube intubation and single lung ventilation. Depending on surgeon preference, patients are either placed in 30 degrees reversed Trendelenburg position with arms abducted or in lateral decubitus position. The former approach allows bilateral ETS to be performed without the need to reposition the patient halfway through the procedure. Bilateral ETS are usually performed in the same session, and patients are discharged later on the same day or day after. The introduction of needlescopic instruments allow for even smaller incisions. Technical details of port placement and 2-port or 3-port approaches vary depending on patient anatomy and surgeon preference. The 2-port approach is more commonly used. Success rates have been quoted in multiple studies to be above 90%, with complications, excluding CH, at 5.7–9.7%, and 1.9–2.7% requiring further post-operative intervention such as chest drain insertion or re-exploration [12, 18]. Serious complications that have been reported include pneumothorax (1%), hemothorax (1%), chylothorax (1%), bradycardia and Horner's syndrome (0.7–3%) secondary to damage to stellate ganglion [15]. Rarely, permanent bradycardia has been reported in patients post sympathectomy. The guidelines therefore discourages sympathectomy for patients with preoperative baseline pulse rate of less than 55 per minute. Cases of pacemaker dependent bradycardia have been reported and patients should be warned of risk of reduced exercise capacity post operation [19]. The reported rate of CH varies in the range of 2.5% to as high as 97% and is the single most significant complication that affects patient satisfaction. In our centre's experience, clinical outcomes after needlescopic thoracic sympathectomy by either cauterization or nerve excision for patients with palmar and axillary hyperhidrosis were excellent. At 16-month follow up, there was no recurrence of hyperhidrosis, and 5% developed CH that did not warrant further intervention.

Despite the ultra-minimal invasive nature of needlescopic VATS, chronic postoperative wound sequelae over thoracic incisions were reported to affect 31.4% of patients in a series [20]. In another study, residual wound pain, numbness and paresthesia were also reported in around 40% of patients [21]. Over 15% of patients also experienced residual shoulder joint dysfunction and paraesthesia. In our series, the rate of paraesthesia was 50% post needlescopic sympathectomy, with 17.6% of patients experiencing the symptom 12 months post-surgery [22].

Uniportal Thoracic Endoscopic Sympathectomy

One stage bilateral uniportal sympathectomy can be safely and successfully performed, and is increasingly practiced around the world. Studies have shown uniportal surgery has benefits over conventional ETS in terms of less post-operative pain, better aesthetics and shorter operative time. Furthermore, the efficacy and rates of CH are not inferior to conventional ETS.

Many different methods of uniportal surgery have been reported [22, 23]. The majority of cases are done under general anesthesia with double lumen intubation and single-lung ventilation. Patients can be positioned in the semi-sitting position with 90 degrees abduction of the upper limbs or the lateral decubitus position. The Semi-Fowler's position is desirable as this allows bilateral surgery without readjustment of position and can facilitate improved intraoperative upper posterior chest wall exposure via inferior displacement of lung by gravity. The use of CO_2 insufflation to aid in the collapse of lung is commonly used, but insufflation pressure should be kept below 6–8 mmHg to avoid haemodynamic compromise. A single incision is made over the anterior axillary line around third to fourth intercostal space lateral to the pectoralis major muscle bilaterally, and the length of the incision is around 8 mm to 1 cm. Other reports have utilized incisions at the mid axillary line. Various instruments have been reportedly used for uniportal sympathectomy, and the number of instrument inserted into the incision also varies. The initial report utilized a modified pediatric urology cystoureteroscopy for the bilateral procedure [23]. Subsequently, Rocco described the technique of using conventional endoscopic instruments such as the 3 mm thoracoscope and 5 mm endoscopic dissector to accomplish the sympathectomy. However, this requires insertion of two instruments into a small incision which may result in fencing and undesirable movements of the endoscope. The use of single incision laparoscopic surgery port (SILS) port may be considered which can accommodate up to three endoscopic instruments via a flexible multichannel access port.

An alternative to the traditional endoscopic instruments is the use of Vasoview Hemopro 2 dissector for sympathectomy (Fig. 6). Originally designed for endoscopic vein harvesting, the multifunctional single instrument module allows uniportal sympathectomy without the need to fit multiple instruments into one small incision [24]. The instrument consists of a 7 mm high resolution endoscope, a parallel working channel for the Hemopro 2 dissector, a built in CO_2 gas insufflation channel and retractable lens cleaning system all incorporated

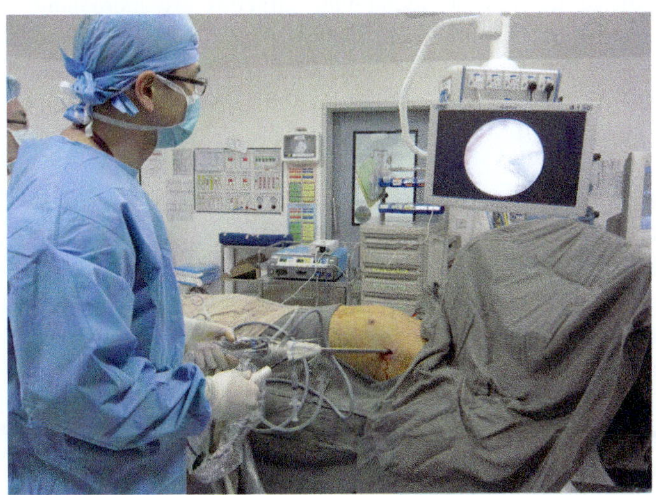

Fig. 6 Single port endoscopic sympathectomy with Vasoview device

into the 12 mm diameter Vasoview device. The design of the Hemopro 2 grasper and scissors contain unique thermostatic designs which can reduce collateral thermal tissue damage during cutting and cauterization (Video 2).

So far no direct comparisons have been made between different uniport techniques. Chest drains are not necessary postoperatively unless there is extensive adhesiolysis or minor lung parenchymal injury. Withdrawal of endoscopic suction device while the patient is on inspiratory hold via manual ventilation can minimize post-operative pneumothorax.

Results of uniportal surgery have been encouraging. In a series of 130 patients undergoing uniport ETS for palmar hyperhidrosis, there was 100% symptom resolution, with reported quality of life improvement in over 90%. The rate of CH was 19%, and none of the patients experienced residual pain during follow-up on postoperative day 7. The major complication rate was 0.35%. Mean operation time was 38 min with mean hospital stay of 1.1 days [25]. Another study reported 97% of patients with two point reduction in the hyperhidrosis severity score after receiving uniport ETS of mixed methods and approach with Vasoview or paediatric GAAB neuroendoscopes. Out of the 100 patients, only 13% required analgesics during the first week following their surgery [26]. In our centre, 16 patients underwent Vasoview bilateral VATS sympathectomy for severe palmar hyperhidrosis. All procedures were successful with resolution of hyperhidrosis in all patients. Mean operative time was 56 min for bilateral procedures, and there were no conversion to larger incisions. Mean post-operative stay was <1 day and the post operation VAS pain score at discharge was 1.8 [27]. In a study comparing uniportal ETS and 2-port ETS, Chen et al. found uniportal ETS to be equally safe and effective as conventional ETS, with less postoperative pain and shorter operative time (39.5 vs 49.7 min) [28]. While more stringent studies are needed to substantiate the benefit of uniportal ETS over conventional ETS, with the maturation of the uniport technique, surgeons are increasingly comfortable in practicing uniport surgery. Patients should be adequately consented to be able to choose between conventional ETS and uniport ETS depending on available expertise [29].

Nonintubated Uniportal Sympathectomy

Carillo et al. reported the novel technique of nonintubated bilateral uniportal sympathectomy in 2015 in an outpatient setting. The first cases of awake thoracoscopic sympathectomy were performed in 2005 by Elia via the two port approach, since then small scaled studies have shown the safety and effectiveness of non-intubated awake thoracoscopic sympathectomy [30]. Carillo's technique involves putting the patient in a semi-Fowler's position with both arms abducted [31]. Oxygenation is provided via a venturi mask with oxygen 3–4 L/min. Controlled infusion of propofol is administered with additional sedation by midazolam and remifentanil. Local anesthesia is injected and a 8 mm skin incision is created in the anterior axillary line at the level of the third intercostal space. An open pneumothorax is created via the insertion of a flexible trocar, and the lung is collapsed. Local anesthesia is injected into both sides of the sympathetic chain at the level of T3. The parietal pleura is incised and the sympathetic chain is cauterized down to reach the rib periosteum. The nerve bundle of kuntz is also divided. A chest tube connected to suction is inserted into the pleural cavity after hemostasis with the patient in full inspiration. The drain is removed once chest X-ray in the recovery show no significant pneumothorax. The patient was discharged 6 h after surgery on the same day, with clinic follow up showing dry hands.

Non intubated VATS surgery provides numerous advantages over intubated surgery. Most noteworthy is the avoidance of complications relating to endotracheal tube insertion such as airway trauma, barotrauma during mechanical ventilation, neuromuscular blockade and relatively slow pulmonary recovery. To date, no randomized controlled trial is present to prove the superiority of the non intubated approach, but it is believed to enhance post operative recovery, leading to earlier discharge.

Main contraindications of non-intubated thoracic surgery include hemodynamic instability, morbidly obese patients, expected dense and extensive pleural adhesions, non-compliant patients, and contraindications to regional anesthesia such as coagulopathy. This approach should only be adopted provided there is an experienced anesthetist who can immediately secure the airway and intubate the patient (even in lateral decubitus position) in the event of complications.

Embryonic Natural Orificial Transumbilical Endoscopic Surgery (ENOTES)

Zhu et al. reported their experience of transumbilical thoracic sympathectomy in 148 patients with an ultrathin flexible endoscope. The reported advantage of embryonic natural orifice transumbilical endoscopy surgery in which the umbilicus is used as the port of entry, is the elimination of wounds and incisions over the chest wall which is the main cause behind chronic postoperative pain, numbness or paraesthesia. Patents with cardiopulmonary disease, and history of pulmonary or abdominal surgeries are excluded from ENOTES. After placing the patient under general anesthesia and double lumen intubation, a 5 mm incision was made over the umbilicus. Pneumoperitoneum was achieved at 10 mmHg CO_2 under the guidance of an ultrathin gastroscope and the thoracic cavity was entered via the muscular pars of the diaphragmatic dome with a 5 mm needle knife. T3 ganglionectomy was performed with a hot biopsy forceps for patients with palmar hyperhidrosis; and T3 + T4 ganglionectomy performed for patients with palmar and axillary hyperhidrosis. Accessory fibres and nerves of Kuntz were then cauterized up to 2 cm lateral of the ganglion. In their series of 148 patients successfully treated for palmar hyperhidrosis, the average hospital stay was 1 day and the mean operation time was 43 min. No major complications were reported. The rate of CH was around 22.3 % in 4 years follow-up. Overall resolution of palmar hyperhidrosis was 98% and axillary hyperhidrosis at 74.6%. At 14 months follow-up, 97% of the patients remained symptom free, and almost all the patients were satisfied with the cosmetic results of the surgery [32]. In a comparative study between ENOTES and needlescopic sympathectomy, ENOTES was found to be comparable with VATS sympathectomy in terms of efficacy and complications. Despite the longer operative time (56 vs 40 min), patients underwent ENOTES had reduced post-operative pain and paresthesia at all-time intervals. There was no report of intra-abdominal complications around 1.4 years follow-up [33, 34].

The true value of ENOTES and its added benefit over conventional or uniport ETS remains to be investigated. Studies with larger sample size and longer follow-up are needed to address issues such as added risk of intra-abdominal complications so as to allow surgeons and patients a more accurate measurement of ENOTES's overall value. Nonetheless, ENOTES may represent an alternative for patients who do not wish to have thoracic incisions or have had previous surgery around the chest.

Subxiphoid Uniport Technique

Chen et al. described the first case of single incision subxiphoid thoracoscopic ablative sympathectomy for bilateral hyperhidrosis [35]. This was the first reported bilateral sympathectomy via the subxiphoid approach. The patient was put in a reverse Trendelenburg position with double lumen intubation. Under general anesthesia, a single 2 cm subxiphoid incision was made followed by blunt finger dissection to access the pleural cavity. A 10 mm zero degree thoracoscope was inserted through the incision to explore the pleural cavity. The Sympathetic trunk was identified at the T2 and T3 level and cut with electrocautery. Residual air was evacuated from the thoracic cavity at the end of the procedure with the lungs inflated maximally. Total operative was 60 min and the patient was discharged the next day with resolution of hyperhidrosis at 6 months of follow up. The reported advantage of this approach is the absence of scars in the chest wall and there is no need to traverse the abdominal cavity. The subxiphoid approach, similar to the ENOTES should offer patients with another option in experienced hands, but its superiority is not established over VATS approach.

Conclusion

Uniportal pericardial window and sympathectomy have proven to be safe and effective with good results in terms of symptom improvement and recovery [36].

Shorter incisions and single port access minimize access trauma and further reduces patient discomfort and pain post operatively. There is increasing interests in natural orifice access surgery and alternative access single incision surgery such as the subxiphoid approach, which holds promise in further improving patient care. The emergence of non-intubated uniportal surgery also helps develop outpatient based thoracic surgery, increasing the appeal of lifestyle surgery such as sympathectomy to younger patients. Ultimately, the introduction of uniportal thoracic surgery, along with its evolving techniques, should improve the quality of life of patients with debilitating conditions such as pericardial effusion and primary hyperhidrosis.

References

1. Ng CS, Lau KK, Gonzalez-Rivas D, et al. Evolution in surgical approach and techniques for lung cancer. Thorax. 2013;68:681.
2. Li WW, Lee TW, Lam SS, et al. Quality of life following lung cancer resection: video-assisted thoracic surgery vs thoracotomy. Chest. 2002;122:584–9.
3. Ng CSH. Uniportal VATS in Asia. J Thorac Dis. 2013;5:S221–5.
4. Lau RW, Ng CS, Kwok MW, et al. Early outcomes following uniportal video-assisted thoracic surgery lung resection. Chest. 2014;145(Suppl 3):A50.
5. Gonzalez-Rivas D, Paradela M, Fernandez R, et al. Uniportal video-assisted thoracoscopic lobectomy: two years of experience. Ann Thorac Surg. 2013;95:426–32.
6. Rocco G, La Rocca A, La Manna C, et al. Uniportal video-assisted thoracoscopic surgery pericardial window. J Thorac Cardiovasc Surg. 2006;131:921–2.
7. Song IH, Yum SW, Choi WS, et al. Clinical application of single incision thoracoscopic surgery: early experience of 264 cases. J Cardiothorac Surg. 2014;9:44.
8. Rocco G, Martucci N, La Manna C, et al. Ten-year experience on 644 patients undergoing single-port (uniportal) video-assisted thoracoscopic surgery. Ann Thorac Surg. 2013;96:434–8.
9. Ng CSH, Wong RHL, Lau RWH, Yim APC. Minimizing chest wall trauma in single port video-assisted thoracic surgery. J Thorac Cardiovasc Surg. 2014;147(3):1095–6.
10. Kotzareff A. Resection partielle de trone sympathetique cervical droit pour hyperhidrosis unilateral. Rev Med Suisse Romande. 1920;40:111–3.
11. Kux F. The endoscopic approach to the vegetative nervous system and its therapeutic possibilities: especially in duodenal ulcer, angina pectoris, hypertension, diabetes. Dis Chest. 1951;20(2):139–47.
12. Askari A, Kordzadeh A, Lee GH, Harvey M. Endoscopic thoracic sympathectomy for primary hyperhidrosis: 16-year follow up in a single UK centre. Surgeon. 2013;11:130–3.
13. Atkinson LD, Forde-Thomas NC, Fealey RD. Endoscopic transthoracic limited sympathotomy for palmar – plantar hyperhidrosis: outcomes and complications during a 10-year period. Mayo Clin Proc. 2011;869:721–9.
14. Bell D, Jedynak D, Bell R. Predictors of outcome following endoscopic thoracic sympathectomy. ANZ J Surg. 2014;84(1–2):68–72.

15. Cerfolio RJ, De Campos JR, Bryant AS, et al. The society of thoracic surgery expert consensus for the surgical treatment of hyperhidrosis. Ann Thorac Surg. 2011;91:1642–8.
16. Chou SH, Kao EL, Lin CC, Chang YT, et al. The importance of classification in sympathetic surgery and a proposed mechanism for compensatory hyperhidrosis: experience with 464 cases. Surg Endosc. 2006;20:1749–53.
17. Licht PB, Ladegaard L, Pilegaard HK. Thoracoscopic sympathectomy for isolated facial blushing. Ann Thorac Surg. 2006;11:59–62.
18. Plas EG, Fugger R, Herbst F, et al. Complications of endoscopic thoracic sympathectomy. Surgery. 1995;118:493–5.
19. Lai CL, Chen WJ, Liu YB, et al. Bradycardia and permanent pacing after bilateral thoracoscopic T2 sympathectomy for primary hyperhidrosis. Pacing Clin Electrophysiol. 2001;24:524–5.
20. Hutter J, Miller K, Moritz E. Chronic sequels after thoracoscopic procedures for benign diseases. Eur J Cardiothorac Surg. 2000;17:687–90.
21. Steegers MA, Snik DM, Verhagen AF, et al. Only half of chronic pain after thoracic surgery shows a neuropathic component. J Pain. 2008;9:955–61.
22. Sihoe AD, Cheung CS, Lai HK, et al. Incidence of chest wall paresthesia after needlescopic video-assisted thoracic surgery for palmar hyperhidrosis. Eur J Cardiothorac Surg. 2005;27:313–9.
23. Lardinois D, Ris HB. Minimally invasive video-endoscopic sympathectomy by use of a transaxillary single port approach. Eur J Cardiothorac Surg. 2002;21:67–70.
24. Ng CSH, Yeung ECL, Wong RH, et al. Single-port sympathectomy for palmar hyperhidrosis with Vasoview HemoPro 2 endoscopic vein harvesting device. J Thorac Cardiovasc Surg. 2012;144(5):1256–7.
25. Ibrahim M, Menna C, Andreettti C, et al. Bilateral single port sympathectomy: long term results and quality of life. Biomed Res Int. 2013;2013:348017.
26. Kujipers M, Klinkenberg TJ, Bouma W, et al. Single port one-stage bilateral thoracoscopic sympathicotomy for severe hyperhidrosis: prospective analysis of a standardized approach. J Cardiothorac Surg. 2013;8:216.
27. Ng CSH, Lau RWH, Wong RHL, et al. Single port Vasoview sympathectomy for palmar hyperhidrosis: a clinical update. J Laparoendosc Adv Surg Tech A. 2014;24(1):32–4.
28. Chen YB, Ye W, Yang WT, et al. Uniportal versus biportal video-assisted thoracoscopic sympathectomy for palmar hyperhidrosis. Chin Med J. 2009;122(13):1525–8.
29. Ng CSH, Lau RWH, Wong RHL, et al. Evolving techniques of endoscopic thoracic sympathectomy: smaller incisions or less? Surgeon. 2013;11:290–1.
30. Elia S, Guggino G, Mineo D, et al. Awake one stage bilateral thoracoscopic sympathectomy for palmar hyperhidrosis: a safe outpatient procedure. Eur J Cardiothorac Surg. 2005;28:312–7; discussion 317.
31. Carillo Gerardo AO, Carretero Miguel AC, Barreiro LP, et al. Nontintubated bilateral single port thoracoscopic sympathectomy in the context of an outpatient program, the least invasive management for hyperhidrosis surgery. Ann Translat Med. 2015;3(22):357.
32. Zhu LH, Du Q, Chen L, Yang S, et al. One-year follow-up period after transumbilical thoracic sympathectomy for hyperhidrosis: outcomes and consequences. J Thorac Cardiovasc Surg. 2014;147(1):25–8.
33. Zhu LH, Chen L, Yang S, et al. Embryonic NOTES thoracic sympathectomy for palmar hyperhidrosis: results of a novel technique and comparison with the conventional VATS procedure. Surg Endosc. 2013;27(11):4124–9.
34. Zhu LH, Chen WS, Chen L, et al. Transumbilical thoracic sympathectomy: a single-centre experience of 148 cases with up to 4 years of follow-up. Eur J Cardiothorac Surg. 2016;49:i79–83.
35. Chen J-T, Liao C-P, Chiang H-C, et al. Subxiphoid single-incision thoracoscopic bilateral ablative sympathectomy for hyperhidrosis. Interact Cardiovasc Thorac Surg. 2015;21:119–20.
36. Rocco G. Endoscopic VATS sympathectomy: the uniportal technique. Multimed Man Cardiothorac Surg. 2007;2007(507):MMCT S.2004.000323. https://doi.org/10.1510/MMCTS.2004.000323.

Uniport Anterior Mediastinal Surgery

Ching Feng Wu and Diego Gonzalez-Rivas

Abstract

Most anterior mediastinal tumors, such as thymoma, are indolent in the growth phase but they are potentially malignant in their clinical course due to neighboring organ invasion, pleural dissemination, and occasional systemic metastasis. Surgical resection should be considered for this kind of mediastinal tumor. Video-assisted thoracoscopic surgery (VATS) has been widely used for mediastinal tumor resection since over 20 years (Yim AP, Kay RL, Ho JK, Chest 108:1440–3, 1995). A series of literatures has demonstrated its safety and that its oncological outcome is not inferior to sternotomy procedure (Shiono H, Kadota Y, Hayashi A, et al., Surg Laparosc Endosc Percutan Tech 19:424–7, 2009; Zahid I, Sharif S, Routledge T, et al., Interact Cardiovasc Thorac Surg 12:40–6, 2011). With the improvement of surgical skills and instruments, uniport VATS has achieved the same operation indication as multiport VATS. Although such an approach for a mediastinal tumor is feasible and may be preferable, caution must be exercised in some patients due to the difficulty of dissecting the involved vessels.

Electronic Supplementary Material The online version of this chapter (https://doi.org/10.1007/978-981-13-2604-2_9) contains supplementary material, which is available to authorized users.

C. F. Wu
Minimally Invasive Thoracic Surgery Unit (UCTMI), Clinical Fellow at Coruña University Hospital, Coruña, Spain

Division of Thoracic and Cardiovascular Surgery, Department of Surgery, Chang Gung Memorial Hospital, Taoyuan, Taiwan

D. Gonzalez-Rivas (✉)
Department of Thoracic Surgery, Shanghai Pulmonary Hospital, Tongji University School of Medicine, Shanghai, China

Department of Thoracic Surgery and Minimally Invasive Thoracic Surgery Unit (UCTMI), Coruña University Hospital, Coruña, Spain
e-mail: diego@uniportal.es

Introduction

In surgery for anterior mediastinal lesion resection, the standard approach is still trans-sternal or thoracotomy. However, the safety and oncological outcome of video-assisted thoracoscopic surgery (VATS) has been proven in a series of papers over the last 20 years [1–3]. The advantages of this operation approach include less pain in the early postoperative period, less pulmonary function impairment, better cosmetic results and total avoidance of the risk of disruption or infection of the sternotomy wound. In recent years, VATS has seen an evolution in the following aspects: (1) reduction of the number of working ports [4, 5] (2) non intubation surgery [6]. Uniport VATS emerged and became the less invasive alternative to multiport VATS. Gradually the technique was adopted by thoracic surgeons around the world who expanded its use in thoracic surgery, including segmentectomy, lobectomy, sleeve lobectomy and so on [7–9].

This chapter attempts to provide a clinically useful step and management approach for uniport anterior mediastinal mass resection based on previously published literatures and our own experience [10, 11]. Although written specifically with anterior mediastinal mass in mind, the operative principles are applicable for all kinds of single port surgery.

Operation Preparation (Fig. 1)

Choice of the side for entrance is a matter of safe complete removal of anterior mediastinal tumor or the thymus and perithymic fatty tissue from diaphragm to cervical area. The comparison of choosing either side for entrance is listed as Table 1. After we chose the side for entrance, the operation preparation is as follows: patients with anterior mediastinum tumor, are positioned in a 30 degree semi-supine position on the operating table with a roll placed beneath the shoulder and the ipsilateral arm held abducted over a padded L-screen in order to expose the axilla area (Fig. 1). Patients are intubated with double

D. Gonzalez-Rivas et al. (eds.), *Atlas of Uniportal Video Assisted Thoracic Surgery*,
https://doi.org/10.1007/978-981-13-2604-2_9

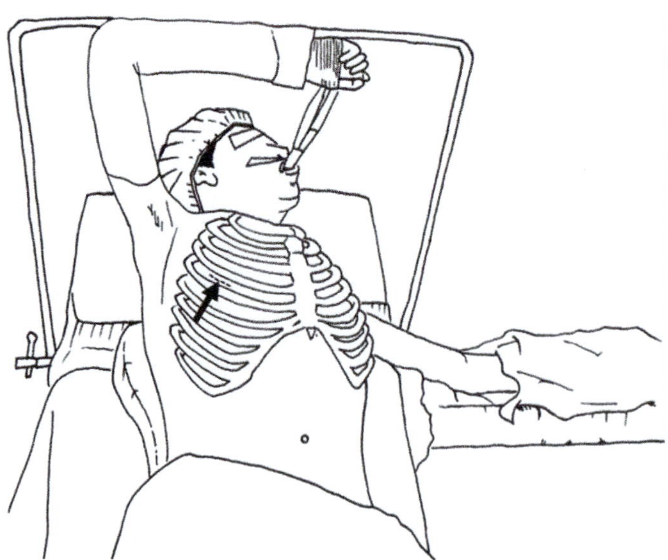

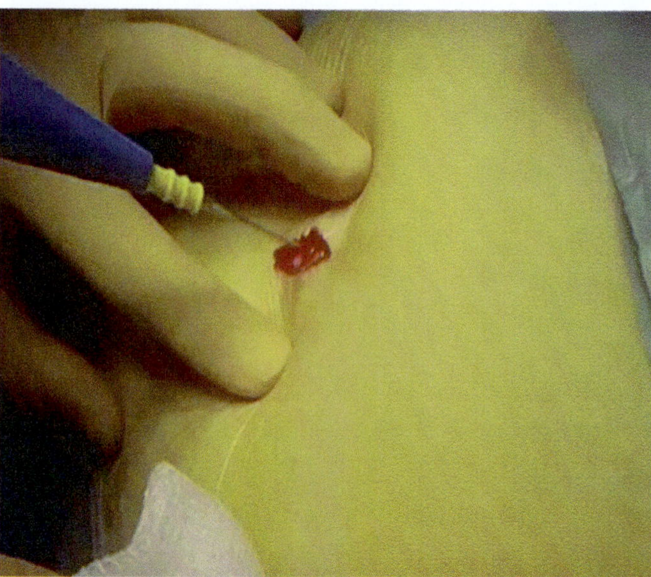

Fig. 1 Operation preparation and wound incision site: a 2–3 cm incision is placed initially in the fourth or fifth intercostal space at the anterior axillary line

Table 1 Comparison of right side and left side approach

	Right side approach	Left side approach
Advantage	1. Obvious anatomic landmark (superior vena cava) 2. More easier to dissect the confluence of innominate vein 3. Ergonomic for right hand dominant surgeon	1. Easier to dissect the left side dominant anterior mediastinal tumor
Disadvantage	1. Hard to see the left side phrenic nerve	1. No obvious anatomic landmark 2. Hard to dissect the confluence of innominate vein

lumen endotracheal tube. One lung ventilation provides proper visualization and space for the operation. Operator and first assistant (cameraman) all stand at the same side. The high resolution video monitors are arranged in front of the operator so that the surgeon and first assistant have a direct and unobstructed view of the monitors. Some surgeons prefer to have a better pleural cavity exploration by CO_2 insufflations in multiport VATS. However, it is very difficult for operator to do the same thing in uniport VATS because uniport VATS has only one utility. It is very difficult to make a complete sealed environment unless surgeons use SILS™ port kit. However, SILS™ port kit sometimes may limit range of motion of instruments due to the innate restrictions of intercostal space.

Creation of the Wound (Fig. 1)

Choosing the incision position is the determining step of the operation. Proper creation of the incision wound optimizes visualization and offers the best angle for instruments to perform resection. Depending on the location of the target lesion, a 2–3 cm incision is placed initially in the fourth or fifth intercostal space at the anterior axillary line. For total thymectomy or if the target lesion is located above the confluence of the innominate vein and superior vena cava, the fourth intercostal space is the best choice (Fig. 1). Otherwise, we select the fifth intercostal space for the wound incision. The operator may use their finger to confirm whether there is pleural symphysis or not after the wound creation. If pleural symphysis is found, the endoscope can be put through the wound carefully and a harmonic scalpel or electric hook can be used to release it away from wound. This maneuver could increase the operator's instrument working space without injury to the lung tissue. A rubber wound retractor might help the operator to have a better operation view. However, if pleural symphysis is found upon entering the chest cavity, we recommend doing pneumolysis first and then placing the wound protector after completing pneumolysis because the wound retractor might hinder the instrument manipulation during the pneumolysis procedure. A 30 degree high resolution lens is better than a 0 degree lens due to the better panoramic view of the whole operation field. A wider view could provide more detail of nearby structures, such as nerves or blood vessels, which should not be injured during surgery.

Detaching the Anterior Mediastinal Tissue from the Pericardium (Fig. 2)

With the position described above, the operator can easily find the target lesion in the anterior mediastinum (Fig. 2a). Use the non dominant hand to manipulate the suction tube or lymph node grasper and the dominant hand to grasp the harmonic scalpel or electric hook (Fig. 2b). First, initiate the dissection plane between the thymus tissue and the pericardium from the inferior border of the thymus. The thymus tissue is easily detached from this plane and moved superiorly unless the tumor has invaded the pericardium. Then, the operator can incise the mediastinal pleura anterior to the phrenic nerve until the confluence of the innominate vein and superior vena cava with electric hook or harmonic scalpel (Fig. 2c). After finishing this procedure, the dissection procedure is continued to keep the target lesion or thymic tissue from the pericardium (Fig. 2d). This method provides an obvious landmark and allows clear visualization of the dissection line between thymus tissue and vessels.

Ligating the Thymic Vein, Retrieving the Bilateral Horns of Thymus (Fig. 3)

Following the plane between the innominate vein and the thymus (Fig. 3a), divide the mediastinal pleura anteriorly along the length of the internal mammary artery/vein at the

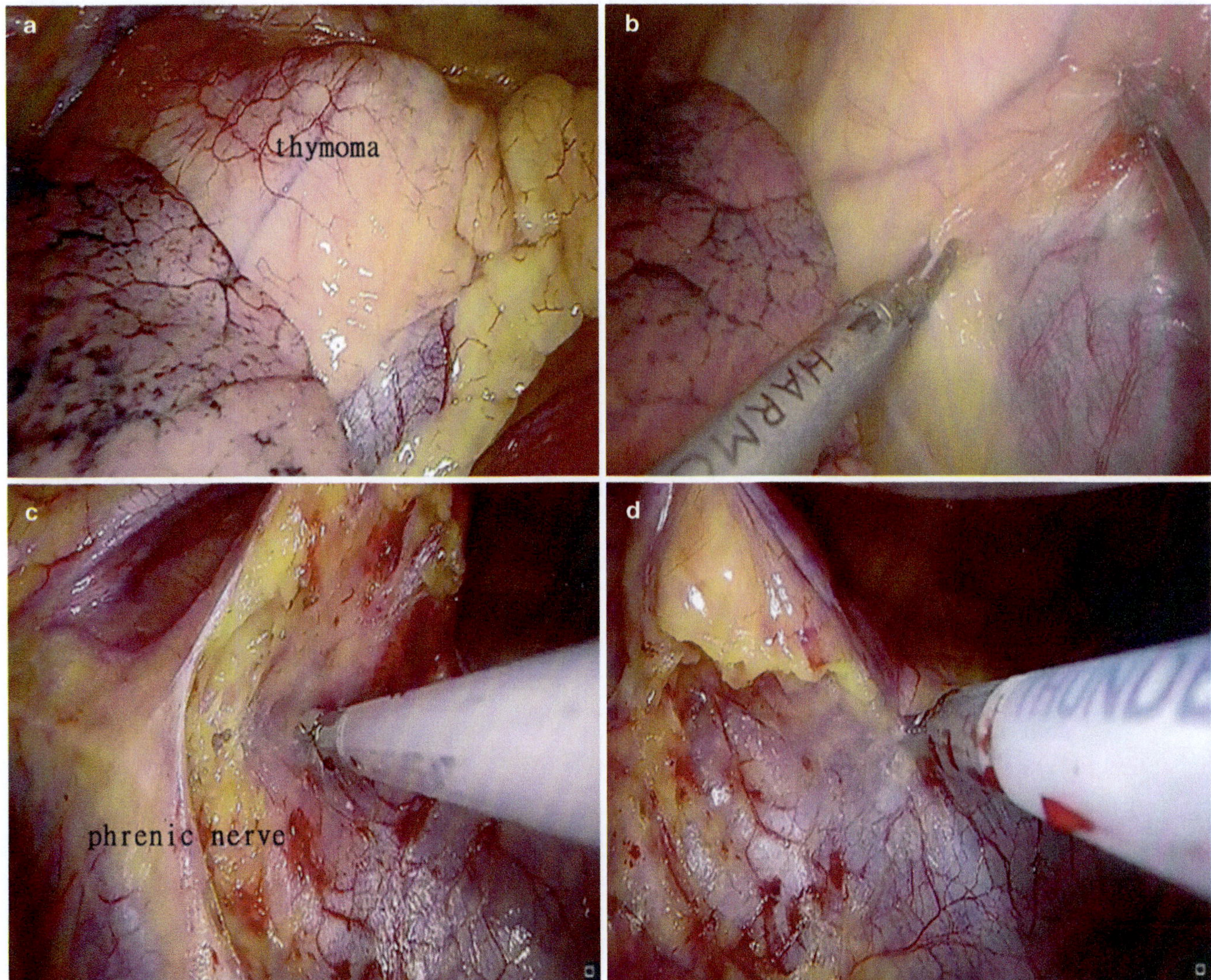

Fig. 2 Detachment of anterior mediastinal tissue from pericardium (**a**) confirm the anterior mediastinal target lesion (**b**) begin to dissect the lower border of thymic tissue (**c**) open the mediastinal pleura anterior to the phrenic nerve (**d**) detach thymic tissue away from pericardium

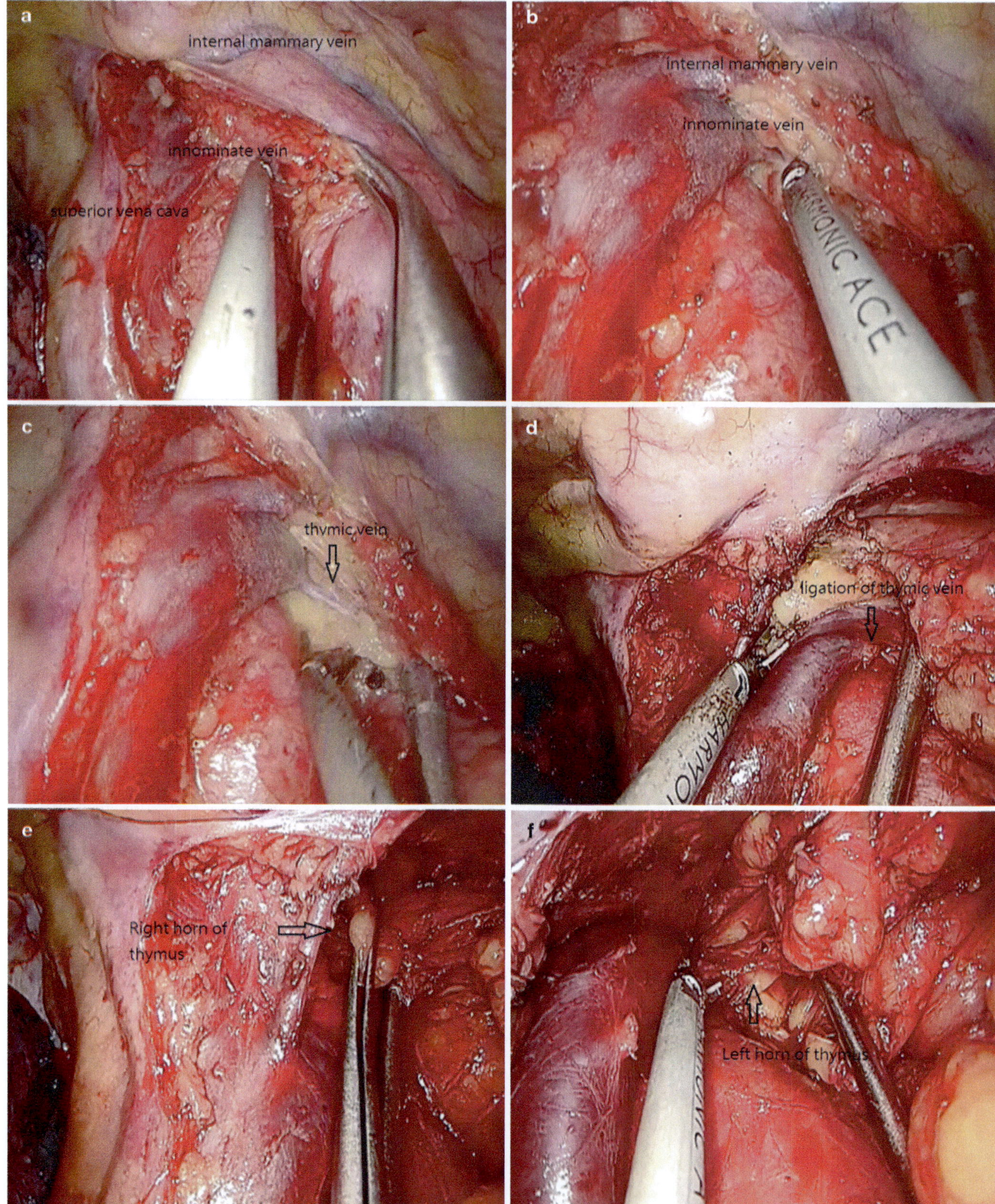

Fig. 3 Ligating the thymic vein, retrieving the bilateral horns of thymus (**a**) localizing the surgical plan of the innominate vein and thymus (**b**) opening the mediastinal pleura below the internal mammary vein (**c**) finding thymic vein (**d**) Ligating the thymic vein with harmonic scalpel (**e**) grasping the right horn of thymus gently (**f**) retrieving the left horn of thymus

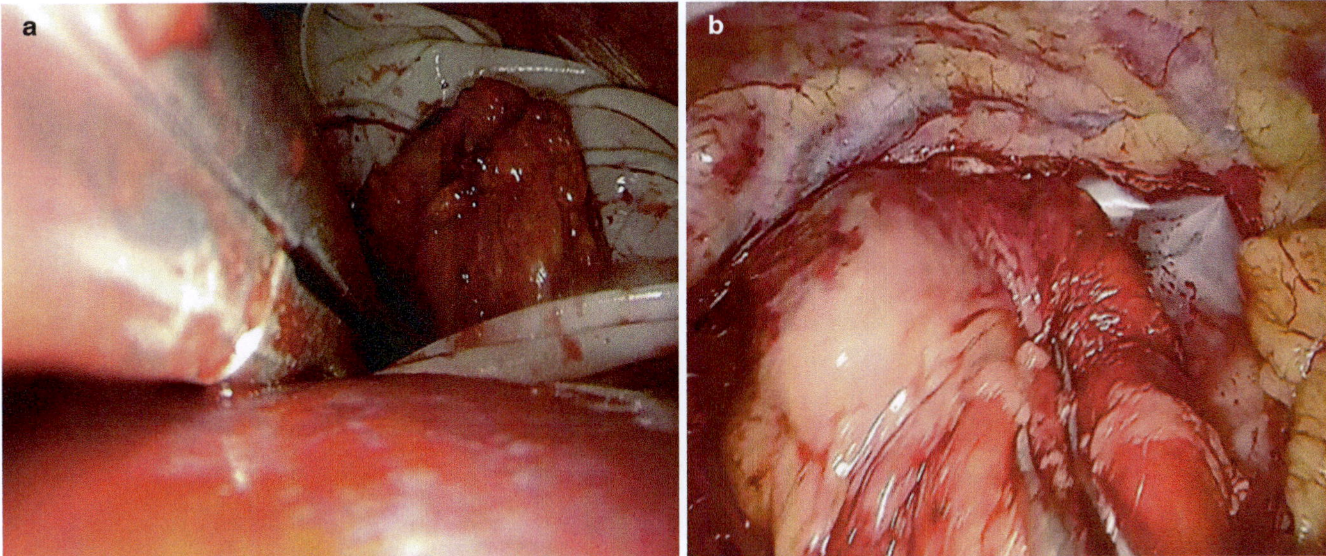

Fig. 4 Extracting the specimen: placing the endobag into the chest cavity under throacoscope and gently grasping the specimen into the surgical glove (**a**) or endobag (**b**)

level of the sternum (Fig. 3b). Then tracing the innominate vein, the thymic vein can be found (Fig. 3c). Finding the thymic vein or drainage vessels from the innominate vein is very important. If the operator doesn't notice it, unexpected bleeding could result, or even cause catastrophic injury to the innominate vein. Gentle traction on the thymic gland also aids in better exposure of the innominate vein and drainage vessels, giving the operator complete control over the thymic vein and feeding vessels from the innominate vein, allowing him to divide the thymic vein and drainage vessels with hemoclips or harmonic scalpel (Fig. 3d). If there is no clear visualization between the innominate vein and thymus tissue, using vascular loop to encircle the innominate vein first could help to deal with any unexpected bleeding episode. After division of the thymic vein or drainage vessels from the innominate vein, we continue to open the mediastinal pleura below the internal mammary vein until the left side pleura. Crossing the innominate vein, exposure of the right horn of thymus is best achieved with gentle downward traction on the thymus tissue and careful dissection with lymph node grasp or suction tube for counter-traction (Fig. 3e). After liberating the right horn of thymus, we release the left horn of thymus with the same method (Fig. 3f). Sometimes, there are arterial branches from the internal mammary in this region, which we can divide by harmonic scalpel or hemoclips. During the whole operation, our primary concern should be to avoid injury to the phrenic nerve of the left side, especially in Myasthenia Gravis patients. If possible, not opening the left side pleura will decrease the possibility of injury to the left side phrenic nerve. If the anterior mediastinal tumor is not thymoma, such as teratoma, pericardium cyst and so on, en block resection of the tumor is enough (Case 1) (Fig. 4).

Extracting the Anterior Mediastinal Tumor (Fig. 4)

After completing the dissection, an endobag is introduced into the thoracic cavity under thoracoscope. Then, using lymph node grasp the specimen is placed into the surgical glove (Fig. 5a) or endobag (Fig. 5b). When grasping the specimen, the operator should pay attention not to squeeze the capsule of the specimen. Once the operator has ensured that the specimen is totally in the endobag, it can be extracted from the chest wall and sent for further pathological examination.

How to Deal with Visceral Pleural Adhesion and Bleeding Episode (Fig. 5)

Sometimes, we might encounter anterior mediastinal tumor with visceral pleural adhesion. If the adhesion is not tight to the visceral pleura, doing pneumolysis first provides a better operating view for the following procedure. If pleural symphysis is found around the wound, use the finger or instruments under endoscope to release it. If the adhesion is tight to the visceral pleura, wedge resection of the adhesive lung tissue first should help to shorten the operation time and afford a better visualization (Fig. 6a, b). Bleeding episode may occur when trying to separate the thymic vein or feeding

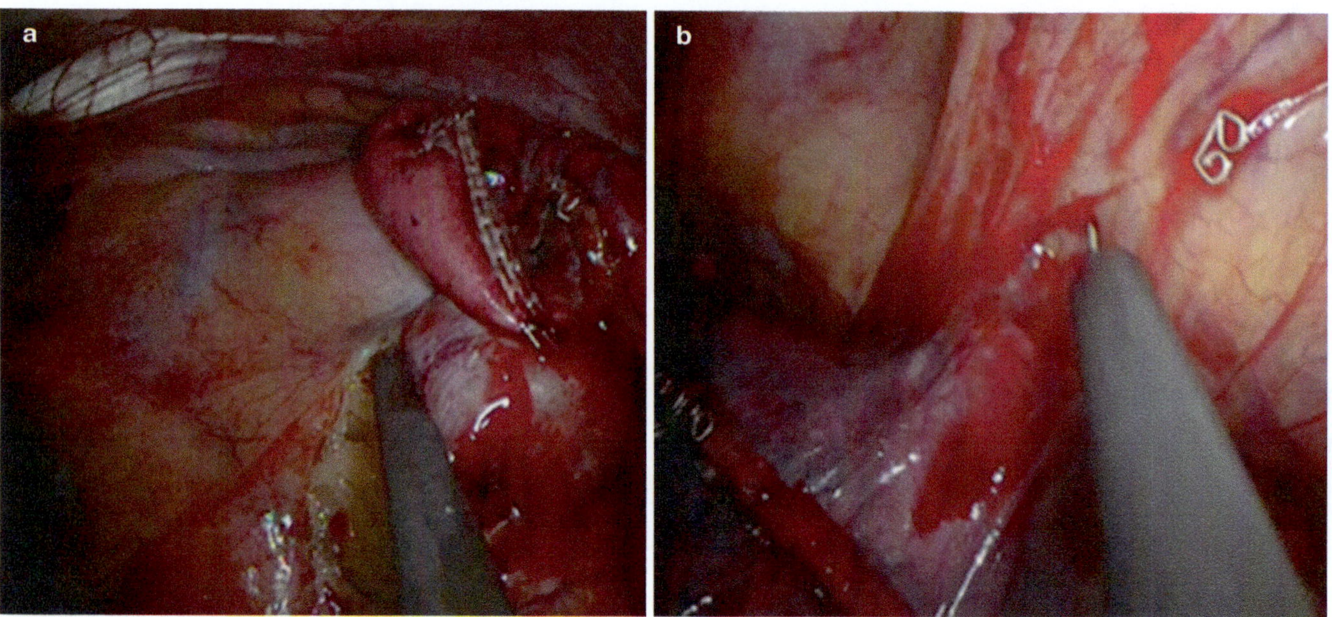

Fig. 5 Dealing with visceral pleural adhesion (**a**) wedge resection for tight adhesion to visceral pleura (**b**) pneumolysis for loose visceral pleura adhesion

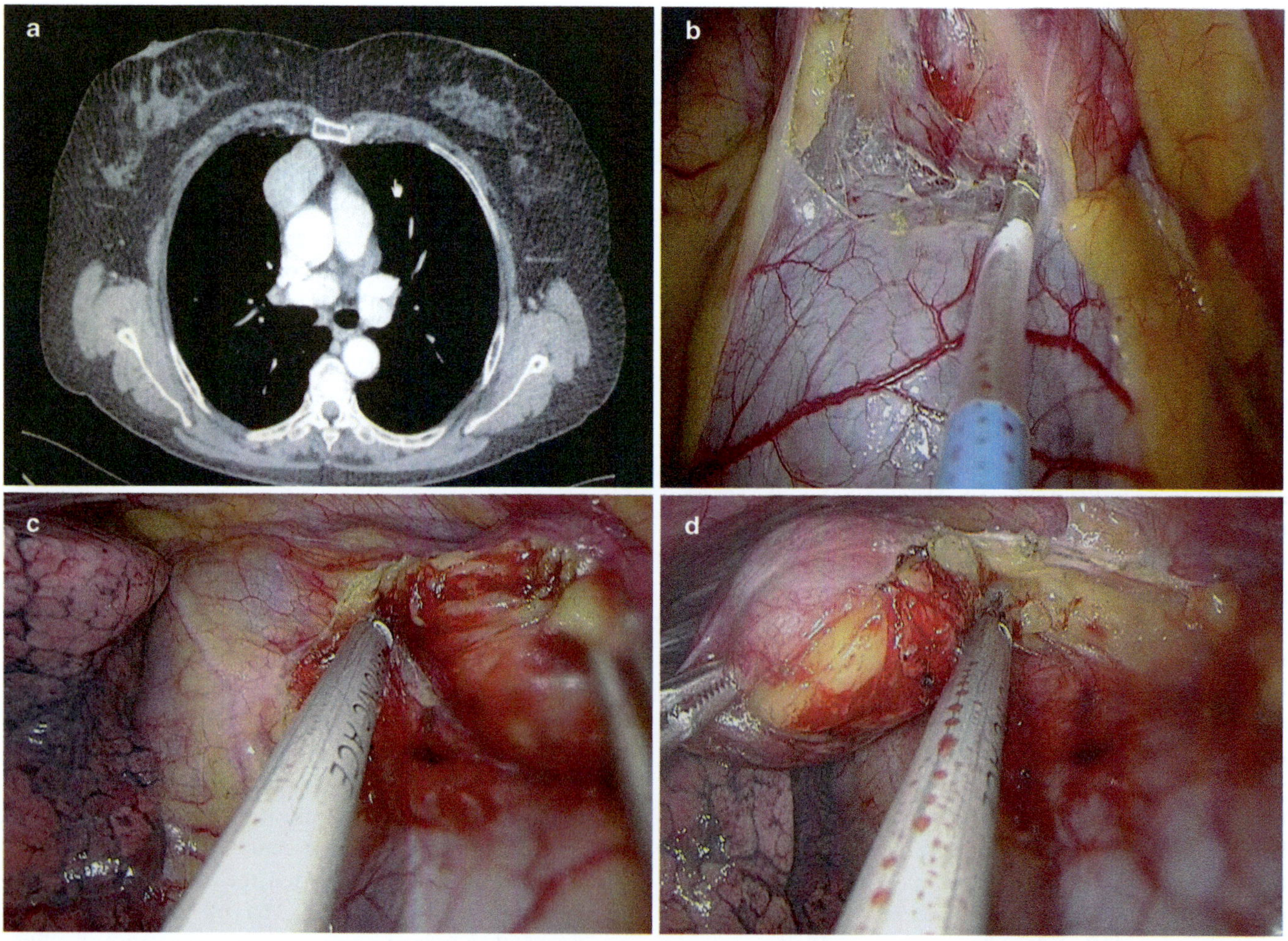

Fig. 6 (**a**) CT image of tetratoma (**b**) using electric cautery or hook to open mediadtianl pleura, (**c**) and (**d**) using harmonic scapel to do an en block resection of antermediastinal tumor resection

vessels from the innominate vein. In such an event, one should keep calm and first quickly compress the bleeding area with grasp or gauze. If you find only thymic vein is injured during dissection, try to ligate it with hemolick or hemoclick. If the innominate vein is injured, a well-experienced single port surgeon could try to encircle it and use tourniquet to reduce blood loss volume while trying to repair the bleeding area. However, if it is hard to perform the procedure mentioned above or operator's experience is not good enough to control the bleeding, or if the patient's vital signs are unstable, do not hesitate to open the wound and convert to open surgery. Surgeons could shift endoscope surgery to anterior thoracotomy or sternotomy fairly quickly. Whether anterior thoracotomy or sternotomy is necessary depends on the bleeding points. If surgeons injury the innominate vein when they try to dissect the plane of bilateral thymic horn, it is better to do sternotomy than anterior thoractomy to control the bleeding because the bleeder usually are located at the ceiling of operation view field. Sternotomy might provide better operation view for surgeons to control the bleeder.

Case Demonstration

- Case 1: Anterior mediastinal tumor en block resection: Tetratoma (Fig. 6)
- Case 2: Uniport total thymectomy (Video 1)
- Case 3: Bleeding episode in anterior mediastinal tumor resection (Video 2)

Discussion

Proponents of minimally invasive surgery have emphasized its benefits, including reduced blood loss during the operation, less pain in the early postoperative period, less compromised pulmonary function, and better cosmetic results. The true connotations of minimal invasive surgery is not only reduce the size of wound but also the inner trauma of patients. Ng et al. found VATS patients could preserve better immune function than thoracotomy patients [11]. Technically, uniport VATS is the less invasive alternative to multiport VATS. Soon after, we might get the comparison result of multiport VATS and singe port VATS in immune response to see whether this new technique indeed to bring less injury to the patients.

In addition, on the effectiveness of long term oncological result, we still lack of long term results to prove it is better or at least not inferior to multiport VATS. However, with the increasing popularity of this new technique, Some articles tried to compare the short term clinical outcome of uniport and multiport VATS. Young et al. find uniport VATS might have a clinical effect in reducing postoperative pain in acute stage (within 72 h) [12]. For uniport VATS mediastinal tumor resection, Wu et al. have proved its benefit in causing less pain sensation and shorter post operation hospital stay in retrospective study [13]. But, due to the weakness of methodology, a larger, prospective study proving the advantages of uniport VATS with more solid and objective evidence is needed. With regard to long term oncological outcomes in thymoma, a paramount issue is the occurrence of postoperative MG or tumor recurrence. Since single port surgery is a relatively new procedure, there is still a lack of associated published literatures to support it. However, based on the same oncological treatment principle, the long term outcomes of uniport VATS might not be inferior to multiple port VATS within the foreseeable future.

References

1. Yim AP, Kay RL, Ho JK. Video-assisted thoracoscopic thymectomy for myasthenia gravis. Chest. 1995;108(5):1440–3.
2. Shiono H, Kadota Y, Hayashi A, et al. Comparison of outcomes after extended thymectomy for myasthenia gravis: bilateral thoracoscopic approach versus sternotomy. Surg Laparosc Endosc Percutan Tech. 2009;19(6):424–7.
3. Zahid I, Sharif S, Routledge T, et al. Video-assisted thoracoscopic surgery or transsternal thymectomy in the treatment of myasthenia gravis? Interact Cardiovasc Thorac Surg. 2011;12(1):40–6.
4. Rocco G, Martin-Ucar A, Passera E. Uniportal VATS wedge pulmonary resections. Ann Thorac Surg. 2004;77:726–8.
5. Suda T, Hachimaru A, Tochii D, et al. Video-assisted thoracoscopic thymectomy versus subxyphoid single port thymectomy: initial result. Eur J Cardiothorac Surg. 2016;49(Suppl 1):i54–8. Epub 2015 Oct 14. https://doi.org/10.1093/ejcts/ezv338.
6. Gonzalez-Rivas D, Bonome C, Fieira E, et al. Non-intubated video-assisted thoracoscopic lung resection: the future of thoracic surgery? Eur J Cardiothorac Surg. 2016;49(3):721–31.
7. Gonzalez-Rivas D, Fieira E, Mendez L, et al. Single port video assisted thoracoscopic anatomic segmentectomy and right upper lobectomy. Eur J Cardiothorac Surg. 2012;42C(6):169–71.
8. Gonzalez-Rivas D, Paradela M. Fieira single incision video-assisted thoracoscopic lobectomy: initial results. J Thorac Cardiovasc Surg. 2012;143:745–7.
9. Gonzalez-Rivas D, Fieira E, Delgado M. Uniportal video-assisted thoracoscopic sleeve lobectomy and other complex resections. J Thorac Dis. 2014;6(Suppl 6):S674–81.
10. Wu CF, Gonzalez-Rivas D, Wen CT, et al. Single port video-assisted thoracoscopic mediastinal tumor resection. Interact Cardiovasc Thorac Surg. 2015;21(5):644–9.
11. Ng CS, Wan IY, Yim AP. Impact of video-assisted thoracoscopic major lung resection on immune function. Asian Cardiovasc Thorac Ann. 2009;17(4):426–32.
12. Young R, McElnay P, Leslie R, et al. Is uniport thoracoscopic surgery less painful than multiple port approaches? Interact Cardiovasc Thorac Surg. 2015;20:409–14.
13. Wu CF, Gonzalez-Rivas D, Wen CT, et al. Comparative short-term clinical outcomes of mediastinum tumor excision performed by conventional VATS and single port VATS: is it worthwhile? Medicine (Baltimore). 2015;94(45):e1975. https://doi.org/10.1097/MD.0000000000001975.

Uniportal Posterior Mediastinal Surgery

Luis Angel Hernandez-Arenas, Yang Yang, Zhu Yu-Ming, Gening Jiang, and Diego Gonzalez-Rivas

Abstract

The Uniportal Transthoracic approach for posterior mediastinal tumours is a succinctly described technique, it is feasible and safe, and offers a good view and exposure of the operating field in the posterior mediastinum. A 3–4 cm incision is made in the fourth, fifth or sixth intercostal space depending on the location of the lesion at the level of the anterior axillary line. A 5 mm or 10 mm, 30° high definition video camera is always used. The Uniportal VATS approach can be used for diagnostic procedures or complete excision of the posterior mediastinal tumours. In this chapter we explain how to perform the dissection and resection of the posterior mediastinal tumours by uniportal approach.

Electronic Supplementary Material The online version of this chapter (https://doi.org/10.1007/978-981-13-2604-2_10) contains supplementary material, which is available to authorized users.

L. A. Hernandez-Arenas
Department of Thoracic Surgery, University Hospitals Birmingham NHS Foundation Trust, Birmingham, UK

Department of Thoracic Surgery, Shanghai Pulmonary Hospital Affiliated to Tongji, University School of Medicine, Shanghai, China

Y. Yang · Z. Yu-Ming · G. Jiang
Department of Thoracic Surgery, Shanghai Pulmonary Hospital Affiliated to Tongji, University School of Medicine, Shanghai, China

D. Gonzalez-Rivas (✉)
Department of Thoracic Surgery, Shanghai Pulmonary Hospital, Tongji University School of Medicine, Shanghai, China

Department of Thoracic Surgery and Minimally Invasive Thoracic Surgery Unit (UCTMI), Coruña University Hospital, Coruña, Spain
e-mail: diego@uniportal.es

Anatomy

The posterior mediastinum is the potential space along each side of the vertebral column and adjacent to the proximal portion of the ribs, divided from the remainder of the extra-pleural intrathoracic cavity by imaginary lines. The posterior mediastinum is bordered by the following thoracic structures:

- *Lateral*: Mediastinal pleura (part of the parietal pleural membrane).
- *Anterior*: Pericardium.
- *Posterior*: T5–T12 vertebrae.
- *Roof*: Imaginary line extending between the sternal angle (the angle formed by the junction of the sternal body and manubrium and the T4 vertebrae.
- *Floor*: Diaphragm (Table 1).

Incidence and Pathophysiology

Posterior mediastinal tumours make up about 22–30% of all tumours of the mediastinum. They tend to be neural in origin (74–94%) and arise from sympathetic ganglion cells (ganglioneuroma, ganglioneuroblastoma or neuroblastoma) or from nerve sheaths (schwannoma or neurofibroma). Neurogenic tumours are benign in 70–80% of the patients [1] the remaining 25% of posterior mediastinal tumours consist of a plethora of rare tumours, including lymphoma, teratomas and sarcomas, amongst others. Moreover, lesions arising externally to the mediastinum may extend into the posterior compartment and appear as posterior mediastinal tumours.

In children aged 0–10 years, they tend to be malignant, most commonly neuroblastoma. In the second decade of life, benign tumours, such as neurofibromas ganglioneuromas, and rarely schwannomas, are more common [2].

D. Gonzalez-Rivas et al. (eds.), *Atlas of Uniportal Video Assisted Thoracic Surgery*,
https://doi.org/10.1007/978-981-13-2604-2_10

Table 1 Shows the posterior mediastinal contents

Posterior mediastinal contents
Oesophagus
Arteries – Descending aorta with its branches
Veins – Azygos – Hemizygos – Accessory hemizygos
Nerves – Vagus – Splanchnic nerves
Thoracic duct
Lymph nodes

Clinical Manifestation and Diagnosis

Approximately, 40% of mediastinal masses are asymptomatic, and are discovered incidentally on routine imaging examination. Symptoms are generally due to compression or direct invasion of surrounding mediastinal structures or due to paraneoplastic syndromes. Symptoms may include chest pain, cough, dyspnoea or neurological abnormalities. Asymptomatic patients are more likely to have benign lesions; whereas symptomatic patients are more often malignant [3].

The gold standard diagnostic test for patients with posterior mediastinal tumours is a CT scan of the thorax. When extension into the spinal column or cord is suspected, MRI is the investigation of choice, since it has the ability to differentiate the spinal cord from other soft tissue tumours within the spinal canal and therefore detect associated spinal cord pathology.

Transthoracic uniportal VATS approach for diagnosis and treatment of posterior mediastinal lesions is a safe and feasible procedure. We recommend starting the learning curve of uniportal VATS approach with these types of procedures (Figs. 1 and 2).

Surgical Technique

Patients Position

- Under general anaesthesia, a double lumen endotracheal tube is inserted, alternatively, a bronchial blocker may be utilised to achieve single-lung ventilation.
- The patient is placed in a lateral decubitus position. The operating table flexion point is located between the iliac crest and the costal margin. Alternatively, a pillow is placed under the chest at the level of the subxiphoid process to widen the intercostal spaces on the operative side (Fig. 3).

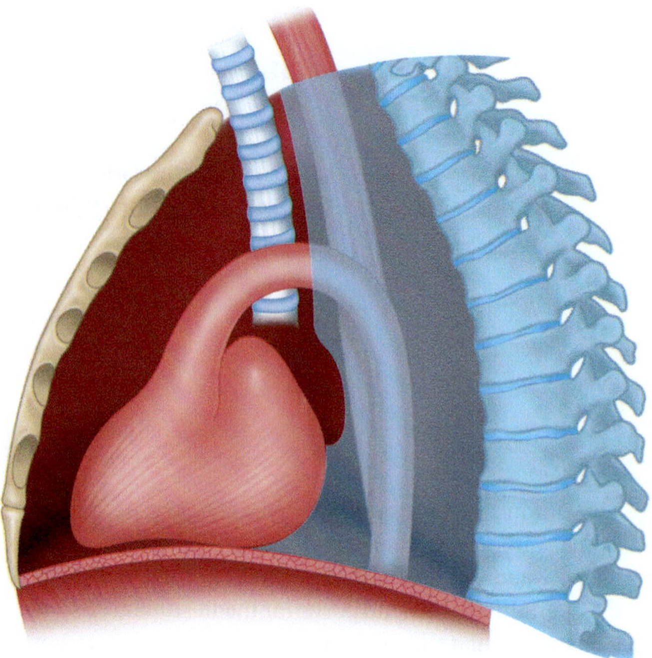

Fig. 1 Shows the limits of the posterior mediastinal

- The arms are extended and the upper arm is supported with pillows or a padded armrest and soft rolls or a beanbag is used to secure the patient on the table.
- A surgeon and an assistant are positioned in front of the patient, the scrub nurse and the screen are placed behind the patient. Alternatively a surgeon and a scrub nurse are positioned in front of the patient, with an assistant standing at the back and a screen placed at the head of the patient.

Incision Placement

A 3–4 cm incision is made in the fourth, fifth or sixth intercostal space at the level of the anterior axillary line to obtain a better view of the posterior mediastinum. The serratus muscle and the intercostal muscles are divided and the pleura is opened. The level of the incision is chosen depending of the position and location of the lesion. A wound protector can be used at the discretion of the surgeon, A 5 mm or 10 mm, 30° video camera and VATS instruments are always used (Fig. 4).

Surgical Technique (Video 1)

- The camera and the instrumentation are placed through the same incision. It is very important to keep the camera in the superior side of the wound and always use bimanual instrumentation (Fig. 5).

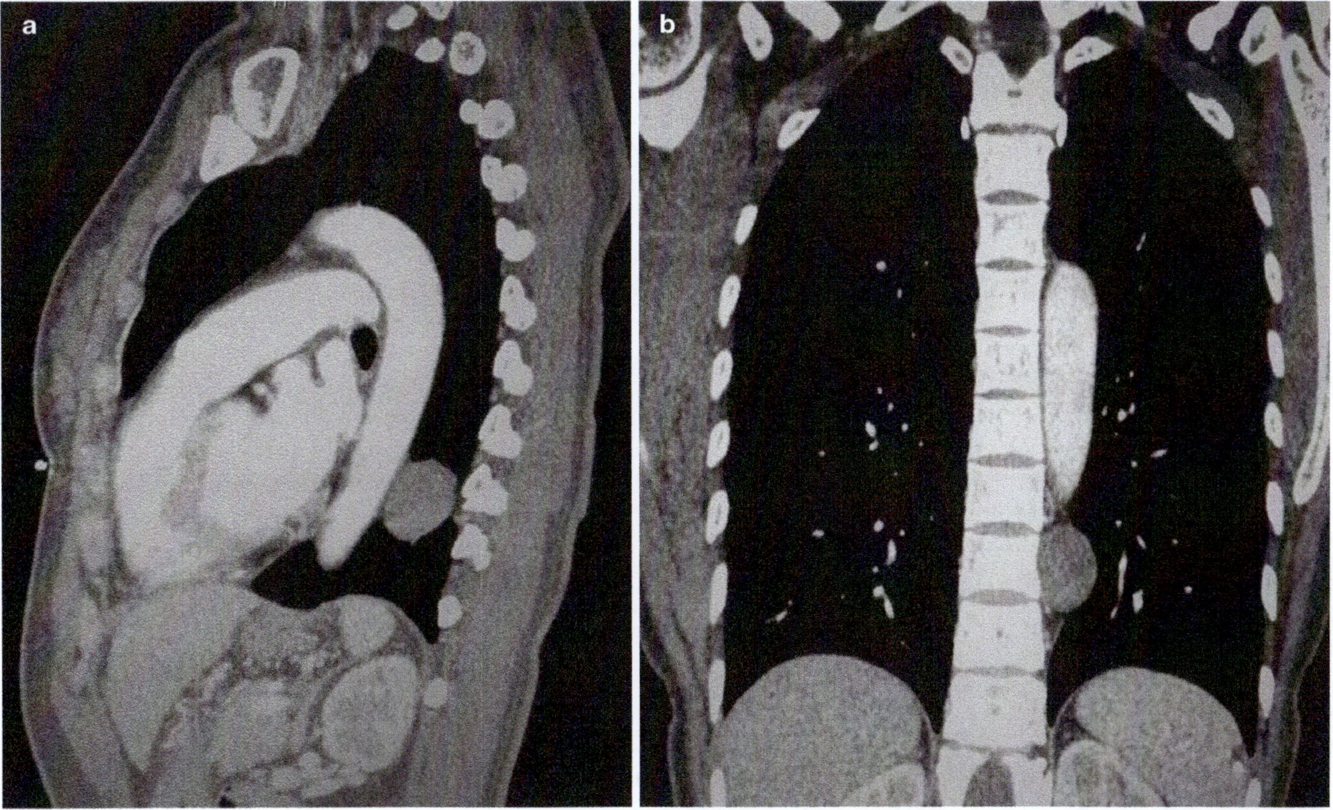

Fig. 2 Shows a chest CT scan with left posterior mediastinal tumour. (**a**) sagital view, (**b**) coronal view

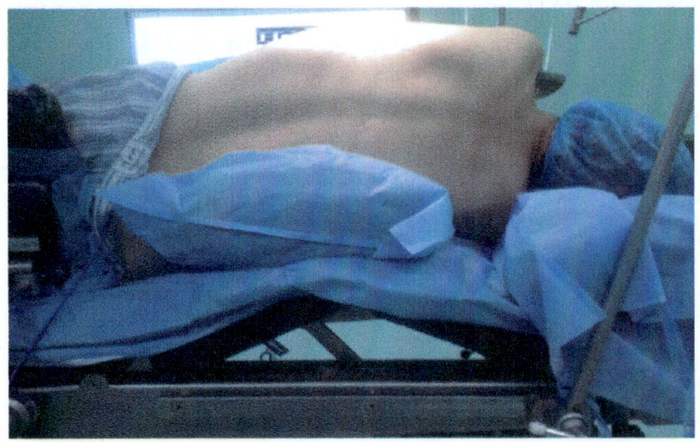

Fig. 3 Position of the patient

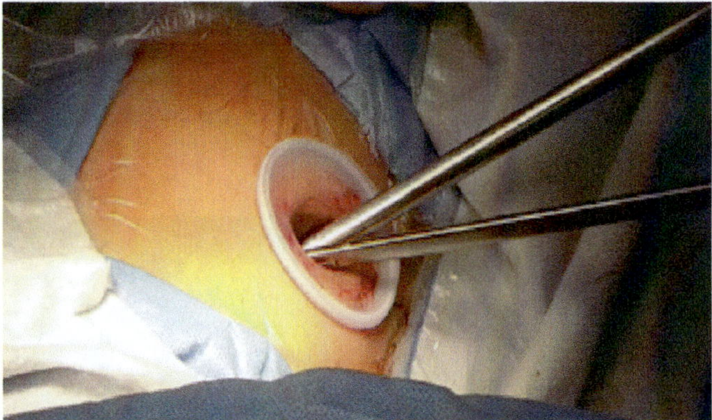

Fig. 4 Incision placement with wound protector

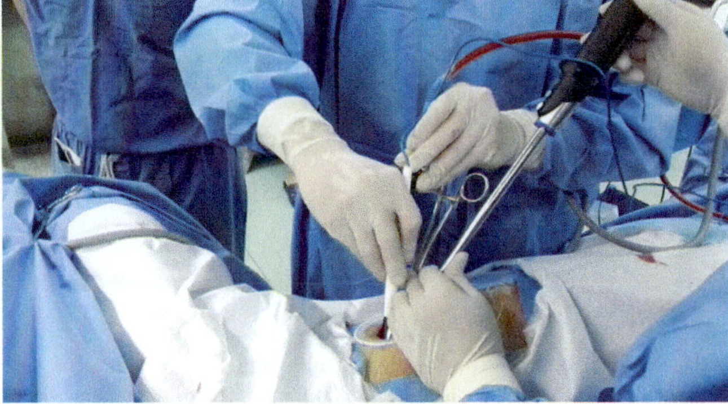

Fig. 5 Bimanual instrumentation through the same incision, with camera in the upper side of the wound

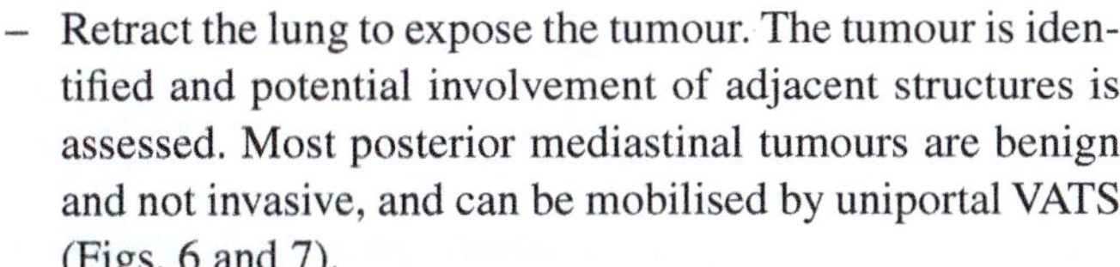

- Retract the lung to expose the tumour. The tumour is identified and potential involvement of adjacent structures is assessed. Most posterior mediastinal tumours are benign and not invasive, and can be mobilised by uniportal VATS (Figs. 6 and 7).

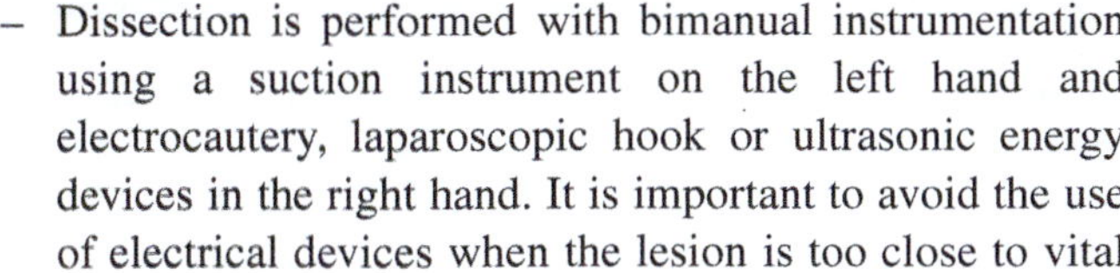

- Dissection is performed with bimanual instrumentation using a suction instrument on the left hand and electrocautery, laparoscopic hook or ultrasonic energy devices in the right hand. It is important to avoid the use of electrical devices when the lesion is too close to vital

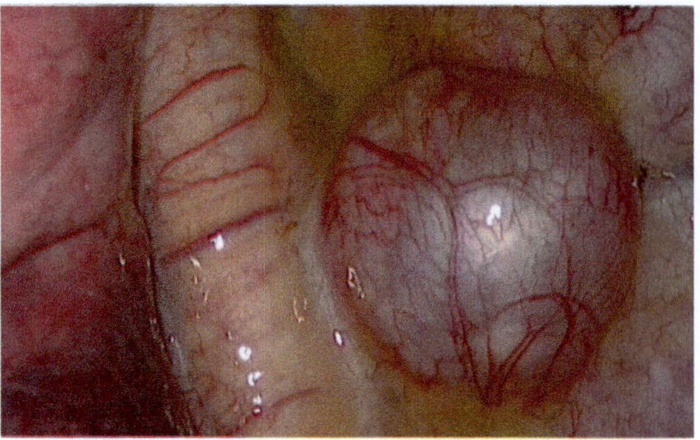

Fig. 6 Posterior mediastinal tumour exposed near to the aorta after the lung was retracted with thoracoscopic grasper

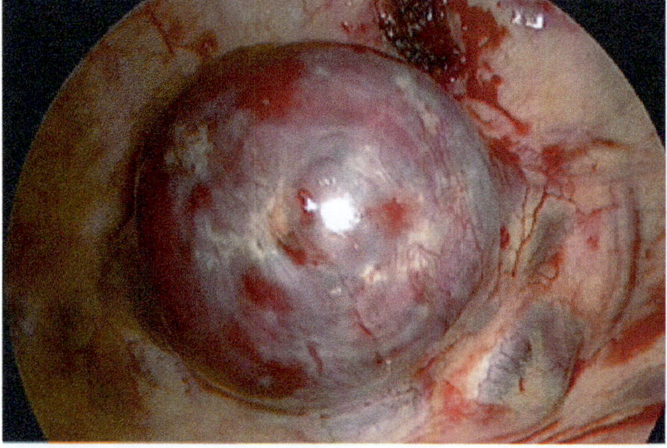

Fig. 7 Lymphoma imitating a posterior mediastinal tumour. Diagnosis was confirmed with intraoperative biopsies with frozen section

neural structures such as stellate ganglion, recurrent laryngeal nerve or phrenic nerve (Fig. 8).

- The pleura is incised circumferentially around the tumour with a reasonable edge to achieve an adequate margin and the rim of the pleura can be used for grasping to facilitate resection of the lesion (Fig. 9).
- Careful dissection helps to expose the base of the lesion and create a plain between the lesion and the prevertebral fascia (Fig. 10).
- Additional retraction can be achieved by gentle manipulation of the tumour with a blunt tipped instrument or suction (Fig. 11).
- Haemostasis is always maintained with electrocautery or ultrasonic devices for small vessels, but for larger vessels we recommend the use of endo clips (Fig. 12).
- After the tumour has been completely excised it is placed in an endocatch bag to minimise the risk of seeding the tract with tumour cells (Fig. 13).
- Sometimes the incision needs to be slightly enlarged if the lesion is too big to avoid trauma to the intercostal nerve.

Discussion

For benign posterior mediastinal tumours complete resection by thoracoscopic surgery is the preferred approach. The Uniportal VATS approach is a feasible and safe technique for diagnostic procedures or complete excision of the posterior mediastinal tumours trough one incision with the same clinical and surgical outcomes as conventional VATS [4]

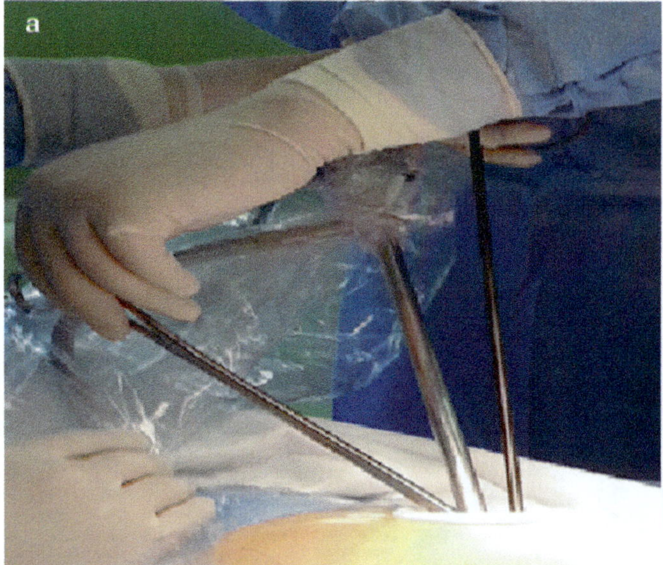

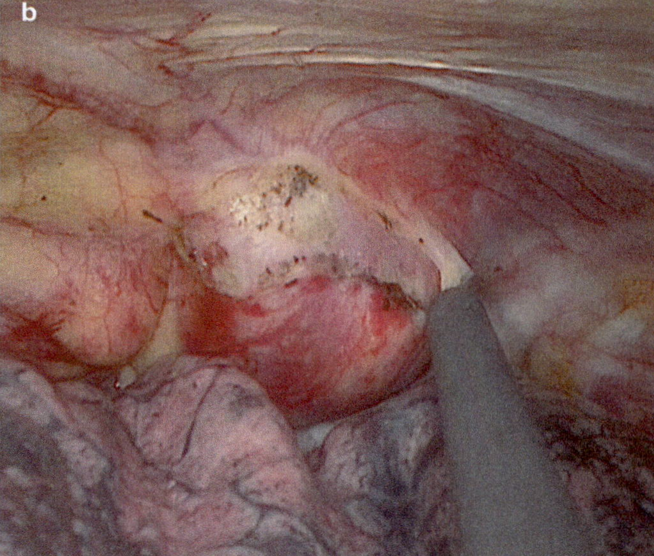

Fig. 8 (**a**) Dissection is performed with bimanual instrumentation. (**b**) Simultaneous image inside the thorax, thoracoscopic grasper in left hand and in this case laparoscopic hook in right hand starting the dissection of schwannoma

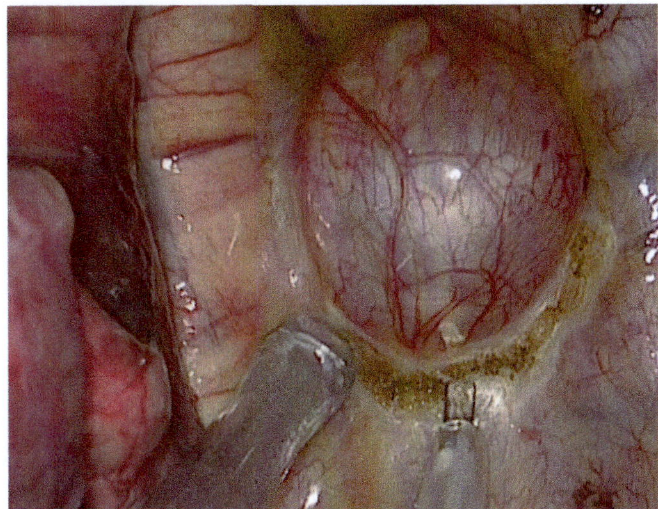

Fig. 9 Pleura incised circumferentially around the tumour with electrocautery achieving and adequate margin

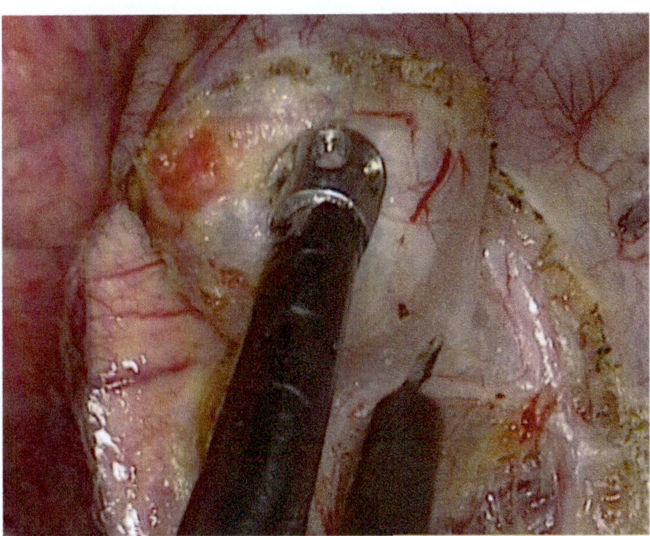

Fig. 11 Additional retraction achieved with suction in left hand and dissection of posterior mediastinal tumour with laparoscopic hook in right hand

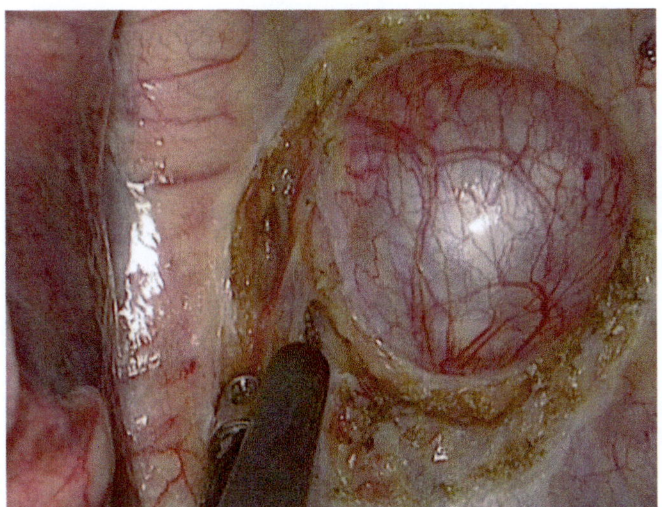

Fig. 10 Exposing the base of the lesion and creating a plain between the lesion and the prevertebral fascia and aorta with laparoscopic hook

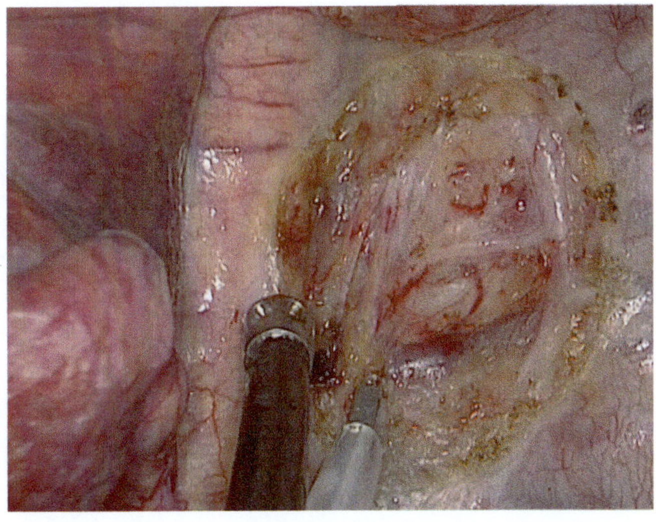

Fig. 12 Correct haemostasis with electrocautery after complete excision of posterior mediastinal tumour

offering to the patient a less invasive procedure and better cosmetic result.

The resection of a benign posterior mediastinal tumours with no invasion is one of procedures that we recommend for the surgeons who wants to move to the Uniportal VATS approach facilitating the learning curve for major lung resections.

Also the uniportal approach is useful in special situations when a combined one stage resection is carried out by a multispecialty team (thoracic surgeons and neurosurgeons or orthopaedics) such as the Dumbbell tumour with spinal canal extension and in the case of the schwannoma [5].

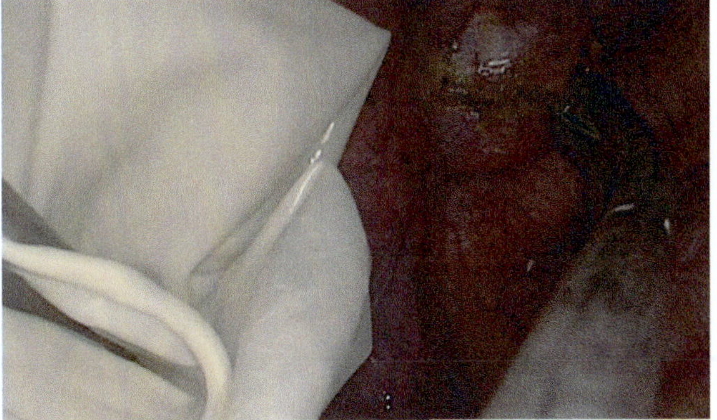

Fig. 13 Shows the extraction of the posterior mediastinal tumour with the help of a surgical globe

References

1. Ronson RS, Duarte I, Miller JI. Embryology and surgical anatomy of the mediastinum with clinical implications. Surg Clin N Am. 2000;80:157–69.
2. Reed M. Technique of thoracoscopic resections of posterior mediastinal tumours. Oper Tech Thorac Cardiovasc Surg. 2010;15(2):114–24.
3. Divisi D, Battalgia C, Crisci R, Giusti L. Diagnostic and therapeutic approaches for masses in the posterior mediastinum. Acta Biomed Ateneo Parmense. 1998;69(5–6):123–8.
4. Wu CY, Heish MJ, Wu CF. Single port VATS mediastinal tumor resection: Taiwan experience. Ann Cardiothorac Surg. 2016;5(2):107–11.
5. Shadmehr MB, Gaisser HA, Wain JC, Grillo HC, Bor LE. The surgical approaches to dumbbell tumors of the mediastinum. Ann Thorac Surg. 2003;76(5):1650–4.

Subxiphoid Mediastinal Resections

Takashi Suda

Abstract

We previously developed a surgical technique called subxiphoid single-port thymectomy to excise the thymus through a single opening made below the xiphoid process. This procedure is facilitated by creating adequate space for surgery by inducing compression of bilateral lungs and the mediastinum by means of CO_2 insufflation. We previously reported a comparative study of the early outcomes after VATS thymectomy and single-port thymectomy performed at our hospital from January 2005 to December 2014. Subxiphoid single-port thymectomy takes the same amount of operative time as VATS thymectomy via a lateral thoracic approach, but results in less blood loss and enables earlier termination of postoperative analgesics. This method offers an excellent cosmetic outcome with just one 3-cm incision in the abdomen and is the most minimally invasive form of thymectomy that avoids sternotomy and intercostal nerve injury. Investigation of the safety of this procedure and long-term therapeutic outcomes for myasthenia gravis and anterior mediastinal tumors is necessary.

Introduction

Thymectomy for myasthenia gravis and anterior mediastinal tumors is a more minimally invasive form of surgery than conventional median sternotomy. Cooper et al. [1] reported on transcervical thymectomy via a cervical incision. This method is an excellent minimally invasive surgical procedure that does not involve sternotomy or thoracostomy, thus causing no pain or paralysis. However, this approach has not been widely adopted due to its technical complexity and difficulties in securing the surgical field. Video-assisted thoracoscopic (VATS) thymectomy is a type of minimally invasive thymectomy that is currently used widely when operating via a lateral thoracic approach. VATS thymectomy via a lateral thoracic approach was first reported for the treatment of thymoma in 1992 [2] and for the treatment of myasthenia gravis in 1993 [3]. In 2003, robot-assisted thymectomy via a lateral thoracic approach was reported [4], and its good long-term outcomes were recently reported [5]. However, unilateral lateral thoracic approaches make it difficult to confirm the location of the contralateral phrenic nerve and secure the visual field in the neck. Moreover, pain or paralysis after intercostal nerve injury is common at the site of port insertion because the incision is made through the intercostal space [6].

The subxiphoid approach was reported as the "infrasternal approach" in 1999 [7]. Similar to transcervical thymectomy, this approach is an excellent minimally invasive surgical procedure because there is no requirement of a sternotomy or thoracostomy, although the procedure remains challenging due to difficulties in securing the surgical field. In addition, there is interference between bilateral forceps and the camera during surgery. We reported cases of single-port thymectomy that was facilitated by creating adequate space for surgery by inducing compression of bilateral lungs and the mediastinum by means of CO_2 insufflation (Fig. 1) [8]. We operated via a subxiphoid approach using instruments for single-port surgery. This method offers an excellent cosmetic outcome with just one 3-cm incision in the abdomen and is the most minimally invasive form of thymectomy that avoids sternotomy and intercostal nerve injury.

Electronic Supplementary Material The online version of this chapter (https://doi.org/10.1007/978-981-13-2604-2_11) contains supplementary material, which is available to authorized users.

T. Suda (✉)
Division of Thoracic Surgery, Fujita Health University School of Medicine, Toyoake, Aichi, Japan
e-mail: suda@fujita-hu.ac.jp

D. Gonzalez-Rivas et al. (eds.), *Atlas of Uniportal Video Assisted Thoracic Surgery*,
https://doi.org/10.1007/978-981-13-2604-2_11

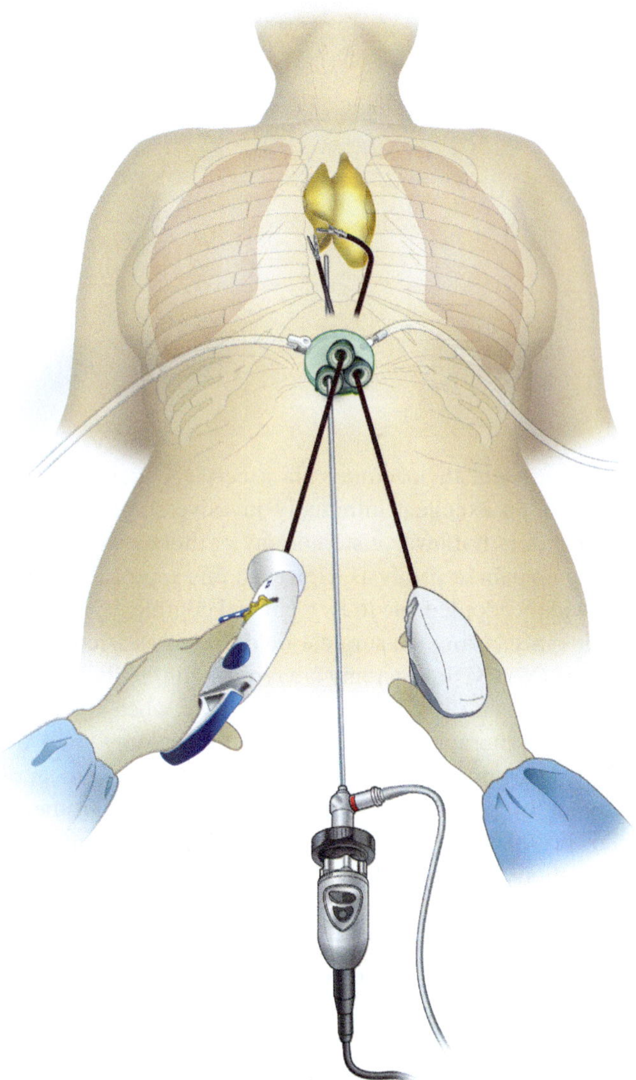

Fig. 1 Subxiphoid single-port thymectomy. The thymus is resected from a single wound in the subxiphoid region

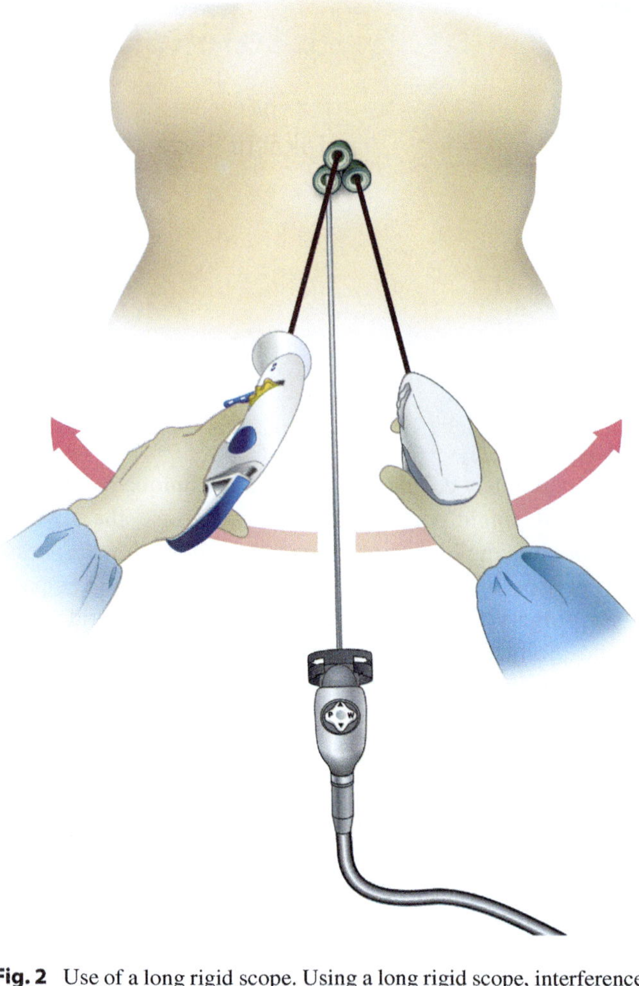

Fig. 2 Use of a long rigid scope. Using a long rigid scope, interference between the surgeon's hands can be prevented

Operative Technique of Subxiphoid Single-Port Thymectomy

Instruments for Subxiphoid Single-Port Thymectomy

There are many types of ports available for single-port surgery. To date, we have used the SILS™ Port (Covidien, Mansfield, MA, USA), X-gate (Akita Sumitomo Bakelite Co., Akita, Japan), and GelPOINT Mini (Applied Medical, Rancho Santa Margarita, CA, USA). The GelPOINT Mini uses a port platform made of gel, which reduces interference between forceps by preventing the child ports from becoming excessively immobilized. This feature makes the GelPOINT Mini the most appropriate port for subxiphoid single-port thymectomy.

We used the 36-cm SILS™ Clinch (Covidien, Mansfield, MA, USA), which is a forceps for single-port surgery that bends at the tip, and one of the SILS™ Hand Instruments, as the forceps the surgeon holds in his/her left hand. It is also vital to use a vessel-sealing device in this surgery; therefore, we used a bipolar vessel-sealing device without cavitation of the tip of the instrument. The 37-cm LigaSure™ Maryland (Covidien, Mansfield, MA, USA), with a tip shape appropriate for ablative surgeries, is the most suitable for this surgical technique. The shape of the thorax sometimes prevents the tip of the LigaSure™ from reaching the posterior surface of the sternum. In such cases, the thymus is detached from the posterior surface of the sternum using monopolar forceps with a flexible tip or scissors. For the camera scope, we used a rigid scope of 5-mm diameter with 30° view. Using a long rigid scope, we were able to prevent interference between the surgeon's hands (Fig. 2). To safely perform this surgery, a camera head that offers clear images must be used, even when employing a 5-mm diameter scope.

Patient Selection

Single-port thymectomy is the least invasive thymectomy approach because it does not require the sternotomy and does not cause intercostal nerve injury. However, a disadvantage of single-port thymectomy is that it offers poor maneuverability. It is not easy to suture through a single wound in the subxiphoid region. Due to its minimal invasiveness, we believe single-port thymectomy is indicated in cases of thymoma without invasion and cases of myasthenia gravis without tumors. Single-port thymectomy can also be used to perform partial lung resection when a tumor has invaded the lungs. Dual-port thymectomy [9], which facilitates surgical operability by adding another intercostal port to the single-port thymectomy procedure, or trans-subxiphoid robotic thymectomy [10], which uses the Da Vinci robotic surgical system (Intuitive Surgical, Sunnyvale, CA, USA) are indicated in cases of suspected pericardial invasion. This is because suturing is required to compensate for the pericardial defect. In cases of cardiac, great vessel, and left brachiocephalic vein invasion, a median sternotomy is generally performed; however, dual-port thymectomy or trans-subxiphoid robotic thymectomy can potentially be used if invasion has spread to part of the left brachiocephalic vein. The decision regarding which technique to use, i.e., single-port thymectomy, dual-port thymectomy, trans-subxiphoid robotic thymectomy, or median sternotomy, should be made according to the extent of invasion in cases of thymoma invasion to adjacent organs.

Anesthesia Management

All surgeries are performed under general anesthesia. One-lung ventilation is performed as mechanical ventilation management using a double-lumen endotracheal tube when the thymoma is presumed to invade the lungs. However, bilateral lung ventilation by means of a single-lumen endotracheal tube is sufficient when combined pulmonary resection is not required. CO_2 insufflation displaces both lungs; therefore, it does not interfere with surgical operations. In our set-up for mechanical ventilation, we ensure that positive end-expiratory pressure is avoided by performing pressure-limited ventilation that provides the minimum airway pressure necessary to maintain adequate ventilation.

Operative Positioning

The patient is placed in the supine position with legs spread and both arms placed alongside the trunk. The extent of disinfection is extended to the neck and bilateral lateral thoracic regions to allow for conversion from midline sternotomy to dual-port thymectomy (described below). The surgeon stands between the patient's legs and the endoscopist operates the camera from a standing position to the right of the patient. A monitor is placed at the cranial end of the patient. The surgeon may create distance from the port in use by standing between the patient's legs, but this is not a problem once surgical operations actually commence.

Surgical Technique (Video 1)

The procedure is initiated with a 3-cm transverse incision made along the Langer line 1 cm caudal to the subxiphoid region. A mediastinal incision has the advantage that the wound can be easily widened in an inferior direction, particularly in the case of large tumors and following intramediastinal resection of a thymoma or during thymectomy. Caution is required, as the forceps cannot easily reach the posterior surface of the sternum when the skin incision is made too close to the xiphoid process. The site at which the xiphoid process attaches to the rectus abdominis is dissected to reach the posterior surface of the xiphoid process, and the thymus is blindly and digitally dissected from the posterior surface of the sternum. Thereafter, a 5 mm to 1 cm incision is made into the rectus abdominis fascia and a space is created to insert a single surgical port without opening the peritoneum. If the peritoneum is opened, surgical operation becomes difficult as a result of pneumoperitoneum caused by CO_2 insufflation; however, surgery is still possible. There is no need to dissect the xiphoid process. A single port containing three child ports is inserted into the subxiphoid wound (Fig. 3).

Next, we insufflated CO_2 at a pressure of 8 mmHg. At this point, only foamy, cord-like material is visible because the rear surface of the sternum has not yet been detached. The thymus is then detached from the posterior surface of the sternum using the LigaSure™. The positive pressure

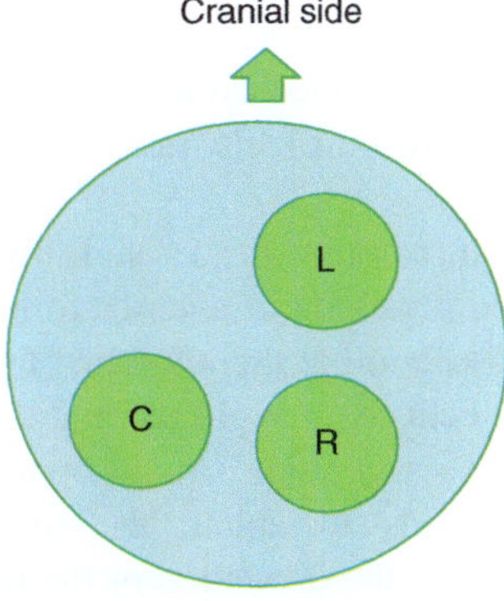

Fig. 3 Insertion position of the child ports. C: Camera port, L: Port for the surgeon's left hand, R: Port for the surgeon's right hand (mainly used as a vessel-sealing device)

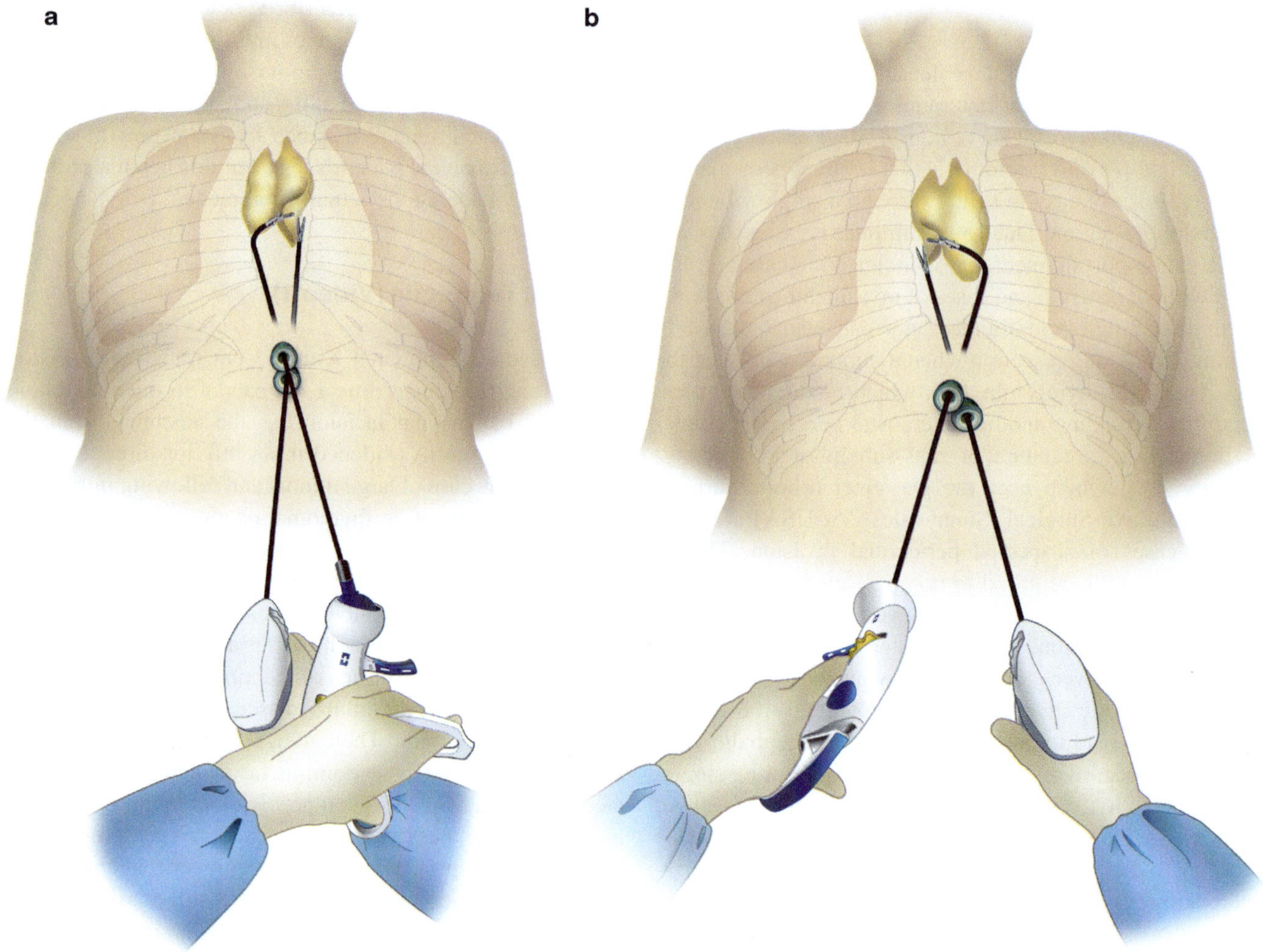

Fig. 4 The single-port surgical technique. To detach the right lobe of the thymus, the thymus is pulled toward the left side of the patient by directing the forceps to the left (**a**), whereas to detach the left lobe, the thymus is pulled toward the right side of the patient by directing the forceps to the right (**b**). At this time, it is necessary for the surgeon to cross hands (b)

resulting from CO_2 insufflation widens the space around the posterior surface of the sternum, as it is detached. The thymus is then separated from the sternum up to the neck. Next, bilateral mediastinal pleurae are opened to gain access to the bilateral thoracic cavities. It is also possible to perform surgery without opening the mediastinal pleurae, although caution is advised due to the difficulty in confirming the location of the phrenic nerves.

The pericardial adipose tissue and thymus are then detached from the pericardium anterior to bilateral phrenic nerves. For the dissection of the left lobe of the thymus, the left-hand forceps bent to the right and the thymus is pulled toward the patient's right side. At this point, the surgeon crosses his/her hands to ablate the thymus with the LigaSure™. Next, for the dissection of the right lobe of the thymus, the left-hand forceps bent to the left and the thymus is pulled toward the patient's left side. There is no need for the surgeon to cross his/her hands during this step (Fig. 4).

It is important that the surgeon is sufficiently proficient at using grasping forceps for single-port surgery to perform this technique.

We start detaching the thymus from the caudal end and dissect the thymic veins last. This is because the thymus is easier to dissect if pulled laterally due to the fact that the thymic veins are dissected tangentially from the subxiphoid wound (Fig. 5).

The inferior pole of the thymus is detached from the pericardium to expose the peripheral and central aspects of the thymus around the left brachiocephalic vein and to expose the confluence of the left and right brachiocephalic veins.

We then move on to operating on the neck. The thin membrane covering the thymus is dissected. The right internal thoracic vein is not usually divided; however, it can be divided if it interferes with surgical manipulation. The superior pole of the thymus is grasped with the forceps and pulled caudally to retract the left brachiocephalic vein and

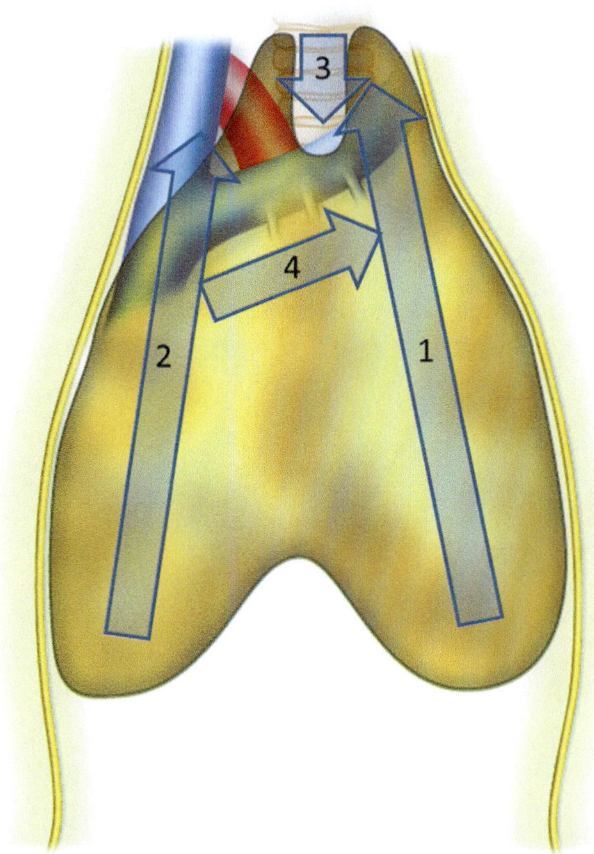

Fig. 5 Our surgical procedure. After opening bilateral visceral pleurae, (1) the surgery starts from the left inferior pole of the thymus by detaching the thymus from the pericardium and by exposing the peripheral side of the thymus at the left brachiocephalic vein. (2) The right inferior pole of the thymus is then detached from the pericardium along the right phrenic nerve to expose the center of the thymus around the left brachiocephalic vein and the confluence of the left and right brachiocephalic veins. (3) The two superior poles of the thymus are detached from the thyroid to expose the cranial end of the left brachiocephalic vein. (4) The thymic veins are divided with the vessel-sealing device and the thymectomy is completed. We dissect the thymic veins last. This is because the thymus is easier to dissect if pulled laterally due to the fact that the thymic veins are dissected tangentially from the subxiphoid wound

improve the field of view of the neck. The superior pole of the thymus and adipose tissue in the neck are detached from the right brachiocephalic vein on the right, the thyroid superiorly, the brachiocephalic artery and trachea dorsally, and the medial aspect of the left brachiocephalic vein on the left. Care must be taken not to injure the inferior thyroid vein in this area. The thymic veins sometimes flow into the left brachiocephalic vein from a region of the thymus more cranial to the left brachiocephalic vein; thus, caution is required. The thymus is pulled toward either side to expose the left brachiocephalic vein. Because the path of the thymic vein is tangential to the vessel sealing system, the course of the thymic vein will run in a transverse direction on lateral traction of the thymus, which allows the vessel sealing system to separate the vein from the brachiocephalic vein. And then resection of the thymus is completed. The resected thymus is placed in a bag. The thymus is then removed from the body via the subxiphoid wound. A straight, 20 Fr drain is inserted into the subxiphoid wound before closure.

Tips for Surgery

The tip of the LigaSure™ sometimes interferes with the camera scope and does not go where intended. When performing single-port surgery, the camera scope and forceps cross over each other within the surgical port. The position of the LigaSure™ tip in the surgeon's right hand differs greatly depending on whether the route of insertion of the LigaSure™ passed over or under the camera scope or the forceps in the surgeon's left hand. This route can be modified when the surgeon feels that the LigaSure™ is not advancing in the intended direction. Furthermore, interference by instruments can be reduced by modifying the position of the camera scope using the camera scope's oblique view or by attempting to retract the camera with the zoom function.

Managing Hemorrhage

If there is hemorrhage from the brachiocephalic vein, it is first compressed using the thymus or a cotton swab for thoracoscopic surgery. If compression hemostasis is not achieved, the procedure is rapidly converted to a median sternotomy. If compression hemostasis is possible, a TachoSil® (Takeda Austria GmbH, Linz, Austria) sponge or other hemostatic agent is used. An additional port can be inserted above the fifth or sixth intercostal clavicle midline of the right precordium if hemorrhage occurs, irrespective of the surgical procedure used. This allows more favorable manipulation and is also good for performing hemostatic procedures.

Subxiphoid Thymectomy (Dual-Port Thymectomy)

In single-port thymectomy, all instruments are inserted via a single port, which has the disadvantage of complicating surgical techniques due to interferences among the various instruments. As a result of the poor maneuverability during single-port surgery in the field of abdominal surgery in recent years, both surgeries that do not require a single port and reduced port surgery have come under review. We previously reported dual-port thymectomy, which improved

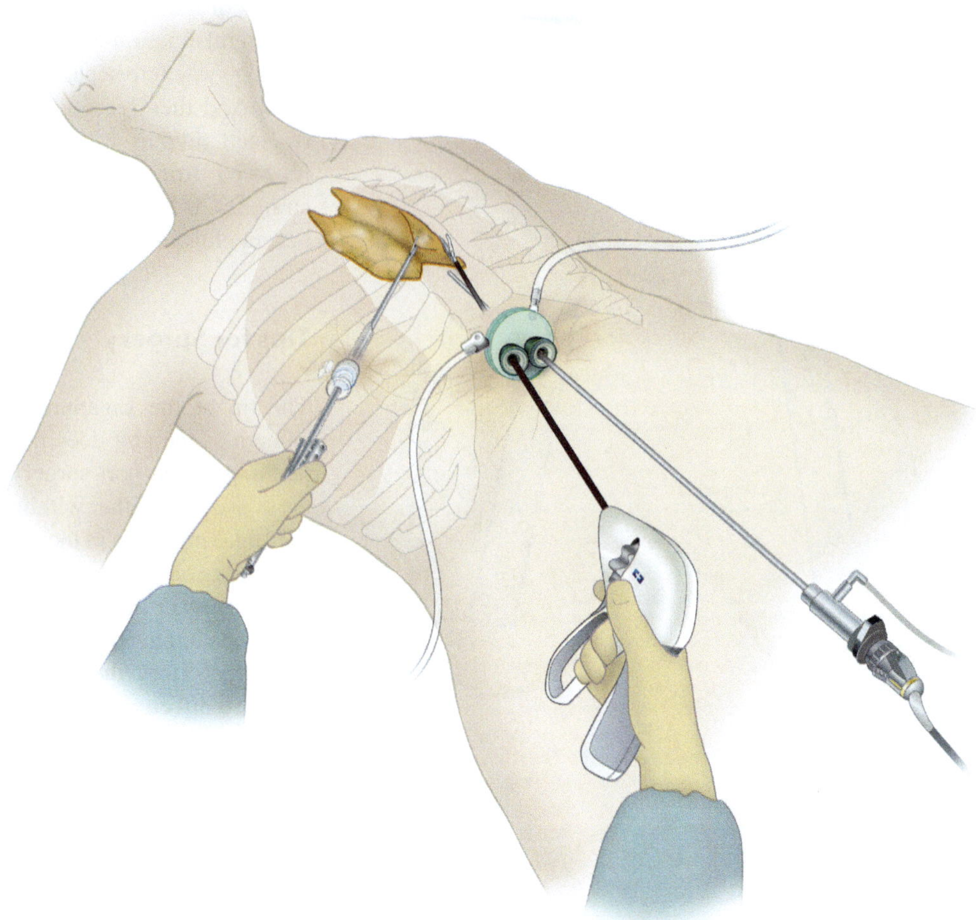

Fig. 6 Subxiphoid thymectomy (dual-port thymectomy). Compared with single-port thymectomy, dual-port thymectomy has an additional port in the right fifth intercostal space to improve operability

the operability of the single-port thymectomy procedure by adding another port in the right fifth intercostal space [9] (Fig. 6). Dual-port thymectomy can result in intercostal nerve injury because the thymus is approached via an intercostal space; however, surgery is easier than that during single-port thymectomy because there is little interference between the forceps in both of the surgeon's hands. It is recommended to start with this method when initially performing thymectomy from the subxiphoid region without an instructor.

The procedure starts with a single-port surgery. The surgeon stands between the patient's legs and the endoscopist operates the camera from a standing position to the right of the patient (Fig. 7). The procedure is identical to that used during single-port thymectomy until bilateral thoracic cavities are opened. A 5-mm port is then inserted toward the neck above the fifth or sixth intercostal space along the midclavicular line on the right anterior chest wall. Next, the surgeon moves to the patient's right side to perform the surgery and the endoscopist operates the camera from a standing position between the patient's legs. The camera scope and LigaSure™ can be inserted via the intercostal port instead of the subxiphoid port.

Postoperative Management

The patient is woken from anesthesia and the endotracheal tube is removed in the operating room. The drain is removed on postoperative day 1. The patient is usually discharged on postoperative day 3. We routinely administer oral analgesics for 1 week postoperatively.

Results

In January 2015, instead of performing thymectomy that does not require combined resection of other organs via a median sternotomy, we started performing VATS thymectomy using a unilateral or bilateral lateral thoracic approach. From March 2011, we switched from VATS thymectomy to single-port thymectomy, using an approach via a single 3-cm skin incision in the subxiphoid region.

I present the early outcomes after performing 62 successive cases of single-port thymectomy for anterior mediastinal tumors or myasthenia gravis by single surgeon at Fujita Health University Hospital from March 2011 to April 2016. Data are presented as mean ± standard deviation. In two

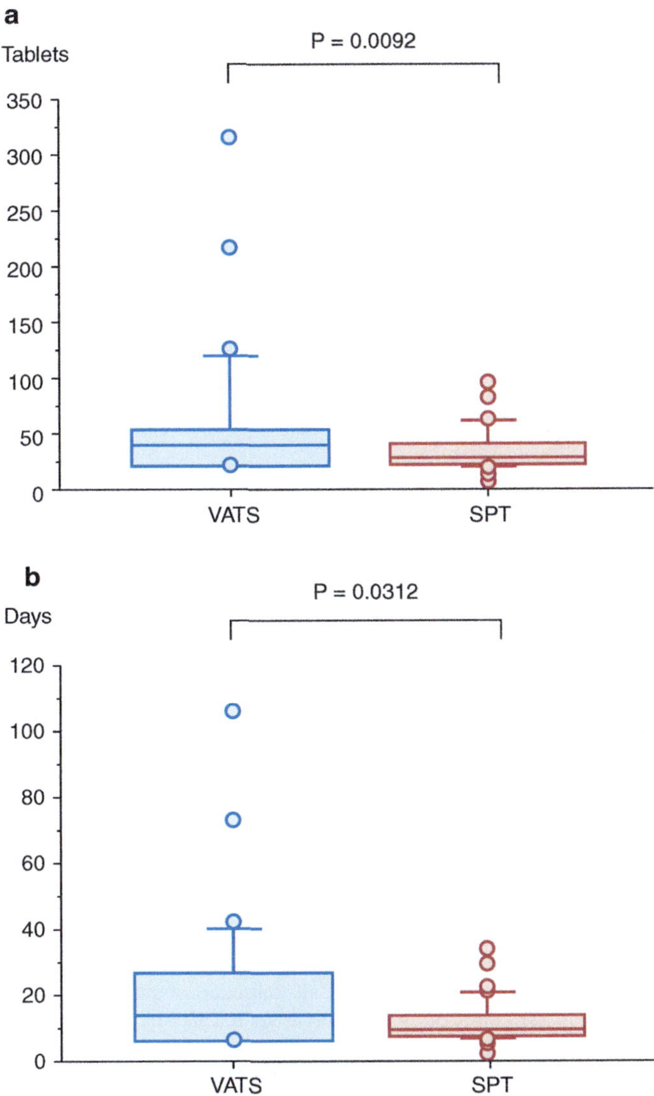

Fig. 7 (**a**) The dose of postoperative oral analgesics used (tablets) was significantly greater in the VATS thymectomy group than in the subxiphoid group. (**b**) The period of postoperative oral analgesics use (days) was significantly longer in the VATS thymectomy group than in the subxiphoid group. (From Suda T, Hachimaru A, Tochii D, et al. Video-assisted thoracoscopic thymectomy versus subxiphoid single-port thymectomy: initial results. Eur J Cardiothorac Surg. 2016;49:i54–i58)

cases (3.2%), the tumor was adherent to one side of the lung, which required simultaneous partial lung resection using a stapler inserted via a subxiphoid port. In four cases (6.4%), the procedure was converted to dual-port thymectomy intraoperatively after surgical operability was found to be challenging. Difficulties included an excessive amount of adipose tissue, pectus excavatum, a hemorrhagic thymic hemangioma, and an iatrogenic pericardial incision. No cases required conversion to median sternotomy. The mean surgical duration was 130.5 ± 46.8 min, mean blood loss was 4.9 ± 3.91 g, and mean hospital stay was 4.3 ± 3.8 days. No intraoperative complications, including intraoperative bleeding, occurred. After surgery, left phrenic nerve paralysis was observed in two cases (3.2%) and transient paroxysmal atrial fibrillation was observed in one case (1.6%). No deaths occurred.

We previously reported a comparative study of the early outcomes after VATS thymectomy (n = 35) and single-port thymectomy (n = 46) performed at our hospital from January 2005 to December 2014 [11]. In this study, no difference in surgical duration (minutes) was observed between the VATS thymectomy group and subxiphoid group [median: 150.0 min (25th and 75th percentiles: 128.0 and 202.0 min) versus 139 min (25th and 75th percentiles: 108.0 and 174.0 min), respectively; p = 0.0853]. Meanwhile, blood loss (g) was greater in the VATS thymectomy group than in the subxiphoid group [median: 20.0 g (25th and 75th percentiles: 3.0 and 50.0 g) versus 2 g (25th and 75th percentiles: 2.0 and 3.0 g), respectively; p < 0.0001], and the postoperative hospital stay (days) was longer in the VATS thymectomy group than in the subxiphoid group [median: 5.0 days (25th and 75th percentiles: 4.0 and 7.0 days) versus 4.0 days (25th and 75th percentiles: 3.0 and 5.0 days), respectively; p = 0.0008]. The dose of postoperative oral analgesics used (tablets) was also significantly greater in the VATS thymectomy group than in the subxiphoid group [median: 41.0 tablets (25th and 75th percentiles: 21.0 and 53.0 tablets) versus 28 tablets (25th and 75th percentiles: 21.0 and 40.0 tablets), respectively; p = 0.0092; Fig. 7a]. In addition, the period of postoperative oral analgesics usage (days) was significantly longer in the VATS thymectomy group than in the subxiphoid group [median: 14.0 days (25th and 75th percentiles: 7.0 and 26.8 days) versus 10 days (25th and 75th percentiles: 7.0 and 13.0 days), respectively; p = 0.0312; Fig. 7b].

Discussion

Thymectomy has traditionally been performed via a median sternotomy. However, cutting into the sternum presents the risk of sternal osteomyelitis as a serious complication in patients with myasthenia gravis, who take immunosuppressive agents or steroids. Moreover, the incision into the anterior chest wall is esthetically unappealing. Recently, less invasive approaches have been selected in cases of thymectomy for thymomas and myasthenia gravis. VATS thymectomy performed via a lateral thoracic approach is a procedure used in a majority of facilities and involves the use of robot-assisted surgery. While VATS thymectomy has the advantage of not requiring transection of the sternum, it also has its disadvantages. One disadvantage is the difficulty in confirming the location of the contralateral phrenic nerve and securing the surgical field of view of the neck. Furthermore, when operating via a lateral thoracic approach, pain and paralysis from intercostal nerve injury are common and persist for several months in the regions consistent

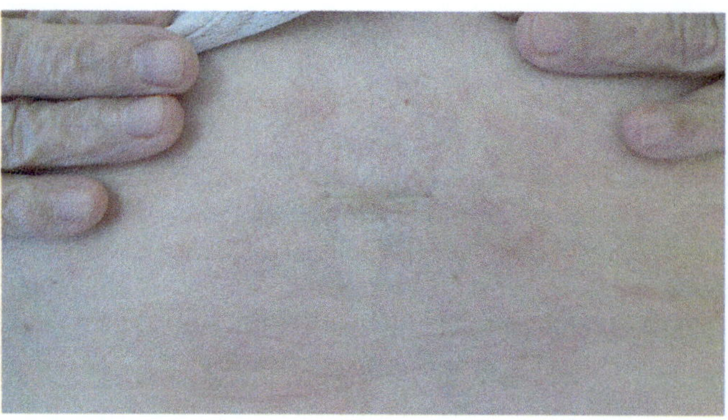

Fig. 8 Wound following single-port thymectomy. (From Suda T, Sugimura H, Hattori Y. Single port thymectomy - A step towards "scarless" thymectomy to replace robotics? (reply) Ann Thorac Surg. 2012 Dec;94 (6):2176–7)

with at least three port wounds. This is because surgical instruments pass through the intercostal space [6]. This pain and numbness can be permanent in the form of post-thoracotomy pain syndrome (PTPS) [12, 13]. As shown in Fig. 7, we encountered some cases of PTPS in the VATS thymectomy group that required long-term use of analgesics. By contrast, single-port thymectomy results in no intercostal nerve injury and requires only small doses of analgesics for a short period of time because there is no need to pass through the intercostal space. Moreover, the wound after single-port thymectomy is esthetically superior [14] (Fig. 8). The subxiphoid approach has recently been used during lung resection, including pulmonary lobectomy, due to its low invasiveness [15, 16]. This approach is expected to be further disseminated as a thoracic surgery approach that does not cause intercostal nerve injury. The disadvantage of single-port surgery is the operability. In this approach, all instruments are inserted via a single port, which results in interference among instruments and poor operability. In addition, this procedure also involves a learning curve; we are currently capable of performing thymectomy in less than 2 h in many cases. If a single-port, robotic surgical system is developed in the coming years, then operability during single-port thymectomy would improve. At present, we perform dual-port thymectomy or trans-subxiphoid robotic thymectomy in cases that require suturing, and we indicate median sternotomy in cases that require angioplasty.

To date, we have encountered two cases (2.9%) of postoperative phrenic nerve paralysis. In one case, the paralysis was temporary and the patient recovered after surgery. In the other case, the mediastinal pleurae were not opened, which made confirmation of the left phrenic nerve difficult, resulting in injury. In endoscopic surgery, the range of visibility is small; it is thus important to always check the location of the phrenic nerve to prevent phrenic nerve injury.

Conclusions

Subxiphoid single-port thymectomy is a minimally invasive surgical approach that takes the same amount of time as VATS thymectomy via a lateral thoracic approach, but results in less blood loss and enables earlier termination of postoperative analgesics. This approach has clear advantages for patients, such as its minimal invasiveness and superior esthetic outcome; therefore, this technique should be mastered by surgeons through sufficient training. Going forward, we will need to investigate the long-term therapeutic outcomes of single-port thymectomy for myasthenia gravis and thymomas.

Conflict of Interest None declared.

References

1. Cooper JD, Al-Jilaihawa AN, Pearson FG, et al. An improved technique to facilitate transcervical thymectomy for myasthenia gravis. Ann Thorac Surg. 1988;45(3):242–7.
2. Landreneau RJ, Dowling RD, Castillo WM, et al. Thoracoscopic resection of an anterior mediastinal tumor. Ann Thorac Surg. 1992;54(1):142–4.
3. Sugarbaker DJ. Thoracoscopy in the management of anterior mediastinal masses. Ann Thorac Surg. 1993;56:653–6.
4. Ashton RC Jr, et al. Totally endoscopic robotic thymectomy for myasthenia gravis. Ann Thorac Surg. 2003;75:569.
5. Ruckert JC, et al. J Thorac Cardiovasc Surg. 2011;141:673.
6. Kehlet H, Jensen TS, Woolf CJ. Persistent postsurgical pain: risk factors and prevention. Lancet. 2006;367(9522):1618–25.
7. Kido T, Hazama K, Inoue Y, et al. Resection of anterior mediastinal masses through an infrasternal approach. Ann Thorac Surg. 1999;67:263–5.
8. Suda T, Sugimura H, Tochii D, Kihara M, Hattori Y. Single-port thymectomy through an infrasternal approach. Ann Thorac Surg. 2012;93(1):334–6.
9. Suda T, Ashikari S, Tochii D, et al. Dual-port thymectomy using subxiphoid approach. Gen Thorac Cardiovasc Surg. 2014;62(9):570–2.
10. Suda T, Tochii D, Tochii S, Takagi Y. Trans-subxiphoid robotic thymectomy. Interact Cardiovasc Thorac Surg. 2015;20(5):669–71.
11. Suda T, Hachimaru A, Tochii D, et al. Video-assisted thoracoscopic thymectomy versus subxiphoid single-port thymectomy: initial results. Eur J Cardiothorac Surg. 2016;49:i54–8.
12. Kirby TJ, Mack MJ, Landreneau RJ, Rice TW. Lobectomy—video-assisted thoracic surgery versus muscle-sparing thoracotomy: a randomized trial. J Thorac Cardiovasc Surg. 1995;109(5):997–1001.
13. Furrer M, Rechsteiner R, Eigenmann V, Signer C, Althaus U, Ris HB. Thoracotomy and thoracoscopy: postoperative pulmonary function, pain and chest wall complaints. Eur J Cardiothorac Surg. 1997;12(1):82–7.
14. Suda T, Sugimura H, Hattori Y. Single port thymectomy – a step towards "scarless" thymectomy to replace robotics? (reply). Ann Thorac Surg. 2012;94(6):2176–7.
15. Suda T, Ashikari S, Tochii S, Sugimura H, Hattori Y. Single-incision subxiphoid approach for bilateral metastasectomy. Ann Thorac Surg. 2014;97(2):718–9.
16. Liu CC, Wang BY, Shih CS, Liu YH. Subxiphoid single-incision thoracoscopic left upper lobectomy. J Thorac Cardiovasc Surg. 2014;148(6):3250.

Part III

Parenchymal Lung Diseases

Uniportal Treatment for Spontaneous Pneumothorax

Alessandro Brunelli and Cecilia Pompili

Abstract

Video-assisted thoracoscopic surgery is the surgical treatment of choice for spontaneous pneumothorax. Most recently, this technique has been made even less invasive by the use of the single-port technique. Uniportal VATS treatment of spontaneous pneumothorax has been shown to be superior to traditional VATS in terms of pain and long-term paraesthesia, while ensuring the same efficacy in terms of prevention of recurrences.

We describe herein the technique of uniportal VATS bullectomy and pleurodesis, summarizing the principle steps of the procedures and the evidence from the literature.

History

The surgical management of spontaneous pneumothorax (SP), using a video-assisted thoracoscopic (VATS) approach performed through a single skin incision, was first described by Rocco et al. [1, 2] in 2004. Since then several authors have published their series and this technique has been widely adopted worldwide for this type of operation. The use of high definition endoscopes and special articulating instruments has facilitated the diffusion of this approach improving its performance and safety.

Electronic Supplementary Material The online version of this chapter (https://doi.org/10.1007/978-981-13-2604-2_12) contains supplementary material, which is available to authorized users.

A. Brunelli (✉)
Department of Thoracic Surgery, St. James's University Hospital, Leeds, UK

C. Pompili
Leeds Institute of Cancer and Pathology, University of Leeds, Leeds, UK

Principles

Uniportal VATS for SP follows the same principle as of the traditional three-port VATS for this condition. Both the American College of Chest Physicians and the British Thoracic Society guidelines recommend the surgical treatment of pneumothorax in case of recurrence after the first episode and in general when the first episode is not resolving (persistent air leak) despite conservative management or presents as hypertensive pneumothorax [3, 4]. These guidelines recommend the performance of a combination of bullectomy and a pleurodesis procedure (pleurectomy, mechanical pleurodesis, or talc pleurodesis). Although, the current guidelines do not explicitly recommend the use of VATS approach over thoracotomy, a recent paper form the Epithor provided a snapshot of the current surgical practice showing that 87% of patients surgically treated for SP were submitted to VATS rather than thoracotomy [5]. Many authors have shown that VATS is associated with lower postoperative morbidity, shorter hospital stay and reduced pain [6–8]. The use of uniportal VATS has been shown to further reduce the surgical impact with favorable results in terms of pain and speed of recovery [2, 9], which makes this approach ideal for treating a benign condition.

Anesthesia

The anesthetic technique used for uniportal VATS bullectomy does not differ from that used for any other major thoracic surgical procedure. Induction is performed intravenously and endobronchial intubation takes place following administration of a non-depolarizing neuromuscular blocking drug. Maintenance is with an inhalational agent.

Single-lung ventilation is necessary to provide an adequate operating exposure. The successful endobronchial tube position is confirmed with a flexible bronchoscope before the patient is turned to the lateral position.

D. Gonzalez-Rivas et al. (eds.), *Atlas of Uniportal Video Assisted Thoracic Surgery*,
https://doi.org/10.1007/978-981-13-2604-2_12

The patient is positioned in the lateral decubitus position and the table is flexed at the level of the 5th–6th intercostal space to increase the spreading of the intercostal spaces for access. In addition, flexing the table drops the pelvis away increasing mobility the camera and other surgical instruments introduced from the surgical incision.

Following completion of the bullectomy and any pleurodesis procedure and positioning of the chest tube the operated lung parenchyma is re-inflated. Extubation should be accomplished in the operating room and post-operative care is monitored in a dedicated thoracic ward.

Surgical Technique

As with all uniportal procedures, both the surgeon and assistant are positioned anterior to the patient. Ideally, two monitors are used, one on each side of the patient, to allow the entire team to follow the progress of the operation. Usually, the assistant holds the thoracoscope, but at times the surgeon may guide the camera, while the assistant retracts.

After prepping the patient in the standard fashion, the single surgical incision is performed at the level of the mid-axillary line on the sixth or seventh intercostal space. The incision is typically 2.5 cm long on the skin (Fig. 1). However, the incision on the intercostal space is usually made 1 cm longer in each direction to optimize access within the space, which facilitates the movement of the instruments through the single port and reduces the leverage of the instruments on the uppermost rib (minimizing trauma to the corresponding intercostal nerve).

The single port represents the inlet for both the thoracoscope and for all the other operative instruments (Fig. 2). The use of a wound protector device is optional. If a trocar used to insert the thoracoscope, it is retracted along the stem, in order to increase the space and maximize the movement of the instruments. Alternatively, the scope may be carefully placed without a port.

After the creation of the single port a 5-mm 30-degree thoracoscope is introduced. With the use of a peanut mounted on a long clamp, the lung is gently retracted and inspected for target lesions (blebs or bullae). The entirety of the visceral pleura should be inspected from the apex to the base of the

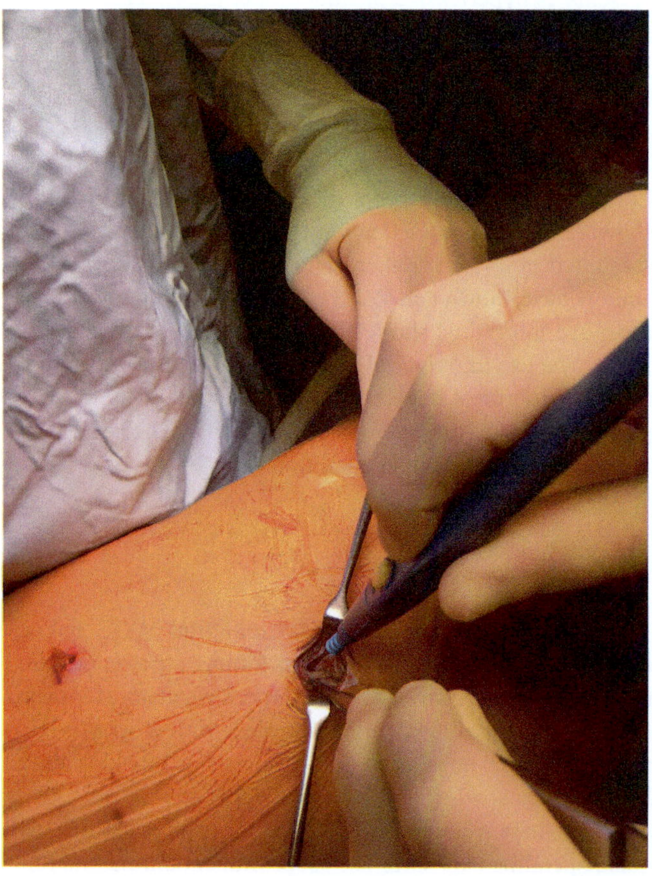

Fig. 1 Single port incision for uniportal VATS bullectomy is usually 2–2.5 cm long and performed at the level of the 5th–6th intercostal space along the mid-axillary line

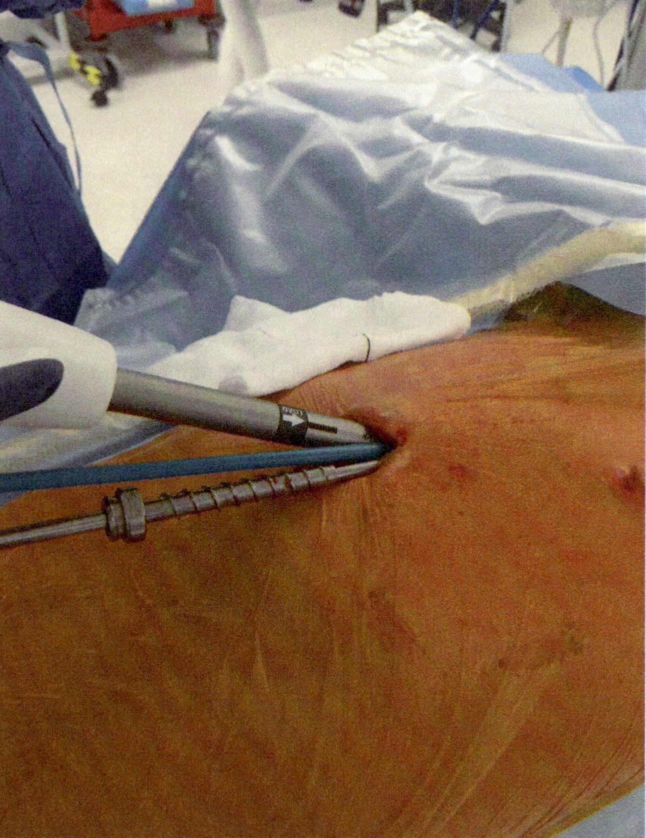

Fig. 2 A typical phase of the operation when all three instruments necessary to perform the wedge resection are inserted through the single incision (camera, lung grasper and stapler)

lung. In case of female patients, the diaphragm should also be explored to rule out foci of endometriosis or defects associated with catamenial pneumothorax. In case of an operation for persistent air leak, the source of air leak should be identified as the primary target for resection.

In most of the cases the area containing blebs is located at the apex of the upper lobe or in the superior segment of the lower lobe. The first step of the procedure is therefore the performance of a bullectomy by wedge resection. The wedge resection is performed by introducing a special endoscopic lung grasper to adequately suspend the lung at the level of the target area. Following lung suspension, an articulating endostapler is introduced through the single incision, usually between the camera and the grasper and advanced up to the target area. The lung parenchyma is pulled and fed in between the jaws of the stapler, which is applied to complete the wedge resection. I generally prefer to use a 45 mm medium thickness stapler, which I find more versatile and easy to accommodate even within small chests. Multiple applications of the stapler are usually needed to perform the bullectomy (Video 1).

The final component of the procedure—also essential—is the performance of the pleurodesis procedures of choice: pleurectomy or mechanical pleurodesis with talc poudrage reserved for unusual cases (Video 2).

At the conclusion of the procedure a chest tube is positioned using the single thoracic access and the lung is re-inflated.

Outcome

Several authors have compared uniportal VATS versus traditional three port VATS for the surgical management of SP, but there are no randomized trials comparing the two techniques. Most of the studies found that uniportal VATS was superior in terms of early postoperative pain score [2, 9, 10] and long-term residual paresthesia [2, 9] compared to three-port VATS.

Salati and coll [9] found that uniportal VATS was also associated with a shorter hospital stay (1 day shorter compared to three-port VATS) and with a reduced hospital cost (390 Euro less expensive than three port VATS).

A recent meta-analysis pooling together data from 17 studies comparing uniportal versus three-port VATS for the management of SP confirmed these findings [11]. A total of 988 patients were aggregated (502 uniportal VATS vs. 486 three port VATS) and compared. The authors found that there was no postoperative mortality recorded in any of the analyzed series and there was no difference in terms of SP recurrence rate between the two techniques (uniportal: 4.3% vs. three port: 4.8%; $p = 0.45$). Similarly, they were no differences in operative time, hospital stay and chest tube duration after surgery between the two approaches. The most important differences after uniportal VATS compared to three port VATS were a significant reduction in postoperative pain scores at 24 h (3.57 vs. 4.49, <0.0001) and at 72 h (2.41 vs. 2.91, $p < 0.0001$), and a reduced incidence of long term paresthesia (uniportal 19% vs. three port 58%, $p < 0.0001$).

Conclusion

In conclusion, based on personal experience and the evidence from the literature, uniportal VATS treatment of SP is a safe and feasible technique, which is able to contribute to reduce postoperative pain and discomfort of the patients while maintaining the same long-term efficacy in preventing recurrences as the three-port approach.

References

1. Rocco G, Martin-Ucar A, Passera E. Uniportal VATS wedge pulmonary resections. Ann Thorac Surg. 2004;77(2):726–8.
2. Jutley RS, Khalil MW, Rocco G. Uniportal vs standard three-port VATS technique for spontaneous pneumothorax: comparison of post-operative pain and residual paraesthesia. Eur J Cardiothorac Surg. 2005;28(1):43–6.
3. MacDuff A, Arnold A, Harvey J, BTS Pleural Disease Guideline Group. Management of spontaneous pneumo-thorax: British Thoracic Society Pleural Disease Guideline 2010. Thorax. 2010;65(Suppl 2):ii18–31.
4. Baumann MH, Strange C, Heffner JE, Light R, Kirby TJ, Klein J, et al. Management of spontaneous pneumothorax. ACCP Delphi Consensus Statement. Chest. 2001;119:590–602.
5. Pagès PB, Delpy JP, Falcoz PE, Thomas PA, Filaire M, Le Pimpec Barthes F, Dahan M, Bernard A. Videothoracoscopy versus thoracotomy for the treatment of spontaneous pneumothorax: a propensity score analysis. Ann Thorac Surg. 2015;99(1):258–63.
6. Barker A, Maratos EC, Edmonds L, Lim E. Recurrence rates of video-assisted thoracoscopic versus open surgery in the prevention of recurrent pneumothoraces: a systematic review of randomised and non randomised trials. Lancet. 2007;370:329–35.
7. Waller DA, Forty J, Morritt GN. Video-assisted thoracoscopic surgery versus thoracotomy for spontaneous pneumothorax. Ann Thorac Surg. 1994;58:372–6;discussion 376–7.
8. Joshi V, Kirmani B, Zacharias J. Thoracotomy versus VATS: is there an optimal approach to treating pneumothorax? Ann R Coll Surg Engl. 2013;95:61–4.
9. Salati M, Brunelli A, Xiumè F, Refai M, Sciarra V, Soccetti A, Sabbatini A. Uniportal video-assisted thoracic surgery for primary spontaneous pneumothorax: clinical and economic analysis in comparison to the traditional approach. Interact Cardiovasc Thorac Surg. 2008;7(1):63–6.
10. Chen PR, Chen CK, Lin YS, Huang HC, Tsai JS, Chen CY, Fang HY. Single-incision thoracoscopic surgery for primary spontaneous pneumothorax. J Cardiothorac Surg. 2011;6:58.
11. Qin SL, Huang JB, Yang YL, Xian L. Uniportal versus three-port video-assisted thoracoscopic surgery for spontaneous pneumothorax: a meta-analysis. J Thorac Dis. 2015;7(12):2274–87.

Uniportal Bullectomy for Emphysematous Bullous Lung Disease

Fernando Vannucci

Abstract

Bullous disease can occur alone or in conjunction with lung emphysema. Bullae vary in size and the term "giant bulla" is used when lesions exceed one-third of the hemithorax. Giant bullae may impair lung function and cause respiratory symptoms—mainly dyspnea and low exercise tolerance—negatively impacting patient's quality of life. Bullous disease can lead to complications such as pneumothorax, infection and bleeding. Therefore, surgical treatment of bullous disease through bullectomy is indicated when complications occur or when giant bulla are associated to respiratory symptoms. An increasing giant bulla can also be considered for surgical resection, even when asymptomatic. The surgical aim is to remove the giant bullae, allowing expansion of the remaining lung, in order to restore respiratory function. Patients with large bullae and normal underlying lungs are those who accomplish the best results, but surgery should not be denied to emphysematous patients until a preoperative assessment is made to properly outline risks/benefits.

Uniportal video-assisted thoracic surgery is a feasible and safe method to perform bullectomy, with results at least comparable to other techniques, leading to symptoms resolution, improved lung function and better quality of life. This chapter will focus on this approach and its technical details.

Electronic Supplementary Material The online version of this chapter (https://doi.org/10.1007/978-981-13-2604-2_13) contains supplementary material, which is available to authorized users.

F. Vannucci (✉)
Department of Thoracic Surgery, Hospital Federal do Andaraí, Rio de Janeiro, RJ, Brazil

Department of Thoracic Surgery, Hospital Central da Polícia Militar, Rio de Janeiro, RJ, Brazil

Introduction and a Brief Historical Remark

The development of surgery for bullous disease is strongly connected to the rise of the surgery for lung emphysema in general. This history dates back the early twentieth century, when the first interventions were described, with poor and unsustainable results [1]. Throughout the following years, with increasing knowledge of the pathophysiology of the disease, most of the surgical procedures have been abandoned and the options have been dramatically narrowed [2–4]. Lung bullectomy, lung transplantation and lung reduction volume surgery have stood over time and nowadays are more precisely indicated to eligible patients, according to their clinical, functional and radiological presentations [2–4]. Even though there are several technical options available—each one with its own advantages and drawbacks—this chapter will focus specifically on the aspects concerning the minimally invasive bullectomy by means of uniportal video-thoracoscopic technique.

Terminology and Basic Pathophysiology

Historically, there have always been some misunderstandings regarding the nomenclature of air-filled lung lesions. In 1991, Klingman and coworkers [5] published a paper to review and define these terms, in order to clarify and unify their classification. Within the context of chronic obstructive pulmonary disease (COPD), *emphysema* is recognized as the abnormal and permanent enlargement of the air spaces distally to the terminal non-respiratory bronchioles, with disruption of alveolar structure and consequent loss of normal acinar architecture. *Bulla* is an air-filled space lined by a fibrous wall and totally surrounded by lung parenchyma. Bullae are usually acquired lesions formed secondary to alveolar tissue destruction, occurring frequently associated—but not necessarily—to emphysema. When a bulla is large enough to occupy one third or more of the hemithorax, it is characterized as "giant

D. Gonzalez-Rivas et al. (eds.), *Atlas of Uniportal Video Assisted Thoracic Surgery*, https://doi.org/10.1007/978-981-13-2604-2_13

bulla". *Blebs* are subpleural air collections caused by superficial alveolar rupture. The air dissects and remains entrapped within the visceral pleural layer, forming the so-called bleb. Blebs are acquired lesions; mostly seen in lung apex and their rupture are the cause of primary spontaneous pneumothorax. Blebs usually tend to occur independently from emphysema. Lung *cysts* can be congenital or acquired. Congenital cysts usually have bronchial origin, arising from abnormal branching of the embryonic tracheobronchial bud. They are lined by bronchial epithelium and usually filled with liquid/mucus produced by these bronchial cells. Acquired lung cysts usually are thin-walled air spaces that remain after a local injury to the previous normal lung tissue. As described, acquired cysts and bullae are located within the lung parenchyma, counting on a continuous wall. When this wall is thicker than three millimeters, these lesions are then called *cavities*, which usually occur in the presence of infection and reflect a variable degree of inflammatory reaction.

The studies of Morgan and coworkers [6] have proved that there is no valvular mechanism involved in bullae formation; Ting and colleagues [7] have shown that there is no significant pressure gradient between the surrounding lung and the growing bulla. These studies have demonstrated that the bulla is initially formed in an area of alveolar destruction, indeed; but its enlargement is more related to a "preferential ventilation" of this area. This preferential ventilation can be explained by the relatively preserved force of elastic recoil of the parenchyma around the bulla, which retracts the normal lung tissue around the bulla away from it, favoring bulla's distention. As it distends, the compliance within it becomes relatively increased if compared to the "non-bullous" remaining parenchyma, and thus the airflow is preferentially directed to the bulla instead of the surrounding lung. So, the final result is the progressive enlargement of the bulla due to airflow redistribution.

Chronic cigarette smoking is the leading cause of lung emphysema and lung bullous disease, but both can also be caused by less common conditions such as alpha-1 antitrypsin deficiency, immune and/or genetic disorders or even be cryptogenic/idiopathic in young male smokers, in whom the remaining lung appears to be absolutely normal. It is also valid to highlight that, even though emphysema is quite prevalent among smokers, the occurrence of giant bullae is rare.

Clinical Manifestations and Evolution

When symptoms are present, dyspnea is, by far, the most common clinical complaint and its severity will depend mainly on the bullae size, the existence and extension of underlying COPD, as well as the occurrence of secondary complications. Although a patient with a giant bulla may be asymptomatic, when it exists, at least some degree of dyspnea is expected. Cigarette smoking history is present in the majority of cases. Regardless the presence of complications, other clinical manifestations secondary to emphysema, such as cough, fatigability and exercise intolerance may coexist [8].

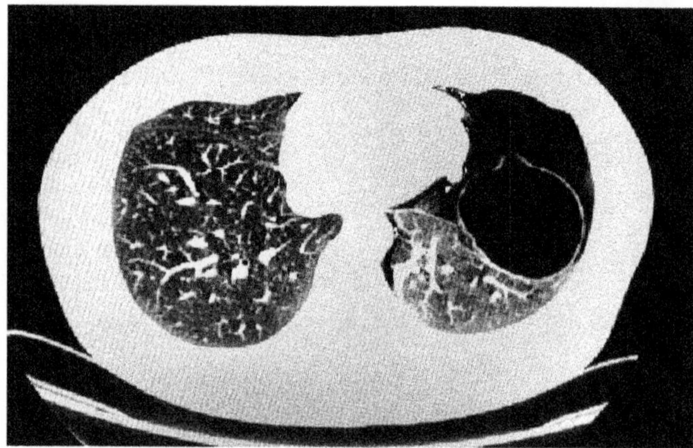

Fig. 1 Pneumothorax secondary to the rupture of a bulla located at the left lower lobe

The initial presentation of giant bullous disease can also be through the existence of complications, with their wide range of clinical manifestations. The most frequent complication described is pneumothorax [8], as seen in Fig. 1. Bulla infection [9, 10] can also occur, with risk of secondary empyema [11]. Less frequently, bleeding can be observed, as hemoptysis [8] or hemopneumothorax [11]. An even more unusual, but possible complication, is the development of cancer at the bulla wall [12, 13].

The natural history of giant bullous disease tends to be similar to the evolution of the underlying COPD. If acute complications do not appear over the years, a gradual worsening of the lung function is expected with time as the disease progresses, especially when smoking habit is kept. Even though some rare reports of bullae reduction and complete resolution exist [14, 15], silent giant bullae are likely to grow and eventually become symptomatic.

Surgical Indications and Preoperative Assessment

A patient with giant bullous disease can be referred to the thoracic surgeon in three main scenarios: (1) asymptomatic patient with an incidental finding of giant bulla in a chest X-ray and/or CT scan; (2) symptomatic patient usually referring dyspnea, with a giant bulla observed in a chest X-ray or CT scan; and (3) symptomatic patient presenting with a complication secondary to giant bullous disease. The most common surgical indication is in a dyspneic patient with a giant bulla occupying space within the chest cavity (≥30%) and compressing an underlying non-emphysematous lung. These patients have variable portions of normal lung parenchyma, which do not ventilate due to the presence of an adjacent bulla, and are those who are more prone to benefit from the surgical resection of the non-functioning bullous lesion. After a careful preoperative workup, surgery may be indicated with good early outcomes in selected and well-prepared patients [16, 17].

While some authors [18] recommend surgery only when symptoms and/or complications develop, others [19] consider reasonable to justify surgical treatment for giant bullae in cases that the lesion occupies more than 50% of the chest cavity and shows evidence of underlying lung collapse, or when a bulla enlargement is clearly detected over the time. We agree with this latter rationale, but always taking into consideration the benefit/risk ratio for each individual patient.

All patients should be thoroughly evaluated and prepared prior to surgical treatment, including mandatory smoking cessation, as the risk of complications and death is unequivocally higher in active smokers. In our opinion, active smoking is the only absolute contraindication to elective bullae surgical resection. Through a multidisciplinary approach, all efforts to help patients quit smoking at least 8 weeks before any surgical procedure should be encouraged. The same multidisciplinary basis is essential to implement a pulmonary rehabilitation program for about 6 weeks [18], in which respiratory physiotherapy and optimized medical treatment by a clinical pulmonologist can help patients to go to surgery at their best pulmonary condition possible.

Among preoperative imaging studies, the high-resolution chest computed tomography scan (CT) is the most important exam. It gives the surgeon all the information needed to plan the surgical resection—number of bullae, their size, location and anatomic relations can be accurately assessed, as shown in Figs. 2 and 3. Additionally, the condition of the underlying compressed lung parenchyma can be estimated and reconstruction techniques can also be useful. If necessary, the study can be complemented by chest CT Angiography scan (Angio-CT), which contributes to define more precisely the relationship between bullae and major pulmonary blood vessels (see Fig. 4). Chest X-rays are routinely used and can be important tools to assess the ability of the underlying lung to re-expand. This can be estimated by comparing recent X-rays with older ones, in which the lung might be seen more expanded than it is presently [20]. If older exams are not available, full inspiration and expiration X-rays can be done to compare if the underlying lung adjacent to bullae shows any sign of airflow, which could predict some re-expansion capacity.

Ventilation/Perfusion scintigraphy is another useful method in preoperative workup. It quantitatively measures lung function, taking into consideration the relative contribution of each lung region.

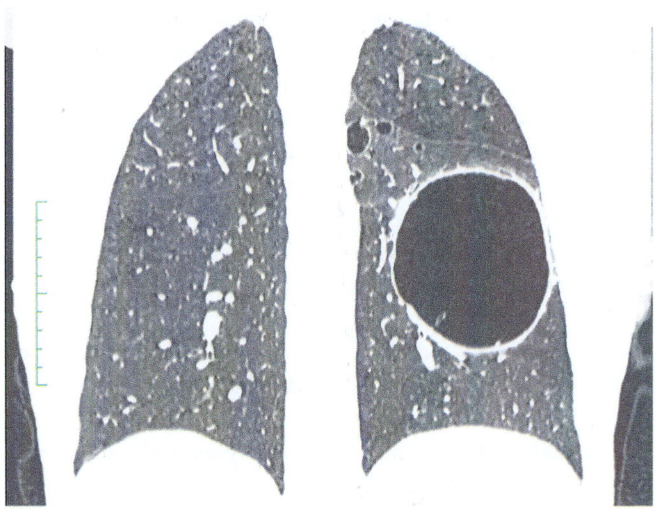

Fig. 3 Coronal chest CT-scan view of the same case shown in Fig. 2. In this image, additional small bullae can be seen at the superior segment of the same lobe

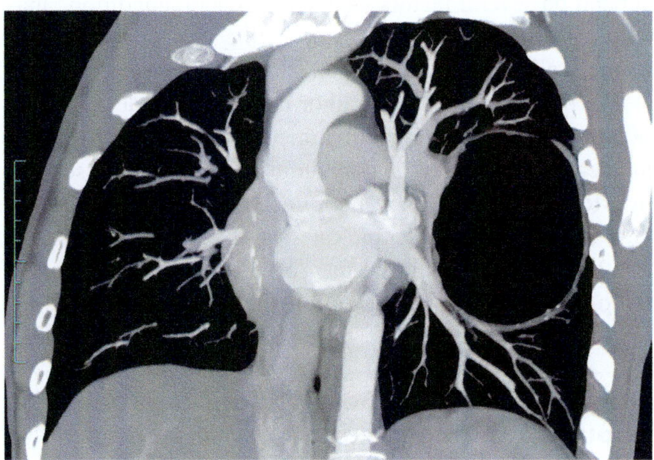

Fig. 4 Same case shown in Figs. 2 and 3. CT-scan angiography in a coronal plane, showing the anatomic relation between the giant bulla and the left pulmonary bronchovascular structures

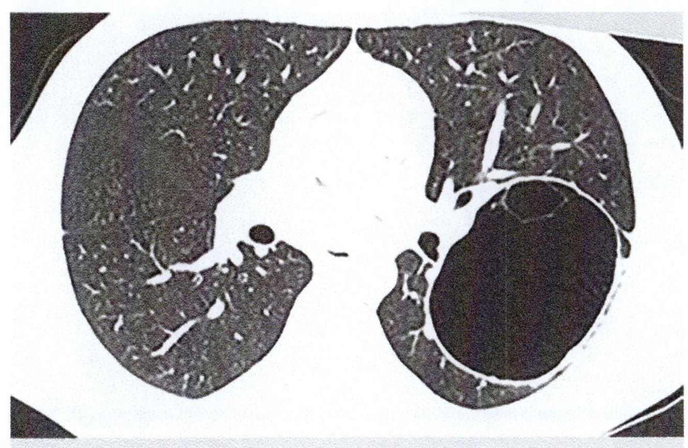

Fig. 2 Axial view of a chest CT-scan showing a giant bulla in the left lower lobe

Pulmonary function tests (PFT's) are also important for an adequate patient selection for surgical treatment. Spirometry, diffusion capacity (DLCO), arterial blood gases and calculation of lung volumes and capacities by whole body plethysmography are the tests that should be done in every surgical candidate [18, 21]. Thus, it is important to stress that none of these tests alone has the strength enough to be considered an absolute predictor of failure or success, nor to be assumed as an isolated factor that could contraindicate surgery.

Surgical Treatment: Options Overview

The mainstay of surgical treatment of giant pulmonary bullous disease is surgical resection. It can be carried out by classic open surgery, by video-assisted thoracic surgery (VATS) [10, 19, 22, 23] or a combination of both approaches [8]. Our approach of choice is by means of single-port access (uniportal VATS), but the chosen approach will ultimately depend on several factors—patient's general condition, anatomic distribution and extension of the disease, the instruments available and the surgeon's experience.

For patients who are too ill or unstable to undergo resection but still need surgical treatment, a less aggressive alternative can be the intra-cavitary drainage, originally described by Monaldi in 1947 [24], but quite modified since then [9, 25]. The use of endoscopic one-way bronchial valves is a non-surgical approach that may offer an even less invasive option for patients who are unfit to elective surgery [26].

Surgical Treatment: General Considerations About Giant Bullectomy

The surgical indication for bullae resection is based on clear objectives and they are all interconnected. These goals are: (1) the removal of giant bullae (which are non-functioning and "space-occupying" lesions), sparing the non-bullous lung parenchyma as much as possible; (2) promote full expansion of the remaining lung; (3) prevent or treat possible complications related to the bullae. Theoretically, these aims tend to contribute to an ultimate improvement of lung function, symptoms resolution and to a better quality of life after surgery.

In general, the use of dual-lumen endotracheal anesthesia is most often used for bullectomy. Local anesthesia under sedation without tracheal intubation has been growing considerably in thoracic surgery and could bring some advantages in selected patients who are suitable to the technique [27, 28]. Regardless the anesthetic approach, we strongly recommend the use of preemptive local anesthesia through multiple intercostal blocks routinely. Besides that, an efficient postoperative analgesic regimen for these patients is vital to optimize and sustain the lung expansion, so the risk of air leak, atelectasis and respiratory infections can be minimized. Moreover, a multidisciplinary postoperative care is also an essential part of the treatment, including early mobilization measures, an aggressive respiratory physiotherapy and an efficient tracheobronchial toilet, whenever needed.

The Uniportal VATS Approach for Bullectomy

Giant bullectomy has been proved to be feasible by means of uniportal VATS [29]. For unilateral bullectomies, our approach of choice is by uniportal VATS, through a 3–4 cm incision in the fifth or sixth intercostal space, between the anterior and middle axillary line. The patient is positioned in full lateral decubitus, with chest elevation using hard cushions to widen the intercostal spaces. We prefer to use a 5 mm thoracoscope, with 30-degree angulation. The monitor is placed next to the patient's head, so the surgeon stands in front of the patient, whereas the camera assistant stands in the back (Figs. 5 and 6). The monitor in this position allows

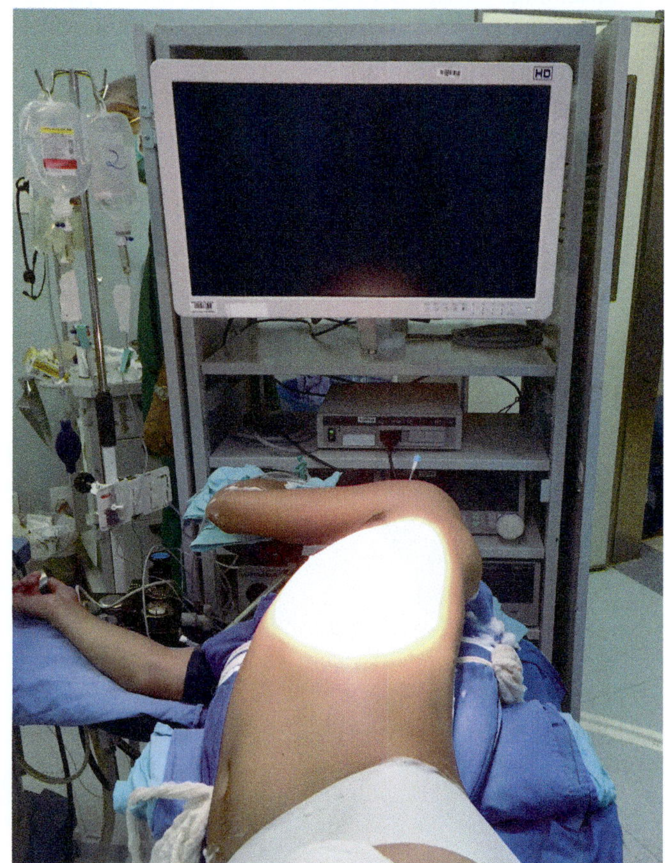

Fig. 5 Patient's position for a left sided uniportal VATS approach. The monitor in this position allows surgeon and camera assistant to work both ergonomically, one at each side of the table

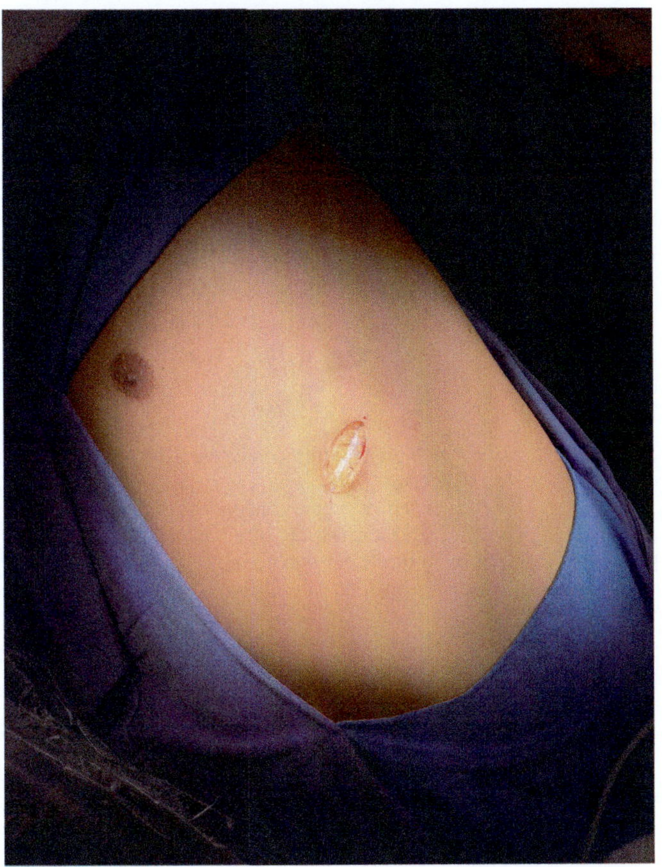

Fig. 6 In this case, the choice was to place the incision at the sixth intercostal space because the bulla was located at the left lower lobe, as shown in Figs. 2, 3, and 4

better ergonomics for the surgical team, but it's important to ensure that the anesthesiologist has full access to the patient's head.

When entering the pleural cavity, care must be taken not to perforate the bulla before checking its real position and its relations with surrounding anatomic structures. Besides that, cautious intraoperative handling of lung tissue is advised to avoid lacerations that could be troublesome, particularly in emphysematous patients. The approach to the bulla itself will depend majorly on its size, location and relation with the underlying lung tissue. Lesions with a narrow neck are easier to resect and they can be simply ligated or stapled at their base. The resection of broad based bullae is technically more demanding and sometimes may lead to more extensive dissection or, in a minority of cases, larger resections. If the lesion is in contact with the interlobar fissure or any other major vascular/bronchial structure (Figs. 2, 3, and 4), the bulla can be isolated through careful dissection (see Video 1).

Following the basic principle of preserving the lung parenchyma as much as possible, anatomic resections such as lobectomies are performed only if absolutely necessary,

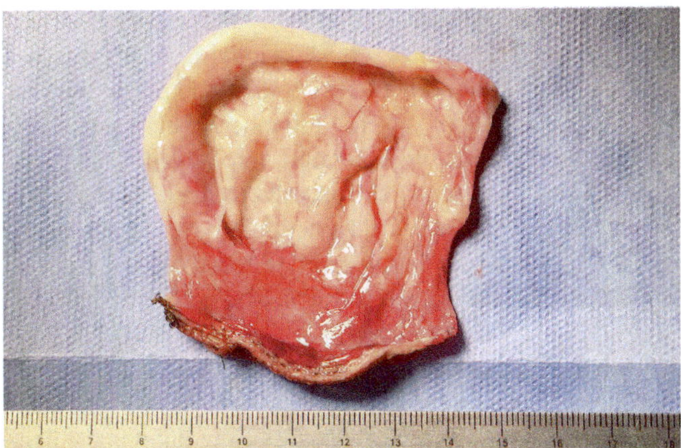

Fig. 7 Surgical specimen removed thoracoscopically: resected bulla with a strip of healthy underlying lung tissue included in the specimen. This figure is about the same case shown in Fig. 1

when the bullectomy alone cannot be accomplished due to anatomic conditions. In our opinion, it is reasonable and preferable to leave a small portion of the bulla capsule unresected, instead of removing a surrounding healthy lobe from a patient in whom the surgery was originally intended to improve lung function.

Irrespective of the bulla's implantation base on the lung, whenever possible it is advisable to include a small strip of normal lung tissue above the stapler (within the surgical specimen), so the staple line lies over a normal tissue (as shown in Fig. 7), in order to lower the risk of air leaks.

If the bulla is too big or too distended to be properly grasped and dissected, it can be punctured and deflated to allow its better handling. Special attention must be paid if the bulla has became liquid-filled due to an infection, situation in which all fluid must be carefully aspirated to prevent contamination of the pleural cavity. Another alternative to shrink large bullae that remain over distended is to use energy devices such as cautery, laser or radiofrequency ablation [30]. Beyond the bulla shrinking itself, this maneuver can enhance the view and allow the identification of the exact limit between the bulla and the underlying lung.

The bulla resection is performed using endoscopic staplers. Once all the needed dissection is accomplished and the bulla is free of adhesions, it is pulled up and away from adjacent structures with graspers while the stapler is inserted and placed according to the identified boundaries between the lesion, the underlying lung and the surrounding structures (see Video 2). Stapler's angulation may be used at the surgeon's own convenience, in order to guarantee the most regular and smooth resection possible, so the lung does not become excessively distorted or twisted.

Following the bullectomy, all the dissection area and staple lines must be checked for bleeding and/or air leaks.

Considering the condition of the underlying lung parenchyma, the local surgical findings, the occasional need for a larger resection and/or a more extensive dissection, the surgeon may decide to adopt several intraoperative strategies to reduce the risk of postoperative prolonged air leaks. According to this rationale, it is valid to mention that reinforced buttressed staples can be helpful in exceedingly fragile lung tissue, which is more prone to prolonged air leak and, when necessary, sealants can also be useful to minimize the risk of this complication.

Additional procedures can also be adopted to ensure complete lung expansion and avoid the persistence of residual spaces. Pleural tent [31, 32], release of the pulmonary ligament, phrenic nerve anesthetic block and postoperative suction on the chest tubes [33] can be beneficial in this setting and should be used judiciously.

If the bulla is associated to pneumothorax as a complication and the surgery is indicated to treat it, depending on the location of the bulla, as well as on the conditions of the underlying parenchyma, the surgical resection of the bulla can be followed by pleural abrasion or pleurectomy, according to the surgeon's judgment and considering the subsequent risk of additional episodes in the future. With the same objective, suction on the chest tubes can also be applied in these cases [33].

Results and Outcomes

Operative mortality after thoracoscopic bullectomy varies in different series from zero to 12% [21]. The most common complication is, by far, prolonged air leak. Both morbidity and mortality tend to be higher in patients with emphysematous underlying lung.

The impact of bullectomy on pulmonary function and on postoperative quality of life can be dramatic early after surgery and the best results are observed in patients with giant bullae compressing normal underlying lungs. This impact is measured through pulmonary function tests (with significant improvement in DLCO, FEV1 and other parameters), symptoms relieve/resolution and better scores in questionnaires dedicated to assess postoperative quality of life.

Even if no evidences of bullae recurrence is noticed, many patients may present a slow, but progressive worsening in lung function and dyspnea years after surgery. Particularly those patients with COPD/emphysematous lungs may return to preoperative levels of lung function and dyspnea in about 4–5 years after surgery [16]. Due to this possible functional worsening and also because the increased risk of lung cancer adjoining a pulmonary bulla is considerably higher [23], these patients must be kept in a strict long-term follow-up strategy.

Summary and Conclusion

When the bullectomy is indicated to ameliorate dyspnea and lung function, the proper selection of patients is even more crucial than when the surgical indication is based on the occurrence of complications related to the bullae. Within the context of minimally invasive surgery and all its benefits, uniportal VATS is a feasible, safe and reproducible method to carry out giant bullectomies, with results (at least) comparable to open surgery (if not better), leading to symptoms resolution, improved lung function and better quality of life.

Acknowledgments *Conflict of Interest Statement*: The author has no conflicts of interest to declare.

Consent: This chapter shows pictures and videos of two cases operated by our group. Written informed consent was obtained from both patients for publication of the selected material.

References

1. Knudson RJ, Gaensler EA. Surgery for emphysema. Ann Thorac Surg. 1965;1(3):332–62.
2. Meyers BF, Patterson GA. Chronic obstructive pulmonary disease. 10: Bullectomy, lung volume reduction surgery, and transplantation for patients with chronic obstructive pulmonary disease. Thorax. 2003;58(7):634–8.
3. Deslauriers J. History of surgery for emphysema. Semin Thorac Cardiovasc Surg. 1996;8(1):43–51.
4. Cooper JD. The history of surgical procedures for emphysema. Ann Thorac Surg. 1997;63(2):312–9.
5. Klingman RR, Angelillo VA, DeMeester TR. Cystic and bullous lung disease. Ann Thorac Surg. 1991;53(3):576–80.
6. Morgan MD, Edwards CW, Morris J, et al. Origin and behaviour of emphysematous bullae. Thorax. 1989;44(7):533–8.
7. Ting KY, Klopstock R, Lyons HA. Mechanical properties of pulmonary cysts and bullae. Am Rev Respir Dis. 1963;87:538–44.
8. Krishnamohan P, Shen R, Wigle DA, et al. Bullectomy for symptomatic or complicated giant lung bullae. Ann Thorac Surg. 2014;97:425–31.
9. Lee KH, Cho SJ, Ryu SM, et al. Fluid-filled giant bulla treated with percutaneous drainage and talc sclerotherapy: a modified Brompton technique. Korean J Thorac Cardiovasc Surg. 2012;45:134–7.
10. Taniguchi Y, Fujioka S, Adachi Y, et al. Video-assisted thoracoscopic bullectomy for an infectious giant bulla with the concomitant use of the perioperative intracavity fluid suction. J Thorac Cardiovasc Surg. 2009;137:249–51.
11. Potapenkov MA, Shipulin PP. Surgical treatment of complicated bullous pulmonary emphysema. Grud Serdechnososudistaia Khir. 1993;4:39–42.
12. Hirai S, Hamanaka Y, Mitsui N, et al. Primary lung cancer arising from the wall of a giant bulla. Ann Thorac Cardiovasc Surg. 2005;11:109–13.
13. Venuta F, Rendina EA, Pescarmona EO, et al. Occult lung cancer in patients with bullous emphysema. Thorax. 1997;52:289–90.
14. Shanthaveerappa HN, Mathai MG, Byrd RP Jr, et al. Spontaneous resolution of a giant pulmonary bulla. J Ky Med Assoc. 2001;99:533–6.

15. Scarlata S, Cesari M, Caridi I, et al. Spontaneous resolution of a giant pulmonary bulla in an older woman: role of functional assessment. Respiration. 2011;81:59–62.
16. Palla A, Desideri MT, Rossi G, et al. Elective surgery for giant bullous emphysema – a 5-year clinical and functional follow-up. Chest. 2005;128:2043–50.
17. Pearson MG, Ogilvie C. Surgical treatment of emphysematous bullae: late outcome. Thorax. 1983;38:134–7.
18. Greenberg JA, Singhal S, Kaiser LR. Giant bullous lung disease: evaluation, selection, techniques, and outcomes. Chest Surg Clin N Am. 2003;13:631–49.
19. De Giacomo T, Venuta F, Rendina EA, et al. Video-assisted thoracoscopic treatment of giant bullae associated with emphysema. Eur J Thorac Surg. 1999;12:753–7.
20. Kayawake H, Chen F, Date H. Surgical resection of a giant emphysematous bulla occupying the entire hemithorax. Eur J Cardiothorac Surg. 2013;43:e136–8.
21. Schipper PH, Meyers BF. Surgery for bullous disease. In: Person FG, Patterson GA, Cooper JD, editors. Thoracic & esophageal surgery. Philadelphia: Churchill Livingstone Elsevier; 2008. p. 631–52.
22. Ng CSH, Yim AP. Video-assisted thoracoscopic surgery (VATS) bullectomy for emphysematous bullous lung disease. Multimed Man Cardiothorac Surg. 2005;2005(425):mmcts.2004.000265. https://doi.org/10.1510/mmcts.2004.000265.
23. Van Bael K, La Meir M, Vanoverbeke H. Video-assisted thoracoscopic resection of a giant bulla in vanishing lung syndrome: a case report and short literature review. J Cardiothorac Surg. 2014;9:4.
24. Monaldi V. Endocavitary aspiration: its practical applications. Tubercle. 1947;28:223–8.
25. Shah SS, Goldstraw P. Surgical treatment of bullous emphysema: experience with the Brompton technique. Ann Thorac Surg. 1994;58:1452–6.
26. Santini M, Fiorelli A, Vicidomini G, et al. Endobronchial treatment of giant emphysematous bullae with one-way valves: a new approach for surgically unfit patients. Eur J Cardiothorac Surg. 2011;40:1425–31.
27. Gonzalez-Rivas D, Bonome C, Fiera E, et al. Non-intubated video-assisted thoracic surgery: the future of thoracic surgery? Eur J Cardiothorac Surg. 2016;50:925–6.
28. Ng CSH, Ho JYK, Zhao Z-R. Spontaneous ventilation anaesthesia: the perfect match for thoracoscopic bullectomy? Eur J Cardiothorac Surg. 2016;50:933.
29. Mazzella A, Izzo A, Amore D, et al. Ann Ital Chir. 2016;87(ePub pii):S2239253X16024816.
30. Sagawa M, Maeda T, Yoshimitsu Y, et al. Saline-cooled radiofrequency coagulation during thoracoscopic surgery for giant bulla. Eur J Cardiothorac Surg. 2014;46:737–9.
31. Venuta F, De Giacomo T, Rendina EA, et al. Thoracoscopic pleural tent. Ann Thorac Surg. 1998;66:1833–4.
32. Kawachi R, Matsuwaki R, Tachibana K, et al. Thoracoscopic modified pleural tent for spontaneous pneumothorax. Interact Cardiovasc Thorac Surg. 2016;23:190–5.
33. Pompili C, Xiumè F, Hristova R, et al. Regulated drainage reduces the incidence of recurrence after uniportal video-assisted thoracoscopic bullectomy for primary spontaneous pneumothorax: a propensity case-matched comparison of regulated and unregulated drainage. Eur J Cardiothorac Surg. 2016;49:1127–31.

Hookwire Localization of Pulmonary Nodules in Uniportal VATS

Ze-Rui Zhao and Calvin S. H. Ng

Abstract

In the era of uniportal thoracoscopic surgery, deep pulmonary nodules can be hard to visualize or palpate, creating an increasing demand for adjuvant modalities to localize the lesion preoperatively. Computed tomography-guided hookwire implantation has been widely adopted by thoracic surgeons due to its feasibility and high success rate. However, procedure-associated complications such as pneumothorax and wire dislodgement can cause patient discomfort or even localization failure, occasionally rendering a thoracotomy inevitable. Several measures have been proposed for optimizing the hookwire technique, including replacing the tip of the hook with a spiral helix, using a soft filament suture as a substitute for the rigid metallic tail of the wire, and use of a hookwire in combination with other localization methods such as the injection of a radionuclide marker. Centralization of the hookwire placement and simultaneous resection performed inside the hybrid theater may resolve the wire-associated complications and provide a promising, cost-effective solution in the future.

Introduction

The advent of video-assisted thoracoscopic surgery (VATS) is associated with faster postoperative recovery and lower morbidity compared with standard thoracotomy procedures. Uniportal VATS has gained in popularity in recent years by reducing the number of access ports to only one incision, conferring potential merits such as reduced postoperative pain and aesthetic superiority compared to conventional approaches [1–3]. However, the disadvantage of uniportal VATS lies in the difficulty in localizing deep sub-pleural nodules, which are frequently neither visible nor palpable due to their part-solid density or the limitation associated with the small incision. Hookwire placement is currently one of the most commonly-used preoperative localization methods for pulmonary nodules, allowing surgeons to identify the target nodules during minimally-invasive treatment. In this article, we discuss the technique, indication, efficacy, complications, and technical limitations of this localization procedure and highlight several methods for further improving the technique to provide a higher success rate.

Technique

Hookwire insertion is normally accomplished in a radiology suite under the guidance of computed tomography (CT) on the same day as, and prior to, the operation. A classical hookwire system comprises a 21-gauge, 10-cm-long cannula and a 20-cm-long calibrated monofilament wire with a 1-cm thorn that is preloaded inside the tip of the cannula (Somatex Medical technologies GmbH, Germany). The direction of hookwire insertion is usually requested to be via an anterior approach or lateral approach rather than posterior approach wherever possible, to minimize interference by the wire, to provide best surgical approach for the surgeon to the lesion, and to allow often the shortest route for wire access [4] (Fig. 1). However, occasionally the posterior approach is the only route for the wire (Fig. 2). The needle puncture site is selected after the CT scan, and the distance between the puncture site and the center of the nodule is also measured. After sterilization of the puncture site and administration of a local anesthetic, the tip of the cannula that houses the hookwire is advanced gradually through the chest wall and the

Electronic Supplementary Material The online version of this chapter (https://doi.org/10.1007/978-981-13-2604-2_14) contains supplementary material, which is available to authorized users.

Z.-R. Zhao · C. S. H. Ng (✉)
Division of Cardiothoracic Surgery, Department of Surgery, Prince of Wales Hospital, The Chinese University of Hong Kong, Hong Kong SAR, China
e-mail: calvinng@surgery.cuhk.edu.hk

D. Gonzalez-Rivas et al. (eds.), *Atlas of Uniportal Video Assisted Thoracic Surgery*,
https://doi.org/10.1007/978-981-13-2604-2_14

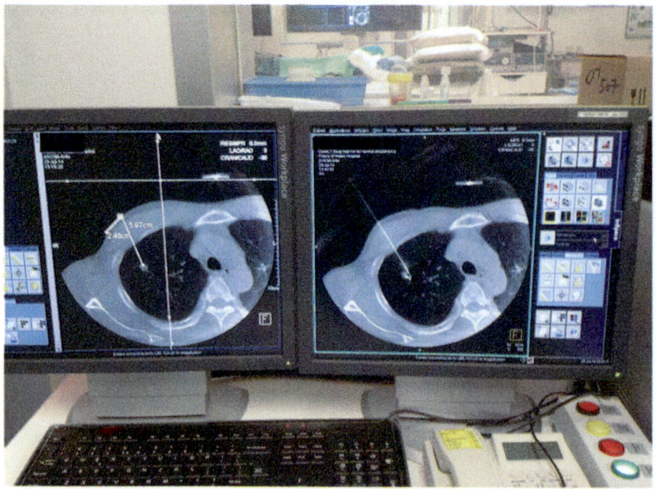

Fig. 1 Hookwire inserted into a deep lesion within the right upper lobe from antero-lateral direction following measurement of the approach vector and distance on the CT scan image

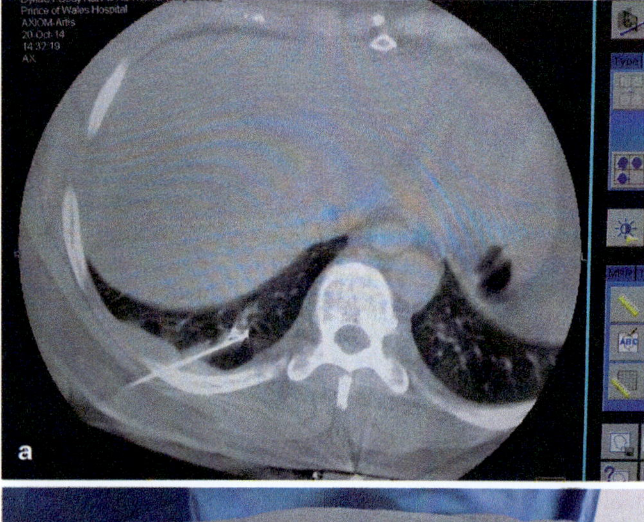

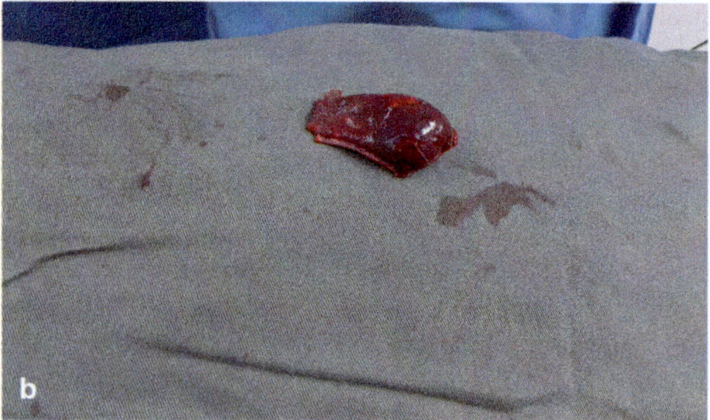

Fig. 2 (**a**) Hookwire insertion from posterior approach with post procedure CT scan. (**b**) Lesion wedged out by uniportal VATS approach using combination of curved (EndoGIA Radial Reload Tristaple™, Covidien Medtronic, USA) and straight staples

pulmonary parenchyma under sequential CT guidance. To avoid compromising its integrity, it is suggested that the tip is inserted into the lesion to a depth of 2 cm [5]; however, this remains controversial since other previous studies recommended placing the wire directly into the nodule to provide a stable anchor [6]. After the tip is placed in a proper position, the outer cannula needle can be withdrawn carefully and the horn of the hookwire is released and anchored to the parenchyma surrounding the nodule. Blood pressure, respiration rate, and the arterial oxygen saturation of the patient should be monitored during the procedure. The wire extending outside the chest wall is positioned carefully on the skin and covered by sterile dressings. The patient is then transferred to the ward to await surgery or directly to the operating room (OR) after localization.

Double-lumen endobronchial intubation is used with general anesthesia in the OR. A 2–3 cm incision is made in the fourth intercostal space to the anterior axillary line, with the patient lying in a lateral decubitus position. An Alexis type wound retractor may be used, and for very small incisions, the retractor may experience difficulty in retrieval at the end of the procedure. A thick suture such as O-Silk tie placed around the inner ring of the retractor would greatly facilitate its removal (Video 1). The location of the hookwire is then inspected through the thoracoscope. Gentle manipulation of the tail of the hookwire outside the chest cavity allows traction of the target pulmonary nodule in a certain direction that facilitates the wedge resection via an endostapler; hence, surgeons may not require concurrent use of other retraction forceps, which would occupy the space of the sole incision [4]. The specimen is then placed in a specimen bag and sent for frozen section diagnosis (Video 2). Whenever necessary, Uniportal VATS lobectomy and lymphadenectomy can be performed by enlarging the incision to 3–5 cm [7]. An air leak test under water is performed at the end of surgery and a 24 F chest tube is inserted towards the apex and placed in the posterior aspect of the incision.

Indication and Efficiency of Hookwire Localization

Although it is up to the surgeon's own judgment to evaluate whether a localization technique is required, Suzuki et al. [8] noted that an indeterminate nodule ≤10 mm in size should be considered for adjuvant marking when the distance between it and the pleura is ≥5 mm. For ground-glass opacity (GGO) lesions of part-solid density without pleural involvement, the indication for a localization procedure may be extended even if they are sizeable. The hookwire technique was reported to successfully localize 25 lesions (mean size: 7 mm; range: 4–15 mm) with a mean distance to the pleura of 13 mm (range: 2–31 mm) [9]. In general, the hookwire technique alone was reported to yield localization rates of around 94% in retrospective cohorts [10]. A greater distance to the pleural surface, however, may hamper the success rate of a wire localization. Ciriaco et al. [11] reported two sub-centimeter pulmonary lesions located ≥15 mm beneath the surface that required a thoracotomy after hookwire implantation because of the difficulty in localization. Chen et al. [12] outlined their experience of hookwire placement in five pulmonary lesions of patients that were previously treated by radiotherapy due to breast malignancies, highlighting that the hookwire allows the surgeon to choose an appropriate site for chest wall incision and confidently localize the nodule.

To date, only one randomized controlled trial [6] has compared hookwire versus radio-guided localization, in 50 6–19 mm lesions (mean size: 11 mm); a statistically equivalent performance was demonstrated for both groups. Patients in the radio-guided group (n = 25) received an injection of a radionuclide (technetium-99) under CT guidance, and their lesions were subsequently detected intraoperatively by the gamma probe. The distance from the nodule to the pleural surface was 25 mm in both groups. The hookwire was able to identify 21 out of the 25 lesions (84%) while 24 of the 25 nodules (96%) were successfully localized in the radio-guided group. Of note, both modalities showed superiority to manual palpation, which could only localize 13 lesions out of the entire population. The author claimed that the hookwire technique was efficacious and its complications were mostly due to external technical factors [6].

Complications

As a percutaneous puncture procedure to the visceral pleura, certain complications such as pleuritic pain, pneumothorax, and hemothorax are inevitably encountered with this technique. Of these complications, the most common is pneumothorax, with a rate of 32.1% (54/168) reported by Dendo et al. [5]. Although most patients experience asymptomatic pneumothorax, around 2–4% require chest drainage before surgery [10, 11, 13], and the incidence may increase in emphysema patients. Additionally, the excessively expanding pneumothorax may conversely 'pull out' the barb of the hookwire from the lung. Massive air embolism is a rare complication, observed previously at a rate of 0.6% (1/161) [14]. Furthermore, it has been suggested that this risk can be mitigated by shortening the duration of prolonged lung inflation via a short insertion trajectory for the hookwire system [15].

Hookwire detachment from the mounting site of the pleura results in an unsuccessful localization and may cause VATS to be converted to a thoracotomy. A recent review showed that approximately 2–10% of patients may experience hookwire dislodgement [10]. Mullan and colleagues [16] previously showed that this can occur at three points: first, when the rigid wire tail on the outside moves relative to the chest wall during transportation to the OR; second, when the lung deflates during one-lung-ventilation, mimicking an extensive preoperative pneumothorax; and third, when the surgeon retracts the wire to facilitate resection during the operation. Wire dislodgement occurred in 6 out of 52 (12%) cases without pneumothorax and in 16 out of 48 (33%) cases when a pneumothorax was identified [17]. Although wire dislodgement appeared to be more frequent when the wire was located adjacent to (11/36, 31%) rather than directly inside (11/64, 17%) the nodule [17], the question of whether such intralesion placement would jeopardize the pathological examination remains controversial. a higher incidence of dislodgements was also noted (7/34, 19.6%) when wires were deployed in superficial areas (5.6 ± 5.8 mm; range: 0–18.7 mm) [18].

Technical Limitations

There are some inherently specific anatomic locations that may prohibit the use of hookwire insertion; for example, the lesion may not be easily accessible percutaneously in areas surrounding the apical, diaphragmatic, or mediastinal regions of the lung, because it is either shielded or too dangerous to approach due to its proximity to the great vessels. Besides this, deep lesions (>40 mm beneath the pleural surface) may be a relative contraindication as the potential complications can be devastating [12]. A lesion located at a depth >20 mm to the surface renders it difficult to form an adequate resection margin and these factor should be taken into account when planning hookwire localization [18].

Ways to Improve the Technique

Trajectory Guidance System for Centesis

Usually, radiologists decide the needle puncture site, and the route and direction of needle advancement, based on their own experience. An automatically generated puncturing trajectory provided by the syngo iGuide needle guidance software (Siemens Healthcare AG, Forchheim, Germany), accompanied by a laser cross indicator [19], is believed to have an advantage in aiding the puncturing process under expeditious and accurate guidance without damaging vital structures.

Decreasing the Rate of Dislodgement

Although patients are usually told to breathe and remain as stable as they can after the insertion of a hookwire, friction between the wire and the chest wall cannot be avoided. By cutting the free rigid end of the wire to approximately 2–3 cm, Chen et al. [12] claimed that such a measure may, to some extent, prevent the occurrence of dislodgement. Another method would be to replace the metallic tail of the wire with a soft nylon filament [5], thus reducing the tendency for pulling or pushing of the wire embedded in the parenchyma during transportation. The flexible external-thoracic portion would also allow patients to move freely around the bed and might relieve discomfort. With these modifications, comprising a short hookwire and a suture system, simultaneous double- and triple-wire implantation can be performed successfully [5].

Changing the terminal tip of the wire into a spiral helix could theoretically lead to more stable fixation of the nodule [20]. By rotating the wire counterclockwise, radiologists can pull back the wire if it is placed too deeply into the parenchyma, a process that is easier than with the traditional hookwire. Through this innovation, Eichfeld and colleagues [21] reported their initial experience of successful placement of the spiral wire in 21 out of 22 cases. However, a comparative study between these two types of wires is still warranted.

Dual Localization

Given that relatively superficial lesions may cause a higher incidence of dislodgement, Doo et al. [18] recommended the combined use of a hookwire with a radionuclide for small nodules located at a distance to the pleural surface <20 mm. The radionuclide may serve as an indicator for a clear resection margin and thereby help to identify the lesion in the case of wire dislodgement. Although the time taken to perform the dual localization procedure was reported to be somewhat similar to that of the hookwire alone, the cost-effectiveness of such a dual technique remains questionable.

Simultaneous Localization and Resection

Performing centralization of the wire placement and the VATS procedure inside a single suite has advantages, in terms of saving time as well as providing a reduction in the rate of pneumothorax, wire dislodgement, and patient discomfort. The initial attempt was published by Nakano et al. [22], who reported the use of linear ultrasound-guided hookwire placement in eight out of nine nodules with an average depth below the skin surface of 20 mm, followed by an immediate resection in the same OR. Although this innovation introduces the concept of simultaneous management, it may only be suitable for superficial lesions that are close to the chest wall. Moreover, it could be difficult to localize a GGO lesion under ultrasonography given its air-containing nature.

Owing to the development of intraoperative cone-beam CT (CBCT), hybrid ORs that incorporate CBCT provide unparalleled real-time imaging for guiding the insertion of a hookwire (see Chapter "Future Development and Technologies") [1–3, 23]. In this situation, patients do not have to be transported between the radiology suite and operating theater, thus minimizing discomfort due to pleuritic pain or pneumothorax. More importantly, the rate of wire dislodgement can be reduced. Although the risk of wire detachment during the establishment of one-lung ventilation may still exist, CBCT could re-localize the lesion in the hybrid unit, hence guaranteeing the successful deployment of the hookwire in uniportal VATS [24].

Initial Results of Hookwire Placement in a Hybrid OR

In our initial experience, 32 pulmonary nodules with a mean size of 9.1 ± 4.6 mm were successfully underwent real-time image-guided hookwire placement with subsequent lung resection in the hybrid OR from February 2014 to September 2017. Fifteen (47%) patients were detected to have pneumothorax immediately after hookwire insertion. However, none of them required intervention. The average interval between the end of hookwire insertion and the start of VATS procedure was 41.1 ± 15.0 min. No wire-dislodgement was found in this cohort and the postoperative length of hospital stay was 3.5 ± 2.0 days. These results indicated that real-time image-guided hookwire localization in the hybrid OR setting is safe and effective for surgical resection for small pulmonary nodules [25].

Conclusions

Hookwire placement is efficacious, and is among the most important adjuvant localization techniques for the accurate diagnosis and resection of small pulmonary nodules under Uniportal VATS. The most common complication associated with this technique is pneumothorax, and patients may occasionally require chest drainage. Dislodgement that leads to failure of localization remains the major complication that surgeons try to avoid. Complications can be partially avoided by simultaneously performing the wire insertion and uniportal VATS inside a hybrid OR. The emerging hookwire approach, under a hybrid setting, works perfectly for small peripheral lesions, even for those with a large GGO portion; thus, its potential advantages over the traditional approach warrant further study.

References

1. Ng CS, Lau KK, Gonzalez-Rivas D, Rocco G. Evolution in surgical approach and techniques for lung cancer. Thorax. 2013; 68:681.
2. Ng CS, Rocco G, Wong RH, Lau RW, Yu SC, Yim AP. Uniportal and single-incision video-assisted thoracic surgery: the state of the art. Interact Cardiovasc Thorac Surg. 2014;19:661–6.
3. Zhao ZR, Li Z, Situ DR, Ng CS. Recent clinical innovations in thoracic surgery in Hong Kong. J Thorac Dis. 2016;8(Suppl 8):S618–26. https://doi.org/10.21037/jtd.2016.03.93.
4. Ng CS, Hui JW, Wong RH. Minimizing single-port access in video-assisted wedge resection, with a hookwire. Asian Cardiovasc Thorac Ann. 2013;21:114–5.
5. Dendo S, Kanazawa S, Ando A, Hyodo T, Kouno Y, Yasui K, et al. Preoperative localization of small pulmonary lesions with a short hook wire and suture system: experience with 168 procedures. Radiology. 2002;225:511–8.
6. Gonfiotti A, Davini F, Vaggelli L, De Francisci A, Caldarella A, Gigli PM, et al. Thoracoscopic localization techniques for patients with solitary pulmonary nodule: hookwire versus radio-guided surgery. Eur J Cardiothorac Surg. 2007;32:843–7.
7. Ng CS, Kim HK, Wong RH, Yim AP, Mok TS, Choi YH. Single-port video-assisted thoracoscopic major lung resections: experience with 150 consecutive cases. Thorac Cardiovasc Surg. 2016;64:348–53.
8. Suzuki K, Nagai K, Yoshida J, Ohmatsu H, Takahashi K, Nishimura M, et al. Video-assisted thoracoscopic surgery for small indeterminate pulmonary nodules: indications for preoperative marking. Chest. 1999;115:563–8.
9. Hanninen EL, Langrehr J, Raakow R, Rottgen R, Schmidt S, Pech M, et al. Computed tomography-guided pulmonary nodule localization before thoracoscopic resection. Acta Radiol. 2004;45:284–8.
10. Kidane B, Yasufuku K. Advances in image-guided thoracic surgery. Thorac Surg Clin. 2016;26:129–38.
11. Ciriaco P, Negri G, Puglisi A, Nicoletti R, Del Maschio A, Zannini P. Video-assisted thoracoscopic surgery for pulmonary nodules: rationale for preoperative computed tomography-guided hookwire localization. Eur J Cardiothorac Surg. 2004;25:429–33.
12. Chen S, Zhou J, Zhang J, Hu H, Luo X, Zhang Y, et al. Video-assisted thoracoscopic solitary pulmonary nodule resection after CT-guided hookwire localization: 43 cases report and literature review. Surg Endosc. 2011;25:1723–9.
13. Miyoshi K, Toyooka S, Gobara H, Oto T, Mimura H, Sano Y, et al. Clinical outcomes of short hook wire and suture marking system in thoracoscopic resection for pulmonary nodules. Eur J Cardiothorac Surg. 2009;36:378–82.
14. Suzuki K, Shimohira M, Hashizume T, Ozawa Y, Sobue R, Mimura M, et al. Usefulness of CT-guided hookwire marking before video-assisted thoracoscopic surgery for small pulmonary lesions. J Med Imaging Radiat Oncol. 2014;58:657–62.
15. Horan TA, Pinheiro PM, Araujo LM, Santiago FF, Rodrigues MR. Massive gas embolism during pulmonary nodule hook wire localization. Ann Thorac Surg. 2002;73:1647–9.
16. Mullan BF, Stanford W, Barnhart W, Galvin JR. Lung nodules: improved wire for CT-guided localization. Radiology. 1999;211:561–5.
17. Thaete FL, Peterson MS, Plunkett MB, Ferson PF, Keenan RJ, Landreneau RJ. Computed tomography-guided wire localization of pulmonary lesions before thoracoscopic resection: results in 101 cases. J Thorac Imaging. 1999;14:90–8.
18. Doo KW, Yong HS, Kim HK, Kim S, Kang EY, Choi YH. Needlescopic resection of small and superficial pulmonary nodule after computed tomographic fluoroscopy-guided dual localization with radiotracer and hookwire. Ann Surg Oncol. 2015;22:331–7.
19. Freundt MI, Ritter M, Al-Zghloul M, Groden C, Kerl HU. Laser-guided cervical selective nerve root block with the Dyna-CT: initial experience of three-dimensional puncture planning with an ex-vivo model. PLoS One. 2013;8:e69311.
20. Torre M, Ferraroli GM, Vanzulli A, Fieschi S. A new safe and stable spiral wire needle for thoracoscopic resection of lung nodules. Chest. 2004;125:2289–93.
21. Eichfeld U, Dietrich A, Ott R, Kloeppel R. Video-assisted thoracoscopic surgery for pulmonary nodules after computed tomography-guided marking with a spiral wire. Ann Thorac Surg. 2005;79:313–7.
22. Nakano N, Miyauchi K, Imagawa H, Kawachi K. Immediate localization using ultrasound-guided hookwire marking of peripheral lung tumors in the operating room. Interact Cardiovasc Thorac Surg. 2004;3:104–6.
23. Zhao ZR, Lau RW, Ng CS. Hybrid theatre and alternative localization techniques in conventional and single-port video-assisted thoracoscopic surgery. J Thorac Dis. 2016;8:S319–27.
24. Ng CS, Man Chu C, Kwok MW, Yim AP, Wong RH. Hybrid DynaCT scan-guided localization single-port lobectomy. [corrected]. Chest. 2015;147:e76–8.
25. Yu PSY, Man Chu C, Lau RWH, Wan IYP, Underwood MJ, Yu SCH, et al. Video-assisted thoracic surgery for tiny pulmonary nodules with real-time image guidance in the hybrid theatre: the initial experience. J Thorac Dis. 2018;10:2933–9.

Intraoperative Ultrasound Guidance in Pulmonary Nodule Localization in Uniportal VATS

Gaetano Rocco, Raffaele Rocco, and Marco Scarci

Intraoperative identification of pulmonary nodules has become a challenging endeavor with the increasing refinement of minimally invasive approaches to lung cancer surgery. The identification of the nodule via a thorough palpation of the lung, once possible through open incisions, has been replaced by a combination of imaging and localization techniques which are tailored to the nature of the lesions (i.e., GGO's), let alone their site in the parenchyma [1].

Two main reasons justify the need for intraoperative identification of a lung nodule, namely, providing its cyto-histological assessment and defining the extent of the resection, both crucial factors to surgical planning. The knowledge of the neoplastic nature of the lesion has become of paramount prognostic significance since the introduction of the new adenocarcinoma classification in 2011 [2] and may indeed dictate the type of resection and the concomitant nodal dissection to be carried out [3]. In the near future, the histological ascertainment of a pulmonary nodule will be defined by genome sequencing on liquid biopsy which today has proved its efficacy especially in advanced lung cancer characterized by a significant tumor burden [4]. Currently, hybrid OR suites and electromagnetic navigation marking represent the most recent innovative methods aimed at identifying an intrapulmonary lesion [5]. Time-honored techniques include hook-wire, dye, or radiolabeling localization have proved helpful in experienced hands but have not gained the absolute favor of the thoracic surgical community [1]. The intraoperative use of ultrasound probes to scan the lung parenchyma has been proposed about 15 years ago and only more recently an attempt at codifying this technique has been proposed [6–9]. In 2011, Rocco and coworkers described the resort to ultrasound probing as a routine method of nodule identification during uniportal VATS [10].

Electronic Supplementary Material The online version of this chapter (https://doi.org/10.1007/978-981-13-2604-2_15) contains supplementary material, which is available to authorized users.

G. Rocco (✉)
Service of Thoracic Surgery, Department of Surgery, Memorial Sloan Kettering Cancer Center, New York, NY, USA
e-mail: roccog@mskcc.org

R. Rocco
Division of Thoracic Surgery Mayo Clinic, Rochester, Minnesota, USA

M. Scarci
Thoracic Surgery Unit, S. Gerardo Hospital, Monza, Italy
e-mail: m.scarci@asst-monza.it

Technique (Videos)

In our practice, uniportal VATS is especially used to confirm the suspicion of either primary or secondary lung cancer [10]. Once the single port incision measuring up to 2.5 cm is placed, a thorough thoracoscopic exploration of the chest cavity is performed and the atelectatic status of the lung is assessed. It is of paramount importance to divide the pleuro-pulmonary adhesions that may hinder the compete mobilization of the parenchyma for ultrasound probing (Video 1). The best results for ultrasound localization are obtained with nodules found in the outer third of the lung. Nevertheless, the complete atelectasis of the lung is preferable but not always necessary to identify solid nodules, especially if these are very peripheral in the parenchyma; however, it might be crucial to localize GGO's, as reported by Kondo and colleagues [8]. Careful examination of preoperative imaging is important to guide the ultrasound probe on the nodule-harboring parenchymal area [11]. Once this target area is identified, a laparoscopic 10-mm ultrasound probe (B-K Medical, Herlev, Denmark) [10] is introduced through the single incision along parallel to a 5-mm, 0 or 30 degree videothoracoscope along with an articulating grasper. This laparoscopic ultrasound probing device is characterized by a frequency range of 5–10 MHz, a focal range of 5–95 mm, a 36-degree sector angle, and a contact surface of 30 × 5 mm [10]. The main

D. Gonzalez-Rivas et al. (eds.), *Atlas of Uniportal Video Assisted Thoracic Surgery*,
https://doi.org/10.1007/978-981-13-2604-2_15

feature of this instrument is the articulating head which can be bent at different angles to serve as a finger-like projection adapting to the geometric features of the lung surface, thus mimicking palpation [10]. In fact, the pressure that the articulating head can exert on the lung further facilitates local lung deflation thereby shortening the distance between the nodule and the lung surface (Video 2). The instrument can provide further clues as to the nature of the investigated lesion with the addition of the Doppler mode which demonstrates differences in its vascularization [10]. The area to be inspected is profusely covered with conductive gel which is spread with the light apposition of the ultrasound probe. Once the lesion is identified as an hypoechogenic mass surrounded by highly reflective aerated lung, the distance between its edge and the lung surface can be easily measured on the device (Video 3). This is an important information to help the surgeon placing the endostapler at the base of the cone generated by the suspension of the target area by the articulating endograsper. Depending on the texture of the parenchyma, a blue or green reload is used of a sufficient length to encompass all or most of the wedge resection line. The specimen is retrieved through an endobag and inspected for the presence of the nodule along with its margins (Video 4). Frozen section is usually obtained and the subsequent surgical plan carried out as necessary. A chest drain is placed in the apex through the same incision and connected to water-seal drainage. The entire procedure can be performed with the patient under general anesthesia or in the awake, nonintubated patient depending on the patient's characteristics [12]. The chest drain can be removed on extubation or on the ward provided that no air leakage is detected.

Conflict of Interest The authors disclose no conflict of interest relevant to this work.

References

1. Lin MW, Chen JS. Image-guided techniques for localizing pulmonary nodules in thoracoscopic surgery. J Thorac Dis. 2016;8S:S749–55.
2. Travis WD, Brambilla E, Noguchi M, Nicholson AG, Geisinger KR, Yatabe Y, Beer DG, Powell CA, Riely GJ, Van Schil PE, Garg K, Austin JH, Asamura H, Rusch VW, Hirsch FR, Scagliotti G, Mitsudomi T, Huber RM, Ishikawa Y, Jett J, Sanchez-Cespedes M, Sculier JP, Takahashi T, Tsuboi M, Vansteenkiste J, Wistuba I, Yang PC, Aberle D, Brambilla C, Flieder D, Franklin W, Gazdar A, Gould M, Hasleton P, Henderson D, Johnson B, Johnson D, Kerr K, Kuriyama K, Lee JS, Miller VA, Petersen I, Roggli V, Rosell R, Saijo N, Thunnissen E, Tsao M, Yankelewitz D. International association for the study of lung cancer/American thoracic society/European respiratory society international multidisciplinary classification of lung adenocarcinoma. J Thorac Oncol. 2011;6:244–85.
3. Rocco R, Jones DR, Morabito A, Franco R, La Mantia E, Rocco G. Validation of the new IASLC/ATS/ERS lung adenocarcinoma classification: a surgeon's perspective. J Thorac Dis. 2014;5S:S547–51.
4. Falk AT, Heeke S, Hofman V, Lespinet V, Ribeyre C, Bordone O, Poudenx M, Otto J, Garnier G, Castelnau O, Guigay J, Leroy S, Marquette CH, Hofman P, Ilié M. NGS analysis on tumor tissue and cfDNA for genotype-directed therapy in metastatic NSCLC patients. Between hope and hype? Expert Rev Anticancer Ther. 2017;22:1–5. https://doi.org/10.1080/14737140.2017.1331736.
5. Zhao ZR, Lau RWH, Ng CSH. Hybrid theatre and alternative localization techniques in conventional and single-port video-assisted thoracoscopic surgery. J Thorac Dis. 2016;3S:S319–27.
6. Piolanti M, Coppola F, Papa S, Pilotti V, Mattioli S, Gavelli G. Ultrasonographic localization of occult pulmonary nodules during video-assisted thoracic surgery. Eur Radiol. 2003;13:2358–64.
7. Matsumoto S, Hirata T, Ogawa E, Fukuse T, Ueda H, Koyama T, Nakamura T, Wada H. Ultrasonographic evaluation of small nodules in the peripheral lung during video-assisted thoracic surgery (VATS). Eur J Cardiothorac Surg. 2004;26:469–73.
8. Kondo R, Yoshida K, Hamanaka K, et al. Intraoperative ultrasonographic localization of pulmonary ground-glass opacities. J Thorac Cardiovasc Surg. 2009;138:837–42.
9. Khereba M, Ferraro P, Duranceau A, Martin J, Goudie E, Thiffault V, Liberman M. Thoracoscopic localization of intraparenchymal pulmonary nodules using direct intracavitary thoracoscopic ultrasonography prevents conversion of VATS procedures to thoracotomy in selected patients. J Thorac Cardiovasc Surg. 2012;144:1160–5.
10. Rocco G, Cicalese M, La Manna C, La Rocca A, Martucci N, Salvi R. Ultrasonographic identification of peripheral pulmonary nodules through uniportal video-assisted thoracic surgery. Ann Thorac Surg. 2011;92:1099–101.
11. Nakamoto K, Omori K, Nezu K. Lung Cancer Project Group of West-Seto Inland Sea, Japan. Superselective segmentectomy for deep and small pulmonary nodules under the guidance of three-dimensional reconstructed computed tomographic angiography. Ann Thorac Surg. 2010;89:877–83.
12. Rocco G, Romano V, Accardo R, Tempesta A, La Manna C, La Rocca A, Martucci N, D'Aiuto M, Polimeno E. Awake single-access (uniportal) video-assisted thoracoscopic surgery for peripheral pulmonary nodules in a complete ambulatory setting. Ann Thorac Surg. 2010;89:1625–7.

Videoendoscopic Uniportal Resection of Solitary Peripheral Lung Nodule

Marco Scarci, Fabrizio Minervini, and Gaetano Rocco

Introduction

More than 150,000 solitary pulmonary nodules are diagnosed in the UK annually. If screening with helical-CT scans should be introduced, as suggested by recent articles, this number will considerably escalate [1].

The cornerstone of the pulmonary nodules management is an appropriate pre-operative planning (Graph 1).

The uniportal approach for the resection of nodules has been adopted for over 10 years [2–5] and we believe it should be considered the preferred approach for the management of solitary lung nodule as the one demonstrated in Fig. 1.

Indications

- Uniportal VATS resection is suggested if the suspicion of cancer is high and extension to lobectomy is anticipated.
- If nodules are not suitable for a biopsy, or previous biopsies have been not diagnostic, VATS resection should be advised.
- Last but not least, a clear discussion with the patient is very valuable in order to choose between several options.

Contraindications

- Pleural adhesions making difficult the creation of a pleural space. Even though in experienced hands adhesions can be taken down in a relatively short period of time, the uniportal approach is particularly advantageous in providing the perfect view to facilitate adhesiolysis.
- Even if previous surgery could make VATS biopsy more difficult because of adhesions, it's not considered an absolute contra-indication.
- Concomitant disease which caused a decline of the lung function and physiological reserve making difficult single lung ventilation although we have performed a number of procedure under spontaneous ventilation. The physiological pneumothorax created once the chest cavity is opened is more than adequate to palpate the nodule and resect it safely [6, 7].

Anaesthetic Considerations

- Standard double lumen tube or laryngeal mask in the hands of experienced anesthesiologists. For this approach the anesthesiologist must be able to intubate the patient on the side. Preoperative assessment of airways anatomy is therefore mandatory. Obese patients are not eligible for this procedure as difficult in maintaining adequate gas exchange develops pretty quickly.
- Electric operating table allows flexing the patient at the hip level. The advantage is twofold: maximal separation of the ribs to aid port placement and undisturbed movements of the video camera, especially in female patients. Do not use a bar on the side as this may hinder the mobility of the scope.

Positioning

- The patient should be positioned in the lateral decubitus position and angled at the level of the hips. We adopted the same VATS approach used in minimally invasive lung resections with the surgeon stands anteriorly to the patient and the assistant on the same side. This setup allows both surgeons to share the same view and better coordination between them during the uniportal approach.

M. Scarci (✉)
Thoracic Surgery Unit, S. Gerardo Hospital,
Monza, Italy
e-mail: m.scarci@asst-monza.it

F. Minervini
Department of Thoracic Surgery, McMaster University,
Hamilton, ON, Canada

G. Rocco (✉)
Service of Thoracic Surgery, Department of Surgery,
Memorial Sloan Kettering Cancer Center, New York, NY, USA
e-mail: roccog@mskcc.org

D. Gonzalez-Rivas et al. (eds.), *Atlas of Uniportal Video Assisted Thoracic Surgery*,
https://doi.org/10.1007/978-981-13-2604-2_16

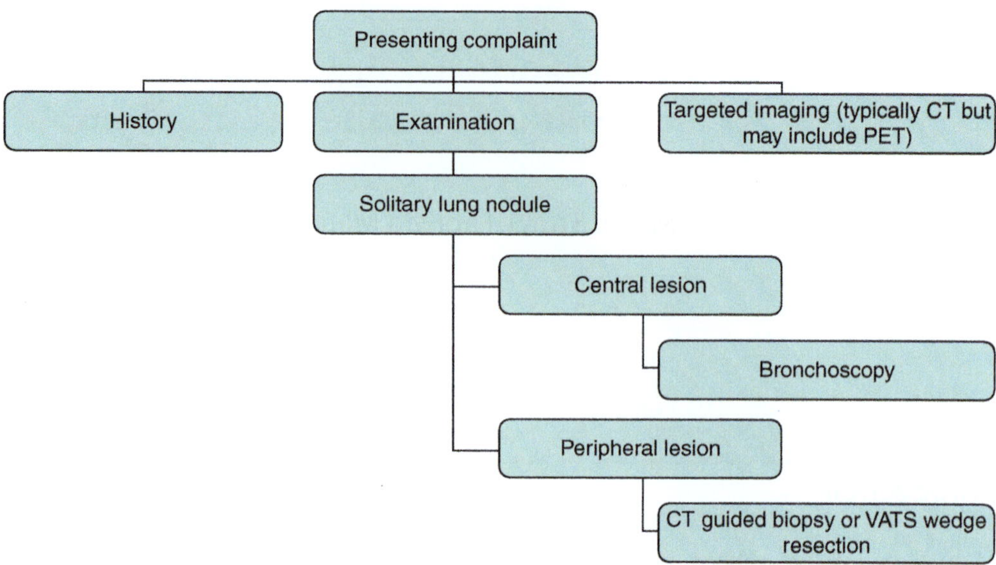

Graph 1 Algorithm for the management of solitary peripheral pulmonary nodule. Pet scanning is a very useful tool and may add decision-making, but is not conclusive in order to differentiate between benign and malignant disease

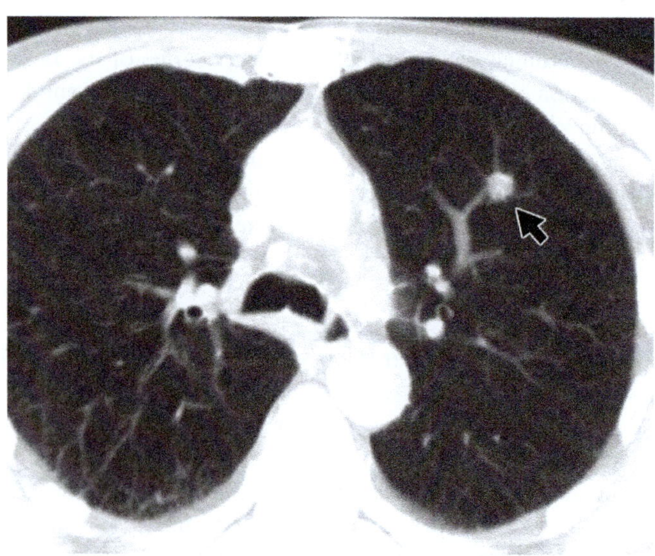

Fig. 1 Pre-operative computerized tomography showing a solitary left upper lobe lesion

Port Placement

- Port placement is standard as for all anatomic lung resection. Our favourite approach when the nodule has a high suspicion of malignancy is a 3–4 cm incision in the fifth intercostal space on the mid-axillary line in front of the latissimus dorsi muscle. This incision allows easy palpation of most areas of the lung and also is the easiest to perform a lobectomy if needed after frozen section. We perform this approach only when the chances of performing a lobectomy are significant, otherwise it might be excessive to make such incision to remove only a small portion of the lung. If conversion is need we simply extend the incision into an anterolateral thoracotomy. As not many muscles are divided this incision is very well tolerated and usually results in lower pain compared to posterolateral thoracotomy.
- In cases when metastatic disease is suspected or a wedge resection is performed with a diagnostic purpose, we prefer to perform one fingerbreadth incision, localized according to the position of the target lesion. If appropriately sited, it is possible to palpate and resect nodules through a very small incision.
- A 30-degree thoracoscope is introduced and the thoracic cavity is carefully inspected. Any visualized effusion should be sampled at beginning of the procedure and sent for histopathology and microbiology. The lung is retracted with VATS graspers and adhesiolysis is performed with electrocautery or, better, energy device if required for manipulation.
- The lesion is identified with atraumatic probing. If the lesion is not easily localised thoracoscopically, the lung can be palpated with a long instrument or with a finger throughout the incision.
- But nonetheless, if it is not possible to localise the lesion, or a safe resection margin can not be obtained, conversion to thoracotomy to get manual palpation should be considered a further operative step.
- Once the lesion is localised, a resection line can be planned below the lesion using forceps. The lung tissue surrounding the lesion is gently lifted with an instrument taking care of avoiding to touch the lesion. A stapler can be introduced throughout the lower part of the incision and staples applied with care. We usually use the graspers to expose the staple line and assist stapler placement. It's crucial to avoid tears of the lung tissue and to maintain at all time the camera in the upper part of the wound, the grasper in the middle and

the stapler in the lower part. This configuration allows the least amount of interference between instruments.

- Once the lesion is successfully resected, the wedge could be removed through the incision with a protective bag in order to prevent spreading of malignant cells and contamination of the thoracic cavity.
- Before the incision is closed, the use of an intercostal nerve block or paravertebral catheter is recommended in order to achieve a better control of the post-operative pain.
- The lung is re-inflated and the incision is closed taking particular care in approximating the muscle layer to avoid air re-entry or fluid leakage from the wound or lung herniation, particularly in thin patients.

In the case of nodules, which are difficult to identify even if with palpation, several localisation methods are available [8, 9].

- *Intra-operative ultrasound*: According to several trials, the identification of a lung nodule using an ultrasound probe introduced through a small trocar is a safe and accurate technique, also allowing the exploration of the surrounding structures [10].
- *Radio-guided localisation*: This method is also described in recent papers with high rates of successful identification of a lung nodule but, at the same time, with higher complication than ultrasound. This method could be complicated by diffusion of contrast into the pulmonary parenchyma [11].
- *Pre-operative techniques*: Several techniques like CT-guided percutaneous dye staining, placement of microcoils, insertion of fiducial markers and hookwire insertion have been reported in the literature in order to identify lung lesions which are difficult to localize [12–14]. However, several complications associated with the above mentioned procedures are reported (bleeding, pneumothorax and severe chest pain).

Even if these techniques are described as safe and accurate, they are dependent on the experience and skill of the surgeon.

If the nodule is deeper than expected, there are several alternative techniques for resection:

1. *Segmental resection*: Useful for lesions in the anterior upper lobe or superior lower lobe/lingula. On the other hand, a larger volume of lung parenchyma than necessary will be resected in case of benign nodules.
2. *Deep stapled nodulectomy*: Involves bi-valving the lung tissue thereby preserving more parenchyma, however, this is often technically difficult to perform.
3. *Nodulectomy with electrocautery*: The nodule is resected by using an electrocauter. The resection line must be stitched to prevent post operative air leak.

Preference Card

- 30 degree video camera
- Endoscopic bag
- Articulating stapler

Results and Discussion

Uniportal videoendoscopic resection has been reported to be a trustable method for the management of solitary lung nodules [2–5, 15, 16]. As discussed earlier, patients with peripheral lesions, highly suspicious for malignancy, should be considered for VATS wedge resection, because of the possibility to inspect the chest cavity and eventually carry out a lobectomy if indicated.

Complications such as miss firing of staplers (although meticulous care and washing in between stapler loads has reduced the incidence of this) or bleeding from staple line may occur and require further manoeuvres to obtain haemostasis. Finally, conversion to three ports-VATS or thoracotomy is not be considered a failure of the uniportal approach, but an additional procedure required to provide a safe resection of the lesion, which is the aim of the surgical procedure.

References

1. Team NLSTR. The national lung screening trial: overview and study design 1. Radiology. 2011;258(1):243–53.
2. Rocco G, Martin-Ucar A, Passera E. Uniportal VATS wedge pulmonary resections. Ann Thorac Surg. 2004;77(2):726–8.
3. Rocco G, Khalil M, Jutley R. Uniportal video-assisted thoracoscopic surgery wedge lung biopsy in the diagnosis of interstitial lung diseases. J Thorac Cardiovasc Surg. 2005;129(4):947–8.
4. Rocco G. VATS lung biopsy: the uniportal technique. Multimed Man Cardiothorac Surg. 2005;2005(121):mmcts.2004.000356.
5. Rocco G, Martucci N, La Manna C, Jones DR, De Luca G, La Rocca A, et al. Ten-year experience on 644 patients undergoing single-port (uniportal) video-assisted thoracoscopic surgery. Ann Thorac Surg. 2013;96(2):434–8.
6. Hung MH, Cheng YJ, Chan KC, Han SC, Chen KC, Hsu HH, Chen JS. Nonintubated uniportal thoracoscopic surgery for peripheral lung nodules. Ann Thorac Surg. 2014;98(6):1998–2003.
7. Hung WT, Hsu HH, Hung MH, Hsieh PY, Cheng YJ, Chen JS. Nonintubated uniportal thoracoscopic surgery for resection of lung lesions. J Thorac Dis. 2016;8(Suppl 3):S242–50.
8. Shi Z, Chen C, Jiang S, Jiang G. Uniportal video-assisted thoracic surgery resection of small ground-glass opacities (GGOs) localized with ct-guided placement of microcoils and palpation. J Thorac Dis. 2016;8(7):1837–40.

9. Han KN, Kim HK, Choi YH. Uniportal video-assisted thoracoscopic surgical (VATS) segmentectomy with preoperative dual localization: right upper lobe wedge resection and left upper lobe upper division segmentectomy. Ann Cardiothorac Surg. 2016;5(2):147–50.
10. Sortini A, Carrella G, Sortini D, Pozza E. Single pulmonary nodules: localization with intrathoracoscopic ultrasounda prospective study. Eur J Cardiothorac Surg. 2002;22(3):440–2.
11. Sortini D, Feo CV, Carcoforo P, Carrella G, Pozza E, Liboni A, Sortini A. Thoracoscopic localization techniques for patients with solitary pulmonary nodule and history of malignancy. Ann Thorac Surg. 2005;79(1):258–62.
12. Chen S, Zhou J, Zhang J, Hu H, Luo X, Zhang Y, Chen H. Video-assisted thoracoscopic solitary pulmonary nodule resection after CT-guided hookwire localization: 43 cases report and literature review. Surg Endosc. 2011;25(6):1723–9.
13. Lenglinger FX, Schwarz CD, Artmann W. Localization of pulmonary nodules before thoracoscopic surgery: value of percutaneous staining with methylene blue. AJR Am J Roentgenol. 1994;163(2):297–300.
14. Mayo JR, Clifton JC, Powell TI, English JC, Evans KG, Yee J, et al. Lung nodules: CT-guided placement of microcoils to direct video-assisted thoracoscopic surgical resection 1. Radiology. 2009;250(2):576–85.
15. Drevet G, Ugalde Figueroa P. Uniportal video-assisted thoracoscopic surgery: safety, efficacy and learning curve during the first 250 cases in quebec, canada. Ann Cardiothorac Surg. 2016;5(2):100–6.
16. Rocco G. History and indications of uniportal pulmonary wedge resections. J Thorac Dis. 2013;5(Suppl 3):S212–3.

Part IV

Uniportal Major Lung Resections

Right Lower Lobe

Eva Fieira Costa, María Delgado Roel, and Marina Paradela de la Morena

Introduction

The uniportal approach, as the three or two-port thoracoscopic procedures, must follow the oncological principles for any major pulmonary resection. The dissection of the hilar structures must be carried out individually, and mediastinal lymphadenectomy must be performed, all through video-visualization with no rib spreading [1,2,3].

General Aspects

The patient is positioned as for conventional VATS, in a full lateral position. The surgeon and the assistant are in front of the patient, so they have the same field of view, improving the coordination between them. The main video monitor must be placed opposite to the surgeon to having a direct view of the monitor across the operative field. However, when a lower lobectomy is performed, the surgeon works in a slight diagonally line inferiorly, so the monitor may be better placed more towards the patient's feet.

The utility incision (3–5 cm), is placed in the fifth intercostal space, in the mid- and anterior axillar lines, relatively anterior on the chest. The proper placement of the incision is crucial to achieve a good access to hilar structures as well as lymph node stations. A wound protector can be useful in order to protect the skin and to optimize access.

The use of specifically designed equipment, although it is not strictly necessary, it is highly recommended. The basics include: a 30-degree video-thoracoscope; long, curved ring graspers; long-curved metallic suction device or a Yankauer sucker; long-tipped electrocautery; long Metzenbaum scissors, sponge holders and endoscopic articulated staplers. The availability of specific devises such as instruments with proximal and distal articulation (coaxial thoracoscopic instruments are preferably), energy devices (ultrasonic dissector-coagulators or bipolar electrocautery devices), vascular clips or curved-tipped endoscopic staplers facilitates the procedure and could improve the learning curve of the uniportal surgeries. Finally, any type of retrieval device (i.e., a plastic bag or a glove) must be available for extraction of the specimens [4,5].

Operative Techniques

When the pleural adhesions are extensive, the surgeon must decided if the lobectomy can be performed by VATS or converting to open-surgery must be properly [6] (Video 1).

Fissure Complete

When the fissure is complete, the surgical sequence is usually as follows: artery, pulmonary ligament, vein, bronchus and fissure.

Once the pleural cavity is explored and the surgeon has checked for the presence or absence of pleural adhesions, the use of tissue graspers or sponges is useful to achieve the correct retraction of the lower and upper lobes, so the major fissure is exposed. The pleura over the interlobar artery must be open and using a scissor or the electrocautery clears the adventitia of the artery (Fig. 1) as well as the lymph nodes located beside; in this manner, not only the complete dissection of the artery is easier, but avoids vascular accidents. If a thick tissue is over the artery, the use of ultrasonic devises could improve the removal of this parenchyma without significant postoperative air leaks, although in those cases the fissureless technique must be the technique of choice.

At this point, once the interlobar artery is identified as well as the middle and lower branches, the section of the

Electronic Supplementary Material The online version of this chapter (https://doi.org/10.1007/978-981-13-2604-2_17) contains supplementary material, which is available to authorized users.

E. F. Costa (✉) · M. D. Roel · M. P. de la Morena
Department of Thoracic Surgery, Coruña Universtity Hospital, A Coruña, Spain

D. Gonzalez-Rivas et al. (eds.), *Atlas of Uniportal Video Assisted Thoracic Surgery*, https://doi.org/10.1007/978-981-13-2604-2_17

lower arterial branches can be performed or the major fissure can be completed. If we prefer to open the fissure first, we can use a clamp, a right-angle dissector or Scanlan® D'Amico mediastinoscopy forceps to achieve the dissection from the hilum to the basilar artery (anterior aspect of the major fissure) and from the sixth segment artery to the posterior pleura, above the intermediate bronchus (posterior aspect), creating a tunnel in each case. A vessel-loop can be useful to improve the pass of the stapler once the tunnel is created. Most patients have an almost complete separation between the middle and the lower lobe, so the anterior aspect of the fissure can be easily opened using the electrocautery or an ultrasonic device. If we prefer a stapler to complete the major fissure anteriorly, the anvil of the forceps must be directed from the hilum to the interlobar artery; careful must be taken in order to prevent vascular accidents in presence of adhesions or lymph nodes during this step; the stapler must be not forced through the tunnel we have created [4].

For the completion of the posterior aspect of the major fissure, the anvil of the stapler must be placed over the surface of the artery and before closing the stapler; the surgeon must check for the correct pass through the created tunnel.

Once the major fissure is completely opened, the dissection of the artery is easier: using a long-curved Metzenbaum scissors or a blunt clamp, the posterior aspect of the artery is

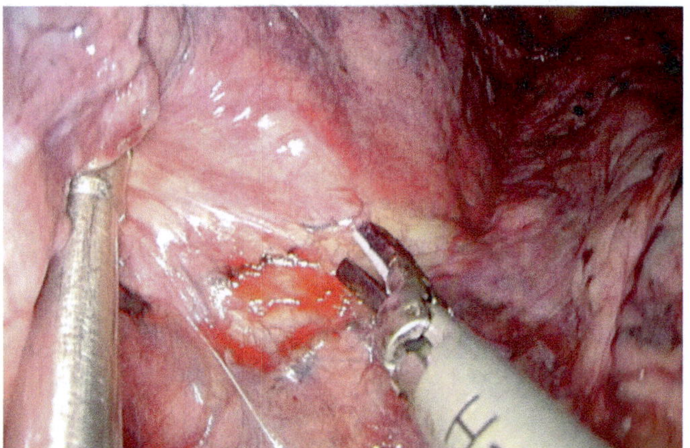

Fig. 1 Exposure of the basilar artery in the major fissure

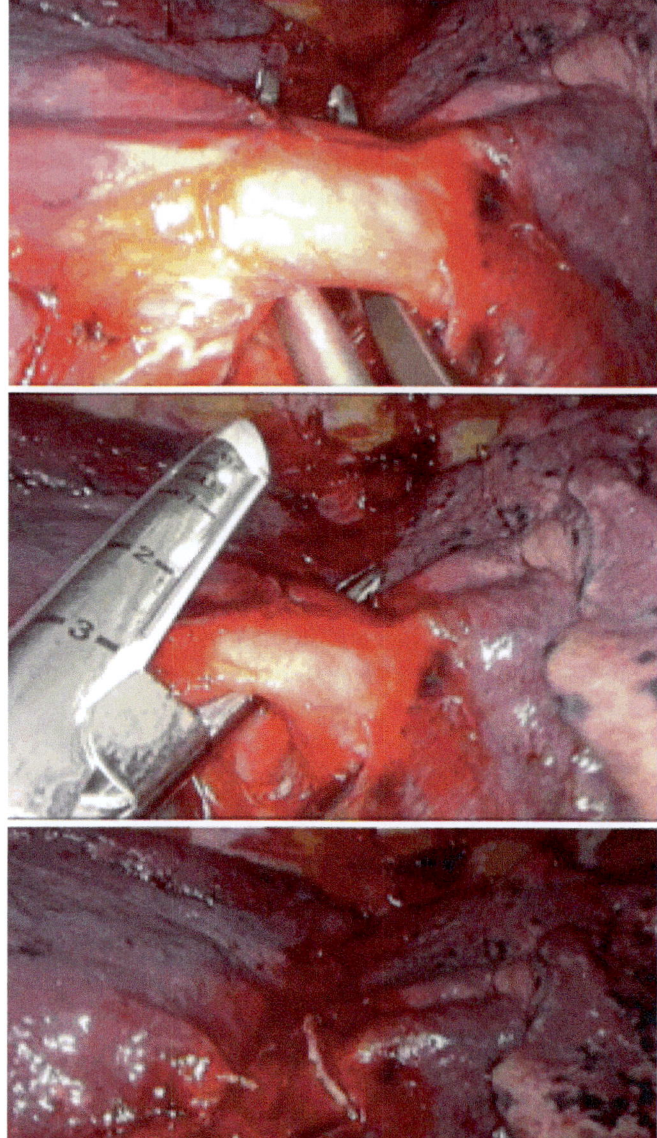

Fig. 2 Transection of the interlobar artery caudally to the right middle lobe arteries

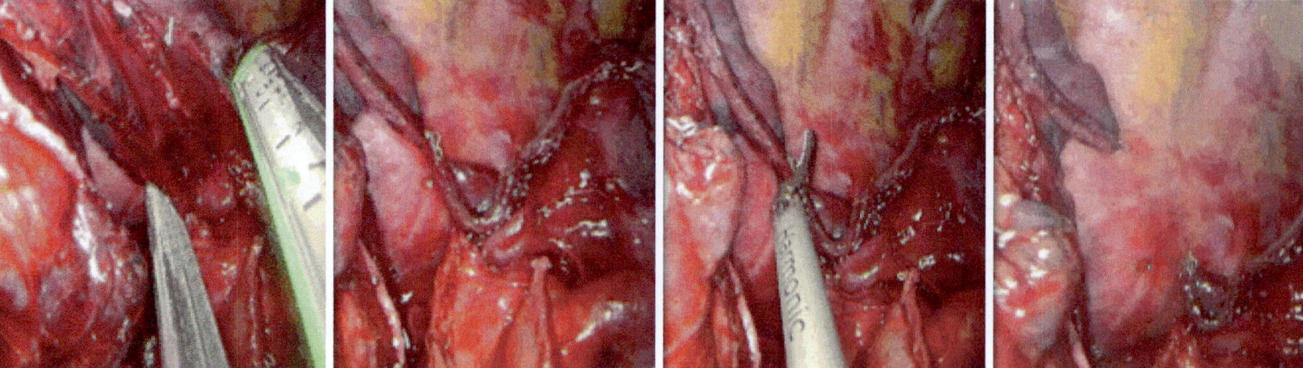

Fig. 3 Complection of the posterior aspect of the major fissure

dissected, releasing tractions or adhesions that may exist between the artery and the bronchus. We can dissected and divide the interlobar artery (Fig. 2) or performed the section of the branches individually; it depends on the size and the distance between them. It is advisable to visualize the middle lobe artery before stapling the basilar branches [7,8].

On many occasions, the superior segmental artery of the lower lobe is divided separately from the basilar branches; it is also important to check for the existence of a recurrent posterior branch for the upper lobe rising from the interlobar artery or the superior segmental artery (more rarely). When the basilar branches and the superior segmental artery are divided individually, the use of vascular clips or ligatures can replace the staplers.

If we prefer not to open the fissure, then the artery is dissected and stapled, so the completion of the fissure remains as the last step (Fig. 3).

After the division of the artery, the pulmonary ligament is taking down at the reflection (Fig. 4) and the lower vein is exposed. The lower lobe is retracted superiorly and the surgical table can be moved into the Trendelemburg position. Sometimes, the use of peanut sponges pulling down the diaphragm may improve the exposure. At this step, the thoracoscope remains in the posterior part of the incision but the assistant must be placed at the right side of the surgeon, closer to the patient's head. During the dissection of the vein, attention should be paid to ensure the entire vein is being dissected (including the superior segmental branches).

At this point, the removal of the mediastinal pleura and fatty tissue including lymph nodes between the distal border of the intermediate bronchus and the superior aspect of the lower pulmonary vein can improve the exposure and dissection of the posterior aspect of the lower vein. If this step is chosen, the lower lobe must be retracted anteriorly with a tissue grasper or a sponge holder (if it was not

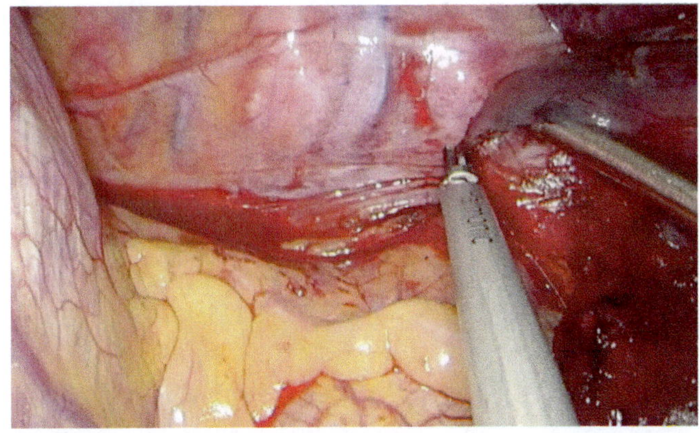

Fig. 4 Section of the pulmonary ligament

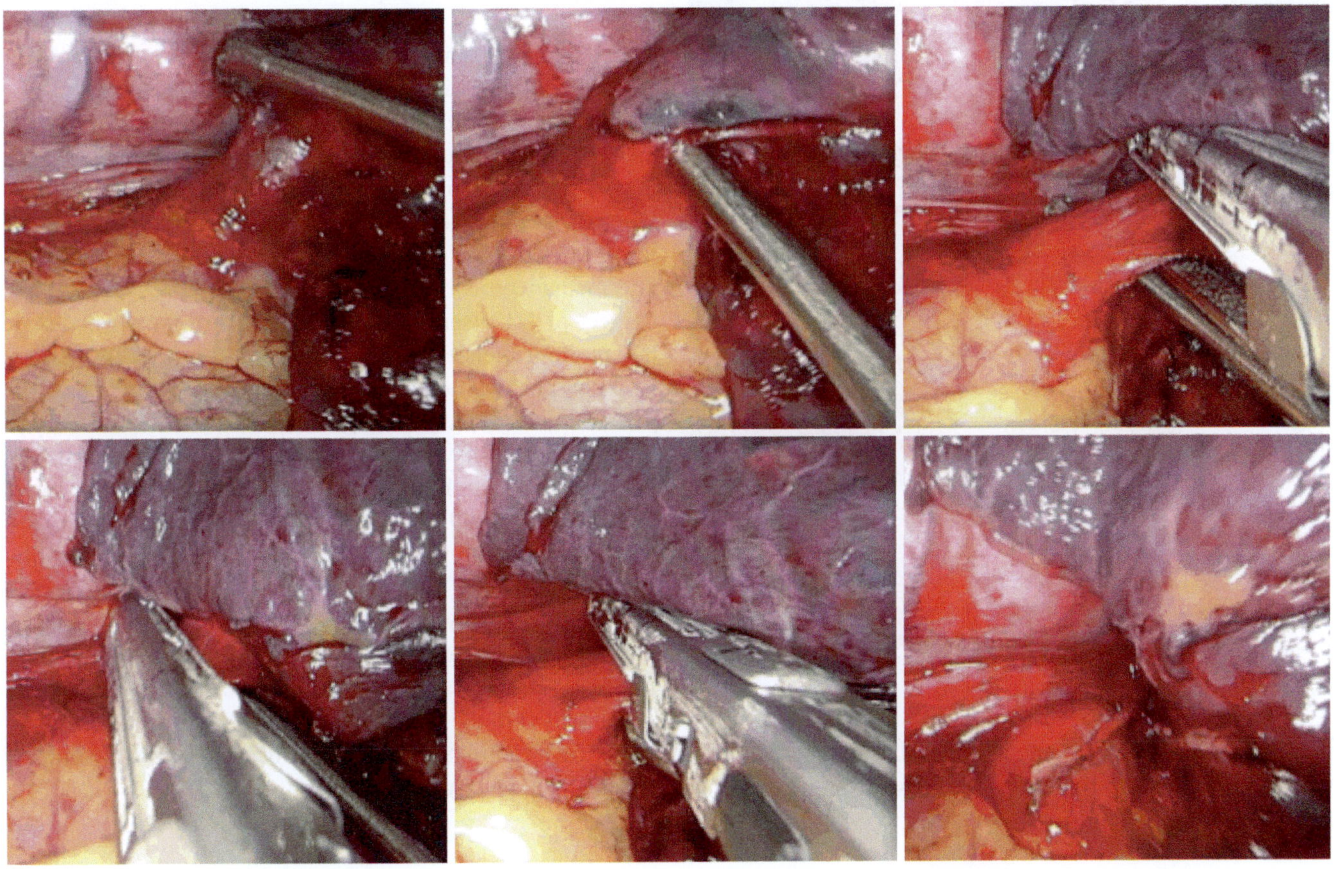

Fig. 5 Exposure, dissection and section of the right lower vein

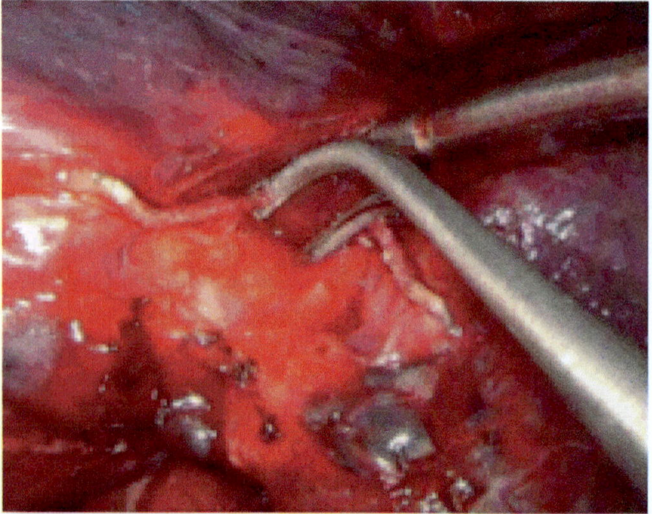
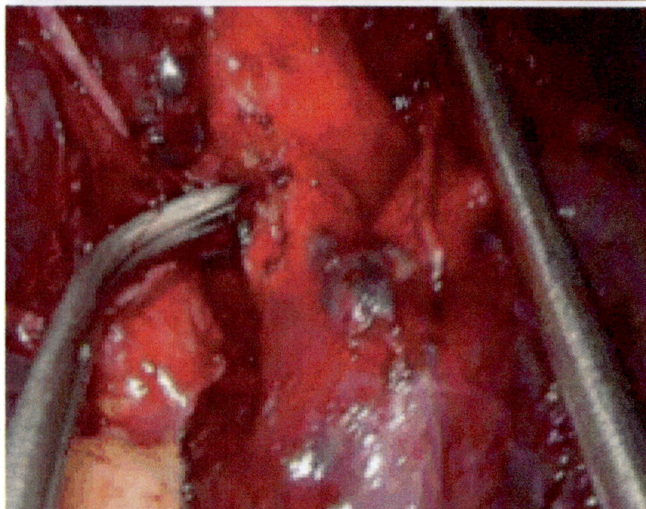
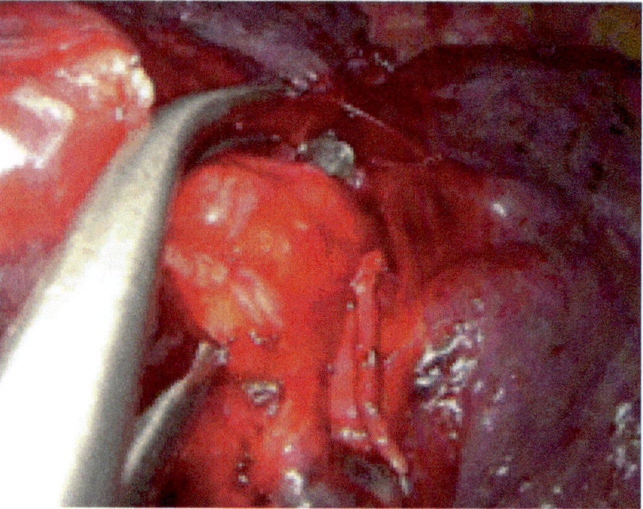

Fig. 6 Dissection of the right lower bronchus

performed before completing the fissure). A blunt clamp or a right-angle dissector is used to pass the lower vein and a vessel-loop can be used to retract the vein and optimize the exposure before stapling (Fig. 5).

When the tumour is located too close to the hilum, an intrapericardial dissection must be performed, due to the short neck of the inferior pulmonary vein.

Finally, the perbronchial tissue is removed and bronchial vessels cauterized if present. The lower lobe is retracted inferiorly into its anatomic position and the dissection of the lower bronchus is performed with a blunt dissector (Fig. 6), making sure the middle lobe bronchus is identified. The stapler is passed through the inferior aspect of the incision (as in almost every step during this lobectomy), *angulated* and closed (Fig. 7).

As the origin of the superior segmental bronchus is almost at the same level than the middle lobe bronchus, the resection line of the stapler to transect the lower lobe bronchus *must be diagonally* [8]. Before firing the stapler, it is mandatory (at least, advisable) to ask for the insufflation of the right lung in order to ensure the middle lobe bronchus is not compromised.

Finally, the surgeon must verify that no adhesions or remaining tissue attaches the lobe and the specimen is then introduced in a surgical bag or glove, to prevent the spread of the disease, and extracted (Fig. 8).

Completion

Once the lobectomy is accomplished, the surgical field is inspected for bleeding and air leaks.

Either mediastinal node sampling or a complete lymphadenectomy should be carried out when a uniportal lobectomy is performed, as for any type of lobectomy (either open or video-assisted lobectomy). Lymph nodes located around the lower lobe bronchus, the interlobar space and above the intermediate bronchus should be dissected. In case with high suspect of N1 disease, the intrapulmonary lymph nodes in the interlobar space must be removed.

An upper mediastinal lymph node dissection should be performed as a rule, although a hilar and interlobar proper lymphadenectomy is more important than upper mediastinal dissection when performing a lower lobectomy. Stations 7, 8 and 9 must be also checked for lymph nodes and removed if present. The technique of uniportal lymphadenectomy is described at Chapter "Uniportal Lymphadenectomy" of this book. A chest tube is placed at the posterior aspect of the incision; usually, we prefer a 24–28 Fr thoracic catheter. At this point, the lung is re-expanded and the surgical incision is closed. We only close the intercostal space if the incision had to be amplified in order to remove the specimen.

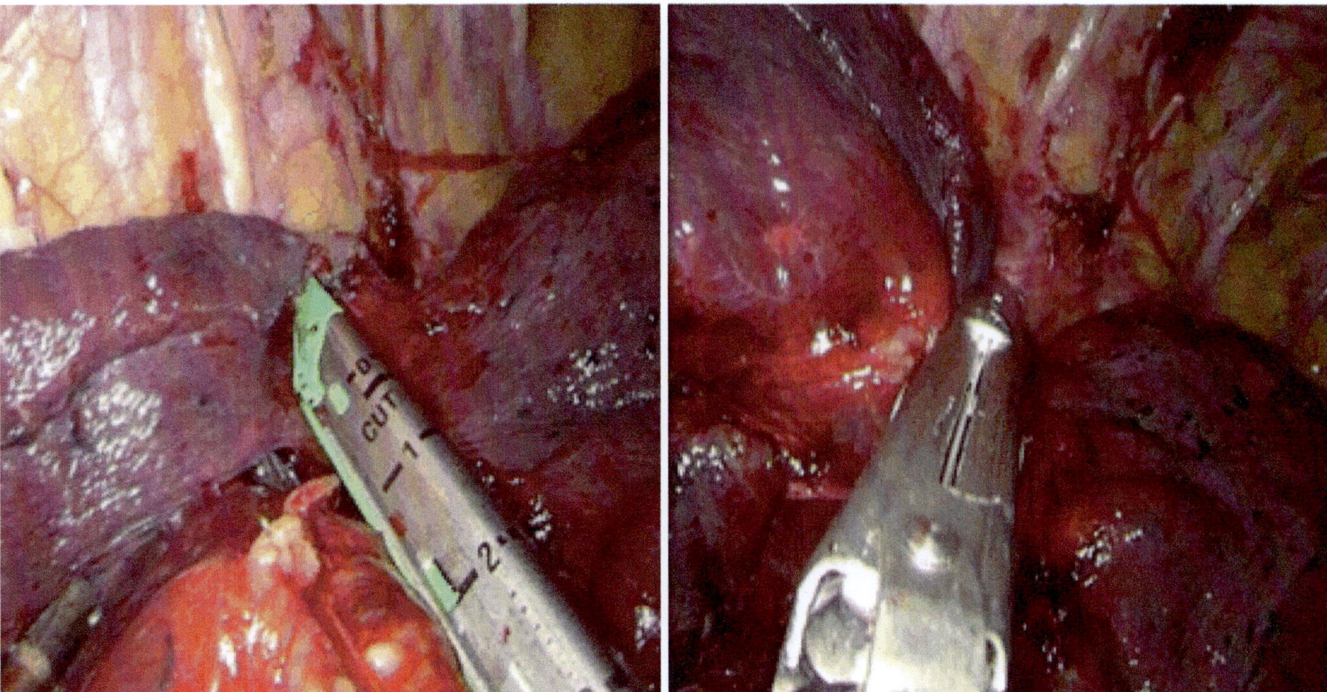

Fig. 7 Transection of the lower bronchus with an angulated stapler

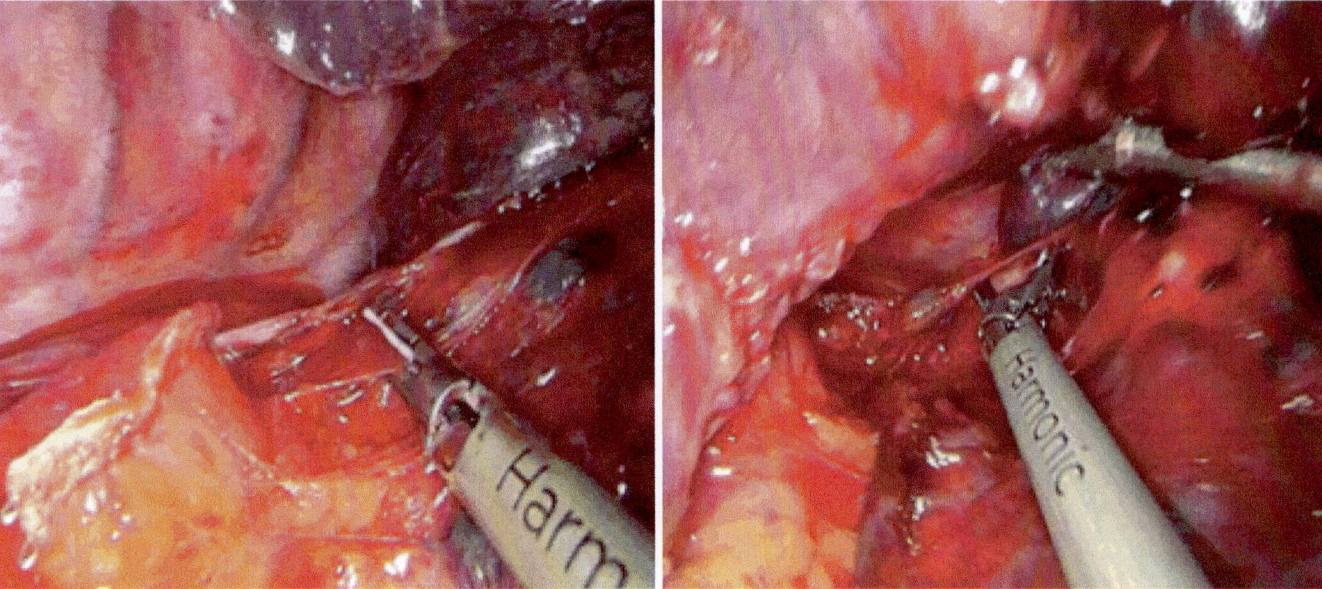

Fig. 8 Removal of tissue attaches

References

1. Fieira Costa E, Delgado Roel M, Paradela de la Morena M, Gonzalez-Rivas D, Fernandez-Prado R, de la Torre M. Technique of uniportal VATS major pulmonary resections. J Thorac Dis. 2014;6(Suppl 6):S660–4. https://doi.org/10.3978/j.issn.2072-1439.2014.10.21.
2. Gonzalez-Rivas D, Fieira E, Delgado M, Méndez L, Fernandez R, de la Torre M. Uniportal video-assisted thoracoscopic lobectomy. J Thorac Dis. 2013;5(Suppl 3):S234–45. https://doi.org/10.3978/j.issn.2072-1439.2013.07.30.
3. Gonzalez-Rivas D, Paradela M, Fernandez R, Delgado M, Fieira E, Mendez L, et al. Uniportal video-assisted thoracoscopic lobectomy: two years of experience. Ann Thorac Surg. 2013;95(2):426–32. https://doi.org/10.1016/j.athoracsur.2012.10.070. Epub 2012 Dec 5.
4. De la Torre M, González-Rivas D, Fernández R, Delgado M, Fieira E, Méndez L. Uniportal VATS lobectomy. Minerva Chir. 2016;71(1):46–60. Epub 2015 Nov 24.

5. Sihoe AD. Uniportal video-assisted thoracic (VATS) lobectomy. Ann Cardiothorac Surg. 2016;5(2):133–44. https://doi.org/10.21037/acs.2016.03.14.
6. Gonzalez-Rivas D. VATS lobectomy: surgical evolution from conventional VATS to uniportal approach. ScientificWorldJournal. 2012; 2012:780842. https://doi.org/10.1100/2012/780842. Epub 2012 Dec 30.
7. Sugarbaker DJ, et al. Cirugía del tórax. 1st ed. Buenos Aires: Médico Panamericana; 2011. ISBN 978-950-06-0142-9.
8. Shields TW, et al. General thoracic surgery. 7th ed. Philadelphia, PA: Lippincott Williams & Wilkins; 2009. ISBN 978-0-7817-7982-1.

Left Lower Lobe Resection

Hyun Koo Kim and Kook Nam Han

Abstract

Lobectomy with systemic lymph node dissection remains the mainstay of surgical treatment of non-small cell lung cancer. The emerging technique of uniportal video-assisted thoracic surgery (VATS) major lung resection may be a promising candidate for a VATS technique with less intercostal pain, a better postoperative course, and comparable oncologic outcomes to conventional VATS lobectomy. This chapter presents the technical details of uniportal VATS resection, specific for lower lobe lesions. Various individual approaches will be determined by the surgeon's experience.

Introduction

Uniportal video-assisted thoracic surgery (VATS) for lung cancer is an alternative technique that is favored by thoracic surgeons because it reduces intercostal pain and minimizes the skin incision, with comparable outcomes. Additionally, it provides feasible options for managing intraoperative events [1–4]. A uniportal VATS approach is conceivable for any procedure in which conventional VATS is possible. The operative sequences and consideration for fissureless cases are similar to the conventional multi-port VATS approach for the left lower lobe.

Electronic Supplementary Material The online version of this chapter (https://doi.org/10.1007/978-981-13-2604-2_18) contains supplementary material, which is available to authorized users.

H. K. Kim (✉) · K. N. Han
Department of Thoracic and Cardiovascular Surgery, Korea University Guro Hospital, Seoul, Republic of Korea
e-mail: kimhyunkoo@korea.ac.kr

Operative Technique

The specific location of the lung lesion and the intraoperative finding of pleural adhesions must be considered by an experienced surgeon before proceeding with this uniportal technique. The unique aspect of left lower lobectomy compared to left upper or right lower lobectomy includes modifying the incision for consideration of the heart and aortic or subaortic lymph node dissection. The patient is usually positioned in the right lateral decubitus with an axillary roll and an armrest to minimize arm stretching (Fig. 1). The location of the port, the surgeon's position, and the sequence of the exposure and division are not always consistent [5–7]. In our experience, we prefer a surgical port with a length of 2–4 cm at the fifth intercostal space in the midaxillary line (Fig. 2a). The surgeon always stands on the right side of the patient and the assistant stands on the left side during the procedure. There are various choices regarding the surgeon and assistant's position [8–10]. The use of a wound retractor also depends on the surgeon's preference (Fig. 2b). The device might be helpful to perform the surgery or to prevent the contamination of the lung cancer [5, 10]. However, some surgeons prefer not to use such devices in order to maximize the instrumental performance. The correct selection of the incision is important in order to expose the hilar structure for left lower lobe resection.

The uniportal VATS approach for left lower lobe resection starts with division of the inferior pulmonary ligament, and subsequently the surgeon can expose the major fissure and pulmonary artery, which can be directly identified through the port (Fig. 3a, b). The procedure is followed with fissure dissection (Fig. 3c). If the major fissure is complete, the sequences of division are usually the artery or pulmonary ligament, vein, and bronchus. From inferior to superior, the arterial trunk to the basilar and superior segments of the lower lobe is identified after fissure dissection (Fig. 3d). If the fissure is incomplete, the artery could be exposed after the vein and bronchus are transected. The fissure should be the last

D. Gonzalez-Rivas et al. (eds.), *Atlas of Uniportal Video Assisted Thoracic Surgery*,
https://doi.org/10.1007/978-981-13-2604-2_18

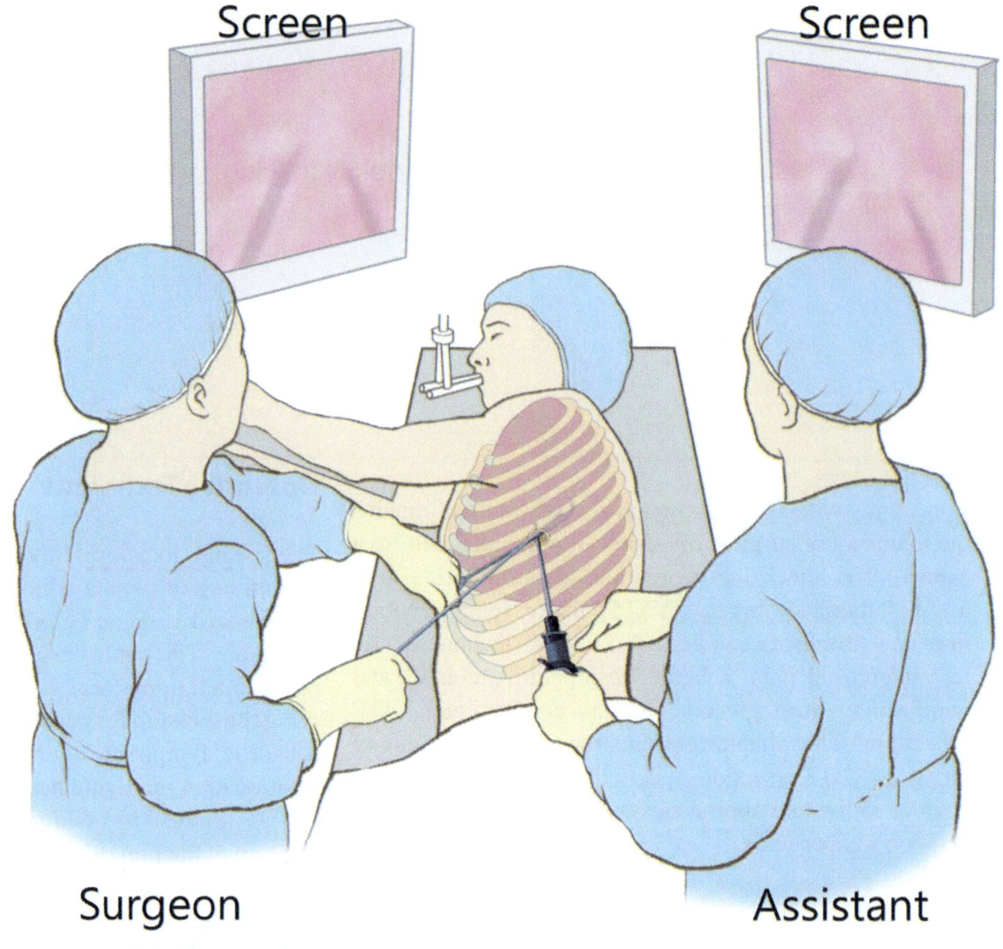

Fig. 1 Operative setting and patient positioning with right lateral decubitus for uniportal video assisted thoracoscopic surgery (left lower lobe resection)

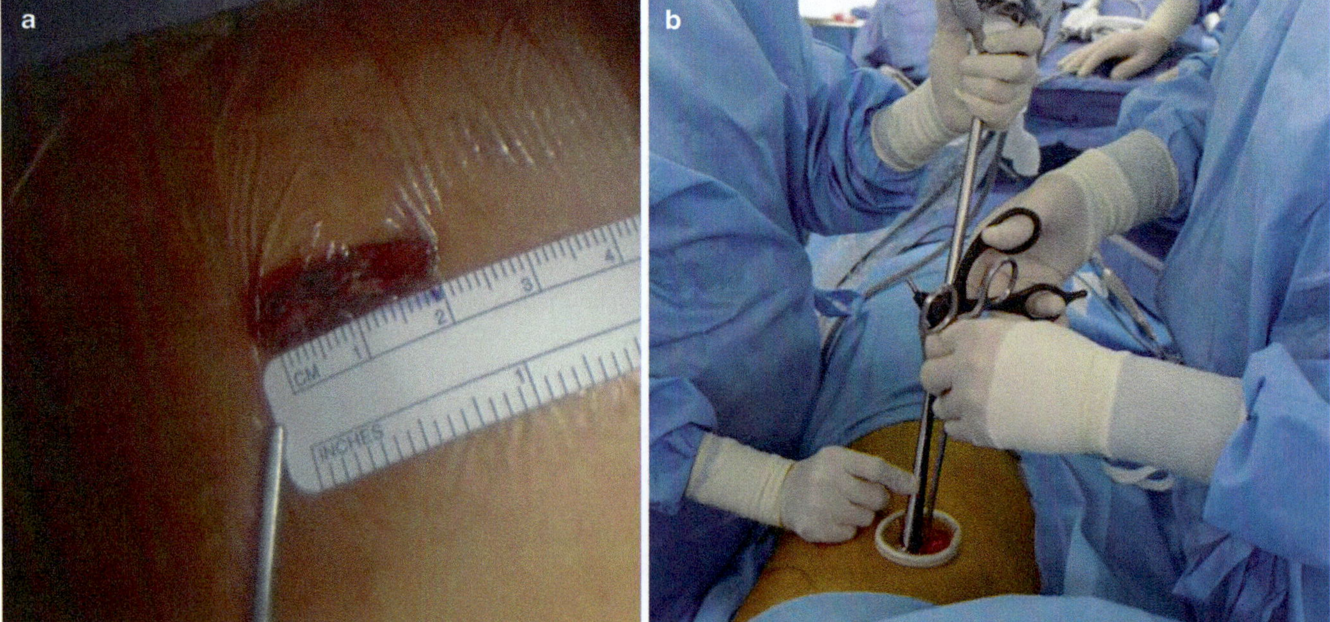

Fig. 2 (**a**) Small (2 cm) skin incision for uniportal VATS for lung resection, (**b**) parallel instrumentation of endoscopic and hybrid devices during uniportal VATS

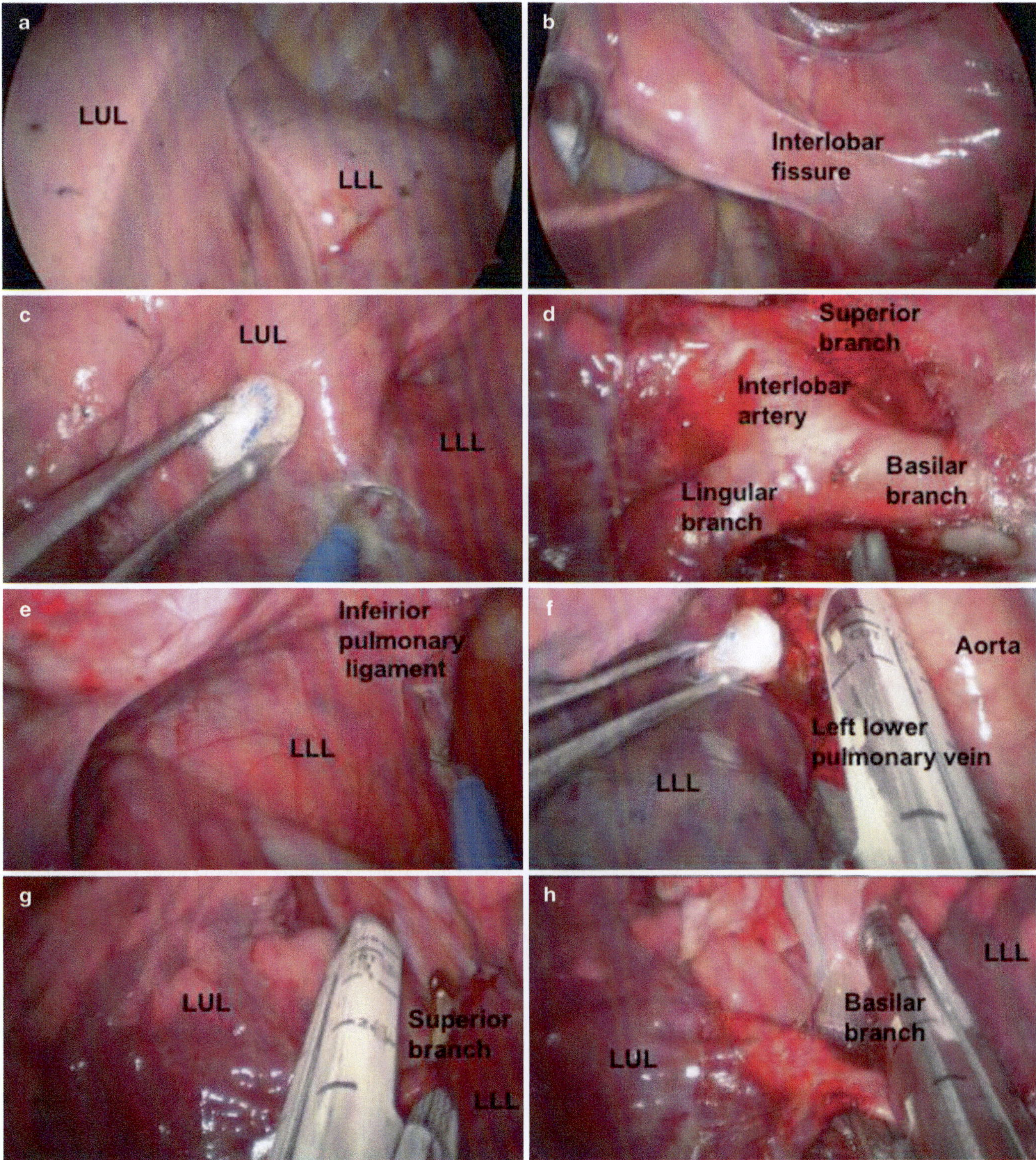

Fig. 3 Uniportal thoracoscopic surgery for left lower resection; (**a** and **b**) major fissure, (**c**) interlobar dissection, (**d**) exposed interlobar pulmonary artery, (**e**) inferior pulmonary ligament, (**f**) stapling the left lower pulmonary vein, (**g**) superior segmental artery of the lower lobe, (**h**) basilar segmental artery of the lower lobe, (**i**) lower lobar bronchus, (**j**) stapling the lower lobar bronchus, (**k**) completed lower lobe resection, (**l**) air leak test by water submersion

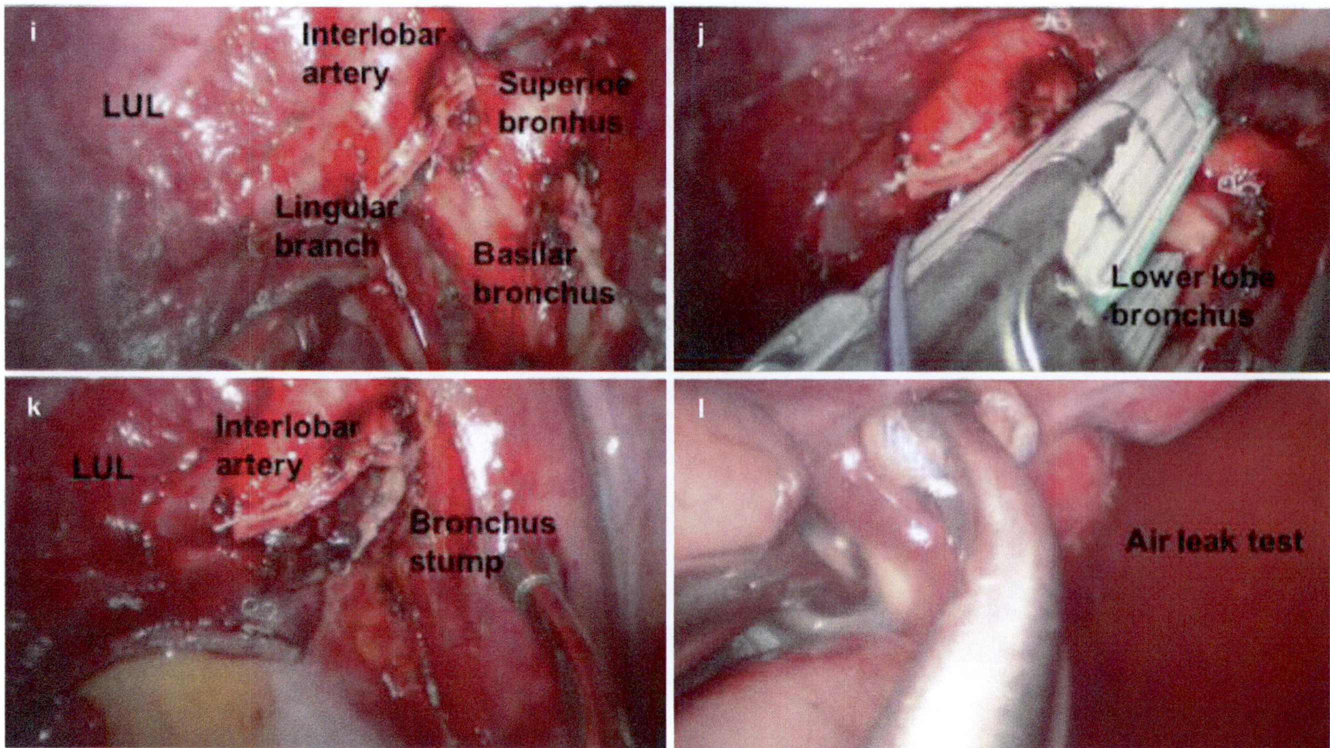

Fig. 3 (continued)

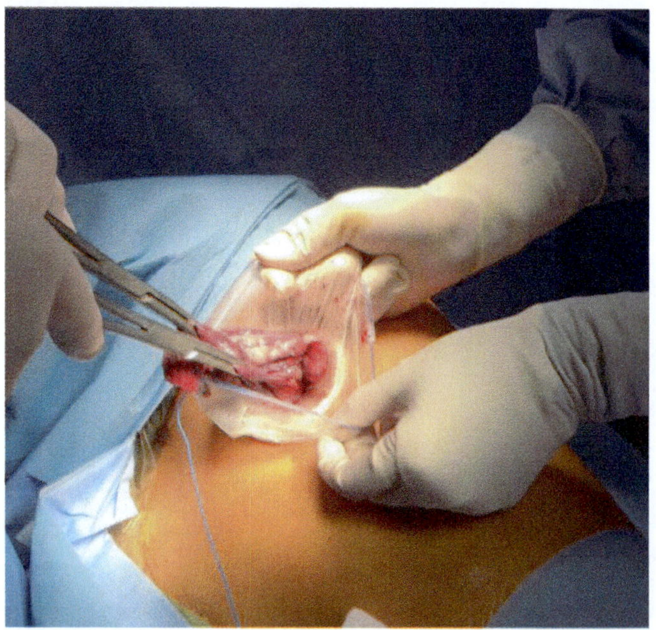

Fig. 4 Retraction of resected specimen with a port inserted wound retractor

step in the fissureless technique to avoid injury of the lingular vascular branch. The lingular arterial branches are identified and should be cautiously spared at this stage. The perivascular lymph nodes should be dissected. For the best surgical views, the lower lobe should be mobilized superiorly by division of the inferior pulmonary ligament (Fig. 3e). Additionally, gentle compression using a sponge stick may be helpful to acquire the space for instrumentation. The inferior pulmonary ligament is identified by the handling of the camera. After the lower lobar veins are identified and isolated, a vascular stapler is inserted for division. Proper mobilization of the lower lobe is important for stapling the lower lobar vein, and the use of a flexible stapler is helpful to pass the tip (Fig. 3f). A guide, such as a Penrose drain, may be helpful in passing the stapler safely. Care must be taken to avoid tension on the vessels, and the surgeon must always assess critical structures before firing the stapler. The segmental branches of the pulmonary artery are encircled and divided with the use of a vascular stapler (Fig. 3g, h). Small vascular branches may be divided with vascular clips if staplers cannot be passed between the vessel and lung parenchyma. The lower lobar bronchus lies directly after the division of the lower lobar trunk of the pulmonary artery (Fig. 3i). The stapler is inserted over the lower lobar bronchus. Inferior traction on the lower lobar bronchus helps to identify posterior structures to avoid injury to the left pulmonary artery. The lower lobar bronchus is divided after lung inflation to ensure that the upper lobar bronchus is not compromised (Fig. 3j). The bronchus division is completed by the use of green or black endostaplers (Fig. 3k, l). The resected specimen can be removed through the same port with gentle traction (Fig. 4, Video 1).

Results

There are no randomized studies comparing the uniportal VATS approach with open thoracotomy or conventional VATS procedures. However, there are early results in several retrospective studies of uniportal VATS lobectomy [1, 4, 11–13]. In this series, there are no described limitations of the uniportal VATS approach as a result of the specific location of the lung lesion. Our preliminary results of uniportal VATS lobectomy in lung cancer also revealed acceptable early results compared to conventional VATS or open thoracotomy. However, results were not available specifically for the left lower lobe. The unique aspect of left lower lobectomy compared to either upper or right lower lobectomy includes modifying the incision for consideration of heart injury during port placement and aortic or subaortic lymph node dissection. In addition, with a recent retrospective study proposing worse prognosis for left lower lobe cancer due to patterns of lymphatic drainage [14–16] even with surgical feasibility of the uniportal VATS approach it is very important to keep in mind the surgical completeness as the principle of lobectomy and mediastinal lymph node dissection, which could achieve acceptable long-term oncologic outcomes via the uniportal VATS approach for left lower lobar lesion. Although there is no available clear evidence of the benefits supporting the uniportal approach, future studies should clarify these questions on long-term intercostal pain, technical issues, and operative safety.

Conclusions

The uniportal VATS approach for left lower lobe resection represents a less invasive approach than conventional multiport VATS and minimizes the postoperative intercostal pain. The proper placement of the incision is crucial for exposing the hilar structures and the mediastinal lymph node in left lower lobectomy. The operative sequences should be modified according to whether the fissure is complete or not. The uniportal approach for left lower lobe resection is a safe and feasible option for benign and malignant lung lesions.

References

1. Ng CS, Kim HK, Wong RH, et al. Single-port video-assisted thoracoscopic major lung resections: experience with 150 consecutive cases. Thorac Cardiovasc Surg. 2016;64:348–53.
2. Rocco G, Martucci N, La Manna C, et al. Ten-year experience on 644 patients undergoing single-port (uniportal) video-assisted thoracoscopic surgery. Ann Thorac Surg. 2013;96:434–8.
3. Ng CS, Lau RW. Single-port VATS: the new paradigm. World J Surg. 2016;40:484–5.
4. Gonzalez-Rivas D, Paradela M, Fernandez R, et al. Uniportal video-assisted thoracoscopic lobectomy: two years of experience. Ann Thorac Surg. 2013;95:426–32.
5. Fieira Costa E, Delgado Roel M, Paradela de la Morena M, et al. Technique of uniportal VATS major pulmonary resections. J Thorac Dis. 2014;6:S660–4.
6. Assouad J, Vignes S, Nakad J, Grunenwald D. Single incision video-assisted thoracic surgery using a laparoscopic port. Ann Thorac Surg. 2011;91:2020–1;Author reply 2021.
7. Chen D, Du M, Yang T. Uniportal video-assisted thoracoscopic lobectomy for lung cancer. J Thorac Dis. 2016;8:1830–3.
8. Chen C-H, Lee S-Y, Chang H, et al. Technical aspects of single-port thoracoscopic surgery for lobectomy. J Cardiothorac Surg. 2012;7:50.
9. Jiang L, Bao Y, Liu M, et al. Uniportal video-assisted thoracoscopic left basilar segmentectomy. J Thorac Dis. 2014;6:1834–6.
10. Sihoe ADL. Uniportal video-assisted thoracoscopic lobectomy. Ann Cardiothorac Surg. 2016;5:133–44.
11. Chung JH, Choi YS, Cho JH, et al. Uniportal video-assisted thoracoscopic lobectomy: an alternative to conventional thoracoscopic lobectomy in lung cancer surgery? Interact Cardiovasc Thorac Surg. 2015;20:813–9.
12. Shen Y, Wang H, Feng M, et al. Single-versus multiple-port thoracoscopic lobectomy for lung cancer: a propensity-matched study dagger. Eur J Cardiothorac Surg. 2016;49(Suppl 1):i48–53.
13. Xie D, Wang H, Fei K, et al. Single-port video-assisted thoracic surgery in 1063 cases: a single-institution experience dagger. Eur J Cardiothorac Surg. 2016;49(Suppl 1):i31–6.
14. Kudo Y, Saji H, Shimada Y, et al. Do tumours located in the left lower lobe have worse outcomes in lymph node-positive non-small cell lung cancer than tumours in other lobes? Eur J Cardiothorac Surg. 2012;42:414–9.
15. Iwasaki A, Shirakusa T, Enatsu S, et al. Is T2 non-small cell lung cancer located in left lower lobe appropriate to upstage? Interact Cardiovasc Thorac Surg. 2005;4:126–9.
16. Ou SH, Zell JA, Ziogas A, Anton-Culver H. Prognostic factors for survival of stage I nonsmall cell lung cancer patients: a population-based analysis of 19,702 stage I patients in the California Cancer Registry from 1989 to 2003. Cancer. 2007;110:1532–41.

Right Middle Lobe

Miao Lin and Li Jie Tan

Compared to traditional VATS, the uniportal has some advantages. It provides a vertical, caudo-cranial perspective which preserves the depth of intraoperative visualization. Besides, the uniportal approach helps the surgeons keep a standard body posture straight facing monitor with minimal neck movement. However, the right middle lobectomy has a problem with uniportal VATS: the surgical approach through intercostal incision is merely vertical to the vessel plane, which leads to a great vary of operation difficulty. Thus, we summerize our experiences of the right middle lobectomy with the uniportal VATS.

A clear understanding of the right middle lobe anatomy is the key element of surgery. The right middle lobe includes two pulmonary segments: lateral and medial segments, which by definition have pulmonary arterial supply from A4 and A5, respectively. A4 and A5 could arise as separate branches or a common trunk from interlobar artery. The middle lobe vein most often joins the right superior pulmonary vein. But a few people has separate middle lobe vein which directly drainage into left atrium or joins the right inferior pulmonary vein. The middle lobe bronchus is more anatomically consistent, and always originate at the medial aspect of the bronchus intermedius.

Before surgery, the patient is kept in a folding knife gesture (with the cranial side raised up and caudal side pushed down) in the true lateral decubitus position (Fig. 1). The arm of the patient should be extended anteriorly and rotated slightly cephalad. Intraoperatively, the surgeon and the assistant stand on the abdominal side of the patient. The assistant stood at the footstool in the caudal side. The screen is placed in front of the operating table.

In uniportal VATS right middle lobectomy, a 3–4 cm incision was made at the fifth intercostal space along the anterior axillary line (Fig. 2). For obese patients with high diaphragms, an incision made at the fourth intercostal space is appropriate. However, the intercostal space for incision is

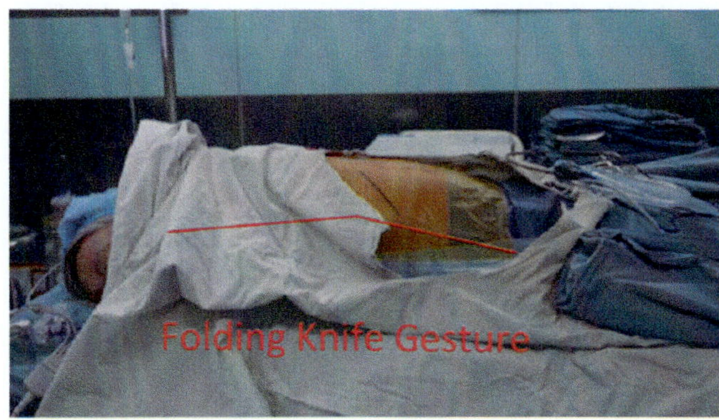

Fig. 1 The folding knife gesture and lateral decubitus position for uniportal middle lobectomy

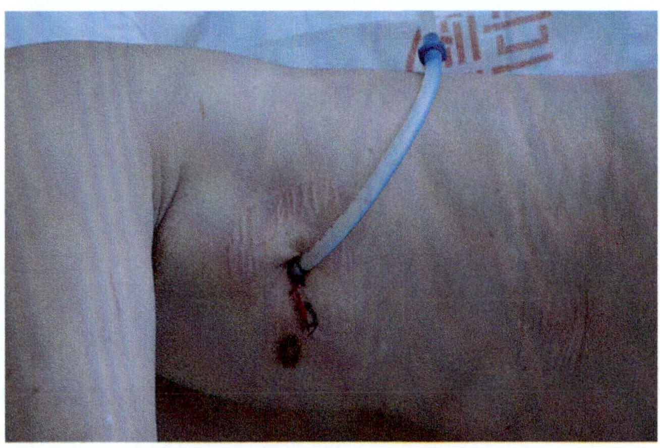

Fig. 2 Surgical incision in uniportal middle lobectomy

Electronic Supplementary Material The online version of this chapter (https://doi.org/10.1007/978-981-13-2604-2_19) contains supplementary material, which is available to authorized users.

M. Lin · L. J. Tan (✉)
Division of Thoracic Surgery, Zhong Shan Hospital, Fu Dan University, Shanghai, China
e-mail: tan.lijie@zs-hospital.sh.cn

D. Gonzalez-Rivas et al. (eds.), *Atlas of Uniportal Video Assisted Thoracic Surgery*,
https://doi.org/10.1007/978-981-13-2604-2_19

still controversial. Surgeon could directly reach the middle lobe vein through the incision made at the fourth or fifth intercostal space. But there would be no space left for a linear cutting stapler, and ligation might be a better choice. Sometimes, the third intercostal space is preferred, so that a linear cutting stapler could be applied. A soft plastic wound protector was applied to the incision without rib-spreading. A 10-mm 30° thoracoscope was introduced in the superior side of the incision during the lobectomy. Other surgical instruments, including the uniportal VATS specialized surgical instruments, the harmonic shear, and the hook electrocautery, were introduced in the inferior part of the incision during the procedure.

Commonly, the middle lobe vein branch is first dissected in uniportal VATS. In the beginning of the surgery, the pleura is divided anterior to the superior pulmonary vein, just posterior to the phrenic nerve. The middle lobe vein branch is identified and dissected circumferentially. The space between the middle lobe branch and the branches to the upper lobe is developed, exposing the beginning of the interlobar portion of the right pulmonary artery. The right middle lobe vein is divided with a linear cutting stapler or between ligatures. During the process of middle lobe vein, surgeon should pay attention to pulmonary vein variations. As mentioned before, some individuals has separate middle lobe vein which joins the left atrium or joins the right inferior pulmonary vein (Video 1).

Part of the fissure is then divided. The pleura overlying the decussation of the interlobar portion of the artery in the fissure is divided and the subadventitial plane of the artery is dissected. The middle lobe arteries arise from the trunk of right pulmonary artery could be observed. It is usually not necessary to do additional dissection of the branches to the upper and lower lobes. And some individuals have only one middle lobe artery. Surgeon could either dissect middle lobe artery or further divide the fissure. If we choose the fissure to manipulate, the plane superior to the middle lobe vein and anterior to the artery need to be first identified using a right angle clamp or a double-action force. Then a linear cutting stapler can help complete the minor fissure. The middle lobe artery is dissected circumferentially, and divided with a linear cutting stapler or between ligatures.

The middle lobe bronchus is always found beneath the middle lobe artery. Lymph nodes around the middle lobe bronchus is removed before closing and dividing by a linear cutting stapler. Preservation of adequate ventilation to the lower lobe should be assessed after closing the middle lobe bronchus and before firing the stapler by asking the anesthesiologist to ventilate the right lung with two to three breaths. Sometimes, the exposure of middle lobe bronchus need medial dissecting of the middle lobe artery to the basilar segments of the lower lobe.

At last, the plane is identified between the middle and other lobes. This major and minor fissure is completed with a linear cutting stapler. If this surgery is a lung cancer therapy, an following appropriate nodal dissection is necessary (Video 2).

There are procedure variation of the operation. The middle lobe vein is always dissected first. But the manipulation order of middle lobe artery, bronchus, and fissure could be altered so as to make the surgery smoothly. Due to the lack of operation space, application of linear cutting stapler seems not easy in uniportal surgery, especially in right middle lobectomy. A traction by silks of target vessel would make the insertion of a linear cutting stapler easier.

Uniportal Video-Assisted Thoracoscopic Right Upper Lobectomy

Diego Gonzalez-Rivas and Marina Paradela de la Morena

Abstract

Video-assisted thoracoscopic surgery (VATS) through a single incision grows increasingly popular in recent years, as a safe and feasible procedure with good postoperative outcomes. The advantages of this approach include direct view to the target tissue avoiding the use of the trocar, anatomic instrumentation and potential less postoperative pain.

The improvements in both endoscopic instruments and surgical skills have allowed to perform not only initial stages but also complex cases with success, following the oncological principles for major pulmonary resection.

However, uniportal VATS lobectomy remains a challenging technique for thoracic surgeons. For the right upper lobectomy, the most complex structure to divide through an uniportal approach is vein of the upper lobe and represents the main reason for conversion to double port technique during the learning curve. Because of this, we usually recommend to divide the upper arterial trunk first. The rest of the operative sequence is similar to the fisureless technique for conventional VATS.

General Aspects

Under general anesthesia and double lumen intubation, the patient is placed in a lateral decubitus position. Coordination between the main surgeon and the assistant is cruzial in order to avoid malposition of instruments and camera. When we described the approach in 2010, the assistant and the surgeon were always positioned on the same side, i.e. anterior to the lateral decubitus patient to have the same vision and more coordinated movements (Fig. 1). However, we have seen after more experience with the technique that for the upper lobes, the position of the assistant on the opposite side to the surgeon is more convenient (the surgeon has more freedom of movements for a better instrumentation and the assistant is more confortable to keep the camera at the upper part of the incision). This distribution offers more space to the surgeon but requires expert assistants (Fig. 2). For lower lobes we still prefer the assistant placed in front of the patient (Fig. 1).

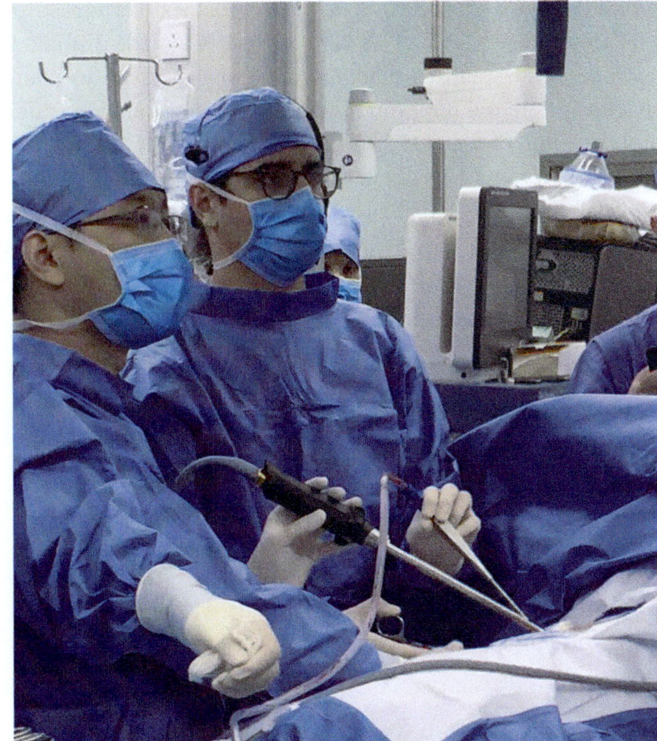

Fig. 1 Surgeon and assistant placed in front of the patient during left lower lobectomy

A 3–4 cm incision is preferably performed at the fourth intercostal space between the middle and anterior axillary line. A wound protector is recommended specially for obese

D. Gonzalez-Rivas (✉) · M. P. de la Morena
Department of Thoracic Surgery, Shanghai Pulmonary Hospital, Tongji University School of Medicine, Shanghai, China

Department of Thoracic Surgery and Minimally Invasive Thoracic Surgery Unit (UCTMI), Coruña University Hospital, Coruña, Spain
e-mail: diego@uniportal.es

D. Gonzalez-Rivas et al. (eds.), *Atlas of Uniportal Video Assisted Thoracic Surgery*,
https://doi.org/10.1007/978-981-13-2604-2_20

patients, sleeve resections or during the lymphadenectomy. In case of adhesion it should be not used to release the lung because the plastic ring inside may diminish angle of instrumentation. The camera should be always placed at the upper part of the incision working with the instruments below. There are several tricks to keep the camera always fixed in the same position such as using a vessel loop, suture, or a tape. By doing this we reduce the fatigue of the assistant and we assure a better stability in the vision during the operation.

Straight instruments are not suitable for the single port VATS technique, so they must be curved in order to avoid interference with the vision. The long curved suction becomes a very useful tool when performing advanced instrumentation. It can be used for many functions such as aspirate, hold, expose, compress, release adhesions, etc.

Tumor location through a single incision may be difficult, especially for small carcinomas with air-bronchogram and absence of pleural dimpling. In these situations, an adequate mobilization of the lung is crucial to perform a delicate tactile exploration. If it is expected that the identification of the neoplasm will be very tedious, CT-guided needle localization by radiologist avoids uncertainty.

Lung exposure is another key-point of uniportal VATS lobectomy. Rotation of surgical table provides a good view of the structures avoiding the excessive traction of the parenchyma. The development of new technology (new staplers, vascular clips, ultrasonic devices), and the use of specific equipment (instruments with double joint articulation) facilitates dissection and division of the vessels during the surgery.

The lobe should be always removed in a protective bag and a lymph node dissection should be performed in lung cancer cases. If a paravertebral blockade was not conducted prior the surgery, the intercostal spaces can be infiltrated with bupivacaine at the end of the operation. Finally, a single chest tube is placed, preferably in the posterior part of the incision.

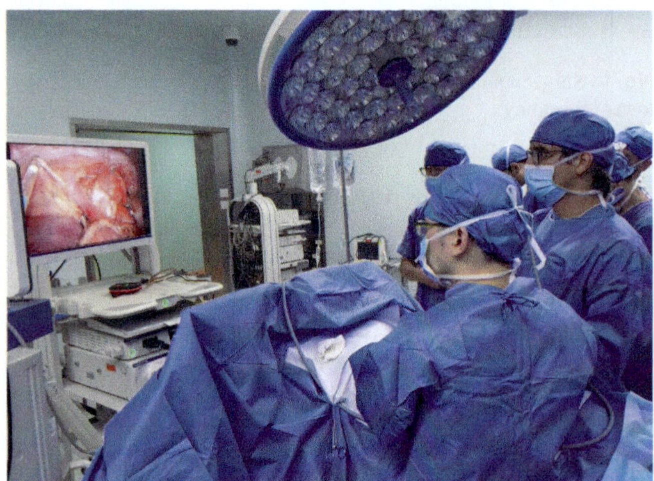

Fig. 2 Position for surgeon (front of the patient) and assistant (back of the patient) during a right upper lobectomy

Operative Technique

The operative sequence for a uniportal right upper lobectomy (RUL) is like the fissureless technique for conventional VATS.

The main steps for a typical RUL are:

1. Identification of the plane between the truncus anterior (Boyden's trunk) and upper vein
2. Dissection and transections of Boyden's trunk
3. Dissection and division of the upper vein identification previous identification of the middle lobe vein
4. Dissection and transection of the upper lobe bronchus previous inflation test
5. Dissection and division of the posterior artery (A2)
6. Division of the anterior and posterior part of the fissure

Although there is not fixed mode in handing the vessels or bronchus of the RUL, we recommend to divided the upper arterial trunk first (Fig. 3). The uniportal view provides a good view to dissect and divide this artery which is normally hidden by the superior vein when we use a 3-port thoracoscopic approach. Once this branch is divided, the vein is more easy to expose and divide. It is recommended to expose the middle lobe vein before starting dissection of upper lobe vein (Fig. 4).

We must also expose and dissect the upper vein widely to optimise the passage of the endostapler (Fig. 5). Taping the vein by using a suture or a vessel loop it a useful trick to enlarge the space behind (Fig. 6). The development of curved-tip stapler technology clearly facilitates the passage of the endostapler to divide the upper vein (Fig. 7).

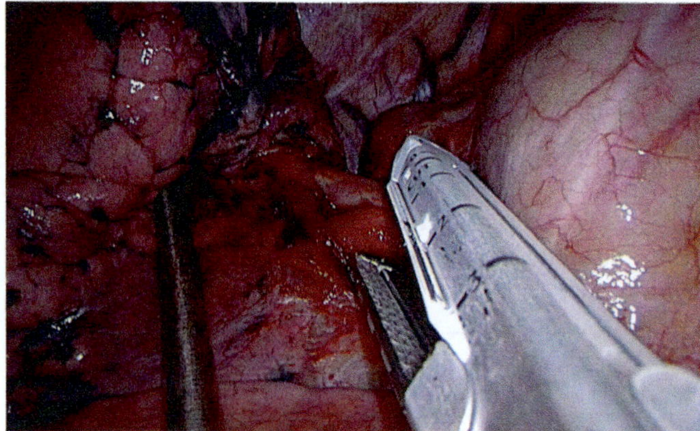

Fig. 3 Division of truncus anterior with a vascular stapler as the first step

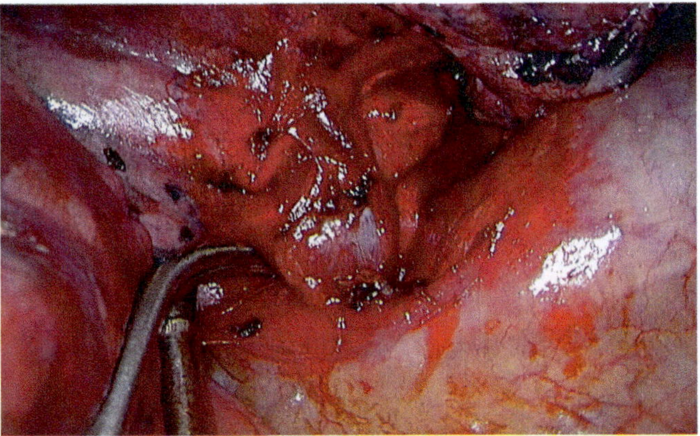

Fig. 4 Identification of middle lobe vein and dissection of upper lobe vein with a right angle clamp

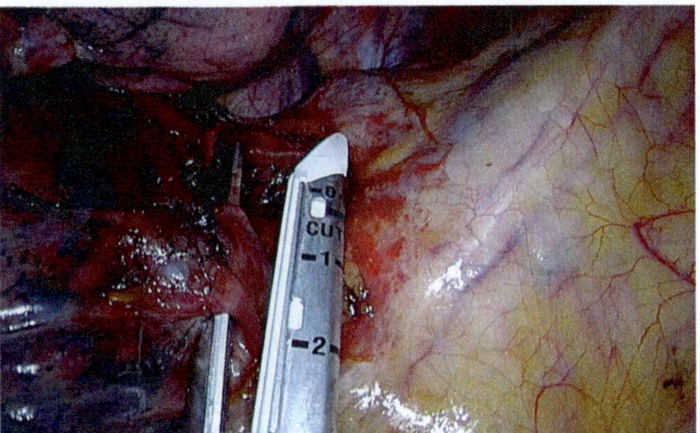

Fig. 5 Division of upper vein with an articulated stapler

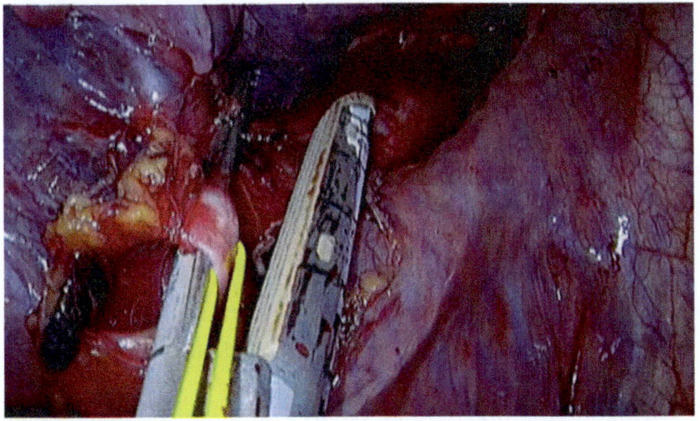

Fig. 6 Insertion of stapler facilitated by vessel loop encircling the vein

The "suction device trick" is very useful for stapling the upper vein and the upper lobe bronchus. After the dissection of the upper vein (Fig. 8) or bronchus (Fig. 9), we should pass the long curved suction device behind the space created by the dissector, while keeping the dissector widely opened. The trick consist to lift up the vein or bronchus upwards with the long curved suction, creating a path through which the stapler is easily introduced.

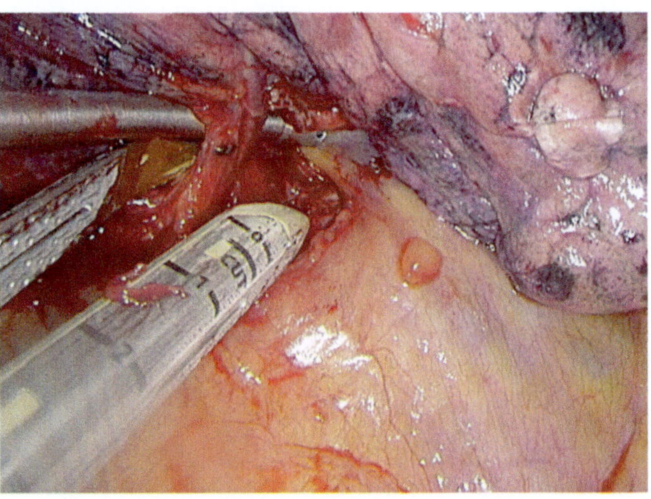

Fig. 7 Division of upper lobe vein by using a curved tip stapler

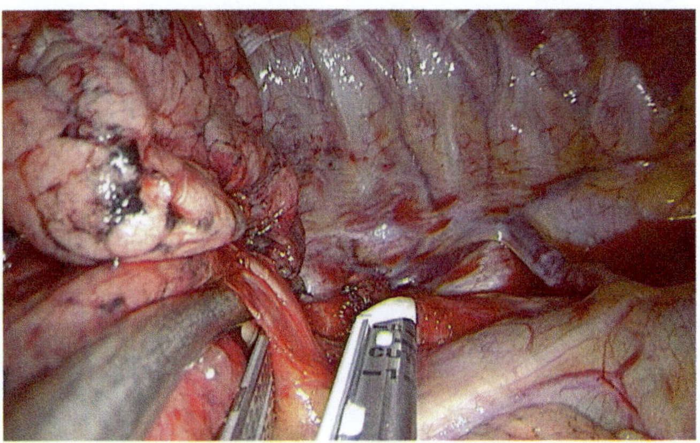

Fig. 8 The "suction device trick" to help the insertion of stapler to divide the upper lobe vein

Another option is to divide the RUL bronchus before the vein. To expose the bronchus we advise to dissect the posterior bifurcation between intermediate bronchus and the upper bronchus by cutting the posterior pleural reflection. Care must be taking when passing the bronchus to avoid damage to the azygous vein or main bronchus. Once the bronchus is divided, we can rotate more the lobe and facilitate the insertion of the endostapler for vein, which is the most difficult structure during uniportal RUL (Fig. 8). The "trick of the suction" protects damage of the posterior artery (A2) when stapling the RUL bronchus (Fig. 9). This maneuver is not recommended to perform on the artery to avoid hematoma or even avulsion due to the traction.

When the angle for insertion of the endostapler for upper lobe vein is still not suitable, it is recommended to open the anterior part of the minor fissure. This maneuver

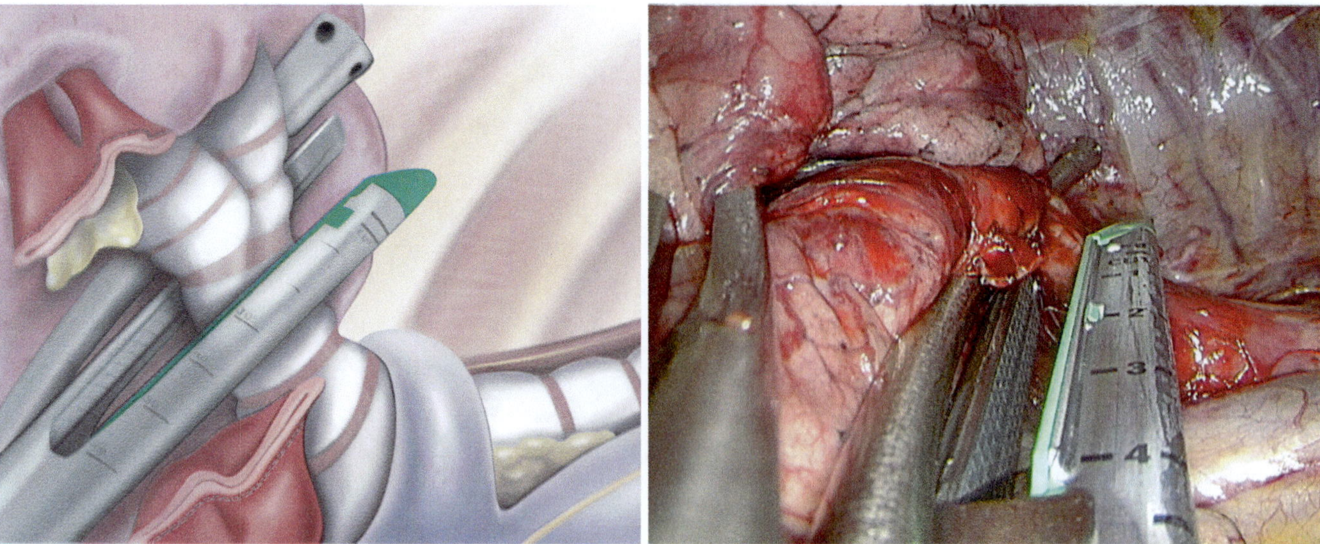

Fig. 9 Drawing and photo showing the long curved suction maneuver during transection of the bronchus

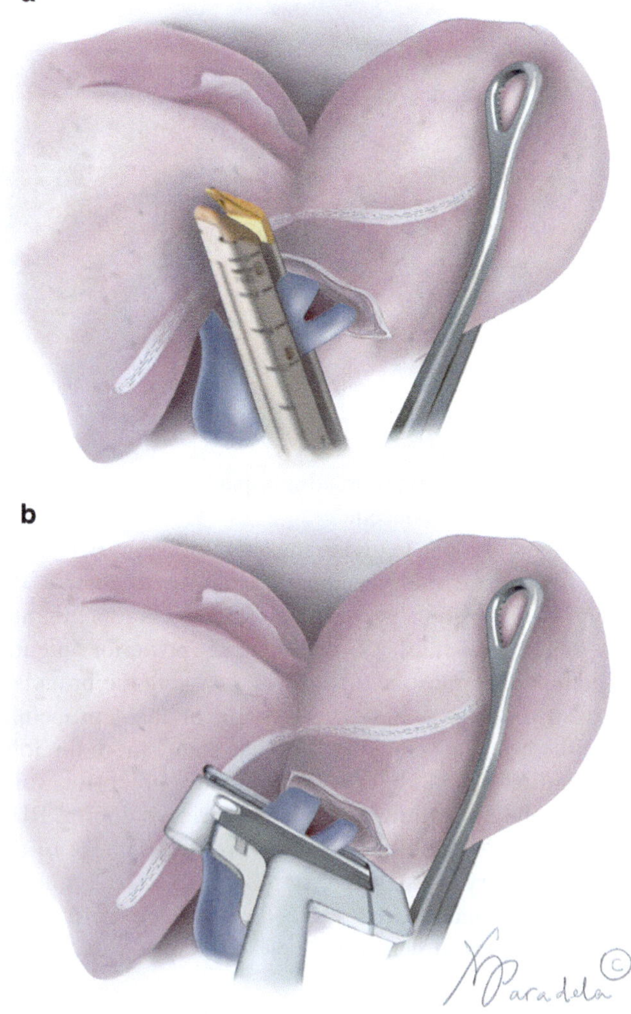

Fig. 10 Unusual options to deal with the upper lobe vein. (**a**) Completion of the anterior part of minor fissure, cranially rotation of the upper lobe and use of the stapler with caudally orientated curved tip angulation. (**b**) Use of TA conventional stapler to transect the vein

is performed by placing the anvil of the endostapler between the middle and upper lobe vein pulling the lung into the jaws of the endostapler. Once the minor fissure is divided, the passage around the upper lobe vein is easier with the tip of the endostapler oriented to the bottom (Fig. 10a). Opening the minor fissure also provides a much better field of vision for the ascending arteries and the RUL bronchus.

If the upper vein is still difficult to divide, the use of two cartridges of a conventional TA stapler may be a effective option, especially for beginners with the technique (Fig. 10b).

We must be careful with the dissection and division of A2 which is the most dangerous branch during a RUL and a frequent reason of bleeding and conversion during the learning curve of VATS. The new generation of vascular polymer clips are a safe alternative to transect this small vessels. We recommend the use of two clips for the proximal part of the vessel (Fig. 11). However, we prefer the use of energy devices for the distal end, in order to avoid displacement of the clips during the mobilization of the upper lobe and to prevent the interference of the clip with the stapler when dividing the fissure.

Another method would be to simply ligate the vessel using ties (with knots secured proximally digitally or with a thoracoscopic knot pusher), and dividing the vessel between ligatures or use energy device for distal division (Fig. 12).

The last step is completion of the fissure. After transecting the vein, artery and bronchus, we continue dividing the fissure with the placement of the endostapler above the interlobar artery, pulling the lobe anteriorly making sure that the middle lobe artery is far from the stapler. All the bronchial and vascular stumps should be kept out from the staplers jaws (Fig. 13).

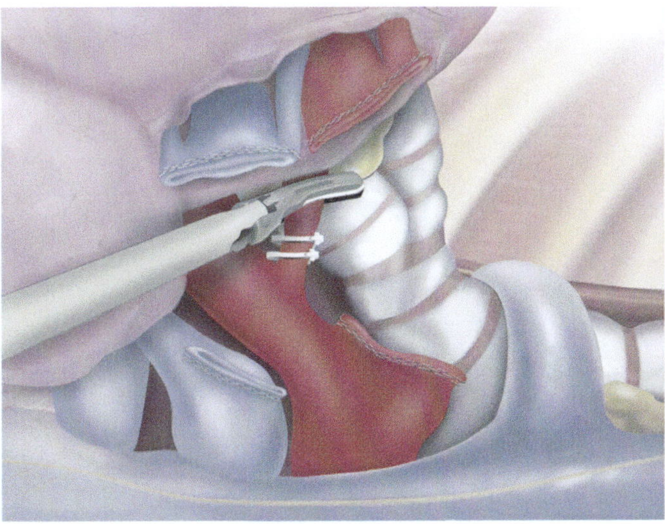

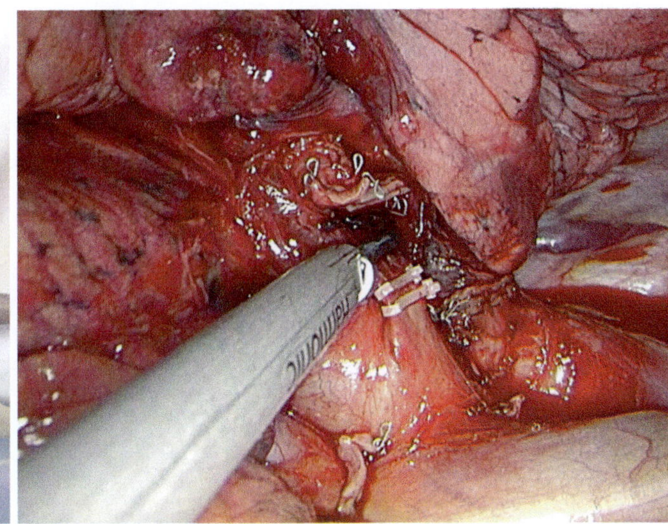

Fig. 11 Drawing and photo showing posterior artery secured with two proximal polymer clips and distally divided with an energy device

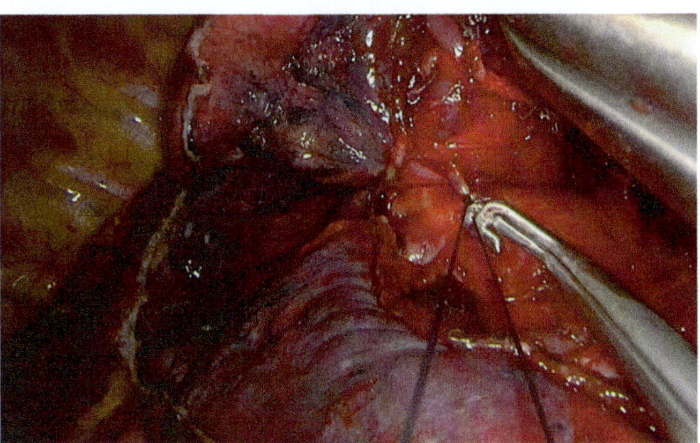

Fig. 12 Posterior artery tied with the help of a thoracoscopic knot pusher

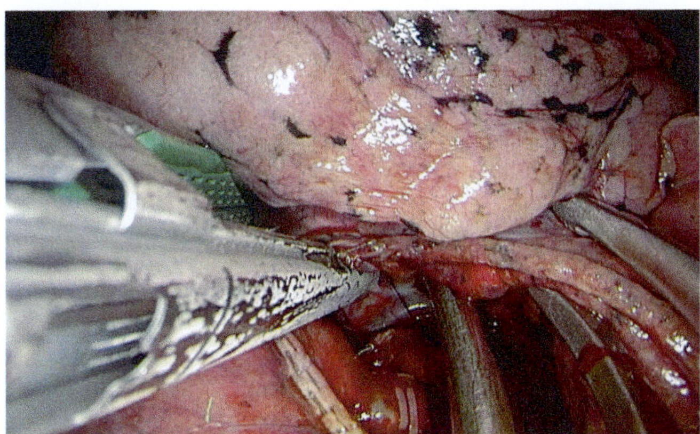

Fig. 13 Completion of the fissure after division of vessels and bronchus (fissureless technique)

Before dividing the fissure it is necessary to see clearly the middle lobe artery and dissect as distal as possible the stump of RUL vein to avoid it being stapled with the fissure.

How to Select the Proper Angle for Stapler Insertion

For a RUL, if we start with the vein and artery in a hilum first approach, we normally retract the lobe to the left, in a caudal direction, so the angle of the stapler should follow the direction of the lung grasper. When we approach the RUL starting the dissection of the vessels in the fissure, the lobe is usually retracted in a cranial position, so the angle for the endostapler will be cranially curved to the grasper retracting the lung.

We recommend to inform the nurse assistant to prepare all the staplers with the angulation according to this rule before the starting the surgery. The endostaplers should always be positioned on the bottom of the wound to allow more stabilization, leaning on the skin and the subcutaneous tissue of the incision.

Uniportal Right Upper Lobectomy

Heron Andrade, Arthur Vieira, and Paula Ugalde Figueroa

Introduction

Over the past two decades, video-assisted thoracoscopic surgery (VATS) has evolved from a diagnostic procedure to a treatment for complex lung cancer cases. VATS is now accepted as a feasible, safe, and effective surgical technique for the treatment of lung cancer [1]. In fact, in current practice guidelines, thoracoscopic surgery is the suggested approach for the treatment of early-stage lung cancer [2, 3]. Decreased blood loss, reduced pain, shorter length of hospital stay, and fewer overall complications are just a few of the many potential benefits of this minimally invasive approach [4]. High-volume centers have not only evolved VATS techniques by performing more complex surgeries using VATS, but have also developed a new approach decreasing the number of incisions to one—the uniportal technique [5–7].

VATS Evolution: From Multiportal to Uniportal

In the early 1990s, video-assisted thoracic procedures were mainly performed through three or more ports. McKenna and colleagues published a series of 1100 VATS lobectomy cases using 3–4 ports with excellent technical results [8]. This paper was considered a landmark for the inclusion of VATS in the thoracic surgery arena. Pushing the boundaries, surgeons from major centers then developed VATS techniques with fewer incisions (fewer ports). D'Amico and colleagues demonstrated the feasibility and safety of VATS using two incisions (one 10-mm port and a working incision of approximately 4 cm) in a series of 500 patients who underwent lobectomy for lung cancer [9]. In 2004, Rocco and colleagues introduced the single-port (uniportal) approach for simple procedures, such as wedge pulmonary resections for the diagnosis of interstitial lung diseases and for the treatment of spontaneous pneumothorax [10]. In 2011, Gonzalez-Rivas and colleagues reported the first lobectomy performed using a uniportal VATS technique [11].

Over the last 5 years, the single-port approach has rapidly gained popularity across Europe and Asia [12]. Li, Akter, and their colleagues demonstrated shorter hospital stays and reduced chest tube drainage with the uniportal technique [13, 14]. However, contradictory results were recently presented in a report from Perna and colleagues, which failed to demonstrate any superiority of the uniportal approach versus a multiple-port approach with regards to postoperative pain, duration of chest tube drainage, length of hospital stay, or the incidence of postoperative complications [15]. Although the methodology of Perna's study has been questioned, it is notable as the first randomized trial to analyze postoperative outcomes according to the number of VATS incisions [16].

Minimally invasive thoracic surgery demands extremely precise movements, a profound knowledge of anatomy, and comfort with specialized equipment to avoid technical complications, especially vascular accidents. Some surgeons believe that it is safer and easier to perform lung surgery through multiple ports; however, there is no data that validates this impression. Because vision is the predominant sense used during a VATS procedure, we believe that the uniportal technique offers a safer approach because the straight, frontal view of the pulmonary hilum elements facilitates a secure dissection. For this reason, the uniportal approach has been our standard VATS approach since January 2014 [7].

The learning curve for proficiency with any VATS procedure can vary according to the complexity of the case, the technical skills of the surgeon, and the surgical volume of both the surgeon and the surgeon's institution. Ideally, the

Electronic Supplementary Material The online version of this chapter (https://doi.org/10.1007/978-981-13-2604-2_21) contains supplementary material, which is available to authorized users.

H. Andrade · A. Vieira · P. U. Figueroa (✉)
Division of Thoracic Surgery, Institut Universitaire de Cardiologie et de Pneumologie de Quebec—Université Laval, Quebec City, QC, Canada
e-mail: paula-antonia.ugalde-figueroa.1@ulaval.ca

D. Gonzalez-Rivas et al. (eds.), *Atlas of Uniportal Video Assisted Thoracic Surgery*,
https://doi.org/10.1007/978-981-13-2604-2_21

surgeon should be able to perform all types of lobectomy and be able to manage an incomplete fissure and pulmonary adhesions. The surgeon's operating time should reach a steady and reasonable duration (for example, less than 3 h). The rate of conversion to thoracotomy should match that seen in the majority of studies in the literature, and intraoperative complications should be comparable with complications that occur using the surgeon's thoracotomy technique. Using VATS lobectomy, even standard cases are technically demanding and have the potential risk of uncontrollable pulmonary hemorrhage. High-volume centers have demonstrated very low rates of complications and conversion to thoracotomy [8, 9]. In our series of 250 uniportal VATS procedures, which included early-stage lung cancer and complex lung resection cases, we converted to thoracotomy in 6.1% of cases [7]. However, when only early-stage lung cancer cases were analyzed, the conversion rate was 2.2% [7].

Indications for Uniportal Lobectomy

Indications for the uniportal lobectomy are the same as those for multiportal VATS. Indications include early-stage (stages I and II) non-small cell lung cancer (NSCLC), infectious disease that results in the destruction or loss of function of a lobe, and pulmonary sequestration.

Contraindications for Uniportal Lobectomy

The contraindications for uniportal lobectomy are mostly relative. With the development of different types of articulated staplers and the experience gained with time, most complex lung resections have been described using uniportal techniques including bronchoplasty, pneumonectomy and arterioplasty [7, 17–19]. The safety of the patient and the comfort of the surgeon must always be the leading factors in determining the surgical approach.

In general, as for any VATS technique, the most common relative contraindication is locally advanced lung cancer. Central tumors invading the pulmonary hilum, tumors invading the chest wall, and tumors invading adjacent structures (such as the vena cava, atrium and aorta) are some examples. Complex pleural adhesions, calcified lymph nodes, and anatomic malformations may also demand the use of more ports or a prophylactic conversion to thoracotomy [20].

Preoperative Planning

Patients should be evaluated regarding their operability and the resectability of their disease. The patient's clinical status determines their operability. Functional evaluation is performed with spirometry to measure preoperative FEV_1 (forced expiratory volume in 1 s) and DLCO (diffusion capacity of the lung for carbon monoxide). Patients with borderline lung function should undergo a cardiopulmonary exercise test to measure peak VO_2 (ventilatory oxygen uptake) and assess possible postoperative complications [2]. Other cardiac exams may be requested depending on the clinical scenario and type of lung resection.

In patients with NSCLC, a complete lung cancer staging is performed with chest computed tomography (CT) scan, positron emission tomography (PET) scan, endobronchial ultrasound (EBUS) or mediastinoscopy, and magnetic resonance imaging (MRI) of the brain [2]. A CT scan with intravenous contrast is extremely useful to evaluate the vascular anatomy, mediastinal and hilar lymph nodes, and the position of the tumor relative to adjacent organs. PET scan is used to evaluate distant and lymph nodal metastasis as well as to identify the metabolic activity of the tumor. EBUS or mediastinoscopy is performed for invasive mediastinal staging [2].

Uniportal Right Upper Lobe Technique for Lung Cancer

Patient Positioning, Uniportal Access, and Lobectomy Overview

We initiate single-lung ventilation under general anesthesia in all our patients. We position the patient in a full lateral decubitus with a breakpoint just above the iliac crest for a hyperextension of the chest. This will enlarge the intercostal spaces facilitating the access to the pleural cavity (Fig. 1). The surgeon and the assistant position themselves in front of the patient, so they will have the same viewing angle, which allows a better coordination of movements inside the chest cavity.

Conventional and dedicated VATS instruments are used along with a 5-mm, 30° camera. A single 3–4 cm incision is made in the fourth intercostal space between the anterior axillary and the median axillary line. In women, we take care to avoid the breast. Access to the pleural cavity is easier when a wound protector is used.

The right upper lobectomy begins with the inspection of the pleural space to ensure resectability of the tumor and the absence of metastatic disease. Subsequently, the following steps are taken to perform the lobectomy through the single port:

1. Ligation of the anterior trunk of the pulmonary artery
2. Transection of right upper lobe bronchus
3. Ligation of right upper lobe pulmonary vein
4. Completion of the fissure
5. Lymphadenectomy

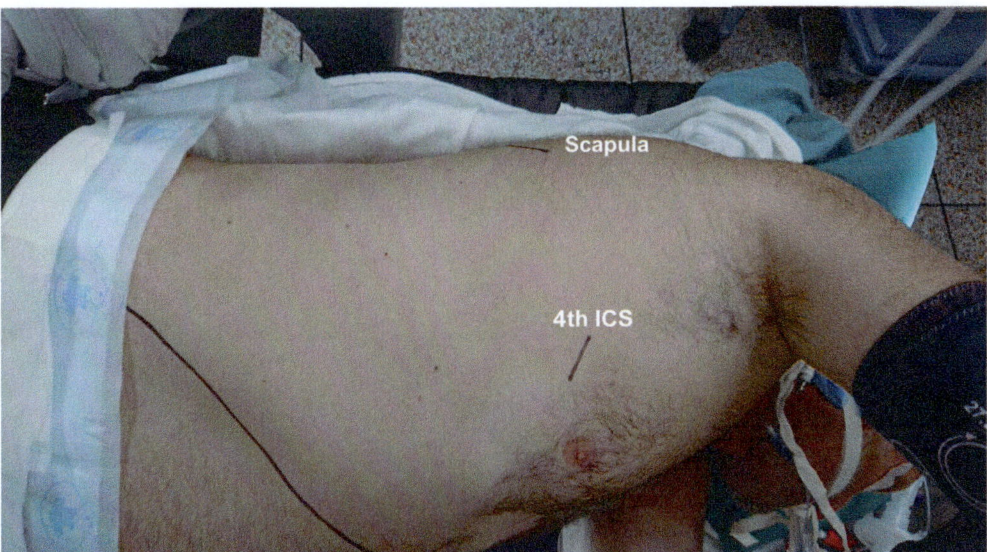

Fig. 1 Patient positioning for a uniportal right upper lobectomy with the scapula and fourth intercostal space (ICS) marked

Ligation of the Pulmonary Artery Anterior Trunk

We position the right upper lobe (RUL) towards the posterior chest wall to expose the anterior and the superior portions of the pulmonary hilum. The mediastinal pleura is opened from the superior pulmonary vein (SPV) towards the posterior portion of the airway. Care is taken to identify the phrenic nerve and the proper plane of dissection between the azygos vein and the superior structures of the pulmonary hilum. The pleura must be dissected all the way to the back wall of the bronchus intermedius (BI), so the carina between the right upper lobe bronchus (RULB) and BI can be identified. This posterior dissection will allow the RUL to be more mobile and allow the RULB to be easily encircled. The dissection can be performed bluntly or with the help of scissors, an electrocautery, or an ultrasonic scalpel. We avoid blunt dissection to decrease bleeding. Repeating the dissection from the SPV towards the airway will progressively expose the SPV, the anterior trunk (AT) of the pulmonary artery and the airway.

With a thoracoscopic dissection instrument, we liberate all adhesions between the SPV and the AT, as well as adhesions between the AT and the airway. It is important to avoid pressure over the artery to prevent hematomas and tearing of the wall of the artery while safely encircling the AT. Hilar and lobar lymph nodes (#10 and #11) can be removed during the vascular dissection and sent for frozen-section analyses. When stapling the AT, only one instrument should be used to apply cranial traction to the lobe. This will result in upright placement of the AT, and the staple device will easily and safely slide behind the artery (Fig. 2). Due to the straight view of the artery afforded by the uniportal approach, it is rarely necessary to articulate the staple device.

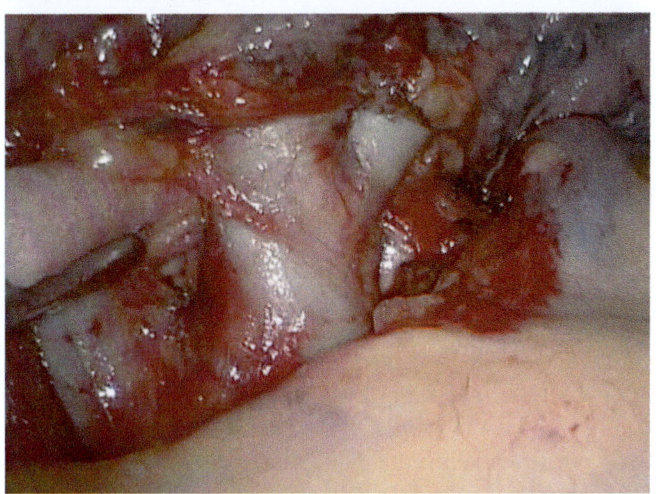

Fig. 2 The dissected anterior trunk (AT) of the pulmonary artery (Boyden's trunk)

Dissection of the Right Upper Lobe Bronchus

The RULB is behind and lateral to the AT. Without changing the position of the instruments, you can proceed with its dissection after the transection of the AT is completed. The RULB can be bluntly dissected with an instrument protecting the pulmonary artery. An interlobar lymph node will be identified at the carina between the RULB and BI. Once this lymph node is removed, the dissection around the bronchus is straightforward, especially if the posterior pleura has been liberated. We apply continuous pressure at the carina of the RULB, towards the posterior chest wall, with a long thoracoscopic blunt dissector. Once we are able to go around the RULB, we release as much of the lung as possible and release the artery from the RULB, so that a staple device can be safely introduced. We usually perform a ventilation test to

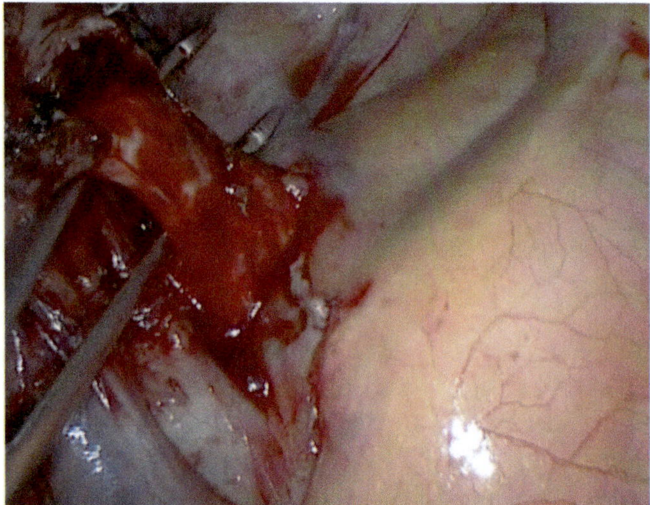

Fig. 3 The dissected right upper lobe bronchus (RULB)

ensure proper stapling. After we transect the RULB, we like to dissect from the bronchial stump towards the BI. This will later facilitate the completion of the fissure (Fig. 3).

Dissection of Right Upper Lobe Vein

Once the AT and the RULB are divided, we reposition the lobe for an anterior dissection. With some posterior traction over the RUL, the superior and inferior pulmonary veins must be identified. In general, the SPV receives the middle lobe vein(s) and the upper lobe vein(s). It is important to identify the proper level of dissection between those two veins to develop the plane that will allow full release the right upper lobe vein (RULV). At the other margin of the RULV, the release must be more delicate because of the proximity between the RULV and the pulmonary artery. Once both borders of the RULV are free, we always pass a vessel loop around the RULV to fully liberate the vein (Fig. 4). Stapling the RULV is the most demanding step of this operation, not only because the vein is directly in front of the working incision, but also because the pulmonary artery is directly behind the vein, which makes it dangerous to pass the staple device around the vein. However, when the vein is largely released from all its adhesions, it becomes mobile and flexible allowing anterior traction with the blade of the staple device for a safe passage around the vein, distant from the artery.

Completion of the Fissure

Once the hilar elements of the lobe have been dissected, the superior lobe should be placed in its anatomic position to allow identification of the fissure. Usually, there is an

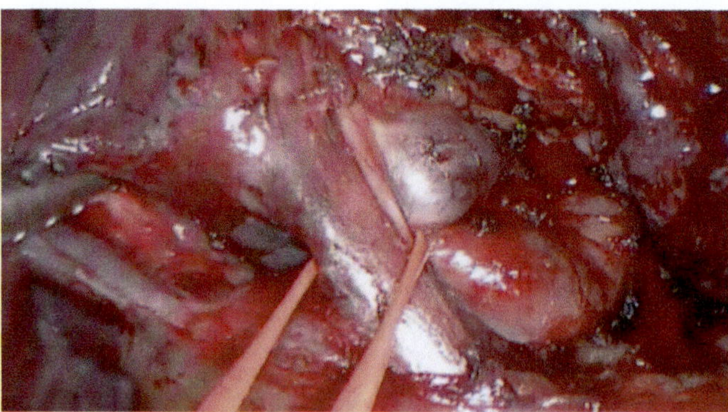

Fig. 4 The dissected right upper lobe vein (RULV), encircled with a vessel loop

outline of the fissure between the lobes, but in the absence of this sign, the middle lobe vein is an important landmark. After placing a couple of staple loads in the minor fissure, the limit between upper and middle lobes will be clearly identified at the pulmonary hilum. We section the parenchyma along the fissure, towards the major fissure, taking care to ensure that the RULB stump stays within the surgical specimen (Fig. 5). It is possible to transect one or two arterial branches (e.g. the posterior ascending artery) along with the fissure (the "*fissureless technique*"). Alternatively, those vessels can be independently ligated with vascular staples.

Lymphadenectomy

We routinely perform hilar and mediastinal lymphadenectomy. We resect the hilar and interlobar lymph nodes when dissecting the hilum and complete the mediastinal lymphadenectomy after the lobectomy. All lymph nodes are sent for frozen-section analysis. When positive lymph nodes are found, we extend the lymphadenectomy.

Final Steps

The lobe can be removed through the uniportal incision if the tumor is smaller than 3 cm, does not infiltrate the visceral pleura, and if a wound protector is used. Otherwise, the resected lobe should be placed inside a disposable bag to avoid contact with the incision or tearing and spillage during removal. We perform an intercostal nerve block intrapleurally from the first to the seventh intercostal space with bupivacaine (0.25%, 3 mL per space) (Fig. 6). Before closing the incision, we insert a 24 F chest tube through the working incision and maintain it in a water seal (Fig. 7). A routine postoperative bronchoscopy is done for airway toilette while the patient is still intubated.

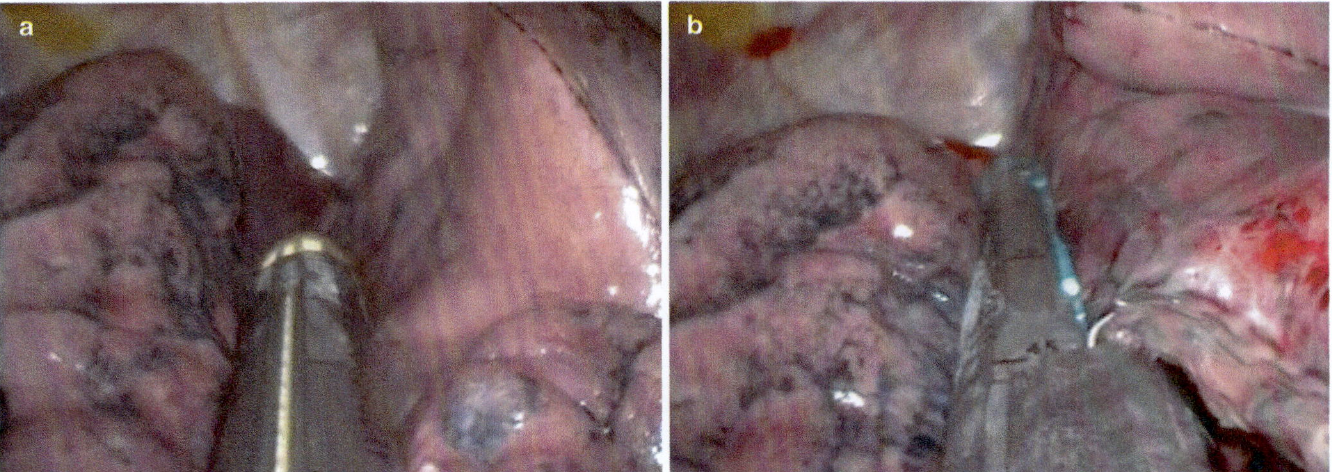

Fig. 5 Stapling the fissure between the upper and middle lobes. (**a**) Stapling the minor fissure; (**b**) Stapling the major fissure

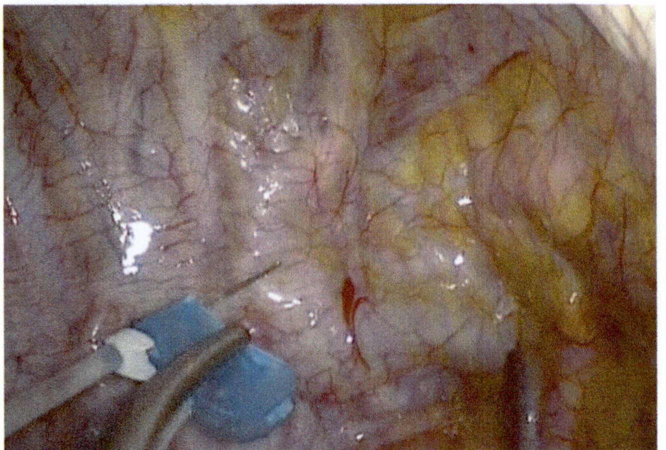

Fig. 6 Intercostal nerve blockade

Postoperative Care

Early ambulation after surgery, efficient analgesia, and respiratory exercises are key steps for the patient's proper recovery. The drain is removed in the absence of an air leak and if the drainage is less than 300 mL in 24 h.

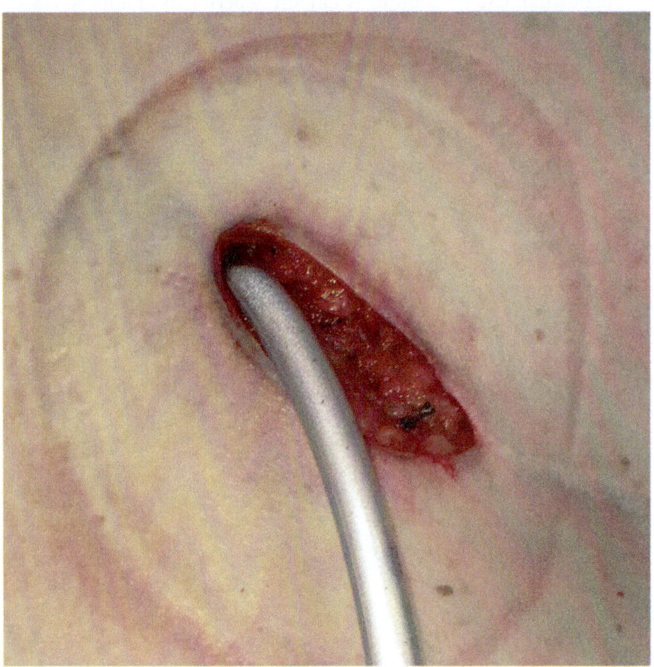

Fig. 7 A 24 F drain inserted into the incision before closure

References

1. Swanson SJ, Herndon JE, D'Amico TA, Demmy TL, McKenna RJ, Green MR, et al. Video-assisted thoracic surgery lobectomy: report of CALGB 39802 – a prospective, multi-institution feasibility study. J Clin Oncol. 2007;25:4993–7.
2. National Comprehensive Cancer Network (NCCN). NCCN Clinical Practice Guidelines in Oncology (NCCN Guidelines®). Non-small cell lung cancer. Version 4.2016. Jan 12, 2016. Abstract available at http://www.ncc.org/professionals/physician_gls/pdf/nscl.pdf.
3. Howington JA, Blum MG, Chang AC, Balekian AA, Murthy SC. Treatment of stage I and II non-small cell lung cancer: diagnosis and management of lung cancer, 3rd ed: American College of Chest Physicians evidence-based clinical practice guidelines. Chest. 2013;143(Suppl 5):e278S–313S.
4. Scott WJ, Allen MS, Darling G, Meyers B, Decker PA, Putnam JB, McKenna RW, Landrenau RJ, Jones DR, Inculet RI, Malthaner RA. Video-assisted thoracic surgery versus open lobectomy for lung cancer: a secondary analysis of data from the American College of Surgeons Oncology Group Z0030 randomized clinical trial. J Thorac Cardiovasc Surg. 2010;139(4):976–83.
5. Kara HV, Balderson SS, D'Amico TA. Modified uniportal video-assisted thoracoscopic lobectomy: Duke approach. Ann Thorac Surg. 2014;98:2239–41.
6. Battoo A, Jahan A, Yang Z, Nwogu CE, Yendamuri SS, Dexter EU, Hennon MW, Picone AL, Demmy TL. Thoracoscopic pneumonectomy: an 11-year experience. Chest. 2014;146:1300–9.
7. Drevet G, Ugalde Figueroa P. Uniportal video-assisted thoracoscopic surgery: safety, efficacy and learning curve during

the first 250 cases in Quebec, Canada. Ann Cardiothorac Surg. 2016;5(2):100–6.
8. RJ MK Jr, Houck W, Fuller CB. Video-assisted thoracic surgery lobectomy: experience with 1,100 cases. Ann Thorac Surg. 2006;81(2):421–5.
9. Onaitis MW, Petersen RP, Balderson SS, Toloza E, Burfeind WR, Harpole DH Jr, D'Amico TA. Thoracoscopic lobectomy is a safe and versatile procedure: experience with 500 consecutive patients. Ann Surg. 2006;244(3):420–5.
10. Rocco G, Martin Ucar A, Passera E. Uniportal VATS wedge pulmonary resections. Ann Thorac Surg. 2004;77:726–8.
11. Gonzalez D, Paradela M, Garcia J, de la Torre M. Single-port video-assisted thoracoscopic lobectomy. Interact Cardiovasc Thorac Surg. 2011;12:514–5.
12. Gonzalez-Rivas D. VATS lobectomy: surgical evolution from conventional VATS to uniportal approach. Sci World J. 2012;2012:780842.
13. Li C, Ma H, He J, Ni B, Xu C, Zhao J. Clinical analysis of thoracoscopic lobectomy in the treatment of peripheral lung cancer with single utility port. Chin J Lung Cancer. 2013;16:487–91.
14. Akter F, Routledge T, Toufektzian L, Attia R. In minor and major thoracic procedures is uniport superior to multiport video-assisted thoracoscopic surgery? Interact Cardiovasc Thorac Surg. 2015;20(4):550–5.
15. Perna V, Carvajal AF, Torrecilla JA, Gigirey O. Uniportal video-assisted thoracoscopic lobectomy versus other video-assisted thoracoscopic lobectomy techniques: a randomized study. Eur J Cardiothorac Surg. 2016;50:411–5.
16. Gonzalez-Rivas D, D'Amico T, Jiang G, Sihoe A. Uniportal video-assisted thoracic surgery: a call for better evidence, not just more evidence. Eur J Cardiothorac Surg. 2016;50(3):416–7.
17. Gonzalez-Rivas D, Fernandez R, Fieira E, et al. Uniportal video-assisted thoracoscopic bronchial sleeve lobectomy: first report. J Thorac Cardiovasc Surg. 2013;145:1676–7.
18. Gonzalez-Rivas D, Delgado M, Fieira E, et al. Double sleeve uniportal video-assisted thoracoscopic lobectomy for non-small cell lung cancer. Ann Cardiothorac Surg. 2014;3:E2.
19. Gonzalez-Rivas D, Delgado M, Fieira E, et al. Uniportal video-assisted thoracoscopic pneumonectomy. J Thorac Dis. 2013;5(Suppl 3):S246–52.
20. D'Amico TA. Operative techniques in early-stage lung cancer. J Natl Compr Cancer Netw. 2010;8:807–13.

Left Upper Lobectomy

Chengwu Liu and Lunxu Liu

Abstract

Uniportal video-assisted thoracoscopic surgery (VATS) is an emerging technique, which can be laid into the spectrum of great efforts achieved in minimally invasive thoracic surgery. Although technical difficulties due to limited access and angulation do exist, great progress has been achieved during the past decade. Uniportal VATS is now widely used to perform different lobectomies, among which left upper lobectomy may be the most technique demanding one. This chapter aims to illustrate methods and techniques for uniportal VATS left upper lobectomy by single direction approach.

Introduction

Uniportal video-assisted thoracoscopic surgery (VATS) was first introduced by Rocco *et al.* in 2004 for simple thoracic procedures such as pleural biopsy, pneumothorax, and lung wedge resection, *et al.* [1]. In 2011, Gonzalez *et al.* reported the first case of uniportal VATS lobectomy [2]. Although complicated cases of sleeve or even double-sleeve lobectomy were reported within very short periods of time [3], there were still many centers in which uniportal VATS lobectomy was not well practiced due to technical difficulties.

Due to limited access and angulation for operation, uniportal VATS lobectomy seemed to be more technique demanding than commonly used multiportal VATS lobectomy. Special methods and strategies were necessary to perform a smooth uniportal VATS lobectomy. As admitted by most thoracic surgeons, left upper lobectomy might be the most technique challenging work compared with other lobectomies. In this chapter, detail techniques of uniportal VATS left upper lobectomy by single direction approach would be described, and other approach would also be mentioned. It might be helpful for facilitating a beginning in practice of this procedure.

Electronic Supplementary Material The online version of this chapter (https://doi.org/10.1007/978-981-13-2604-2_22) contains supplementary material, which is available to authorized users.

C. Liu · L. Liu (✉)
Department of Thoracic Surgery, West China Hospital, Sichuan University, Chengdu, China

Indications and Preoperative Preparation

The indications of uniportal VATS lobectomy are almost equal to multi-portal VATS lobectomy including both benign and malignant pulmonary diseases. The benign indications include, infectious pulmonary diseases such as fungal and/or tuberculosis infections, bronchiectasis, congenital malformations, and so on. All patients underwent routine systemic function assessments, including blood tests and cardiopulmonary function text preoperatively. For cases with malignancy, contrast enhanced computerized tomography (CT) scanning of the thorax and the upper abdomen, CT scanning or magnetic resonance imaging of the brain, bone scintigraphy, and bronchoscopy would be administered to exclude the candidates for curative surgery.

Anesthesia and Analgesia

General anesthesia with double-lumen endotracheal intubation was administered to each patient to accomplish appropriate single lung ventilation. Most patients were extubated immediately after the operation and transferred to the ward while those with severe comorbidities would be transferred to intensive care unit (ICU) for further monitoring. Ropivacaine (7.5 mg/mL) was given to each patient during the wound closure to accomplish extrapleural intercostal nerve block anesthesia. All patients were provided with multidisciplinary analgesia including patient-controlled analgesia (PCA), transdermal and/or oral analgesics, postoperatively.

D. Gonzalez-Rivas et al. (eds.), *Atlas of Uniportal Video Assisted Thoracic Surgery*,
https://doi.org/10.1007/978-981-13-2604-2_22

Positioning

Generally, each patient was placed in a folding knife gesture (with both of the cranial side and caudal side pushed down) in the right lateral decubitus position. During operation, the surgeon and the thoracoscope assistant stand on the abdominal side of the patient while the other assistant stood at the back side of the patient. The thoracoscope assistant stood at a foot-stool to hold the thoracoscope more comfortable and avoid interrupting with the surgeon.

Incision and Instrumentation

During uniportal VATS lobectomy, management of the hilar structures and dissection of the mediastinal lymph nodes (for cases of malignancy) would be the major procedures. Since there would be only one port available, both of the two major procedures should be taken into account cautiously. Appropriate distance between the incision and the operating area and optimal angulation would facilitate the operation. Therefore, the placement of the incision should take both the distance and angle into the consideration. Even though there might be anatomic variation, the left hilum would be close to the level of 4th–5th intercostal space. To provide facilities for procedures around the hilum, upper and lower mediastinal areas, the incision (3–5 cm) was always placed in the fourth intercostal space just anterior to the latissimus dorsi with arms raised anteriorly. A soft plastic wound protector was applied to the incision without rib-spreading (Fig. 1).

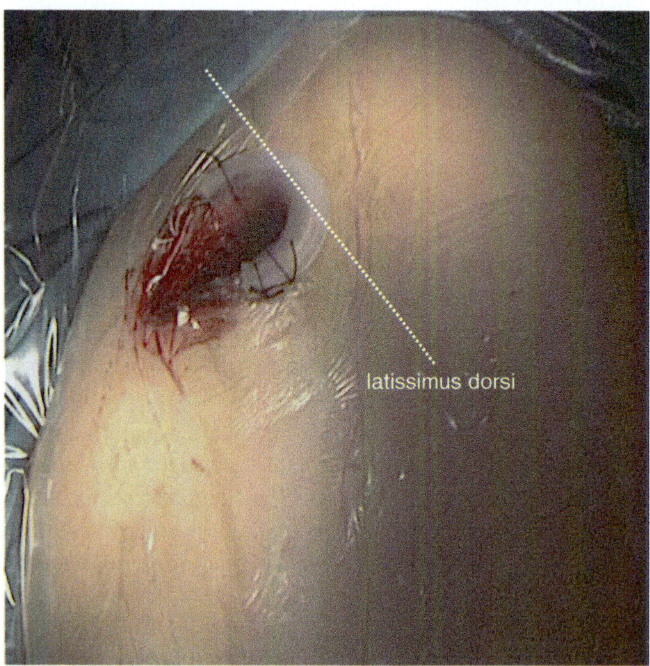

Fig. 1 Incision

The protector would minimize iatrogenic touch during the introduction of instruments to the surgical field, especially in the cases of patients with thick chest wall. A commonly used 10-mm 30 degree thoracoscope was introduced in and placed at the posterior part of the incision during the whole procedure. The main surgical instruments included thin and long ring forceps (double articulated), curved metal endoscopic suction, energy devices (electro-cautery hook and harmonic scalpel), flexible linear stapler, and hem-o-lock.

Thoracic Exploration

The observation view in uniportal VATS differed from traditional multiportal VATS. Since the incision was located at the anterior part of the chest close to the anterior part of the hilum, the posterior and inferior parts of the thoracic cavity were far from the surgical incision. Therefore, the thoracic cavity required careful exploration to identify any unexpected invasion, metastases, and adhesions, which might cause severe bleeding if they were snapped carelessly. Only after confirmation of the resectability should we proceed with the procedure.

Left Upper Lobectomy

"Single Direction" Left Upper Lobectomy

After exploration the procedure generally continued in an anterior approach following the strategy of "single direction". The concept of "single direction" was first proposed by us during triportal VATS lobectomy [4]. Due to different patterns of operation, the strategy of "single direction" used in uniportal was different from that in triportal VATS lobectomy. During triportal VATS left upper lobectomy, the procedure was proceeded in the direction of ventrum-to-dorsum. However, during uniportal VATS left upper lobectomy the direction of procedure was changed, that was from anterior-superior to posterior-inferior. We also named it as "tangential single-direction" strategy (Fig. 2). Although we changed the direction of procedure, the key points of "single direction lobectomy" were still the same, including dissecting from superficial to deep structure, no need of bypass, no repeated turnover of the lobes, and the fissure be divided last. This technique was a fissureless technique. For uniportal VATS left upper lobectomy, the procedure was initiated at the hilum with the first arterial branch (truncus apicoanterior branch) managed first. After that, any structure which came out first would be handled preferentially. An example of sequence of resection was as following: the truncus apicoanterior branch, the superior pulmonary vein, the posterior arterial branches, the left upper bronchus, the anterior

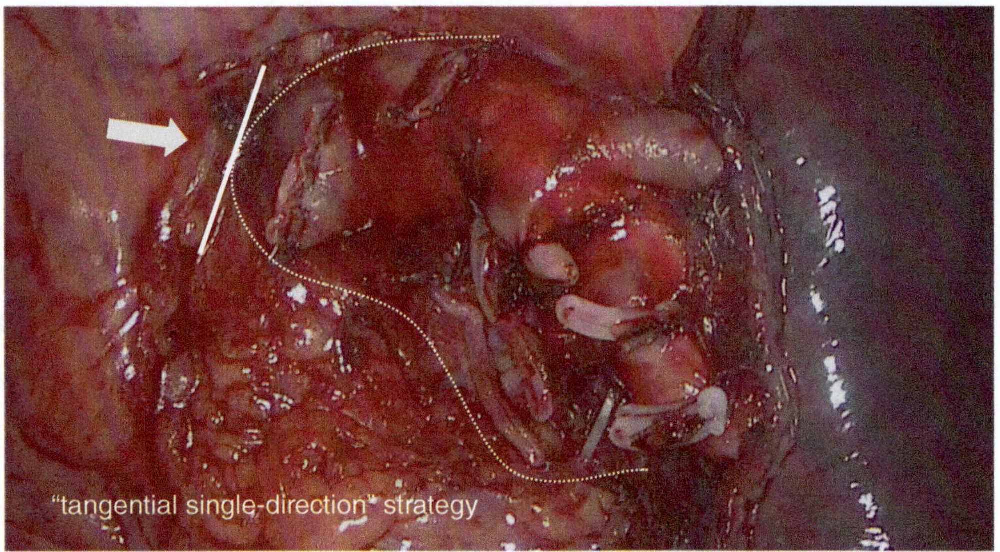

Fig. 2 "Tangential single-direction" strategy

part of the oblique fissure, the lingular branch, and the posterior part of the oblique fissure.

Management of the Truncus Apicoanterior Branch

The left upper lobe was first retracted dorsally using ring forceps. The procedure was initiated with opening of the mediastinal pleura posterior to the phrenic nerve and anterior to the hilar structures. The hilum would be released by dissecting tissues around the hilum up to the upper border of the pulmonary artery trunk and down to the inferior pulmonary vein. Then dissection was performed around the pulmonary artery with the upper lobe retracted toward left posterior costophrenic angle to dissect and transect the truncus apicoanterior branch first.

The left pulmonary artery passed anterosuperiorly along the left main bronchus and branched its first segmental artery before it passed distally and posterosuperiorly over the left upper lobe bronchus and into the interlobar fissure. The procedure continued with dissection of the truncus apicoanterior branch of the upper lobe. It was first dissociated from the surrounding tissues. Sometimes there might be serious lymph node issues. In that case, dissection should be performed carefully to avoid injury to the artery or the bronchus. In serious cases, clamp the left main pulmonary artery in advance would be helpful to avoid massive bleeding. After the lymph nodes been dissociated from the artery, they could be retrieved immediately or pushed to the distal part and would be harvested together with the lobe. After dissection, a modified Kelly forceps would emerge through the space between the branch and the upper lobe bronchus. Then the linear stapler was placed directly or facilitated by a traction belt, which was used for intracavitary overhanging of the branch. The truncus apicoanterior branch would be transected. The truncus apicoanterior branch often arose from the anterior portion of the vessel and sometimes the trunk of it was too short. Therefore, care must be taken when placing the linear stapler to avoid laceration of the vessel especially at the initial part of the branch. Sometimes there might be two separate branches feeding the apical and anterior segments. If the branches were too slender, proximal ligation with silk suture or hem-o-lock might also be methods of choice. After that ultrasonic scalpel would be used to transect them.

Management of the Superior Pulmonary Vein

After the truncus apicoanterior branch been transected, the superior pulmonary vein would emerge as the next target to be managed. Dissection was performed along the upper and lower border of the superior pulmonary vein via hook electro-cautery. A modified Kelly forceps would emerge through the space between the vein and the bronchus lying behind. At last, the linear stapler was placed to transect the superior pulmonary vein. When placing the linear stapler a traction belt either using a silk suture or robber belt might be helpful. We called it as intrathoracic vertical overhanging technique: after the target vein been dissected, the traction belt was used to twine the target and a Kelly forceps was inserted to clamp the belt for overhanging the target vertically; then the linear stapler was inserted and placed appropriately facilitated by changing the traction angle in real time; finally, the traction belt was removed followed by the target been divided [5]. During this process, it's important to identify the inferior pulmonary vein before we transect the superior vein because sometimes there might be no separate inferior pulmonary vein. Generally, the superior pulmonary vein was wide with its upper border overlying the pulmonary artery and its lower border overlying the lower lobe bronchus. Therefore, there should be sufficient length of the venous trunk dissected for better placing the linear stapler.

Management of the Posterior Arterial Branches

After the superior pulmonary vein been transected, the procedure was moved to manage the posterior arterial branches, for which it's often not suitable to place the linear stapler due to limited space or inappropriate angle. Therefore, after dissection they were commonly managed via ligation with silk suture or hem-o-lock and transected by ultrasonic scalpel. The number and diameter of the posterior branches varied among patients. Extreme care must be taken during management of them.

Management of the Left Upper Bronchus

After managing the posterior arterial branches, the procedure would continue with management of the bronchus. With the posterior arterial branches been transected there would be appropriate space and angulation for placement of linear stapler to transect the upper bronchus. As mentioned before the upper border of the bronchus was previously dissected. Then the bifurcate was dissected. During this procedure several notes should be noticed. There were always bronchial feeding arteries running along the upper border of the left main bronchus. Caution should be taken when performing operation in that area. And of course they could be ligated in advance to avoid bothersome bleeding. Lymph nodes located besides the upper border of the upper bronchus would be retrieved or pushed to the distal part. Then the lymph nodes located at the corner between the upper bronchus and the lower bronchus would be meticulously resected. After the upper lobe bronchus became "naked", the modified Kelly forceps was used to pass through the posterior space between the artery and the upper bronchus. A traction belt could be used for facilitating placement of the linear stapler or not. At last, it would be transected by the linear stapler. It must be noted that the stapler should not be placed too far from or too close to the bifurcate to make sure of a perfect stump. If the stump was too short, it might break due to high tension. If the stump was too long, there might be residual cavity left, which provided place for recurrent infection.

Management of the Fissure and the Lingular Arterial Branch

After the upper bronchus been transected, there were only the lingular arterial branch and the fissure left. The anterior part of the fissure would be completed first before we managed the lingular arterial branch. There might be two situations. The first, for cases with complete fissure, the visceral pleura was opened directly using hook electro-cautery or harmonic scalpel to expose the interlobar pulmonary artery. The second, for cases with hypoplastic fissure, a linear stapler was necessitated to complete the fissure. Identification of the lingular branch and the branch feeding the superior segment of the lower lobe was the landmark to continue procedure. Most of time the lingular branch were ligated proximally with silk suture or hem-o-lock and transected via ultrasonic scalpel or transected by linear stapler directly. At last, the posterior part of the fissure was completed by linear stapler. When dissecting the fissure, it's important to make sure that the staple line covered both surfaces of the lung and no remaining parenchymal of the upper lobe would be left after the fire of the staple. Here the lobectomy was completed.

Hybrid Approach Left Upper Lobectomy

Although the strategy of "single direction" fit well with most uniportal VATS lobectomies, we didn't stick to it because there were variations when performing left upper lobectomy. Sometimes we'd also like to use a hybrid approach to complete it. The procedure was generally initiated in the anterior aspect of hilum. The superior pulmonary vein or the truncus apicoanterior branch would be managed first. Following the strategy of "single direction" we'd proceed to the posterior arterial branches. However, if the posterior branches arose from the trunk too far behind, it would be difficult to manage them rounding the left upper bronchus. In such situation we'd choose to continue the procedure in a posterior approach. The left upper lobe would be retracted forward to expose the interlobar fissure. There might be two situations. The first, for cases with complete fissure, the visceral pleura was opened directly to expose the interlobar pulmonary artery. The second, if the fissure was hypoplastic, linear stapler would be used to complete it. The anterior part was often opened first followed by the posterior part. Identification of the lingular branch and the branch feeding the superior segment of the lower lobe was important for the surgeon to continue procedure. The lingular branch and the posterior arterial branches would be managed sequentially. After managing the pulmonary vein and artery, the management of the bronchus would be easy because there would be no impediment left behind when placing the linear stapler. During this process the upper lobe would be pulled up and the connective tissues around the bronchus would be dissected. After the upper lobe bronchus became "naked", it would be transected by the linear stapler. Until here the lobectomy had been completed.

Other Procedure

The specimen was taken out via a self-made protective bag using a common rubber glove, which was cheap, effective, and readily available. The specimen would be sent for frozen-section pathological examination. If the lesion was malignant, systemic mediastinal lymphadenectomy would be performed. When doing this we preferred the method of "non-grasping en bloc mediastinal lymph node dissection" [6]. After checking active bleeding and air leakage, a 28-Fr chest tube with side holes was inserted to the top of the thoracic cavity. The tube was located at the posterior part of the incision. The chest tube would be removed when there was no air leakage and the volume of drainage was less than 300 mL per day postoperatively. Each patient would be discharged with no main complications.

Conclusions

Uniportal VATS left upper lobectomy is a technique demanding operation. Although there might be various methods and techniques among surgeons, optimized procedure and meticulous operation are necessary to complete a good uniportal VATS left upper lobectomy. The strategy of "single direction" fits well with uniportal VATS lobectomy.

References

1. Rocco G, Martin-Ucar A, Passera E. Uniportal VATS wedge pulmonary resections. Ann Thorac Surg. 2004;77:726–8.
2. Gonzalez D, Paradela M, Garcia J, et al. Single-port video-assisted thoracoscopic lobectomy. Interact Cardiovasc Thorac Surg. 2011;12:514–5.
3. Tu CC, Hsu PK. Global development and current evidence of uniportal thoracoscopic surgery. J Thorac Dis. 2016;8:S308–18.
4. Liu L, Che G, Pu Q, et al. A new concept of endoscopic lung cancer resection: single-direction thoracoscopic lobectomy. Surg Oncol. 2010;19:e71–7.
5. Guo C, Liu C, Lin F, et al. Intrathoracic vertical overhanging approach for placement of an endo-stapler during single-port video-assisted thoracoscopic lobectomy. Eur J Cardiothorac Surg. 2016;49(Suppl 1):i84–6.
6. Liu C, Ma L, Guo C, et al. Non-grasping en bloc mediastinal lymph node dissection through uniportal video-assisted thoracic surgery for lung cancer surgery. J Thorac Dis. 2016;8:2956–9.

Left VATS Upper Lobectomy

Marco Scarci, Benedetta Bedetti, Luca Bertolaccini, Ilaria Righi, Davide Patrini, and Roberto Crisci

The left upper lobectomy is probably one of the most difficult to perform by uniportal approach because of the variable vascular anatomy and, sometime, the unfavourable angle to insert staplers. In this chapter we aim to provide a simple guidance on how to safely perform a uniportal left upper lobectomy sharing few tips and tricks.

Patient Positioning

Unlike a thoracotomy, in uniportal VATS surgery correct patient positioning is essential to facilitate surgery. The hip of the patient is at the level of the table break. Such manoeuvre permits maximum separation of the ribs. The chest is then parallel to the floor. Some authors put the upper arm on a gutter, but we believe that such device, whilst providing a better stability to the patient, limits greatly the movement of the thoracoscope. For that reason, we suggest to keep the arms together between two normal pillows. This approach also allows exposure of the forearms should an arterial/venous line becomes necessary and limits the stretching of the brachial plexus thus reducing the risk of iatrogenic injury.

Electronic Supplementary Material The online version of this chapter (https://doi.org/10.1007/978-981-13-2604-2_23) contains supplementary material, which is available to authorized users.

M. Scarci (✉) · D. Patrini
Thoracic Surgery Unit, S. Gerardo Hospital, Monza, Italy
e-mail: m.scarci@asst-monza.it

B. Bedetti
Malteser Hospital, Bonn, Germany

L. Bertolaccini
Department of Thoracic Surgery, AUSL Romagna Teaching Hospital, Ravenna, Italy

I. Righi
IRCSS Cà Granda Maggiore Hospital, Milan, Italy

R. Crisci
Thoracic Surgery Unit, "G. Mazzini" Hospital, University of L'Aquila, Teramo, Italy

It is also of paramount importance to secure the patient to the table in two positions: the hip and the legs. This is because in uniportal VATS the table is tilted to facilitate exposure.

Port Position

We start with the utility incision at the level of the fifth intercostal space, usually in front of the anterior edge of the latissimus dorsi, one intercostal space below an imaginary line between the tip of the scapula and the nipple (Fig. 1). Especially at the beginning of the uniportal experience, a surgeon might be tempted to move the incision to the fourth intercostal space in the hope to facilitate dissection of the

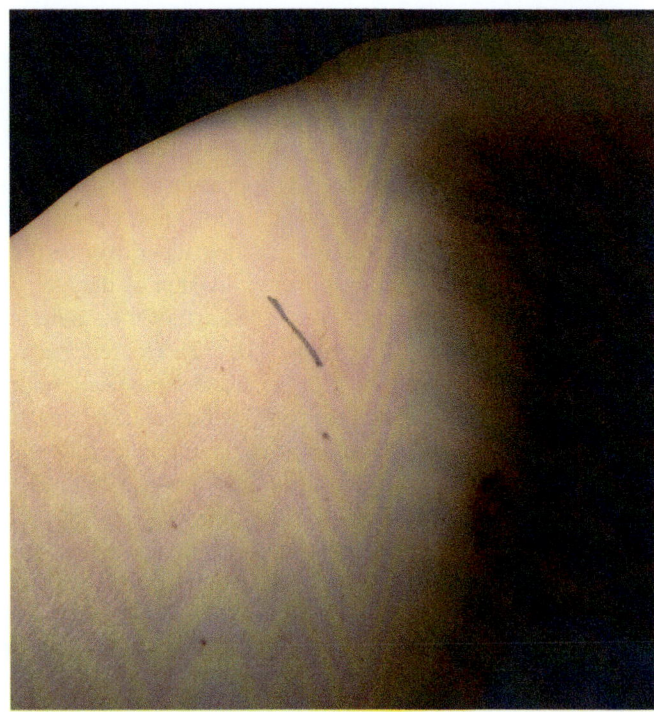

Fig. 1 Patient and port position

D. Gonzalez-Rivas et al. (eds.), *Atlas of Uniportal Video Assisted Thoracic Surgery*,
https://doi.org/10.1007/978-981-13-2604-2_23

artery. Whilst this might be the case, the introduction of the staplers and dissection/division of the superior pulmonary vein becomes very tedious and challenging. We would also recommend keeping the camera, especially with an inexperienced assistant, in the superior part of the incision using an elastic vessel sling clipped to the surgical drapes and passed around the scope.

Even if the creation of the port might seem a trivial procedure, particular care must be taken to avoid oozing from the muscle as, during a lengthy procedure, the blood collecting into the chest will absorb the light and hinder the dissection of the hilar structures. We tend to split the muscles along their fibres.

Procedural Steps

At this point the hemithorax is carefully examined for signs of pleural spread or other conditions that would preclude resectability or a VATS procedure.

We start the dissection incising the inferior pulmonary ligament with an energy device or hook diathermy (when the angle is not favourable for the jaws of the energy device). Care must be taken not to injury the descending aorta which lies immediately behind. The reason for such manoeuvre is threefold: (1) to perform a lymphadenectomy of station 8 and 9, (2) To expose the inferior pulmonary vein to confirm the anatomy and (3) to facilitate further posterior dissection of the hilar structures. The dissection then proceeds anteriorly to identify the superior pulmonary vein and the truncus anterior. There is usually a station 10 lymph node which needs to be removed to facilitate the subsequent division of the vessel. To avoid vascular injuries, we prefer to have a rough idea of the position of the left upper lobe vessels and then proceed with sequential dissection and division clearing the vessels' fascia. Unlike multiport approach, almost always the truncus anterior is dissected and divided first (Video 1). This is especially true if the truncus lies superiorly to the superior edge of the vein. In this case division of the artery first is mandatory to allows the safe passage of the stapler's anvil during division of the vein (Video 2). On few occasions, the artery and vein lie roughly at the same level, with the vein partially obscuring the access to the truncus. In such cases we divide the vein first as passage of the stapler is usually fine. In our view the use of a powered stapler is safer and tends to reduce the chance of vascular injuries.

We use a specifically designed right angle dissector with the tips slightly slanted. This provide excellent visualization of the tips as they pass below the vessels. Particular care must be taken in evaluating the best angle of approach avoiding excessive upward angulation of the tips, which might result in vascular injury.

Although not strictly necessary, especially using curved staplers, it is advisable, at the beginning of the uniportal experience, to encircle the vessels with a silicone vessels loop to aid retraction and safe stapler insertion. Some surgeons use a silk tie as this does not need to be removed and the stapler can fire through it. We would discourage from such approach as removing the silk tie can cause a sawing damage of the vessels' back wall and, if stapled onto the vessel can create a traction point with potential for iatrogenic damage during dissection of further structures.

Once the artery is divided, the inferior and superior border of the upper lobe vein are dissected and encircled. Especially in the case of left upper lobectomy, pulling the vein toward the operator facilitates the passage of the stapler (Video 2). A similar result can be achieved inserting a curved sucker behind the vessel to retract and protect the artery below. To facilitate the retraction of the lung it is possible to divide, if grossly incomplete, the fissure between upper and lower lobe.

Once the vein and the truncus have been divided we continue to divide a further one or two arterial vessels in a clockwise direction. They can be divided between two polymer clips or with staplers. Generally speaking, no hilar structure requires an angulation of the stapler of more than 30 degrees.

We then proceed with the dissection of the fissure. When that is complete it is easy to isolate and divide the lingula branch (Video 3). In case of complex or fused fissure we recommend to avoid dissection through the lung parenchyma, in the open surgery fashion. This creates a bothersome oozing which precludes further dissection. Instead we would recommend taking advantage of the view afforded by the uniportal approach. The anterior portion of the fissure is divided with a stapler, if grossly incomplete, or energy device if thinner, then the pulmonary artery is isolated adopting a bottom-up approach. Behind the two veins, the bifurcation of the bronchi is identified, the pulmonary artery lies just supero-anteriorly. The wall of the artery is followed upward to identify its roof and then a tunnel is created on top of it to allow the passage of the anvil of the stapler (Video 4). In this way the fissure is divided without causing annoying airleak. Eventually the interlobar pulmonary artery is followed backward to identify the lingula branch that is eventually divided.

The division of the lingula and the truncus allow extra mobility of the pulmonary artery, which drops down thus reducing the risk of accidental injury during dissection of the bronchus.

Division of the upper lobe bronchus is the most difficult manoeuvre in a left upper lobectomy. Lymphnodes, if present, are swiped toward the specimen or removed. There are four potential ways to deal with the bronchus:

1. If all the arterial branches are divided, a stapler is inserted across the bronchus which is then easily divided.
2. Another option is to open the bronchus sharply, retract on the stump and to dissect hidden arterial branches and then close the bronchus with a stapler or sutures.

3. Alternatively, it is possible to use a TA stapler if the angle is not favourable (Video 5).
4. Lastly it is possible to run a stapler in the same fashion of the three ports approach, but we would recommend against such technique as the risk of injuring the artery behind is quite high.

Eventually, once all the structures have been divided, the back portion of the fissure is complete front to back with multiple stapler loads. Care must be taken to stay always above the interlobar pulmonary artery. Moreover, it is advisable to pull the lung into the stapler rather than push the stapler through, to avoid the risk of accidental damage to the underlying PA or disrupt arterial stumps.

The lobe is then extracted with an endobag. We use a bag with a rigid aluminium rim that opens up inside the chest. This is anguled in such way to keep the ring parallel to the diaphragm and allow enough space for the bag to open and to insert the lobe. We usually just grab one edge of the lobe flip it inside the bag, then close the bag loop around to avoid spillage.

Further Reading

1. Gonzalez-Rivas D, Fieira E, Delgado M, Mendez L, Fernandez R, de la Torre M. Uniportal video-assisted thoracoscopic lobectomy. J Thorac Dis. 2013;5(Suppl 3):S234–45.
2. Feng M, Lin M, Shen Y, Wang H. Uniportal video-assisted thoracic surgery for left upper lobe: single-direction lobectomy with systematic lymphadenectomy. J Thorac Dis. 2016;8(8):2281–3.
3. Nadal SB, Munoz CG, De Jesus Venegas JJ, Mafe J. Uniportal left upper lobectomy with totally incomplete fissure. CTSnet video article: https://www.ctsnet.org/article/uniportal-left-upper-lobectomy-totally-incomplete-fissure.

Uniportal Video-Assisted Thoracoscopic Segmentectomy

Dong Xie, Konstantinos Marios Soultanis, Xuefei Hu, and Yuming Zhu

Introduction

Anatomic segmentectomies are usually indicated for early staged lung cancer, benign tumors, or pulmonary metastases, when the purpose is resecting the lesion while sparing parenchyma. VATS pulmonary segmentectomy became more popular and achieved through various additional techniques including preoperative localization and the identification of the intersegmental plane. The single-port VATS technique was first pioneered by Rocco and colleagues [1]. Gonzalez-Rivas et al. developed the uniportal technique for VATS major pulmonary resections include the segmentectomies since 2010 [2–5]. In 2016 the Shanghai Pulmonary hospital team published the largest number of uniportal VATS anatomic resections reported in a single institution [6].

Shih et al. compared the early stage outcomes of VATS segmentectomy using a multi-port technique versus a single-port technique. Single-port VATS segmentectomy yielded comparable surgical outcomes to multi-port segmentectomy for primary lung cancer [7]. The anatomic segmentectomies are included intentional operation and compromise operation.

Indication and Preoperative Evaluation

Routine preoperative evaluation included computed tomography (CT) of the chest and upper abdomen, pulmonary function tests, and flexible bronchoscopy. Brain magnetic resonance imaging (MRI), bone scintigraphy and positron emission tomography (PET) scan were carried out if malignant tumor was suspected. Patients with enlarged mediastinal lymph nodes at the CT scan or high SUV uptake at the PET CT were scheduled for mediastinoscopy or transbronchial needle aspiration preoperatively to exclude N2 disease.

Indications for VATS segmentectomy were cT1aN0M0 nodule less than 2 cm in diameter, peripheral location, metastasis from other organs, or benign disease. Calcified lymph nodes and N2 disease were considered a contraindication for segmentectomy. Adhesions, even if extensive, were not a contraindication for a single port segmentectomy.

Operative Technique

General anesthesia with one-lung ventilation is routinely used, although in selected cases a non-intubated VATS. Anesthesia protocol may be applied. The patient is positioned in the lateral decubitus position. The surgeon stands in front of the patient with his assistant standing at the opposite side. The skin in incised at the fourth or fifth intercostal space, between the anterior and midaxillary lines. A wound protector is used to protect the camera from getting repeatedly stained and prevent tumor seeding during the retrieval of the specimen. Visualization is achieved via a 10 mm 30-degree scope. The surgical instruments should be long, thin-shafted, double articulated to facilitate the dissection of the structures.

Upon entering the chest, the nodule is identified, and the entire lung is examined for identification of additional lesions. Articulated stapling devices are preferred over straight ones because they facilitate the transection of the structures even when dealing with difficult angles. The segmental vessels and bronchus are dissected free and severed at their take-off. Small vessels can be tied or ligated with polymer clips and divided with energy devices. The segment is transected at the intersegmental plane, which is usually identified with the inflation of the lung following the division of the segmental bronchus. The air inflated, escapes through the remaining intersegmental bronchi leading to atelectasis of

Electronic Supplementary Material The online version of this chapter (https://doi.org/10.1007/978-981-13-2604-2_24) contains supplementary material, which is available to authorized users.

D. Xie · X. Hu · Y. Zhu (✉)
Department of Thoracic Surgery, Shanghai Pulmonary Hospital, Tongji University School of Medicine, Shanghai, People's Republic of China

K. M. Soultanis
Department of Thoracic Surgery, Hellenic Airforce General Hospital, Athens, Greece

D. Gonzalez-Rivas et al. (eds.), *Atlas of Uniportal Video Assisted Thoracic Surgery*,
https://doi.org/10.1007/978-981-13-2604-2_24

the lung, while the target segment remains inflated. The specimen is retrieved through the incision with or without an endobag. Bi- or tri-segmentectomy is performed when the tumor is close to the intersegmental border.

Mediastinal lymphadenectomy is performed in case of a malignancy except for minimally invasive adenocarcinoma (MIA) and adenocarcinoma in situ (AIS). Lymphadenectomy (systematic lymph node sampling or systematic mediastinal dissection), requires dissection of at least three mediastinal lymph node stations including subcarinal and is carried out with the use of energy devices. A 28 F chest drain is placed at the posterior part of the incision. The pain management protocol includes patient control analgesia (PCA) and oral analgesics if needed.

Lingula-Sparing Left Upper Lobectomy

The branches of left superior pulmonary vein to the upper lobe are exposed by retracting the lung posteriorly, the lingula vein is identified, and the branches for S^{1+2} and S3 are treated with a stapling device (Fig. 1a). Following the division of the vein, the anterior and apical segmental arteries are stapled (Fig. 1b). The posterior segmental artery can be approached either anteriorly or posteriorly and severed with stapler or polymer vascular clips dissected and stapled (Fig. 2a). If a posterior approach is attempted the lung should be retracted anteriorly and the posterior part of the interlobar fissure dissected. Following the division of the vessels, the bronchus for the trisegment is identified and transected (Fig. 2b). The parenchymal resection is then completed by dissection through the intersegmental plane (Fig. 2c).

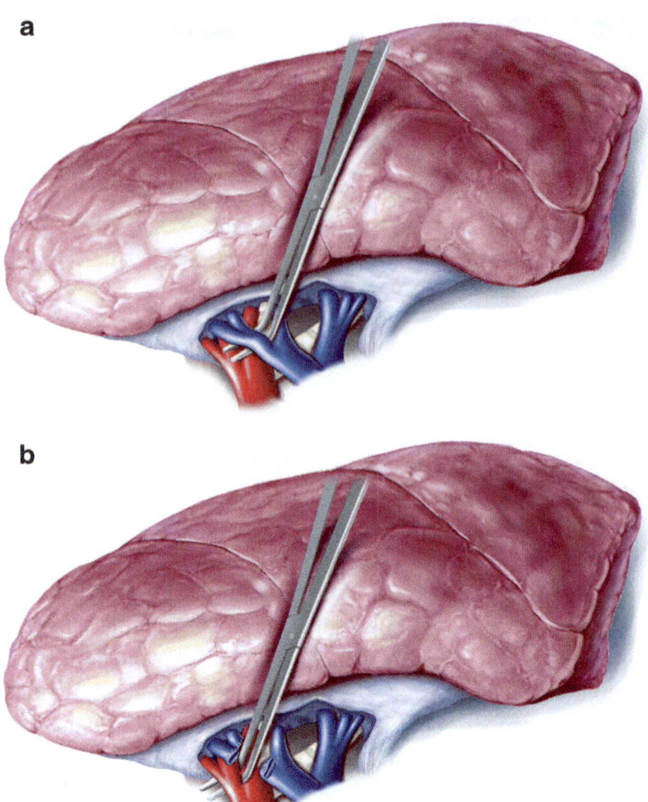

Fig. 1 (**a**) The left upper trisegmental branches of the left superior pulmonary vein. From an anterior view, the upper trisegmental branches of the left superior pulmonary vein are dissected out and stapled. (**b**) Anterior and apical arteries of left upper lobe. The anterior and apical branches of the left pulmonary artery are dissected out and stapled

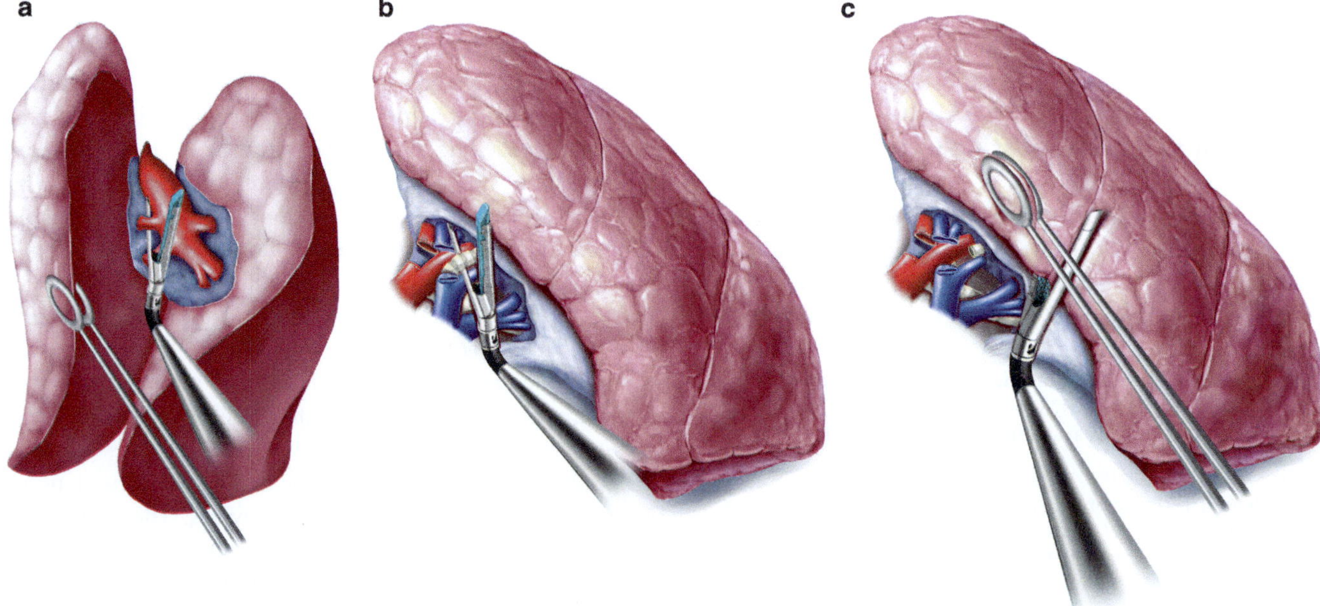

Fig. 2 (**a**) Posterior segmental arterial branch of left upper lobe. The posterior segmental arterial branch of left upper lobe are dissected out and ligated. (**b**) Left upper lobe bronchial anatomy. The segmental bronchus of the left apical trisegment is exposed. (**c**) Completion of intersegmental fissures for left upper trisegment with the stapling device

Lingulectomy

The lingular artery is dissected and stapled or clipped after dissection of the anterior portion of the interlobar fissure (Fig. 3a). The lingular vein is subsequently exposed by posterior retraction of the lung and (after identification of the veins for S^{1+2} and S3) is stapled (Fig. 3b). The lingular bronchus is then identified and transected (Fig. 4a). Lastly the intersegmental plane between the trisegment and the lingula is identified and dissected (Fig. 4b, Video 1).

Superior Segmentectomy (Video 2)

The posterior part of the fissure is dissected, allowing the exposure of the superior segmental artery (a6) which is stapled or clipped (Fig. 5a). The segmental vein is visualized after the artery is stapled by anterior retraction of the lung (posterior approach), and transected (Fig. 5b). The segmental bronchus is then identified either from anteriorly or posteriorly and stapled (Fig. 6a). The parenchymal resection is then completed in the segmental fissure (Fig. 6b). For a superior segmentectomy a completely anterior approach can be followed if the bronchus is treated after the a6, which leaves the vein last. For such an approach the segment should be retracted caudally.

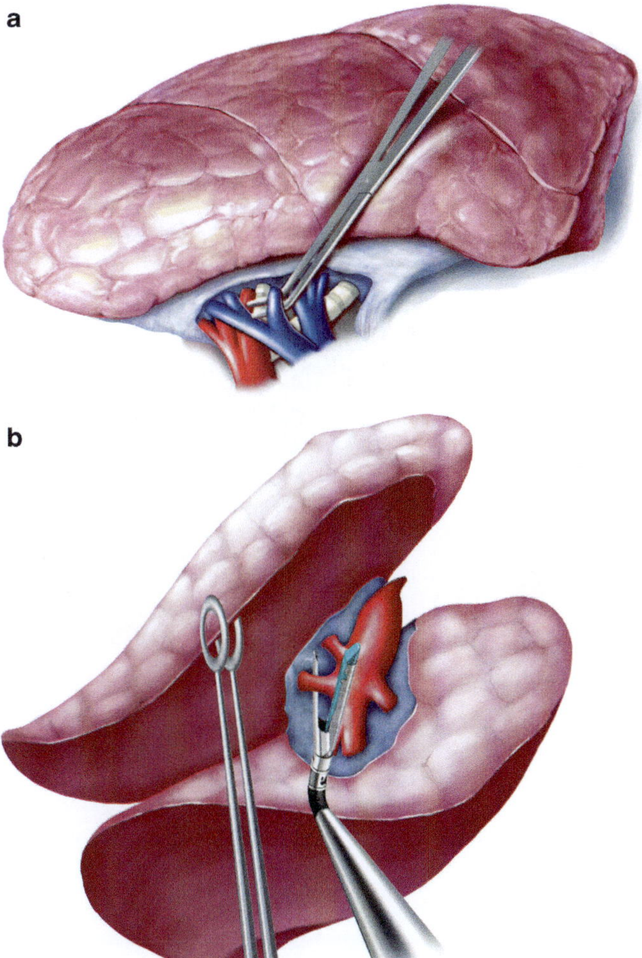

Fig. 3 (**a**) Left lingular segmental vein. The left lingular segmental vein is dissected out and stapled. (**b**) Left lingular segmental artery. The left lingular segmental artery is dissected out and stapled

Basilar Segmentectomy

Removal of four segments in the right lower lobe (S7-S8-S9-S10) or three segments in the left lower lobe (S7-S8-S9), sparing the apical segment (S6) is called basilar segmentectomy. These segments are usually removed together since they have a common bronchial and vascular trunk. The major fissure is dissected first, allowing the exposure of the pulmonary artery. The basilar arterial trunk is dissected free after identification of the a6 and stapled. Similarly, the basilar bronchus is stapled after identification of the superior segmental bronchus (b6), leaving the basilar vein last. When dissecting the fissure, the artery and the bronchus, the retraction should me caudal. For the vein the lung is retracted superiorly. In case of an incomplete fissure the procedure can be carried out in a caudal to cranial direction. The lung is retracted cephaladly and anteriorly, the inferior ligament released, and the basilar vein dissected and stapled after identification of the superior segmental vein (v6). Then, the basilar segmental bronchus is exposed after identification of the middle lobe bronchus (or left upper lobe bronchus for a left basilar segmentectomy) and the b6, dissected and divided. In this approach the middle or left upper lobe bronchus are identified lying just inferiorly and medially to the basilar trunk, while the b6 lies superiorly and laterally. Any lymph nodes encountered should be removed to facilitate the dissection of the structures. Maintaining the same traction (cephalad and anterior) the basilar artery is dissected after identification of the a6 and the middle lobe or lingular artery and stapled. The procedure is completed with the division of the intersegmental border.

Upper Lobe Posterior Segmentectomy (LUL-RUL)

The skin is typically incised at the fifth intercostal space between the anterior and middle axillary line. Anterior and caudal retraction of the lung allows dissection of the interlobar fissure and exposure of the segmental structures. The surgeon and the assistant are positioned in opposite sides as previously described.

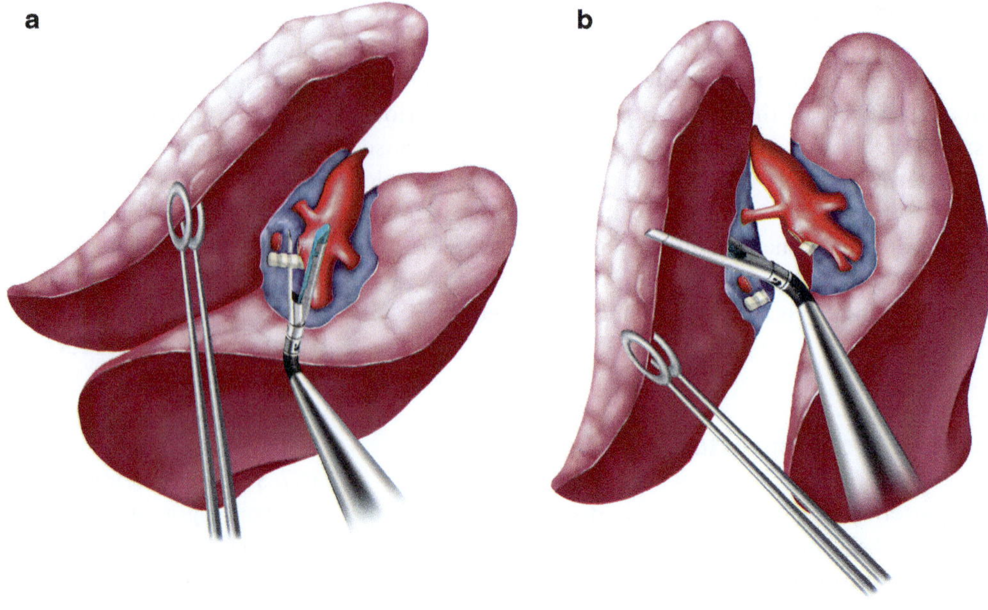

Fig. 4 (**a**) Bronchus of Left lingular segment. The left lingular segmental bronchus is dissected out and stapled. (**b**) Completion of intersegmental fissures for left lingular segment with the stapling device

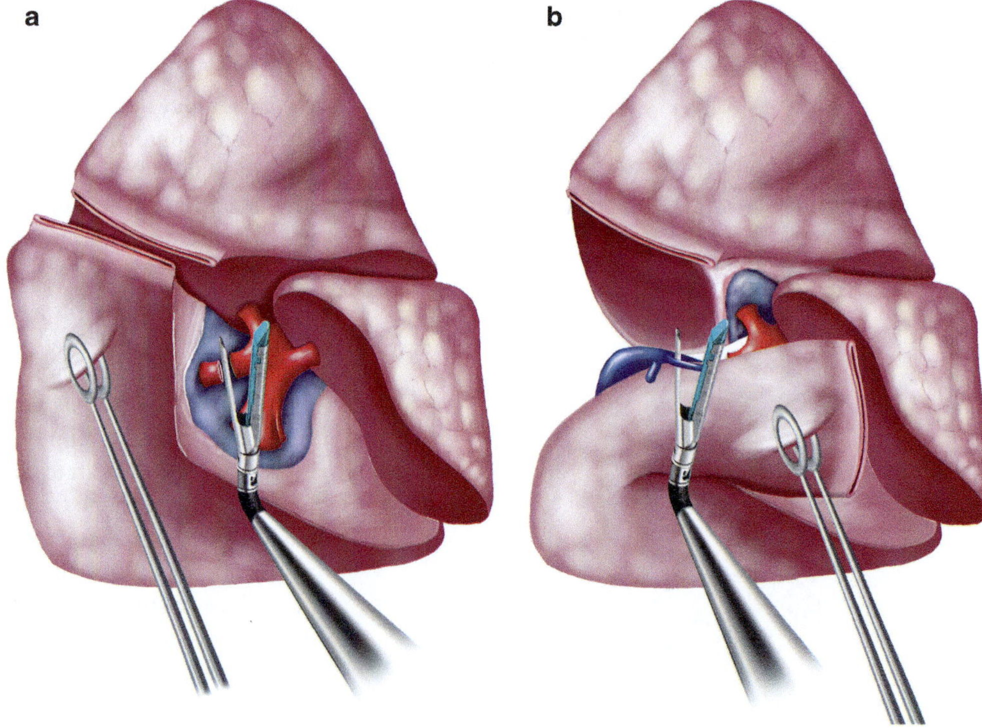

Fig. 5 (**a**) Right lower superior segmental artery. The right lower superior segmental artery is dissected out and stapled. (**b**) Right lower superior segmental vein. The right lower superior segmental vein is dissected out and stapled

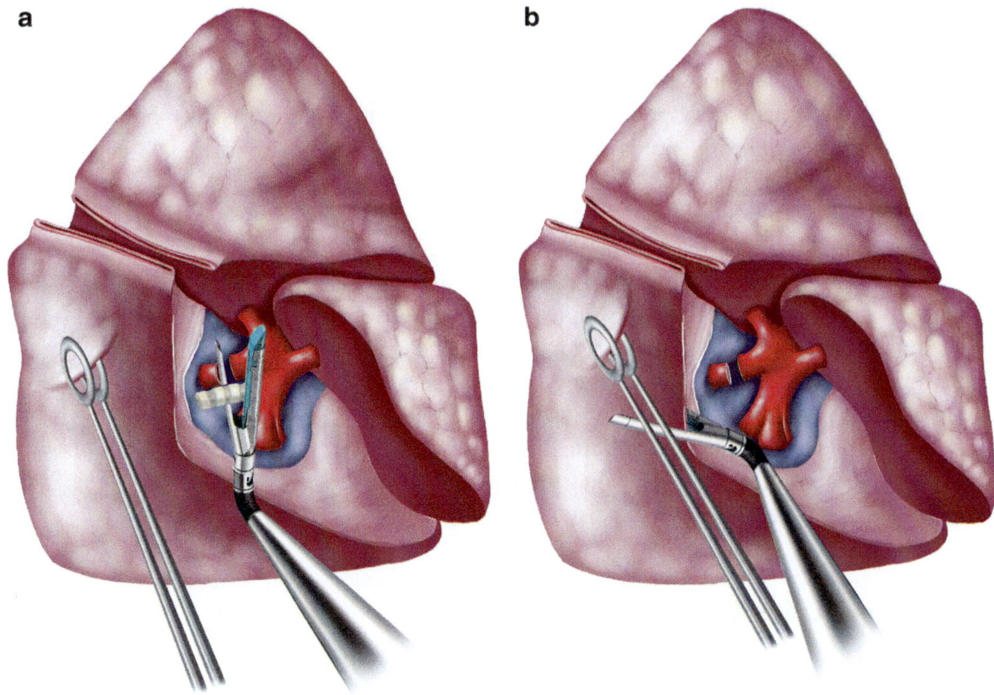

Fig. 6 (**a**) Bronchus of right lower superior segment. The right lower superior segmental bronchus is dissected out and stapled. (**b**) Completion of intersegmental fissures for right lower superior segment with the stapling device

Left Posterior Segmentectomy (It Is Uncommon, Usually in the Left Side the S^{1+2} Are Removed Together)

The superior pulmonary vein is exposed by posterior retraction of the lung and the apical, anterior and lingular tributaries are identified and dissected free using a hook or an energy device. The vein for the posterior segment usually arises from the anterior vein and runs posteriorly. It can be clipped or stapled. Any lymph nodes encountered during this phase are removed. Then the lung is retracted anteriorly, the posterior portion of the fissure is dissected, and the posterior segmental artery identified and clipped or stapled. Grasping the distal stump of the artery facilitates the identification of the segmental bronchus. Usually the posterior segmental bronchus shares a common trunk with the apical, so the dissection should be carried out distally to avoid severing the apical. The procedure is completed with the dissection of the intersegmental border.

Right Posterior Segmentectomy

The transverse and posterior part of the oblique fissure are dissected, allowing the exposure of the central vein and the posterior segmental artery, which lies adjacent to the former. Retracting the lung superiorly and slightly anteriorly, vein tributaries to the posterior segment are identified and clipped. The artery is treated right after. Lymph nodes between the central vein and the posterior segmental artery are removed during this phase. Grasping the distal stump of the artery and maintaining the same traction, dissection is carried out in a cephalad direction until the right upper lobe bronchus is identified. The lymph node encountered at its orifice is removed and the bronchus is dissected distally until the posterior segmental bronchus is identified. In the right side the posterior segmental bronchus usually arises separately. The bronchus is stapled and the segmentectomy is completed with the division of the intersegmental border taking care to include the distal stumps of the severed segmental structures. In case of an incomplete fissure, dissection of the fissure starts at the confluence of the oblique and transverse fissures until the interlobar pulmonary artery is identified. Then the lung is retracted anteriorly, and the posterior mediastinal pleura incised revealing the take-off of the right upper lobe bronchus and the bronchus intermedius. After removal of the lymph node a tunnel is created between the two dissection sites with the use of a snake forceps. A stapler is then used to dissect the fissure and from this point the procedure continues as described above.

Right Upper Lobe Apical-Posterior Segmentectomy

The lung is retracted posteriorly, and the superior pulmonary vein is dissected free. The central and apical vein are identified. The transverse fissure and the posterior part of the oblique fissure are dissected (as described above) and the central vein and posterior segmental artery are exposed. Retraction is now superiorly and anteriorly. Vein tributaries to the posterior segment are clipped before or after the artery is severed. Following the division of the posterior segmental structures, the lung is retracted inferiorly and posteriorly, and the apical vein identified dissected and clipped or stapled. Maintaining the retraction, the apical segmental artery is identified (arising from the truncus anterior), dissected and clipped. Now the apical and posterior segmental bronchi, which arise separately from the right upper lobe bronchus, can be transected together or separately, either from an anterior or posterior approach. Sometimes the apical vein is absent and the vein draining the apical segment arises from the central vein. The intersegmental plane is dissected, taking care to include the distal stumps.

Right Upper Lobe Apical Segmentectomy

For an apical segmentectomy the axis of the operation is directed from anteriorly to posteriorly. The lung is retracted posteriorly and slightly inferiorly, allowing the exposure of the superior pulmonary vein, which is dissected free. The apical and central veins are identified. The apical vein is clipped and severed. Maintaining the retraction, the truncus anterior is dissected, revealing the apical segmental artery, which is dissected and clipped. Subsequently the right upper lobe bronchus is dissected distally until the apical branch is identified, arising as the most superior branch of the trifurcation, dissected and transected. Finally, the intersegmental border is dissected.

References

1. Rocco G, Martin-Ucar A, Passera E. Uniportal VATS wedge pulmonary resections. Ann Thorac Surg. 2004;77(2):726–8.
2. Gonzalez-Rivas D, Paradela M, García J, De la Torre M. Single-port video-assisted thoracoscopic lobectomy. Interact Cardiovasc Thorac Surg. 2011;12:514–5.
3. Gonzalez-Rivas D, Fernández R, Delgado M, et al. Uniportal video-assisted thoracoscopic lobectomy: two years of experience. Ann Thorac Surg. 2013;95:426–32.
4. Gonzalez-Rivas D. Single incision video-assisted thoracoscopic anatomic segmentectomy. Ann Cardiothorac Surg. 2014;3(2):204–7. https://doi.org/10.3978/j.issn.2225-319X.2014.03.05.
5. Gonzalez-Rivas D, Sihoe A. Important technical details during Uniportal video-assisted thoracoscopic major resections. Thorac Surg Clin. 2017;27:357–72.
6. Xie D, Wang H, Fei K, et al. Single-port video-assisted thoracic surgery in 1063 cases: a single-institution experience. Eur J Cardiothorac Surg. 2016;49(Suppl 1):i31–6.
7. Shih CS, Liu CC, Liu ZY, et al. Comparing the postoperative outcomes of video-assisted thoracoscopic surgery (VATS) segmentectomy using a multi-port technique versus a single-port technique for primary lung cancer. J Thorac Dis. 2016;8(Suppl 3):S287–94.

Segmental Resection

Hyun Koo Kim and Kook Nam Han

Abstract

Segmentectomy for lung cancer is usually required in patients with early lung cancer located in the lung periphery. This procedure has been used for the diagnosis of a solid lung nodule, resection of pulmonary metastasis from extrathoracic malignancy, and sometimes for patients with limited cardiopulmonary reserve who cannot tolerate more rigorous procedures than a lobectomy. A less invasive approach (e.g., video-assisted thoracic surgery [VATS]) for segmentectomy is also a viable option, as treatment of lung cancer and mediastinal lymph node dissection by VATS has been reported as a safe and oncologically feasible procedure and might be considered for the initial treatment of small sized lung cancer less than 2 cm, and in low-risk patients.

An uniportal VATS approach for segmentectomy is usually more complex and difficult than for lobectomy. A thoracic surgeon, experienced in the uniportal VATS approach, could achieve acceptable outcomes using appropriate localization techniques and proper division of the intersegmental plane in this limited surgical view. However, the benefit of the uniportal VATS approach is not evident and there is no proven evidence of superiority over the conventional multi-port VATS approach.

This chapter addresses the technical considerations of uniportal VATS segmentectomy and suggests current options for localization and visualization of the segmental plane during the uniportal VATS. In addition, we review the literature supporting the safety and feasibility of uniportal VATS segmentectomy.

Electronic Supplementary Material The online version of this chapter (https://doi.org/10.1007/978-981-13-2604-2_25) contains supplementary material, which is available to authorized users.

H. K. Kim (✉) · K. N. Han
Department of Thoracic and Cardiovascular Surgery,
Korea University Guro Hospital, Seoul, Republic of Korea
e-mail: kimhyunkoo@korea.ac.kr

Introduction

Lung cancer is the leading cause of cancer death worldwide and accounts for more deaths than all other cancers combined [1]. The long-term survival rate is approximately 10–20% despite the recent therapeutic advances, including medical and surgical options, in lung cancer treatment [2]. The recent advent of the lung cancer screening program, with low-dose computed tomography in high-risk populations, has spread worldwide and is currently suggested for those aged 55–74 with a 30 pack-year history of smoking, following National Lung Screening Trial guidelines. However, the criteria for lung cancer screening vary following continued research into populations at risk [3, 4]. As screening program for early lung cancer increases, the incidentally detected solitary pulmonary nodules on chest computed tomography (CT) have become a clinical controversy for physicians [5, 6]. Diagnostic video-assisted thoracic surgery (VATS) resection might be first considered in selected patients if percutaneous biopsy is unavailable [5, 7, 8].

Technical advances in minimally invasive thoracic surgery and localization techniques have enabled us to adopt VATS for segmentectomy, even for non-palpable small ground glass opacity lesions [9–13]. In addition, an uniportal approach has emerged as a less invasive alternative to conventional VATS in thoracic disease, although the benefits of this procedure have not yet been characterized and the approach remains controversial [14, 15]. Nevertheless, this approach seems to be feasible in selected patients [16, 17]. From the uniportal VATS experience in several groups, mostly in Europe and Asia, uniportal VATS seems to be feasible option for current thoracic procedure where VATS techniques are appropriate, including complex resection [18–21].

The uniportal approach is reported to be feasible for VATS segmentectomy, without limitation by the range of lung segment [11, 22, 23]. Gonzalez et al. first reported the feasibility of uniportal VATS segmentectomy in patients with early-stage lung cancer, with potential advantages of

D. Gonzalez-Rivas et al. (eds.), *Atlas of Uniportal Video Assisted Thoracic Surgery*,
https://doi.org/10.1007/978-981-13-2604-2_25

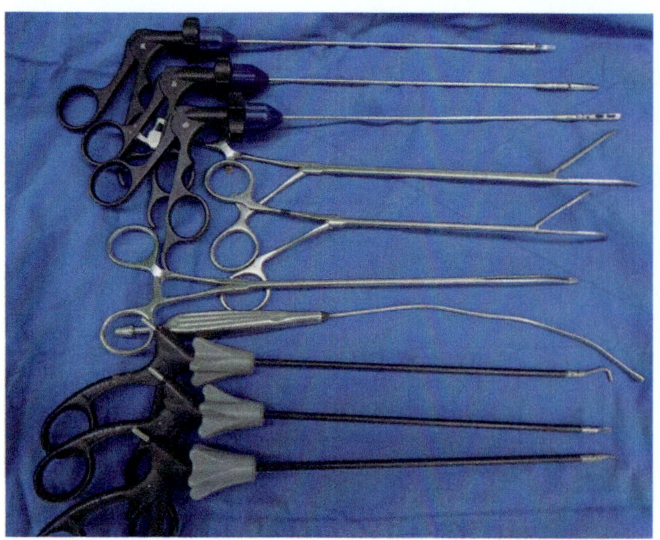

Fig. 1 Endoscopic instruments for uniportal thoracoscopic segmentectomy. 3.3–5 mm diameter mini endoscopic instruments and VATS devices

direct vision to target vessel and less postoperative pain [24]. The patient position and the incision are similar with those for other uniportal procedures. Conventional endoscopic devices can be used and mini-endoscopic devices such as a 3.3 mm diameter camera, endoscopic devices, curved and articulating devices or staplers, energy devices, and vascular clips are more appropriate instruments for procedures through smaller wounds (Fig. 1). The surgical technique and tips for uniportal VATS segmentectomy are described in this chapter. Preoperative localization of the pulmonary lesion during uniportal segmentectomy is mandatory for visualization of the pleural lesion and segmental plane to achieve enough resection margin [25–27].

Localization Technique

Preoperative localization of the pulmonary lesion during uniportal segmentectomy is mandatory for identification of the pleural lesion and the intersegmental plane to achieve enough resection margin. A radiopaque metal, such as hook-wire or fiducials, can be used under CT guidance [13, 28–31]. Direct injection of radiopaque material, such as lipiodol [32, 33] or barium [34], also helps to specify the depth of the lesion before division of the intersegmental plane by intraoperative C-arm fluoroscopy (Fig. 2). A common method used to identify the lung segment during segmentectomy is jet inflation by intraoperative bronchoscopy followed by clamping of the target segmental bronchus [35]. The extent of lymph node evaluation might also be optimized by sentinel lymph node mapping, with tracers such as dyes, radioisotopes, and fluorescence used in patients with clinical node-negative early stage lung cancer (T1a; Fig. 3). Electromagnetic navigational bronchoscopy can be performed before segmentectomy in a hybrid operating room setting [30, 36–38]. Currently, clinically available marking techniques include hook-wire or metallic fiducial placement, intraoperative ultrasonography, dye injection, and navigational bronchoscopy. The following is a review of the techniques for localization and identification of small pulmonary nodules and the intersegmental plane.

Localization Techniques for Small Pulmonary Nodules

Percutaneous Localization

Preoperative localization using hook-wire or microcoils under CT guidance has been reported, in retrospective studies, to yield success rates of up to 90–100% [40–44]. However, there is a reported 24% rate of procedure-related morbidity such as pneumothorax, hemothorax, or air embolism that require chest drain before operation [45, 46]. In addition, approximately 2–10% of the patients experienced hook-wire dislodgement [47–49] between procedure and operation and 2.7% of patients experienced dislodgement with microcoils. During the operation, intraoperative fluoroscopy is needed to find the accurate location of the hook-wire and repeated radiation exposure for the surgeon might be a concern regarding this procedure. However, Hajjar et al. [50] reported that localization using microcoils for deep lung lesion has a much lower rate of dislodgement (2.7%) and lesser morbidity.

Galletta et al. [51] reported on preoperative radio-guided localization using a radiotracer [Technitium-99m (^{99m}Tc) macroaggregates] for small or ground glass opacity pulmonary lesions. They injected the radiotracer near the target lesion under CT guidance and resected the pulmonary lesion by using an endoscopic radioprobe. The modification of ^{99m}Tc macroaggregates with albumin (MAA) enabled localization of the radiotracer in lung parenchyma for more than 18 h after injection. This technique requires no intraoperative fluoroscopy, dislodgement is not a problem, and there is no need for full deflation of the lung, such as during intraoperative ultrasonography. The rate of detection was 95%, which is comparable to other techniques, and a randomized trial comparing hook-wire and radio-guided localization in small lung nodules less than 2 cm showed no significant difference between the success rates of the two techniques [7, 52].

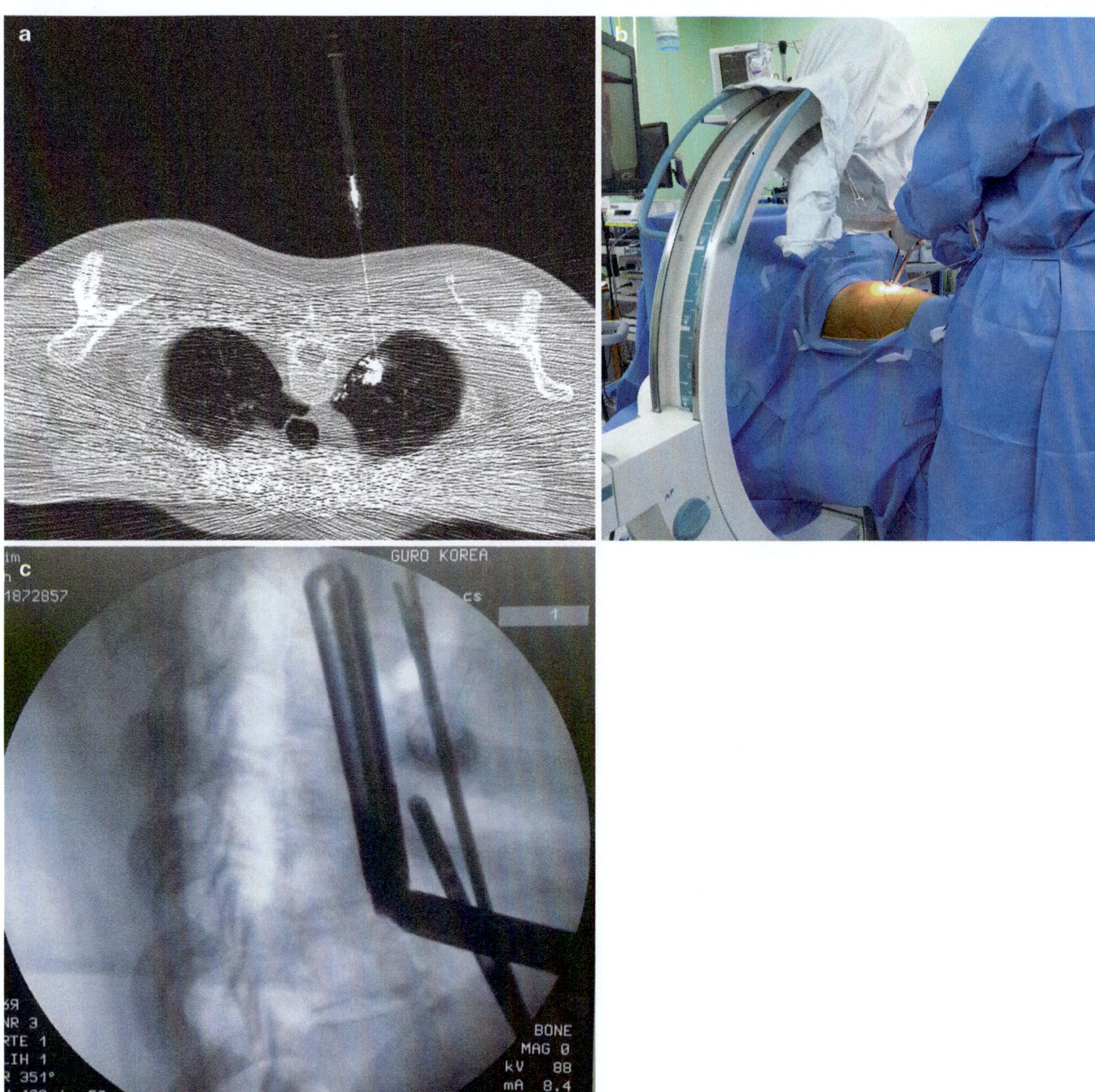

Fig. 2 Dual localization with a hookwire and radiocontrast and uniportal VATS resection using intraoperative C-arm fluoroscopy; (**a**) CT guided dual localization, (**b**) intraoperative C-arm fluoroscopy, (**c**) fluoroscopic images showing the resection margin

Localization with percutaneous injection of a dye or contrast agent is also successful for small lung lesions during VATS resection [53, 54]. However, the technique of percutaneous injection of methylene blue under CT guidance showed a relatively high failure rate of 13% and other disadvantages such as a short interval (<3 h) because of the rapid diffusion rate of dyes [53]. Use of an alternative contrast agent, lipiodol, showed long intervals after injection that could last for 3 months. Furthermore, Watanebe et al. [33] reported a 100% success rate in localization, with low morbidity. Contrast agents (e.g., lipiodol) or radiotracers can be injected alone and detected by fluoroscopy or they can be mixed with colored agents, eliminating the requirement for fluoroscopy [33]. The mandatory use of intraoperative fluoroscopy to detect the metal or radioisotope/radiocontrast might be a concern due to the potential risk of repeated radiation exposure [55–57].

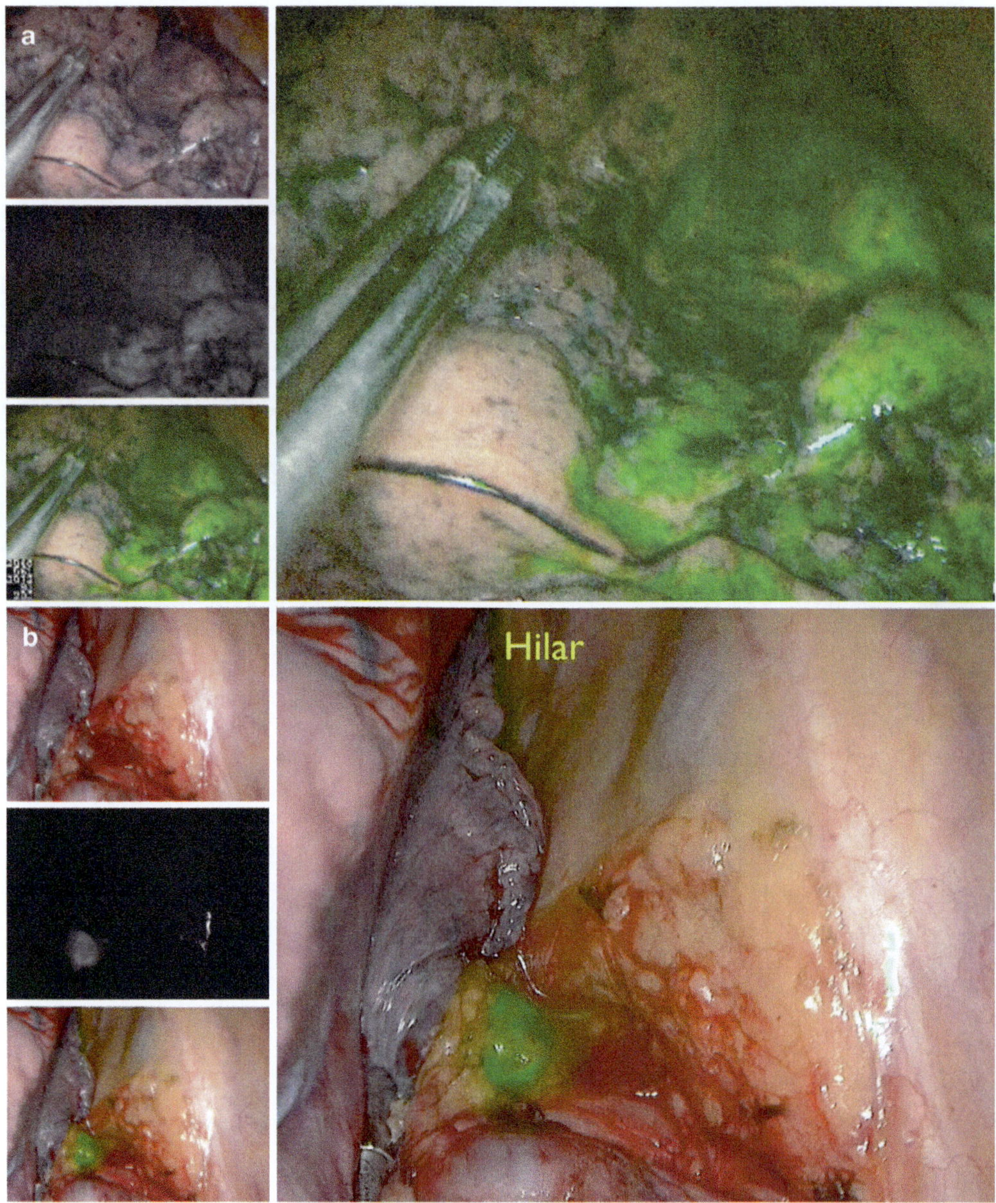

Fig. 3 Fluorescent video system using indocyanine green [39] during segmentectomy; (**a**) identification of the intersegmental plane by intravenous injection of ICG after division of apical posterior segmental artery, (**b**) visualization of the sentinel lymph node by peritumoral injection of ICG during segmentectomy

Intraoperative Localization

Prospective studies using intraoperative pulmonary ultrasonography yield success rates as high as 93%, and the benefit of this technique, described by Khereba et al. [58], is detection of additional nodules, 43% of which were not visualized or palpated previously. This technique may be favored as there are no procedure-related complications, such as those of percutaneous intervention, and no need for intraoperative fluoroscopy, which might be a concern due to accumulated exposure to radiation. Nevertheless, intraoperative ultrasonography needs full deflation of the lung parenchyma during the procedure and the detection rate of nodules depends mainly on the operator's skill, thus requiring steep learning curves.

Recently, the use of electromagnetic navigation bronchoscopy for preoperative localization has been reported by Krimsky et al. [38]. Using both three-dimensional reconstruction of CT scan and guidance of a bronchoscopic probe to target lung lesions under an electromagnetic field, they injected color dyes for intraoperative detection of the lung nodules. Asano et al. [36] reported a 100% success rate with navigational bronchoscopy and injection of barium, using fluoroscopy to detect the target lesion intraoperatively. Miyoshi et al. [30] also reported a 100% success rate with this technique coupled with insertion of microcoils. There was no procedure related complications or adverse events with the transbronchial injection of dye to target the lung lesion.

Although there are various techniques to localize small lung lesions, there have been no prospective or randomized trials comparing methods with each other or versus finger palpation. Currently, the localization techniques using microcoils, radioisotopes aggregates, and hook-wire have higher efficacy and acceptable morbidity [40, 46, 52]. In our study, we reported that the dual localization technique, using a hook-wire and radioisotope (^{99m}Tc-phytate) for small pulmonary nodules, had a success rate of 100%, a 19.4% rate of hook-wire dislodgement, and a 17.6% rate of iatrogenic pneumothorax that required no additional treatment [7].

Identification of the Intersegmental Plane

Preoperatively, 3D reconstruction of the CT scan may help the surgeon to understand the lung segmental anatomy and thus improve surgical performance, even for this anatomically difficult segment [59–62]. Three-dimensional computed tomography images for surgical simulation are a useful option to observe the segmental vascular and bronchial anatomy and thus plan the least invasive segmentectomy. Oizumi et al. [63] reported that VATS segmentectomy, using 3D reconstruction with multiple-detector computed tomography (MDCT) images, had a 98% success rate in 52 patients. For identification of the intersegmental plane, they emphasized the importance of the anatomy of intersegmental and intersegmental veins, and that the intersegmental plane should be dissected along the border of intersegmental veins for complete anatomic segmentectomy. Several authors [59, 64, 65] have reported the use of techniques using computer software for 3D reconstruction of lung segmental anatomy, which can be performed by the thoracic surgeon within several minutes and used intraoperatively using handheld devices.

Intraoperatively, inflation and deflation techniques to delineate the intersegmental plane were introduced by Tsubota [66]. Okada et al. [35] introduced the technique of selective inflation of the involved segment using jet ventilation, which enables more accurate resection of the lung segment in this physiologically inflated state. However, these techniques need a well-experienced bronchoscopist or anesthesiologist to perform super-selection of the segmental bronchus intraoperatively.

Recently, the image-guided technique using fluorescence (indocyanine green; ICG) has been introduced to visualize the intersegmental plane [25, 67–69]. After completion of the segmental vessels and bronchus division, the target lung segment could be visualized on a fluorescence video system by injection of a fluorescent dye to the systemic blood vessel after several seconds [25]. There is an alternative method of direct injection of fluorescence dye to involved segment bronchus by fiberoptic bronchoscopy after division [69]. These techniques might be promising for future image-guided segmentectomy for visualization of the segmental plane to achieve accurate resection. However, they require a special fluorescent video system and need more study before being applied clinically.

Operative Techniques

Right and Left Upper Lobe Apical and Posterior Segments (Fig. 4)

Pulmonary segments in the upper lobe can be divided into three segments; apical, posterior, and anterior segment. Thoracic surgeon should fully understand the segmental anatomy prior to perform uniportal VATS segmentectomy and CT scan is essential to define the segmental anatomy. A 2–4 cm length of incision can be created at the fourth or fifth intercostal space along the mid- or anterior axillary line. The truncus anterior pulmonary artery should be dissected first to expose the apical segmental artery. Surgeon can expose the upper segmental veins by lung traction. The superior branch of pulmonary vein located deep in the posterior part of the central veins.

After division of the apicoposterior segmental artery, the upper lobar segmental bronchus can be dissected in the deep location. Further dissection of peribronchial lymph node can enable us to identify the segmental bronchus of the upper lobe. Frozen evaluation of the perisegmental or perivascular lymph node should be carried out before division of the segmental bronchus. Transection of segmental bronchus can be performed by delineating the segmental plane. Super-selection of target segmental bronchus with a bronchoscope might be used to demarcating the segmental line. The recent method of fluorescent dye (Indocyanine green) for colorful segmental line after segmental vessel division might be a promising one.

However, commonly, the segmental line for parenchymal division is identified by lung inflation-deflation technique. The stapling might be guided only with palpation if there are no available option for localization. Localization technique should be recommended to achieve resection margin for deep lesions. A hook-wire insertion, metal fiducial, radiopaque/contrast, or fluorescent dye materials might be used under percutaneous CT or transbronchial bronchoscopic marking. Electromagnetic navigational bronchoscopic system is an emerging option for less invasive localization. Localized lesions can be detected by fluoroscopy, con-beam CT system, or endoscopic camera available near infrared imaging. A thoracoscope or recent robotic surgery system available near infrared imaging might be a feasible option for detection of the fluorescent dye-marked lesion without radiation exposure of C-arm fluoroscopy or con-beam CT.

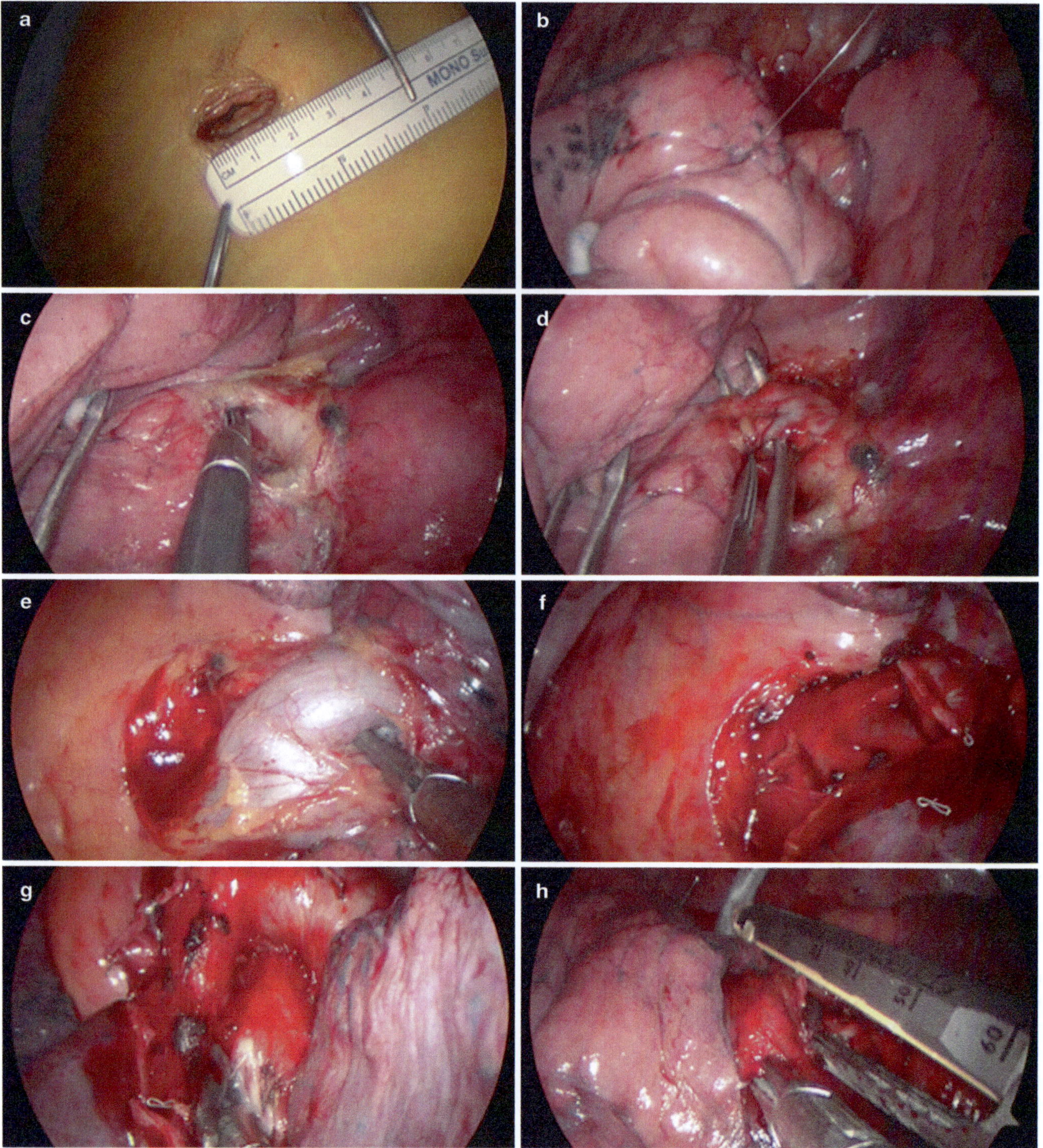

Fig. 4 Uniportal left upper lobe apico-posterior segmentectomy; (**a**) a 2 cm single incision at the fifth intercostal space, (**b**) hookwire localization, (**c**) dissection of the interlobar fissure, (**d**) isolation of the posterior segmental artery, (**e**) identification of the apicoposterior segmental veins, (**f**) apical segmental artery from the upper divisional trunk, (**g**) upper lobe segmental bronchus, (**h**) stapling the apicoposterior segmental bronchus, (**i**) selective jet inflation after clamping the segmental bronchus, (**j**) intersegmental division

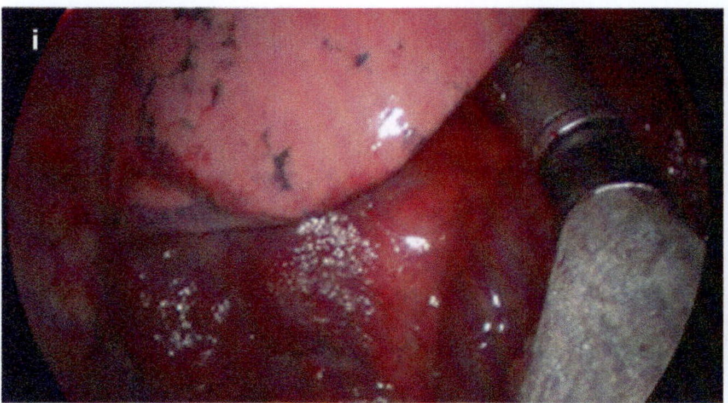

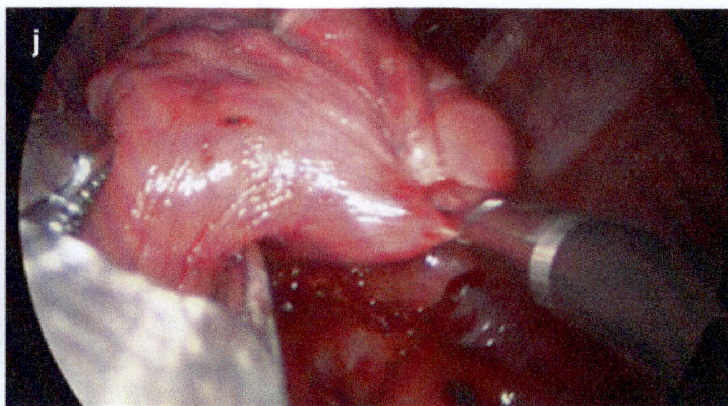

Fig. 4 (continued)

Right and Left Lower Lobe Superior Segments (Fig. 5)

The setting for lower lobe superior segments is not different to those for other segments. We create a 2–4 cm single incision at the fourth or fifth intercostal along the midaxillary line. The interlobar space can be approached directly from the uniportal approach. A major fissure can be dissected by electrocautery or energy devices which might be used to divide an incomplete fissure for parenchymal division if incomplete fissure. The superior segmental vessel can be transected with a stapler or clip and the superior segmental bronchus can be dissected after transection the superior segmental pulmonary artery. Full exposure to interlobar space needs to dissect the superior segmental bronchus and facilitate the dissection superior segmental bronchus from bronchus intermedius. Subcarinal node also can be harvested in these setting. The superior segmental lower pulmonary vein can be dissected by anterior or superior mobilization of the lower lobe and also can be transected with a stapler.

Right and Left Lower Lobe Basilar Segments (Fig. 6)

The basilar branch can be dissected from the major fissure in uniportal view. Full exposure of fissure and interlobar space is essential for the dissection of the basilar branch of pulmonary artery and bronchus. The basilar branch of lower pulmonary vein should be divided with preservation of the superior branch. The demarcating techniques for segmental plane is helpful to preserve the lung parenchyma. Basilar segmentectomy is completed by stapling the segment with careful inspection for injury of remnant bronchovascular structures.

Left Upper Divisional Segment (Tri-segment) (Fig. 7)

The major fissure should be dissected first to approach the upper divisional branches of pulmonary artery. The upper truncal pulmonary artery can be dissected by opening the mediastinal pleura in uniportal view. The lymph nodes should be dissected in interlobar and perivascular space. The upper divisional branch of pulmonary veins can be exposed and dissected with careful mobilization of lung tissue. A soft rubber tape-guided stapling might be needed to minimize the excessive tension to the vascular structure. The upper divisional bronchus can be exposed after pulmonary vessels are transected. Intraoperative bronchoscopy with air inflation and deflation might be used to delineate the segmental plane. After the upper segmental bronchus is divided, inflation techniques are also helpful to divide the intersegmental plane. Sometimes, intraoperative use of c-arm fluoroscopy is needed to achieve adequate resection if the lung lesion lies at the intersegmental border, shown on a preoperative chest image (Video 1).

Left Lingular Segment (Fig. 8)

The major fissure should be dissected to expose the lingular vessels and the lingular vein can be dissected from the upper pulmonary vein with mobilization of the lung in uniportal view. The lingular bronchus can be exposed after division of lingular vein and artery. The lingular artery can be transected by vascular staplers or clips and small branches of interlobar vessels can be divided by clips or energy devices. The inflation-deflation technique is helpful to demarcate the correct segmental line and also to ensure the proper segments of the upper divisional segments. Intraoperative fiberoptic bronchoscopy and C-arm fluoroscopy is also helpful to visualize the correct location of the marking lesion and intersegmental plane during the procedure, if available.

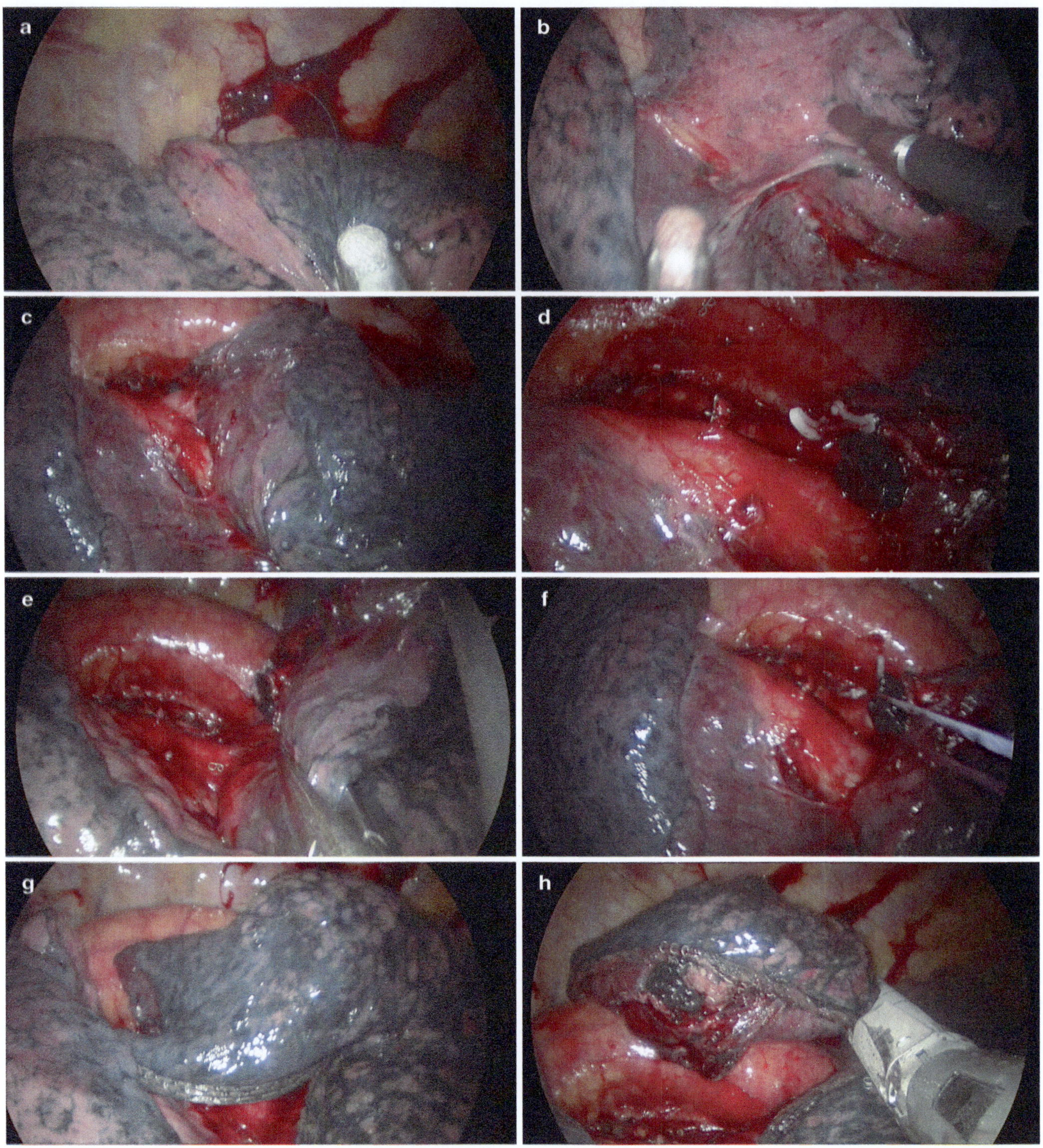

Fig. 5 Uniportal left lower lobe superior segmentectomy; (**a**) localization of the lung lesion at the left lower lobe superior segment, (**b**) dissection of the interlobar fissure, (**c**) identification of the superior segmental artery, (**d**) division of the superior segmental branches, (**e**) identification of the intersegmental plane away from the lesion for adequate resection margin, (**f**) identification of the superior segmental bronchus, (**g** and **h**) intersegmental division

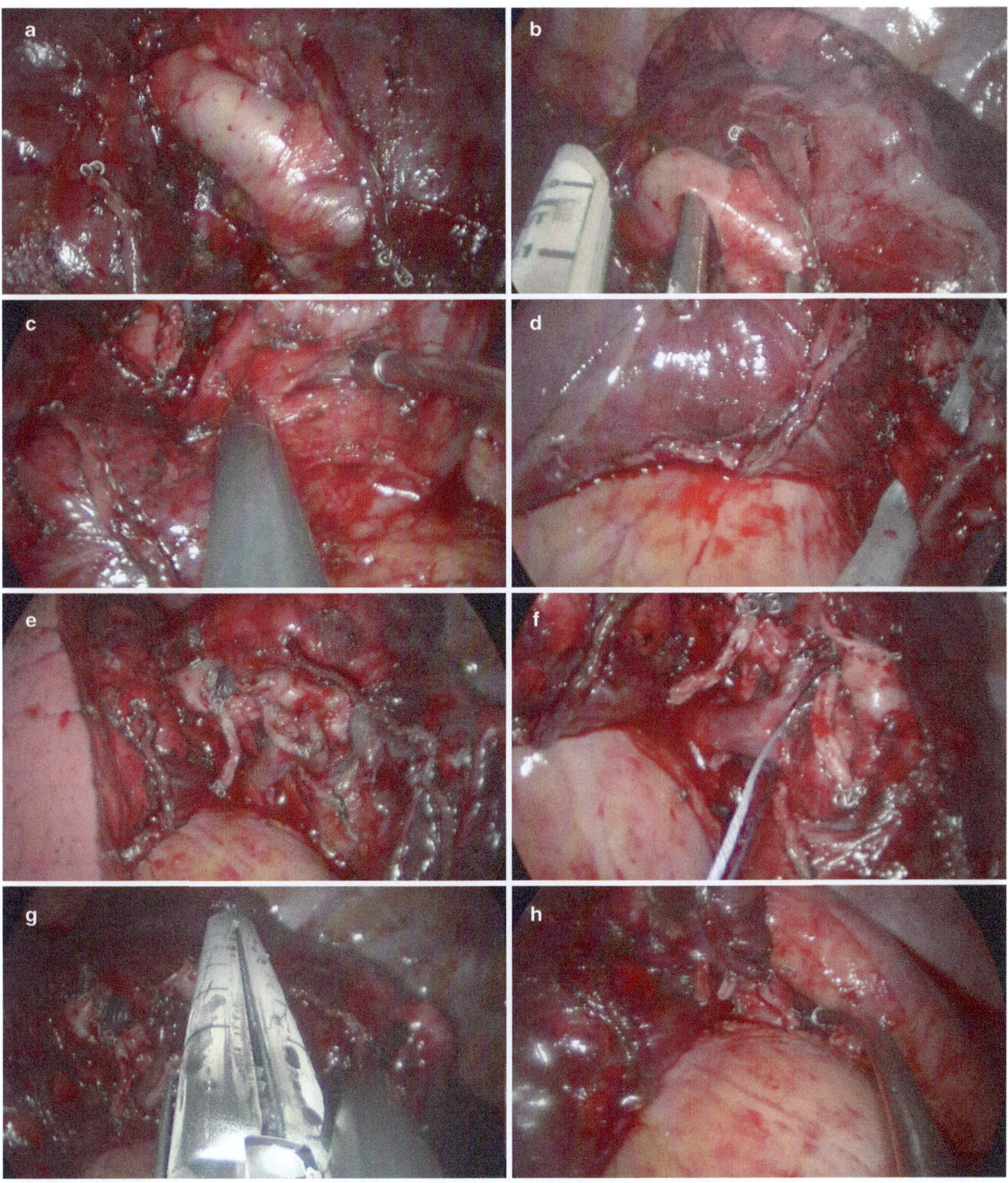

Fig. 6 Uniportal left lower basal segmentectomy; (**a**) exposure of the interlobar artery and basilar artery, (**b**) division of the basilar artery, (**c**) identification of the basilar segmental bronchus, (**d**) division of the basilar bronchus, (**e**) identification of the lower lobar pulmonary veins, (**f**) division of the basilar segmental vein, (**g**) intersegmental division, (**h**) completed basilar segmentectomy

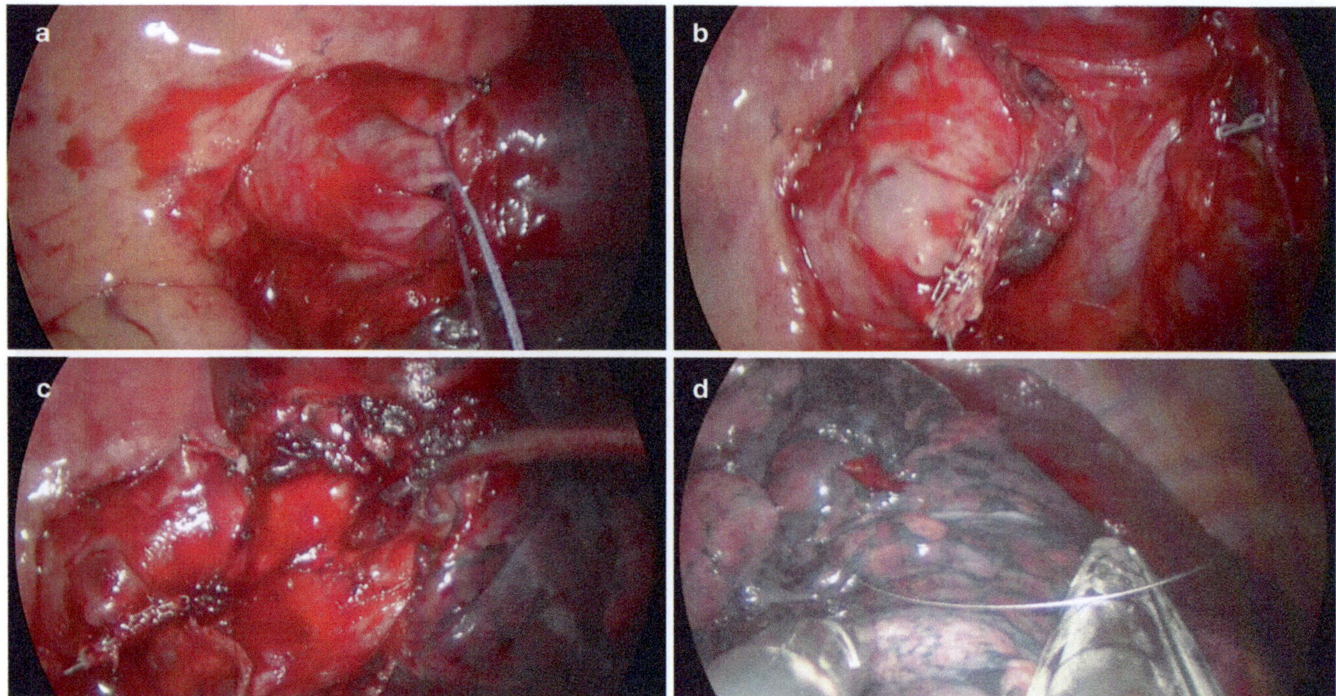

Fig. 7 Uniportal left upper divisional segmentectomy; (**a**) dissection and identification of the upper divisional pulmonary artery, (**b**) transected upper divisional trunk, (**c**) identification of the upper divisional bronchus, (**d**) intersegmental division

Results

There are no randomized trials comparing uniportal VATS and other approaches (conventional multi-port VATs or open surgery) in segmentectomy, or any reports on the lack of long-term oncologic results in lung cancer [18]. These limitations are not widely believed, and only underpowered clinical evidence confirms the clinical superiority over conventional multi-port VATS approach; however, the uniportal VATS approach for segmentectomy seems to be feasible and might be performed in patients with both benign and malignant lung disease [11, 21, 22, 24, 70–73].

Only a few case reports have described operative efficacy and short-term outcomes without comparable outcomes. Gonzalez et al. [24] first reported their experiences of the uniportal VATS segmentectomy performed with lobectomy in a patient with a 1-cm sized pulmonary lesion. They reported 28 consecutive cases with 2-days of hospital stay and reported that the uniportal VATS segmentectomy in early lung cancer might be feasible without long-term oncologic outcomes and clear evidence of superiority in the reduction of postoperative pain [70]. Wang et al. [22, 71] reported their experience of uniportal VATS segmentectomy in 11 patients and showed acceptable result compared with those of 16 patients undergoing the multiport VATS approach. In propensity-matched analysis, they also showed the clinical benefits of the uniportal VATS were less operative time, resection of more lymph nodes, and less blood loss.

Our study also reported on the operative result of 30 consecutive patients with lung cancer or benign lung disease that underwent uniportal VATS segmentectomy [74]. There was no case of conversion to open surgery and the uniportal VATS approach was favorable, with less complications and shorter postoperative stay than those of conventional VATS group. In a following report, comparative results between the uniportal versus multiport approach for VATS segmentectomy in early lung cancer revealed no differences in operation time, the resected lymph nodes, or the intraoperative events. There was a slight reduction in morbidity and postoperative stay in our experience compared to the multiport VATS approach [72].

The potential advantages of adopting the uniportal VATS approach are reduced surgical trauma, less postoperative intercostal pain, and a better postoperative course [18, 75]. For segmentectomy, this technique may be feasible and safe. However, currently these advantages may be limited to procedures carried out by experienced surgeons in a few specialized centers. The criticisms regarding the safety of the surgical performance is unavoidable for adoption of this approach widely by thoracic surgeons [76]. In addition, the presumed benefits of the uniportal approach for segmentectomy in NSCLC have not been proven and are still controversial [77]. The oncologic outcomes should be evaluated in well-designed future clinical studies that include the uniportal approach as one of the less invasive VATS techniques.

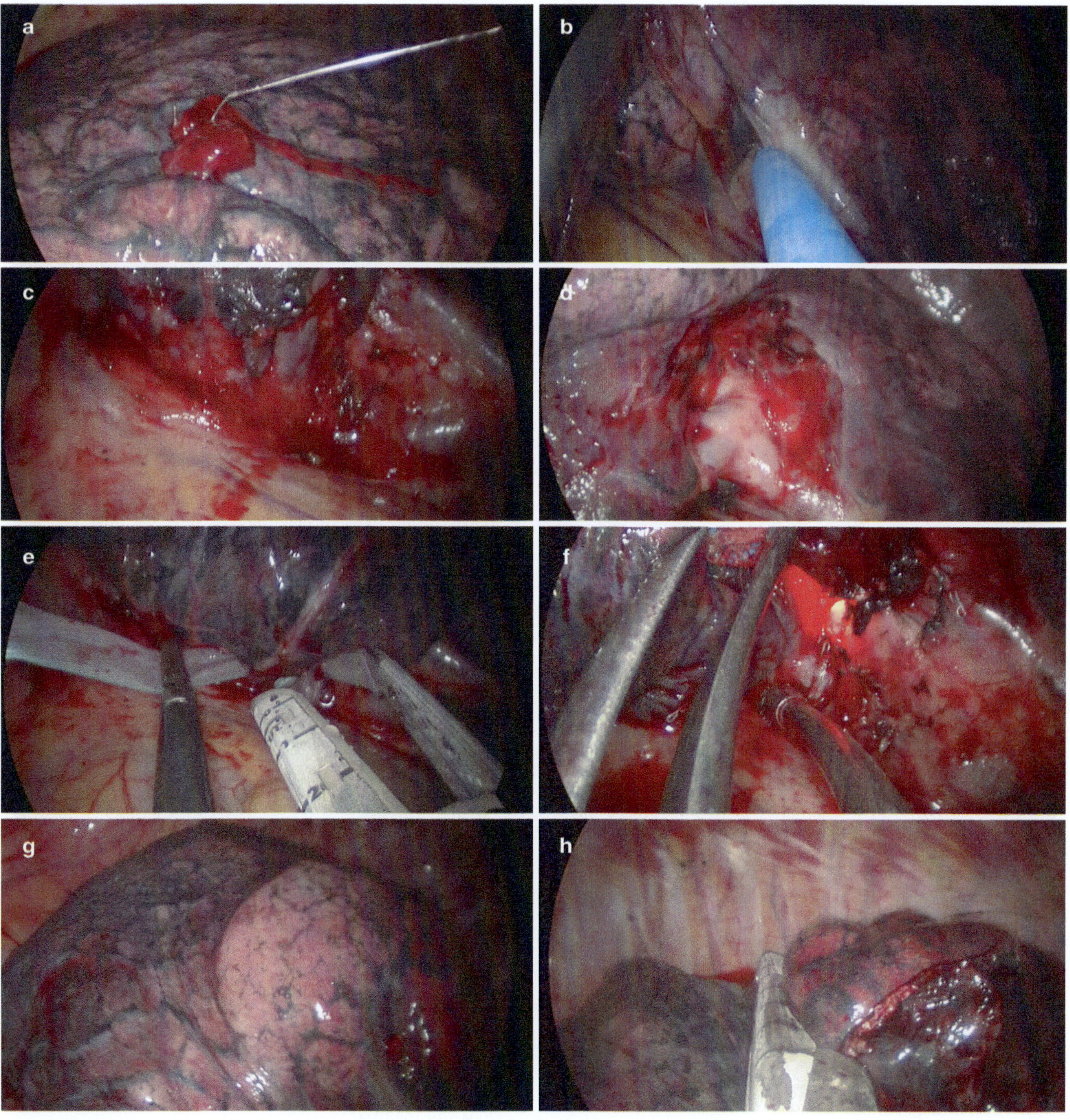

Fig. 8 Uniportal lingular segmentectomy; (**a**) localization with a hookwire at the lingular segmental lesion, (**b**) interlobar dissection, (**c**) identification of the lingular veins, (**d**) identification of the lingular artery from the lower lobar artery, (**e**) lingular vein division, (**f**) identification of the lingular segmental bronchus, (**g**) selective jet inflation to show the intersegmental plane, (**h**) division of the intersegmental plane

Conclusions

We reviewed the uniportal approach for VATS segmentectomy in thoracic disease, which is quite challenging and innovative. With the uniportal approach a full range of lung segmentectomy can be performed, although this technique needs a surgeon's full experience of the uniportal approach from simple procedures to complex anatomic resections. Newer devices for minimally invasive surgery now show promise for improving the technique and could facilitate the rapid progression to the uniportal VATS approach in thoracic disease. As the technology and surgical experience continues to grow, we can refine and address the actual role of the uniportal approach for VATS segmentectomy and the value of minimal resection under minimal incision.

References

1. Ferlay J, Soerjomataram I, Dikshit R, et al. Cancer incidence and mortality worldwide: sources, methods and major patterns in GLOBOCAN 2012. Int J Cancer. 2015;136:E359–86.
2. Institute USNIoHNC. SEER cancer statistics review. Mar 2016.
3. National Lung Screening Trial Research Team, Aberle DR, Adams AM, et al. Reduced lung-cancer mortality with low-dose computed tomographic screening. N Engl J Med. 2011;365:395–409.
4. Jacobson FL, Austin JH, Field JK, et al. Development of The American Association for Thoracic Surgery guidelines for low-dose computed tomography scans to screen for lung cancer in North America: recommendations of The American Association for Thoracic Surgery task force for lung cancer screening and surveillance. J Thorac Cardiovasc Surg. 2012;144:25–32.
5. Takashima S, Maruyama Y, Hasegawa M, et al. CT findings and progression of small peripheral lung neoplasms having a replacement growth pattern. AJR Am J Roentgenol. 2003;180:817–26.
6. Park CM, Goo JM, Lee HJ, et al. Nodular ground-glass opacity at thin-section CT: histologic correlation and evaluation of change at follow-up. Radiographics. 2007;27:391–408.
7. Kim HK, Jo WM, Jung JH, et al. Needlescopic lung biopsy for interstitial lung disease and indeterminate pulmonary nodules: a report on 65 cases. Ann Thorac Surg. 2008;86:1098–103.
8. Sepesi B, Walsh GL. Surgical therapy of ground-glass opacities. Semin Diagn Pathol. 2014;31:289–92.
9. Mogi A, Yajima T, Tomizawa K, et al. Video-assisted thoracoscopic surgery after preoperative CT-guided lipiodol marking of small or impalpable pulmonary nodules. Ann Thorac Cardiovasc Surg. 2015;21:435–9.
10. Sakamoto T, Takada Y, Endoh M, et al. Bronchoscopic dye injection for localization of small pulmonary nodules in thoracoscopic surgery. Ann Thorac Surg. 2001;72:296–7.
11. Han KN, Kim HK, Choi YH. Uniportal video-assisted thoracoscopic surgical (VATS) segmentectomy with preoperative dual localization: right upper lobe wedge resection and left upper lobe upper division segmentectomy. Ann Cardiothorac Surg. 2016;5:147–50.
12. Oh Y, Quan YH, Kim M, et al. Intraoperative fluorescence image-guided pulmonary segmentectomy. J Surg Res. 2015;199:287–93.
13. Doo KW, Yong HS, Kim HK, et al. Needlescopic resection of small and superficial pulmonary nodule after computed tomographic fluoroscopy-guided dual localization with radiotracer and hook-wire. Ann Surg Oncol. 2015;22:331–7.
14. Lau R, Ng C, Kwok M, et al. Early outcomes following uniportal video-assisted thoracic surgery lung resection. Chest. 2014;145:50A-51-50A-52.
15. Gonzalez-Rivas D, Yang Y, Ng C. Advances in uniportal video-assisted thoracoscopic surgery: pushing the envelope. Thorac Surg Clin. 2016;26:187–201.
16. Gonzalez-Rivas D, Paradela M, Fernandez R, et al. Uniportal video-assisted thoracoscopic lobectomy: two years of experience. Ann Thorac Surg. 2013;95:426–32.
17. Rocco G, Martucci N, La Manna C, et al. Ten-year experience on 644 patients undergoing single-port (uniportal) video-assisted thoracoscopic surgery. Ann Thorac Surg. 2013;96:434–8.
18. Zeltsman D. Current readings: redefining minimally invasive: uniportal video-assisted thoracic surgery. Semin Thorac Cardiovasc Surg. 2014;26:249–54.
19. Ng CS, Gonzalez-Rivas D, D'Amico TA, Rocco G. Uniportal VATS-a new era in lung cancer surgery. J Thorac Dis. 2015;7:1489–91.
20. Sekhniaidze D, Gonzalez-Rivas D. Uniportal video-assisted thoracoscopic sleeve resection. Ann Cardiothorac Surg. 2016;5:145–6.
21. Xie D, Wang H, Fei K, et al. Single-port video-assisted thoracic surgery in 1063 cases: a single-institution experiencedagger. Eur J Cardiothorac Surg. 2016;49(Suppl 1):i31–6.
22. Wang BY, Tu CC, Liu CY, et al. Single-incision thoracoscopic lobectomy and segmentectomy with radical lymph node dissection. Ann Thorac Surg. 2013;96:977–82.
23. Gonzalez-Rivas D, Mendez L, Delgado M, et al. Uniportal video-assisted thoracoscopic anatomic segmentectomy. J Thorac Dis. 2013;5(Suppl 3):S226–33.
24. Gonzalez-Rivas D, Fieira E, Mendez L, Garcia J. Single-port video-assisted thoracoscopic anatomic segmentectomy and right upper lobectomy. Eur J Cardiothorac Surg. 2012;42:e169–71.
25. Oh S, Suzuki K, Miyasaka Y, et al. New technique for lung segmentectomy using indocyanine green injection. Ann Thorac Surg. 2013;95:2188–90.
26. Keating J, Singhal S. Novel methods of intraoperative localization and margin assessment of pulmonary nodules. Semin Thorac Cardiovasc Surg. 2016;28:127–36.
27. Chan EG, Landreneau JR, Schuchert MJ, et al. Preoperative (3-dimensional) computed tomography lung reconstruction before anatomic segmentectomy or lobectomy for stage I non–small cell lung cancer. J Thorac Cardiovasc Surg. 2015;150:523–8.
28. Wicky S, Dusmet M, Doenz F, et al. Computed tomography–guided localization of small lung nodules before video-assisted resection: experience with an efficient hook-wire system. J Thorac Cardiovasc Surg. 2002;124:401–3.
29. Heran MKS, Sangha BS, Mayo JR, et al. Lung nodules in children: video-assisted thoracoscopic surgical resection after computed tomography–guided localization using a microcoil. J Pediatr Surg. 2011;46:1292–7.
30. Miyoshi T, Kondo K, Takizawa H, et al. Fluoroscopy-assisted thoracoscopic resection of pulmonary nodules after computed tomography–guided bronchoscopic metallic coil marking. J Thorac Cardiovasc Surg. 2006;131:704–10.
31. Park CH, Hur J, Lee SM, et al. Lipiodol localization for ground-glass opacity minimal surgery: rationale and design of the LOGIS trial. Contemp Clin Trials. 2015;43:194–9.
32. Nomori H, Horio H, Naruke T, Suemasu K. Fluoroscopy-assisted thoracoscopic resection of lung nodules marked with lipiodol. Ann Thorac Surg. 2002;74:170–3.
33. Watanabe K, Nomori H, Ohtsuka T, et al. Usefulness and complications of computed tomography-guided lipiodol marking for fluoroscopy-assisted thoracoscopic resection of small pulmonary nodules: experience with 174 nodules. J Thorac Cardiovasc Surg. 2006;132:320–4.
34. Okumura T, Kondo H, Suzuki K, et al. Fluoroscopy-assisted thoracoscopic surgery after computed tomography-guided bronchoscopic barium marking. Ann Thorac Surg. 2001;71:439–42.
35. Okada M, Mimura T, Ikegaki J, et al. A novel video-assisted anatomic segmentectomy technique: selective segmental inflation via bronchofiberoptic jet followed by cautery cutting. J Thorac Cardiovasc Surg. 2007;133:753–8.
36. Asano F, Shindoh J, Shigemitsu K, et al. Ultrathin bronchoscopic barium marking with virtual bronchoscopic navigation for fluoroscopy-assisted thoracoscopic surgery. Chest. 2004;126:1687–93.
37. Bolton WD, Howe H 3rd, Stephenson JE. The utility of electromagnetic navigational bronchoscopy as a localization tool for robotic resection of small pulmonary nodules. Ann Thorac Surg. 2014;98:471–5;discussion 475–476.
38. Krimsky WS, Minnich DJ, Cattaneo SM, et al. Thoracoscopic detection of occult indeterminate pulmonary nodules using bronchoscopic pleural dye marking. J Community Hosp Intern Med Perspect. 2014;4(1):23084.
39. Turna A, Solak O, Kilicgun A, et al. Is lobe-specific lymph node dissection appropriate in lung cancer patients undergoing routine mediastinoscopy? Thorac Cardiovasc Surg. 2007;55:112–9.
40. Finley RJ, Mayo JR, Grant K, et al. Preoperative computed tomography-guided microcoil localization of small peripheral

pulmonary nodules: a prospective randomized controlled trial. J Thorac Cardiovasc Surg. 2015;149:26–31.
41. Paci M, Annessi V, Giovanardi F, et al. Preoperative localization of indeterminate pulmonary nodules before videothoracoscopic resection. Surg Endosc. 2002;16:509–11.
42. Kanazawa S, Ando A, Yasui K, et al. Localization of pulmonary nodules for thoracoscopic resection: experience with a system using a short hookwire and suture. AJR Am J Roentgenol. 1998;170:332–4.
43. Gossot D, Miaux Y, Guermazi A, et al. The hook-wire technique for localization of pulmonary nodules during thoracoscopic resection. Chest. 1994;105:1467–9.
44. Nakashima S, Watanabe A, Obama T, et al. Need for preoperative computed tomography-guided localization in video-assisted thoracoscopic surgery pulmonary resections of metastatic pulmonary nodules. Ann Thorac Surg. 2010;89:212–8.
45. Dendo S, Kanazawa S, Ando A, et al. Preoperative localization of small pulmonary lesions with a short hook wire and suture system: experience with 168 procedures. Radiology. 2002;225:511–8.
46. Park CH, Han K, Hur J, et al. Comparative effectiveness and safety of preoperative lung localization for pulmonary nodules: a systematic review and meta-analysis. Chest. 2017;151:316–28.
47. Mack MJ, Shennib H, Landreneau RJ, Hazelrigg SR. Techniques for localization of pulmonary nodules for thoracoscopic resection. J Thorac Cardiovasc Surg. 1993;106:550–3.
48. Ciriaco P, Negri G, Puglisi A, et al. Video-assisted thoracoscopic surgery for pulmonary nodules: rationale for preoperative computed tomography-guided hookwire localization. Eur J Cardiothorac Surg. 2004;25:429–33.
49. Miyoshi K, Toyooka S, Gobara H, et al. Clinical outcomes of short hook wire and suture marking system in thoracoscopic resection for pulmonary nodules. Eur J Cardiothorac Surg. 2009;36: 378–82.
50. Hajjar WM, Alnassar S, Almousa O, et al. Thoracoscopic resection of suspected metastatic pulmonary nodules after microcoil localization technique, a prospective study. J Cardiovasc Surg. 2017;58(4):606–12.
51. Galetta D, Bellomi M, Grana C, Spaggiari L. Radio-guided localization and resection of small or ill-defined pulmonary lesions. Ann Thorac Surg. 2015;100:1175–80.
52. Gonfiotti A, Davini F, Vaggelli L, et al. Thoracoscopic localization techniques for patients with solitary pulmonary nodule: hookwire versus radio-guided surgery. Eur J Cardiothorac Surg. 2007;32:843–7.
53. Vandoni RE, Cuttat JF, Wicky S, Suter M. CT-guided methylene-blue labelling before thoracoscopic resection of pulmonary nodules. Eur J Cardiothorac Surg. 1998;14:265–70.
54. Wicky S, Mayor B, Cuttat JF, Schnyder P. CT-guided localizations of pulmonary nodules with methylene blue injections for thoracoscopic resections. Chest. 1994;106:1326–8.
55. Prosch H, Stadler A, Schilling M, et al. CT fluoroscopy-guided vs. multislice CT biopsy mode-guided lung biopsies: accuracy, complications and radiation dose. Eur J Radiol. 2012;81:1029–33.
56. Kim GR, Hur J, Lee SM, et al. CT fluoroscopy-guided lung biopsy versus conventional CT-guided lung biopsy: a prospective controlled study to assess radiation doses and diagnostic performance. Eur Radiol. 2011;21:232–9.
57. Mahesh M. Fluoroscopy: patient radiation exposure issues. Radiographics. 2001;21:1033–45.
58. Khereba M, Ferraro P, Duranceau A, et al. Thoracoscopic localization of intraparenchymal pulmonary nodules using direct intracavitary thoracoscopic ultrasonography prevents conversion of VATS procedures to thoracotomy in selected patients. J Thorac Cardiovasc Surg. 2012;144:1160–5.
59. Iwano S, Yokoi K, Taniguchi T, et al. Planning of segmentectomy using three-dimensional computed tomography angiography with a virtual safety margin: technique and initial experience. Lung Cancer. 2013;81:410–5.
60. Ikeda N, Yoshimura A, Hagiwara M, et al. Three dimensional computed tomography lung modeling is useful in simulation and navigation of lung cancer surgery. Ann Thorac Cardiovasc Surg. 2013;19:1–5.
61. Kanzaki M, Kikkawa T, Shimizu T, et al. Presurgical planning using a three-dimensional pulmonary model of the actual anatomy of patient with primary lung cancer. Thorac Cardiovasc Surg. 2013;61:144–50.
62. Oizumi H, Endoh M, Takeda S, et al. Anatomical lung segmentectomy simulated by computed tomographic angiography. Ann Thorac Surg. 2010;90:1382–3.
63. Oizumi H, Kanauchi N, Kato H, et al. Anatomic thoracoscopic pulmonary segmentectomy under 3-dimensional multidetector computed tomography simulation: a report of 52 consecutive cases. J Thorac Cardiovasc Surg. 2011;141:678–82.
64. Nakada T, Akiba T, Inagaki T, Morikawa T. Thoracoscopic anatomical subsegmentectomy of the right S2b + S3 using a 3D printing model with rapid prototyping. Interact Cardiovasc Thorac Surg. 2014;19:696–8.
65. Onuki T. Virtual reality in video-assisted thoracoscopic lung segmentectomy. Kyobu Geka. 2009;62:733–8.
66. Tsubota N. An improved method for distinguishing the intersegmental plane of the lung. Surg Today. 2000;30:963–4.
67. Pardolesi A, Veronesi G, Solli P, Spaggiari L. Use of indocyanine green to facilitate intersegmental plane identification during robotic anatomic segmentectomy. J Thorac Cardiovasc Surg. 2014;148:737–8.
68. Misaki N, Chang SS, Igai H, et al. New clinically applicable method for visualizing adjacent lung segments using an infrared thoracoscopy system. J Thorac Cardiovasc Surg. 2010;140:752–6.
69. Sekine Y, Ko E, Oishi H, Miwa M. A simple and effective technique for identification of intersegmental planes by infrared thoracoscopy after transbronchial injection of indocyanine green. J Thorac Cardiovasc Surg. 2012;143:1330–5.
70. Gonzalez-Rivas D. Single incision video-assisted thoracoscopic anatomic segmentectomy. Ann Cardiothorac Surg. 2014;3:204–7.
71. Wang BY, Liu CY, Hsu PK, et al. Single-incision versus multiple-incision thoracoscopic lobectomy and segmentectomy: a propensity-matched analysis. Ann Surg. 2015;261:793–9.
72. Han KN, Kim HK, Choi YH. Comparison of single port versus multiport thoracoscopic segmentectomy. J Thorac Dis. 2016;8:S279–86.
73. Lin Y, Zheng W, Zhu Y, et al. Comparison of treatment outcomes between single-port video-assisted thoracoscopic anatomic segmentectomy and lobectomy for non-small cell lung cancer of early-stage: a retrospective observational study. J Thorac Dis. 2016;8:1290–6.
74. Han KN, Kim HK, Lee HJ, Choi YH. Single-port video-assisted thoracoscopic pulmonary segmentectomy: a report on 30 casesdagger. Eur J Cardiothorac Surg. 2016;49(Suppl 1):i42–7.
75. Tamura M, Shimizu Y, Hashizume Y. Pain following thoracoscopic surgery: retrospective analysis between single-incision and three-port video-assisted thoracoscopic surgery. J Cardiothorac Surg. 2013;8:153.
76. Sihoe AD. Reasons not to perform uniportal VATS lobectomy. J Thorac Dis. 2016;8:S333–43.
77. Perna V, Carvajal AF, Torrecilla JA, Gigirey O. Uniportal video-assisted thoracoscopic lobectomy versus other video-assisted thoracoscopic lobectomy techniques: a randomized study. Eur J Cardiothorac Surg. 2016;50:411–5.

Left Uniportal VATS Pneumonectomy

Peter Sze Yuen Yu and Calvin S. H. Ng

Pneumonectomy is usually indicated for more complex or advanced lung cancers, that are centrally located. The decision to proceed with pneumonectomy should not be done lightly as the surgical procedure itself is often considered a disease in itself that can be associated with potentially severe and life-threatening complications [1–3]. A sleeve resection procedure to preserve a lobe should be the operation of choice when circumstances allow [4–6]. The general principles for lung cancer surgery regarding patient having adequate lung function to tolerate the procedure and adequate lung cancer staging is paramount when preparing a patient for pneumonectomy.

Although no definite evidence suggests superiority of minimally-invasive pneumonectomy over open surgery, being an operation which brings significant mortality and morbidity, less incision-related morbidity may result in faster recovery and earlier initiation of adjuvant therapy which may translate into better survival [7]. Furthermore, patients who have undergone pneumonectomy are less likely to be able to complete the adjuvant chemotherapy [8]. The conventional VATS is a safe and feasible approach to pneumonectomy with reported morbidity and mortality of between 0 and 7.5% [9–13], and early limited results suggest that the same applies to uniportal VATS pneumonectomy [14, 15].

Electronic Supplementary Material The online version of this chapter (https://doi.org/10.1007/978-981-13-2604-2_26) contains supplementary material, which is available to authorized users.

P. S. Y. Yu · C. S. H. Ng (✉)
Division of Cardiothoracic Surgery, Department of Surgery,
Prince of Wales Hospital, The Chinese University of Hong Kong,
Hong Kong SAR, China
e-mail: calvinng@surgery.cuhk.edu.hk

Pre-operative Considerations

Being an ultramajor operation, pre-operative discussion and assessment should be done by a multidisciplinary team including Thoracic Surgeons, Pulmonologists, and Oncologists. Assessment of lung function should entail calculation of baseline and predicted-postoperative FEV1 and DLCO, and further physiological tests if necessary. Assessment of cardiovascular risks by the Thoracic RCRI guides further non-invasive tests or aggressive intervention as appropriate at the expertise of cardiologists [16]. Patients should be strongly encouraged to quit smoking at least 4 weeks prior to pneumonectomy. In particular for those with known chronic obstructive airway disease, pre-operative optimization from the respiratory team should be sought.

Operative Strategy

General anaesthesia induction is followed by right sided double lumen endotracheal tube intubation to isolate the left lung. Pre-operative flexible bronchoscopy sputum toileting can be considered, particularly in smokers and those with copious secretions, and specimen sent for culture. Bronchoscopy would also allow a final assessment of the tumour in relation to the airway prior to proceeding with the pneumonectomy. Patient is placed at right lateral decubitus position with operation table flexed to maximize the intercostal spaces as the usual VATS procedures. The skin is disinfected and draped to expose the operative field. Prophylactic antibiotics should be given at least a few minutes prior to making the skin incision.

Careful selection of incision site is of utmost importance to facilitate subsequent exposure and instrumentation. The incision is usually performed at the left fifth intercostal space between the anterior axillary and mid-axillary lines, to allow subsequent more ergonomic endostapler placement across hilar structures. A 2–3 cm incision is made, and an Alexis

D. Gonzalez-Rivas et al. (eds.), *Atlas of Uniportal Video Assisted Thoracic Surgery*,
https://doi.org/10.1007/978-981-13-2604-2_26

type wound retractor is inserted, allowing the insertion of a thoracoscope and VATS lung retraction forceps. The endocameleon thoracoscope (Endocameleon, Karl Storz, Germany) with 0–120 degrees variable angle of vision for viewing is favoured by us. Although the scope is slightly larger, it provides unparalleled viewing directions and angles to facilitate pneumonectomy that is often associated with large immobile bulky tumours. Furthermore, it may reduce chest wall and intercostal nerve trauma by reducing the amount of torque on the single incision site [17–20]. With experience and smaller tumours that are easier to manipulate, a 5 mm 30 degree scope may suffice.

Resectability of the tumor is first confirmed by thoracoscopic inspection of tumor in relation to possible invasion to deep hilar structures, great vessels and heart. Meticulous thoracoscopic exploration of the pleural cavity is performed to identify any pleural metastases or suspected malignant pleural effusion which should be saved for cytology. Pleural lesions should be biopsied and sent for frozen section and if found positive, pneumonectomy should not proceed.

Enlarged or PET-CT positive lymph nodes that may not have been accessible by pre-operative invasive mediastinal lymph node staging, for example at the aorto-pulmonary window, prevascular region, and inferior pulmonary ligament, should be sent for frozen section, and if found positive, in our center, pneumonectomy will not be performed. Following the above inspection and examination, the 2–3 cm single incision can be extended to 4–5 cm, and re-insertion of the Alexis wound protector, for the uniportal VATS left pneumonectomy.

We prefer pneumonectomy in the sequence from the pulmonary veins, main pulmonary artery, then lastly the left mainstem bronchus. The inferior pulmonary vein is exposed by sharp and blunt dissection of the inferior pulmonary ligament, aided by dental pledget mounted on long uniportal VATS instruments, such as node grasper (Scanlan Inc., USA) and angulated diathermy dissector. Some surgeons prefer the use of Harmonic scalpel. After exposure of and freeing the inferior pulmonary vein circumferentially, the lung is retracted cranially, the vein is slung with a thick silk tie and the inferior pulmonary vein can be divided by an endostapler (Videos 1 and 2). Our two preferred staplers for the procedure are Echelon Flex™ Powered Vascular Stapler 35 with Advanced Placement tip (Ethicon, Johnson & Johnson, New Brunswick, NJ, USA) [21] and Endo GIA™ Tristaple™ stapler with curved tip reload (Covidien, Mansfield, MA, USA). Dissection of the connective tissue, hilar mediastinal pleural reflection are continued cranially following inferior pulmonary vein division with diathermy hook or harmonic scalpel.

The left lung is then retracted postero-inferiorly. The anterior and superior mediastinal pleura is opened by combined sharp and blunt dissection to expose the superior pulmonary vein and pulmonary artery. The superior vein is dissected free and thick silk tie is placed round it, followed by division by one of the two aforementioned staplers (Videos 3 and 4). Placing the stapler across the superior pulmonary vein can be difficult in the uniportal setting, and to facilitate better exposure of the superior pulmonary vein, the anterior branches of the pulmonary artery to the left upper lobe may be divided first, to allow passage of the stapler.

The main pulmonary artery may be exposed better by removing aortopulmonary lymph nodes, and with the generous opening of the posterior pleura. We have found that dissecting the deep tunnel between main pulmonary artery and main bronchus can be aided by placing and opening slightly a small uniportal VATS Foerster clamp within the gap between the main pulmonary artery and main bronchus to "retract" open the deep tunnel followed by insertion of node grasper within the clamp for blunt dissection. The main pulmonary artery is also slung by a thick silk tie and then divided by a vascular endostapler (Video 5).

The lung is then retracted anteriorly to exposure the subcarinal space and some dissection of the subcarinal lymph nodes may be done to better expose and mobilize the posterior aspect of the left main bronchus. Gentle traction of the left main bronchus using a vascular sling can expose the left hilar lymph nodes, the prior dissection of which may facilitate subsequent exposure of the subcarinal stations. Dissection of the aortopulmonary lymph nodes can help facilitate mobilization of the superior aspects of the left main bronchus. The bronchus is dissected as proximal as possible, and it is our practice not to completely "skeletonize" it, hoping to maintain its blood supply. We have found the Walker's maneouver of placing a thin nylon tape around the main bronchus to allow traction, particular for heavy bulky tumours, can facilitate a more proximal placement of the endostapler at the left main bronchus. It can then be divided by an endostapler after checking that there is no endobronchial suction catheter present leaving a short bronchial stump. Reinforcement of the bronchial stump with vascular flap, such as intercostal pedicle, may be considered if the patient had prior radiotherapy in the area.

A strong protective specimen bag (LapSac, Cook Medical, USA) is used to wrap the lung to prevent port wound contamination. The specimen is retrieved through the single port. Following irrigation with warm water, systematic lymph node dissection is performed with hook diathermy and Harmonic scalpel. Access to the lymph node stations is usually satisfactory in the absence of the lung. Although thorough lymph node dissection is the corner stone of accurate pathological staging, dissection of the lymph nodes around the aortopulmonary window area should be performed with extra care as to avoid injuring the recurrent laryngeal nerve, which may predispose patients to postoperative silent aspiration, leading to pulmonary complications.

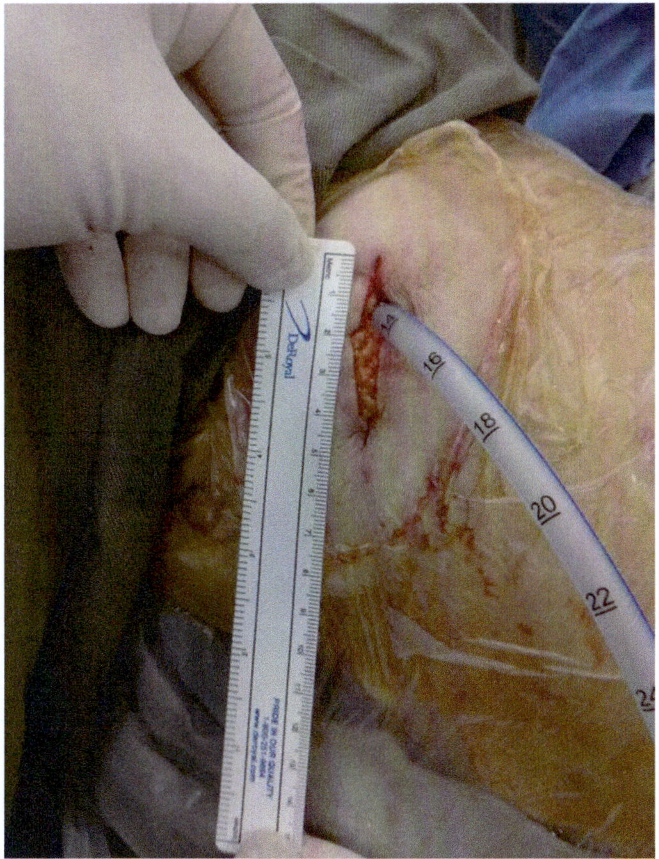

Fig. 1 Left uniportal VATS pneumonectomy wound with chest drain anchored towards the posterior aspect

Meticulous hemostasis is required following pneumonectomy, and the hilar stump is covered by TachoSil® (Baxter, CA, USA), followed by fibrin glue preventing its exposure. Intercostal nerve block is performed. Chest drain is placed through the single incision anchored towards the posterior aspect of the wound, and then the wound closed routinely (Fig. 1).

Postoperative Care

The postoperative care of a patient who have had uniportal VATS left pneumonectomy should be the same as those through other approaches. Reduction in pulmonary vasculature increases the total vascular resistance in the pulmonary circulation, and increases the afterload of the right ventricle. Fluid overload should be avoided in order not to increase the preload of the right ventricle, and to avoid oedema of the remaining lung. We also tend to keep serum potassium above 4.5 milliEquivalents per liter (mEq/L) during the early postoperative period, and aggressively deal with any new onset arrhythmias. Chest drain should not be put on suction to avoid early mediastinal shift which may compromise the systemic venous return and cause obstructive shock. Chest drain is usually removed the next postoperative day should bleeding be no longer a concern. On serial chest X-rays, the hemithorax is expected to have gradual filling of the residual space by fluid. Any sudden decrease in fluid and increase in air content should raise the suspicion of bronchopleural fistula [2].

References

1. Chan EC, Lee TW, Ng CS, Wan IY, Sihoe AD, Yim AP. Closure of postpneumonectomy bronchopleural fistula by means of single, perforator-based, latissimus dorsi muscle flap. J Thorac Cardiovasc Surg. 2002;124(6):1235–6. https://doi.org/10.1067/mtc.2002.127058.
2. Ng CS, Wan S, Lee TW, Wan IY, Arifi AA, Yim AP. Post-pneumonectomy empyema: current management strategies. ANZ J Surg. 2005;75(7):597–602. https://doi.org/10.1111/j.1445-2197.2005.03417.x.
3. Alloubi I, Jougon J, Delcambre F, Baste JM, Velly JF. Early complications after pneumonectomy: retrospective study of 168 patients. Interact Cardiovasc Thorac Surg. 2010;11(2):162–5. https://doi.org/10.1510/icvts.2010.232595.
4. Detterbeck FC, Lewis SZ, Diekemper R, Addrizzo-Harris D, Alberts WM. Executive summary: diagnosis and management of lung cancer, 3rd ed: American College of Chest Physicians evidence-based clinical practice guidelines. Chest. 2013;143(Suppl 5):7S–37S. https://doi.org/10.1378/chest.12-2377.
5. Cusumano G, Marra A, Lococo F, Margaritora S, Siciliani A, Maurizi G, Poggi C, Hillejan L, Rendina E, Granone P. Is sleeve lobectomy comparable in terms of short- and long-term results with pneumonectomy after induction therapy? A multicenter analysis. Ann Thorac Surg. 2014;98(3):975–83. https://doi.org/10.1016/j.athoracsur.2014.04.095.
6. Pan X, Tantai J, Lin L, Cao K, Zhao H. Comparison of short and long-term results between sleeve resection and pneumonectomy in lung cancer patients over 70 years old: 10 years experience from a single institution in China. Thorac Cancer. 2014;5(6):494–9. https://doi.org/10.1111/1759-7714.12116.
7. Lau KKW, Ng CSH, Wan IYP, Wong RHL, Yeung ECL, Kwok MWT, Lau RWH, Wan S, Yim APC, Underwood MJ. VATS pneumonectomy is safe and may have benefits over open pneumonectomy. Interact Cardiovasc Thorac Surg. 2013;17(Suppl 1):S29.
8. Pisters KM, Evans WK, Azzoli CG, Kris MG, Smith CA, Desch CE, Somerfield MR, Brouwers MC, Darling G, Ellis PM, Gaspar LE, Pass HI, Spigel DR, Strawn JR, Ung YC, Shepherd FA, Cancer Care Ontario, American Society of Clinical Oncology. Cancer Care Ontario and American Society of Clinical Oncology adjuvant chemotherapy and adjuvant radiation therapy for stages I-IIIA resectable non small-cell lung cancer guideline. J Clin Oncol. 2007;25(34):5506–18. https://doi.org/10.1200/JCO.2007.14.1226.
9. Sahai RK, Nwogu CE, Yendamuri S, Tan W, Wilding GE, Demmy TL. Is thoracoscopic pneumonectomy safe? Ann Thorac Surg. 2009;88(4):1086–92. https://doi.org/10.1016/j.athoracsur.2009.05.065.
10. Nagai S, Imanishi N, Matsuoka T, Matsuoka K, Ueda M, Miyamoto Y. Video-assisted thoracoscopic pneumonectomy: retrospective outcome analysis of 47 consecutive patients. Ann Thorac Surg. 2014;97(6):1908–13. https://doi.org/10.1016/j.athoracsur.2014.02.022.
11. Tsubota N. Is pneumonectomy using video-assisted thoracic surgery the way to go? Study of data from the Japanese Association for Thoracic Surgery. Gen Thorac Cardiovasc Surg. 2014;62(8):499–502. https://doi.org/10.1007/s11748-014-0400-3.

12. Battoo A, Jahan A, Yang Z, Nwogu CE, Yendamuri SS, Dexter EU, Hennon MW, Picone AL, Demmy TL. Thoracoscopic pneumonectomy: an 11-year experience. Chest. 2014;146(5):1300–9. https://doi.org/10.1378/chest.14-0058.
13. Liu Y, Gao Y, Zhang H, Cheng Y, Chang R, Zhang W, Zhang C. Video-assisted versus conventional thoracotomy pneumonectomy: a comparison of perioperative outcomes and short-term measures of convalescence. J Thorac Dis. 2016;8(12):3537–42. https://doi.org/10.21037/jtd.2016.12.24.
14. Gonzalez-Rivas D, Delgado M, Fieira E, Mendez L, Fernandez R, de la Torre M. Uniportal video-assisted thoracoscopic pneumonectomy. J Thorac Dis. 2013;5(Suppl 3):S246–52. https://doi.org/10.3978/j.issn.2072-1439.2013.07.44.
15. Ng CS, Kim HK, Wong RH, Yim AP, Mok TS, Choi YH. Single-port video-assisted thoracoscopic major lung resections: experience with 150 consecutive cases. Thorac Cardiovasc Surg. 2016;64(4):348–53. https://doi.org/10.1055/s-0034-1396789.
16. Brunelli A, Kim AW, Berger KI, Addrizzo-Harris DJ. Physiologic evaluation of the patient with lung cancer being considered for resectional surgery: diagnosis and management of lung cancer, 3rd ed: American College of Chest Physicians evidence-based clinical practice guidelines. Chest. 2013;143(Suppl 5):e166S–90S. https://doi.org/10.1378/chest.12-2395.
17. Ng CS, Wong RH, Lau RW, Yim AP. Single port video-assisted thoracic surgery: advancing scope technology. Eur J Cardiothorac Surg. 2015;47(4):751. https://doi.org/10.1093/ejcts/ezu236.
18. Ng CS. Single-port thoracic surgery: a new direction. Korean J Thorac Cardiovasc Surg. 2014;47(4):327–32. https://doi.org/10.5090/kjtcs.2014.47.4.327.
19. Ng CS, Wong RH, Lau RW, Yim AP. Minimizing chest wall trauma in single-port video-assisted thoracic surgery. J Thorac Cardiovasc Surg. 2014;147(3):1095–6. https://doi.org/10.1016/j.jtcvs.2013.10.043.
20. Ng CS, Rocco G, Wong RH, Lau RW, Yu SC, Yim AP. Uniportal and single-incision video-assisted thoracic surgery: the state of the art. Interact Cardiovasc Thorac Surg. 2014;19(4):661–6. https://doi.org/10.1093/icvts/ivu200.
21. Ng CS, Pickens A, Siegel JM, Clymer JW, Cummings JF. A novel narrow profile articulating powered vascular stapler provides superior access and haemostasis equivalent to conventional devicesdagger. Eur J Cardiothorac Surg. 2016;49(Suppl 1):i73–8. https://doi.org/10.1093/ejcts/ezv352.

Right Pneumonectomy

Mercedes de la Torre, Eva Mª Fieira, and Marina Paradela

Abstract

Right pneumonectomy is not a frequent major resection in thoracic surgery, with limited indications. In some cases, it may require complex surgery. For this reason we think uniportal VATS right pneumonectomy should only be performed in centers that are experienced in uniportal resections.

In this chapter the surgical technique is well defined step by step, making feasible the removal of the whole lung and putting special attention to the most critical points such us the dissection of the main pulmonary artery.

We consider that the main key points for this surgery are the adequate patient selection (assessment of respiratory and cardiac function, evaluation of comorbidities) and a good planning of the surgical resection (tumour size and localization, tumour relation with hilar structures).

This procedure maintains the uniportal approach advantages, not only during the surgery (direct view to the hilar vessels and tissue) but the patient recovery as well (less pain, early mobilization and reduced hospital stay).

In our experience, Uniportal VATS right pneumonectomy can be considered a feasible and safe procedure.

Indications

Right pneumonectomy has only selected indications and always after discarding that a lesser resection is feasible, such as a lobectomy or a sleeve-resection.

The most frequent is the bronchogenic carcinoma with the following characteristics:

- Tumors involving widely the major fissure, compromising the right upper lobe and the right lower lobe.
- Hilar tumors involving the main right bronchus or the intermediate bronchus but unable to perform a sleeve pulmonary resection.
- Hilar tumors involving the main pulmonary artery.

Contraindications

- Tumors that require an extended resection (chest wall, vertebra, superior vena cava, esophagus or carinal resection).
- Huge mass that limited an appropriate surgical view of the hilum and safe manipulation of the lung.
- Surgeon discomfort.
- Preoperative chemotherapy or radiotherapy are not a definite contraindication.

Historical Review

The first video-assisted thoracoscopic pneumonectomy was described by Craig and Walker in 1995 [1]. In 2012, Gonzalez Rivas performed the first single-incision video-assisted thoracoscopic pneumonectomy, in a patient with a right lower lobe adenocarcinoma involving the upper lobe through the fissure [2].

VATS lobectomy is accepted as a valid treatment for patients with early stages of non-small cell lung cancer. The experience with pneumonectomy is quite different and more limited (Table 1), probably due to the fact that the indication of pneumonectomy implies advanced tumors.

Electronic Supplementary Material The online version of this chapter (https://doi.org/10.1007/978-981-13-2604-2_27) contains supplementary material, which is available to authorized users.

M. de la Torre (✉) · E. M. Fieira · M. Paradela
Coruna University Hospital, A Coruña, Spain
e-mail: mtorre@canalejo.org

D. Gonzalez-Rivas et al. (eds.), *Atlas of Uniportal Video Assisted Thoracic Surgery*,
https://doi.org/10.1007/978-981-13-2604-2_27

Table 1 Previous series of video-assisted thoracoscopic pneumonectomy

Author (year)	No. incisions	Total cases	No. pneumonectomies
Craig and Walker (1995) [1]	3	62	6 (2 right)
Yim et al. (1997) [3]	3	78	6
Roviaro et al. (2004) [4]	3	259	6 (3 right)
Mackenna et al. (2006) [5]	3	1100	14
Congregado et al. (2008) [6]	4	237	22 (13 right)
Gonzalez-Rivas et al. (2011) [7]	3/2	200	6 (1 right)
Batto et al. (2014) [8]	3	107	50
Nagai et al. (2014) [9]	3	2480	47 (9 right)
Augustin et al. (2016) [10]	3	390	6
Gonzalez-Rivas et al. (2014) [11]	1	130	7
Aragon et al. (2014) [12]	1	82	1
Ng et al. (2015) [13]	1	150	2 (left)
Zou et al. (2015) [14]	1	168	1 (left)
Xie et al. (2016) [15]	1	1063	2

Apart from that, several studies have reported the safety of thoracoscopic pneumonectomy and equivalent survival rates compared with thoracotomy.

Patient Selection

Patient selection is very important because right pneumonectomy is a really high-risk surgery, apart from the surgical approach.

It must be considered for non-N2 tumors and after assessing distant metastases, making PET-CT scans mandatory.

Assessment with bronchoscopy of the tumor limits can be performed at the beginning of the surgery in case of endobronchial affectation.

Complete pulmonary function tests, including lung diffusion capacity and a ventilation-perfusion scan, are necessary to define the patient's ability to tolerate a pneumonectomy. Studies of cardiac function to assess ventricular function and to discard pulmonary hypertension are also indicated. Finally, a strict evaluation of patient's comorbidities and performance status is essential.

Sometimes, right pneumonectomy can be an unplanned resection. The intraoperative decision must also be based on this strict patient evaluation.

Surgical Technique

Uniportal VATS pneumonectomy is technically easier to perform than a lobectomy because the fissure does not need to be managed. However, extra care must to be taken during dissection and division of the main artery and the main bronchus.

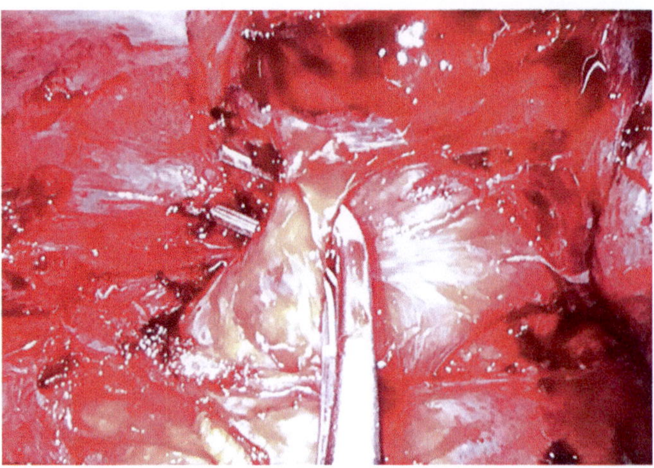

Fig. 1 Disection of the middle lobe vein

Patients are intubated with a double lumen tube and positioned in left lateral decubitus.

The incision is done in the fifth intercostal space in the antero-lateral position, with a length of 4–5 cm.

The first step must be the evaluation of the pleural cavity and the lung, to assess the tumor's resectability and to confirm the need for a pneumonectomy.

For the correct instrumentation, the thoracoscope (10 mm, 30° and high-definition) is placed in the posterior part of the incision while the instruments and the staplers are positioned in the anterior part.

There are two important key points:

- Optimal exposure of the lung to perform the dissection of the structures easier. The lung is retracted with a short or long ring-forceps managed by the assistant.
- Bimanual instrumentation: the surgeon exposes the target tissue with the suction or other ring forceps doing the dissection at the same time.

The lower lobe is retracted cranially to divide the pulmonary ligament and dissect the inferior vein. The lung is then retracted posteriorly, the anterior mediastinal pleural is opened, the middle lobe vein (Fig. 1) and the superior vein (Fig. 2) are dissected and encircled, separately or together. If either one or more veins are invaded by the tumor, the pericardium can be entered and an additional 1–2 cm of vein can be exposed.

To expose the artery, the upper lobe is retracted caudally and posteriorly, the upper mediastinal pleura is open, separating the azygos vein and exposing the superior aspect of the main bronchus. The anterior arterial trunk is dissected (Fig. 3), the anterior aspect of the intermediate trunk is exposed retracting the superior vein and opening the space between the artery and the superior cava vein. It is recommended to remove station 10 lymph nodes to make the main

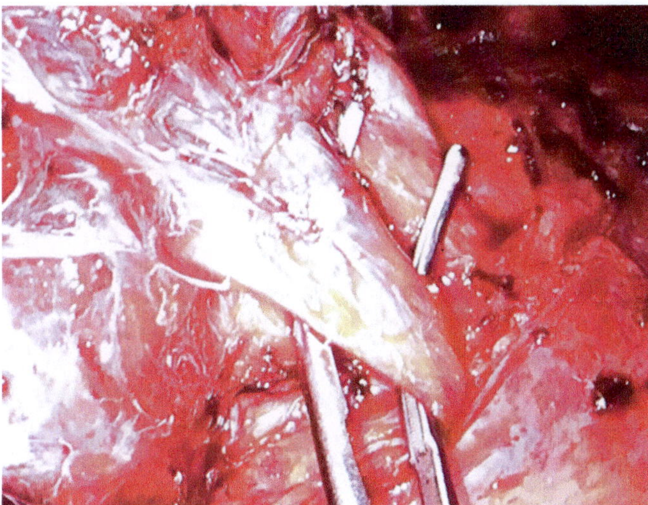

Fig. 2 Disection of the upper lobe vein

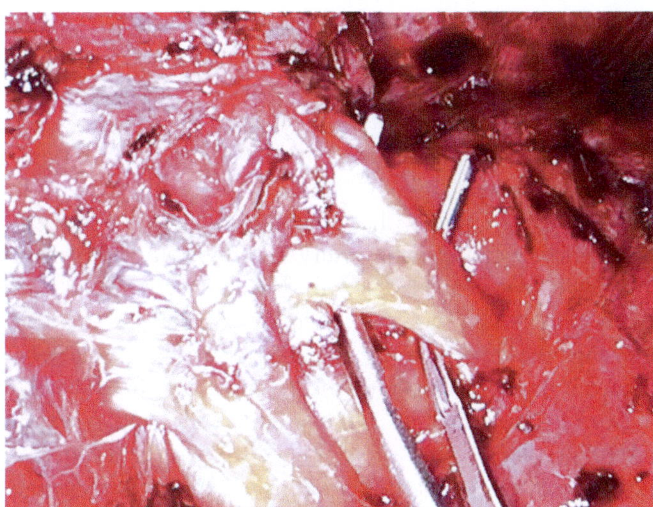

Fig. 3 Disection of the anterior arterial trunk

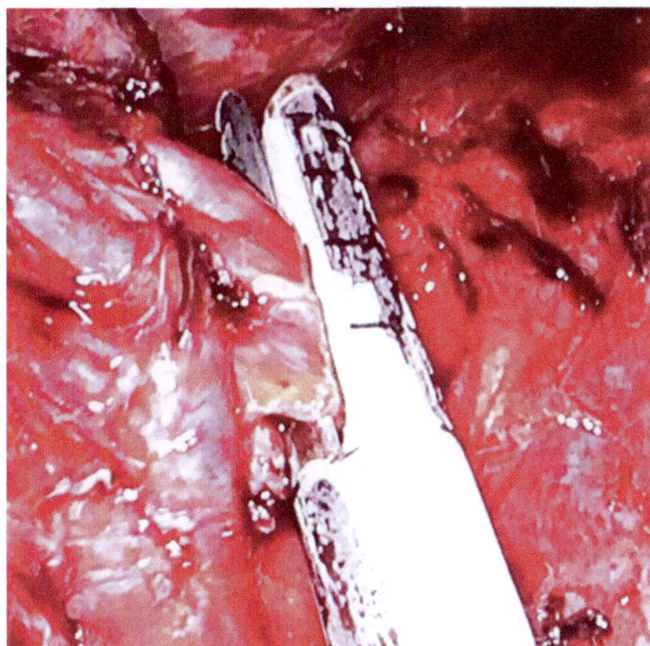

Fig. 4 Division of the anterior arterial trunk

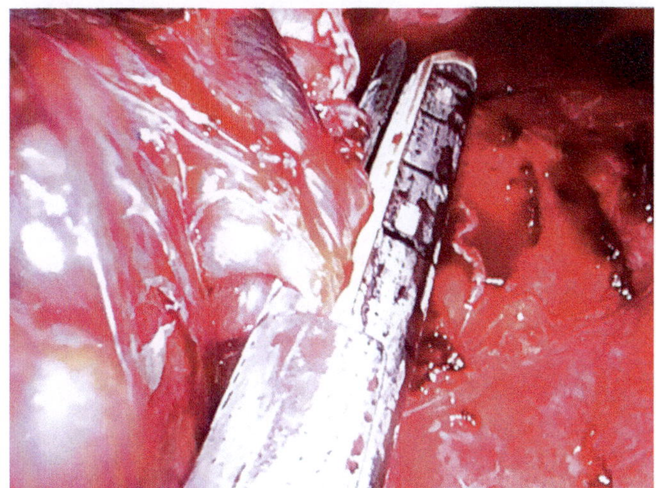

Fig. 5 Division of the upper lobe vein

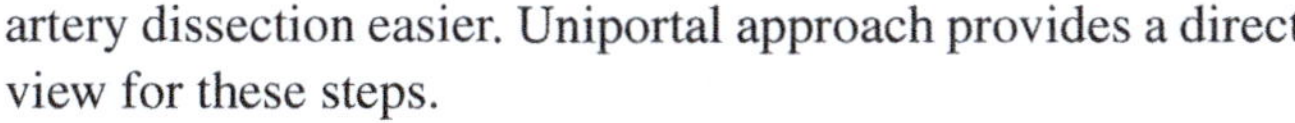

artery dissection easier. Uniportal approach provides a direct view for these steps.

Then, the surgical table is rotated towards the surgeon and the lung is retracted anteriorly (a sponge stick is helpful) to open the posterior mediastinal pleura exposing the pericardium and the posterior aspect of the main bronchus.

The surgical table is returned to the initial position. The upper lobe is retracted caudally and the anterior arterial trunk is divided with a vascular stapler (Fig. 4). This maneuver makes the division of the superior vein easier, also using a vascular endostapler (Fig. 5). This step represents the main difference with the left pneumonectomy, where the whole pulmonary artery is stapled.

The lower lobe is once again retracted cranially to divide the inferior vein following with the middle vein, when it is independent. After that, the hilar tissue is dissected and divided, exposing the inferior aspect of the intermediate arterial trunk. The dissection of this trunk is carefully completed using a right angle clamp or a thoracoscopic dissector and after to encircle it (Fig. 6). We recommend to divide it from the superior aspect to the inferior with a vascular endostapler, retracting the lung backwards (Fig. 7).

The last step is the dissection and transection of the main bronchus (Fig. 8). It is helpful to remove the subcarinal lymph nodes to expose correctly the bronchus and to divide it as close to the carina as possible. For the bronchus division, the

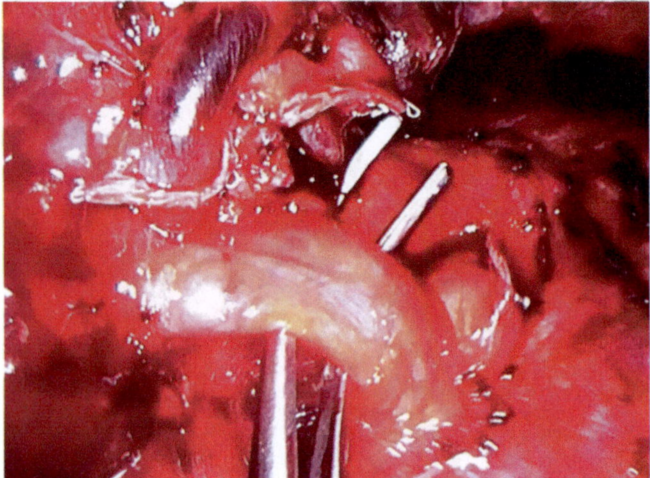

Fig. 6 Dissection of the intermediate arterial trunk

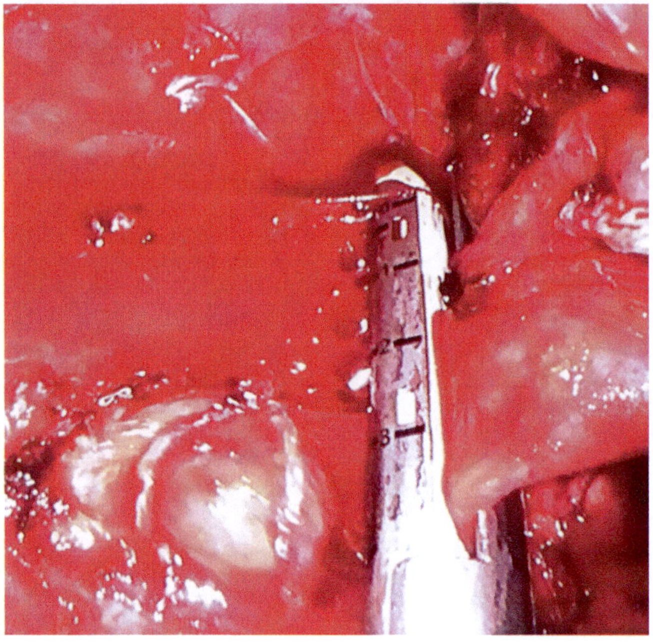

Fig. 7 Division of the intermediate arterial trunk

lung is retracted caudally, respecting the anatomic position of the bronchus and to avoid rotations during its transection. A bronchial endostapler is used.

The whole lung is removed in a protective bag.

In our experience, we don't use bronchial stump coverage. It is known that right pneumonectomy has more risk for bronchopleural fistulae than left pneumonectomy and for this reason many others surgeons recommend to cover bronchial stumps with vascularized tissue, mainly in patients that received neoadjuvant chemotherapy and specially radiotherapy. The intercostal muscle flap and pericardial fat are preferably used.

The pleural cavity should be filled with warm saline to check for bronchial stump air leak.

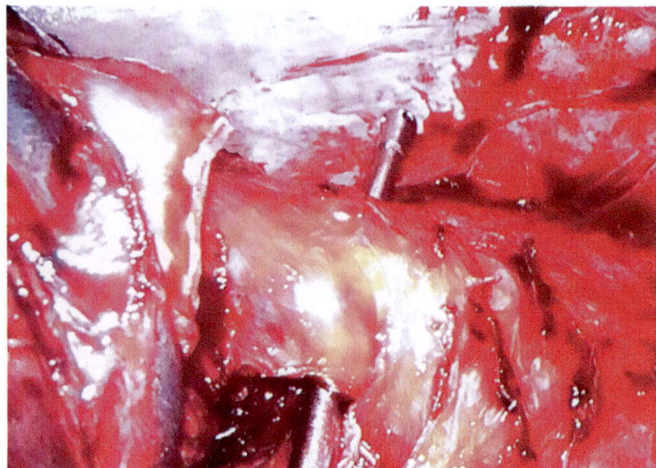

Fig. 8 Dissection of the main right bronchus

Finally, the systematic lymph node dissection is completed.

A single chest tube is placed in the posterior part of the incision or in an independent incision in the seventh intercostal space, depending on the surgeon's choice.

The incision is closed as in a usual uniportal VATS approach.

Special Situations

In case of hilar tumors that adhere to or invade either the boyden trunk or the main artery, the division of the main artery will be necessary. Then, the pneumonectomy can start by dividing the inferior vein, then the middle lobe vein and after that, the superior vein. The anterior pericardium can be opened if it is necessary to divide the superior vein to provide an extra 1–2 cm of length. If the hilum is very fixed, it is very helpful to open the space between the superior cava vein and the main artery, also the pericardium and even to transect the azygos vein and to remove the paratracheal lymph nodes. If the tissue is fibrotic, extra care must be taken. All these maneuvers make the transection of the main right pulmonary artery viable. The last option can be the use of a linear stapler.

In case of big tumors, it might be necessary to enlarge the incision or even to dilate the intercostal space with a rib retractor, removing finally the whole lung. In this situation, we recommend to place the chest tube in another incision and close the intercostal space with a suture.

Discussion

In the last decade, thoracoscopic procedures have expanded in application and popularity to perform more complex operations, such as segmentectomy, bronchoplasty and pneumonectomy.

Video-assisted thoracoscopic surgery pneumonectomy is an uncommon procedure because appropriate candidates are limited and it is difficult to establish the safety of the procedure.

However, both technical and instrumental advances in thoracoscopic surgery, joined to the roll of induction chemotherapy shrinking large tumors more reliable, have enabled to adopt VATS pneumonectomy as a common indication in experienced VATS centers.

Several studies have demonstrated the safety of VATS pneumonectomy [16], reduction in conversion rate with experience, good morbidity and mortality rates and an equivalent impact for local control of advanced lung cancer diseases [8, 9]. One single institutional publication reported equivalent survival for VATS approach compared with thoracotomy [17].

Two points remains the most debated, the maximum tumor size and the vascular involvement. Battoo et al. found that for tumor diameter >7 cm, there was a higher conversion rate. This group emphasized the importance of controlled conversions performed prudently, because delayed conversions were associated with worse outcomes.

The technique of uniportal VATS right pneumonectomy was first described by Gonzalez-Rivas et al. in 2013 [18]. We think the main advantage of uniportal VATS pneumonectomy is the direct view to the hilar structures, especially over the main pulmonary artery. In fact, the main difference compared with two or three-ports VATS right pneumonectomy is the possibility to divide this artery in two trunks, making safer its division. Uniportal VATS provides also a good vision for the dissection and division of the main bronchus. The surgical steps are well defined and we consider previous experience in uniportal VATS lobectomy is mandatory and specific instruments, long and with proximal and distal articulation, are very helpful.

It is important to remember that this approach preserves the principles advantages of minimally invasive surgery for the patients, mainly less postoperative pain, reduced hospital stay and better compliance for adjuvant chemotherapy.

In conclusion, attempting uniportal VATS right pneumonectomy at experienced centers appears safe and must be offered to selected candidates.

References

1. Craig SR, Walker WS. Initial experience of video assisted thoracoscopic pneumonectomy. Thorax. 1995;50:392–5.
2. Gonzalez-Rivas D, De la Torre M, Fernandez R, Garcia J. Single-incision video-assisted thoracoscopic right pneumonectomy. Surg Endosc. 2012;26:2078–9.
3. Yim AP, Liu HP. Thoracoscopic major lung resection-indications, technique, and early results: experience from two centers in Asia. Surg Laparosc Endosc. 1997;7(3):241–4.
4. Roviaro G, Varoli F, Vergani C, Maciocco M, Nucca O, Pagano C. Video-assisted thoracoscopic major pulmonary resections. Technical aspects, personal series of 259 patients, and review of the literature. Surg Endosc. 2004;18:1552–8.
5. Mackenna RJ, Houck W, Fuller CB. Video-assisted thoracic surgery lobectomy: experience with 1100 cases. Ann Thorac Surg. 2006;81:421–6.
6. Congregado M, Jimenez-Merchan R, Gallardo G, Ayarra J, Loscertales J. Video-assisted thoracic surgery (VATS) lobectomy: 13 years experience. Surg Endosc. 2008;22:1852–7.
7. Gonzalez D, De la Torre M, Paradela M, Fernandez R, Delgado M, Garcia J, et al. Video-assisted thoracic surgery lobectomy: 3-years initial experience with 200 cases. Eur J Cardiothorac Surg. 2011;40:21–8.
8. Battoo A, Jahan A, Yang Z, Nwogu CE, Yendumari SS, Dexter EU, et al. Thoracoscopic pneumonectomy: an 11-year experience. Chest. 2014;146(5):1300–9.
9. Nagai S, Imanishi N, Matsuoka T, Matsuoka K, Ueda M, Miyamoto Y. Video-assisted thoracoscopic pneumonectomy: retrospective outcome analysis of 47 consecutive patients. Ann Thorac Surg. 2014;97:1908–13.
10. Augustin F, Maier H, Lucciarini P, Bodner J, Klotzner S, Schmid T. Extended minimally invasive lung resections: VATS bilobectomy, bronchoplasty, and penumonectomy. Langenbeck's Arch Surg. 2016;401:341–8.
11. Gonzalez-Rivas D, Fieira E, Delgado M, Mendez L, Fernandez R, De la Torre M. Is uniportal thoracoscopic surgery a feasible approach for advanced stages of non-small cell lung cancer? J Thorac Dis. 2014;6(6):641–8.
12. Aragon J, Perez I. From open surgery to uniportal VATS: Asturias experience. J Thorac Dis. 2014;6(S6):644–9.
13. Ng CSH, Kim HK, Wong RHL, Yim APC, Mok TSK, Choi YH. Singel-port video-assisted thoracoscopic major lung resections: experience with 150 consecutive cases. Thorac Cardiovasc Surg. 2016;64(4):348–53.
14. Zhu Y, Xu G, Zheng B, Liang M, Wu W, Zheng W, Chen CH. Single-port video-assisted thoracoscopic surgery lung resection: experiences in Fujian Medical University Union Hospital. J Thorac Dis. 2015;7(7):1241–51.
15. Xie D, Wang H, Fei K, Chen CH, Zhao D, Zhou X, et al. Single-port video-assisted thoracic surgery in 1063 cases: a single-institution experience. Eur J Cardiothorac Surg. 2016;49:31–6.
16. Sahai RK, Nwogu CE, Yendumari S, Tan W, Wilding CE, Demmy TL. Is thoracoscopic pneumonectomy safe? Ann Thorac Surg. 2009;88:1086–92.
17. Nwogu CE, Yendumari S, Demmy T. Does thoracoscopic pneumonectomy for lung cancer affect survival? Ann Thorac Surg. 2010;89:S2012–6.
18. Gonzalez-Rivas D, Delgado M, Fieira E, Mendez L, Fernandez R, De la Torre M. Uniportal video-assisted thoracoscopic pneumonectomy. J Thorac Dis. 2013;5(S3):S246–52.

Uniportal Lymphadenectomy

Maria Delgado Roel, Eva Fieira Costa,
Marina Paradela De La Morena, Diego Gonzalez-Rivas,
Ricardo Fernandez Prado, Juan Pablo Ovalle Granados,
and Mercedes De La Torre Bravos

Introduction

Video-assisted thoracic surgery is increasingly being performed by many groups as surgical management for non-small cell lung cancer, only if it is technically possible. The role of this approach is unclear when you perform the lymphadenectomy [1]. On the other hand the number of lymph nodes, stations sampled and lymph node ratio have a direct relationship with a correct pathologic staging, and thus with the prognosis.

With the current experience in VATS in mayor resections published for many groups, we obtain a radical videothoracoscopic mediastinal lymphadenectomy. The results are not inferior and the number of lymph nodes dissected are equivalent to the thoracotomy approach [2, 3].

Uniportal video-assisted thoracic surgery provides us with the best anatomic instrumentation and a direct view. It allows us to perform more complex cases, including a systematic lymph node dissection with a greater number of nodes [4, 5].

Electronic Supplementary Material The online version of this chapter (https://doi.org/10.1007/978-981-13-2604-2_28) contains supplementary material, which is available to authorized users.

M. Delgado Roel (✉) · E. Fieira Costa · M. Paradela De La Morena · R. Fernandez Prado · J. P. Ovalle Granados · M. De La Torre Bravos
Thoracic Surgery Department, Complexo Hospitalario Universitario de A Coruña, A Coruña, Spain

D. Gonzalez-Rivas
Department of Thoracic Surgery, Shanghai Pulmonary Hospital, Tongji University School of Medicine, Shanghai, China

Department of Thoracic Surgery and Minimally Invasive Thoracic Surgery Unit (UCTMI), Coruña University Hospital, Coruña, Spain
e-mail: diego@uniportal.es

Operative Techniques

The Material

It is important to highlight the role of the surgical material in single port technique. With the development of thoracoscopic instruments we improve the instrumentation in a reduced space. Especially with regards to long and double jointed instruments.

Generally, in order to perform de lymphadenectomy we use:

1. Ten millimeter thoracoscope high definition, 30 degree.
2. High definition monitor screen.
3. Long, short and double-jointed curved ring forceps.
4. Long and double-jointed metzembaum scissors.
5. Curved suction.
6. Long and double jointed thoracoscopic dissector.
7. Endopath 5 mm endoscopic peanut (x2).
8. Energy devices.

When we use single port, the camera is placed in the posterior part of the incision [5]. The key for a correct lymphadenectomy in single-port VATS is a good exposition and bimanual instrumentation.

Only three instruments or less are inserted at the same time in most of the lymphadenectomy cases, to avoid the interference between themselves.

If we give more than one use to the different instruments, it helps to avoid changing the instruments during the surgery.

In this way the curved ring forceps are very useful to dissect and to pull the lymph nodes. When it is containing a gauze it is used to push the lung to promote de exposure. We have to try not to grasp too much the lymph nodes with forceps in order to reduce the possibility of breakage.

We use the curved suction and sponge stick to dissect and to expose the structures. The Harmonic scalped makes the haemostasis easier and it is also useful to dissect.

D. Gonzalez-Rivas et al. (eds.), *Atlas of Uniportal Video Assisted Thoracic Surgery*,
https://doi.org/10.1007/978-981-13-2604-2_28

The patient is placed in a semiprone position under general anaesthesia and double-lumen endotracheal tube for single-lung ventilation.

The incision is 3–4 cm long in the fifth intercostal space on the anterior axillary line.

The Technical Aspects in Mediastinal Lymph Node Dissection

Right Paratracheal Space

Group 2R and 4R.

We remove all the mediastinal lymph nodes and fat between the trachea, the cava vein and the azigos vein.

In order to improve the lung exposition we push backwards the lung using a grasper with a gauze, a curved ring forceps or a endoscopic peanut. By moving the table in antitrendelenburg this exposes the paratracheal area, even sometimes after the lobectomy this is enough, and we avoid using more instruments through the incision.

The next step is to open the mediastinal pleural under and above the azygos vein with Harmonic scalped, with the help of a grasper or a curved suction this will enable us to dissect this area. A long endothoracoscopic peanut is very useful to separate the joint between the azygos and the cava vein.

With a small grasper we dissect the lymph nodes package from the cava vein to the trachea, helped by a curved suction. Finally, the use of energy devices facilitate the dissection and it cuts the small lymph nodes vessels, thus reducing the rate of postoperative bleeding (Video 1).

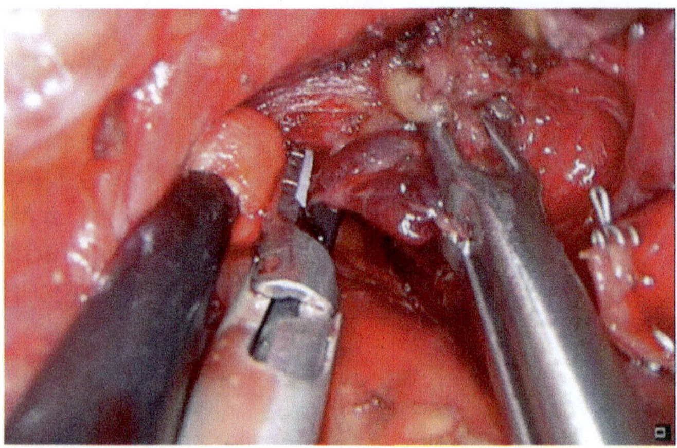

Fig. 1 Left Paratracheal Space Lymphadenectomy

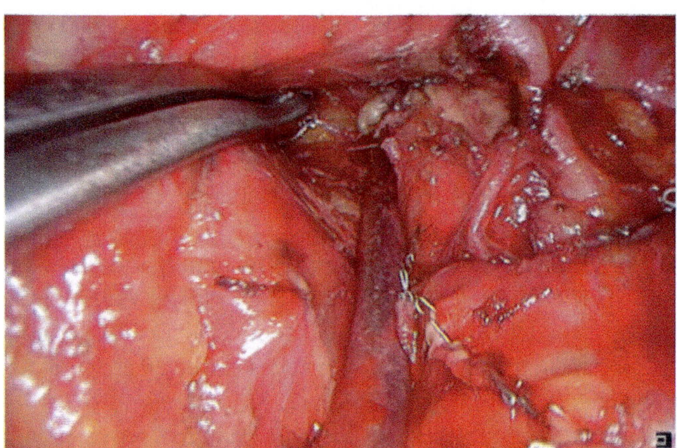

Fig. 2 Left Paratracheal Space Lymphadenectomy

Left Paratracheal Space

It is difficult to dissect lymph nodes at level 4 L. With single port view you can perform a left paratracheal lymphadenectomy under the aortic arch. It is important in this step to avoid injuring the recurrent laryngeal nerve. Usually you have to push the aortic arch and with the harmonic scalpel and the grasper we complete the dissection (Figs. 1 and 2).

The mediastinal pleura is opened with a Harmonic scalpel and it is dissected with the grasper or curved suction. Sometimes the oesophagus is retracted with another sponge stick or even with the curve suction.

We finish with the Harmonic scalpel and remove all the lymph nodes and fat tissues in a bloc (Figs. 3 and 4 and Video 2).

Right Subcarinal Lymphadenectomy

Seven group.

We dissect de lymph nodes below bilateral main bronchus above the lower pulmonary vein and anterior to the oesophagous and the vagus nerve.

Usually the inferior pulmonary ligament is mobilised. We push the lung with a sponge stick to expose the space. When we move the operative table anteriorly we exposes subcarinal space, in this way sometimes the traction to the lung is not necessary.

Left Subcarinal Lymphadenectomy

Seven group.

The most difficult lymphadenectomy is left subcarinal lymphadenectomy, because is the deepest area. Technically it is similar to a right subcarinal lymphadenectomy.

We dissect de lymph nodes below bilateral main bronchus above the lower pulmonary vein and in front of the aorta and the vagus nerve.

We push the lung when it is necessary with a sponge stick to expose the space and we move the operative table anteriorly.

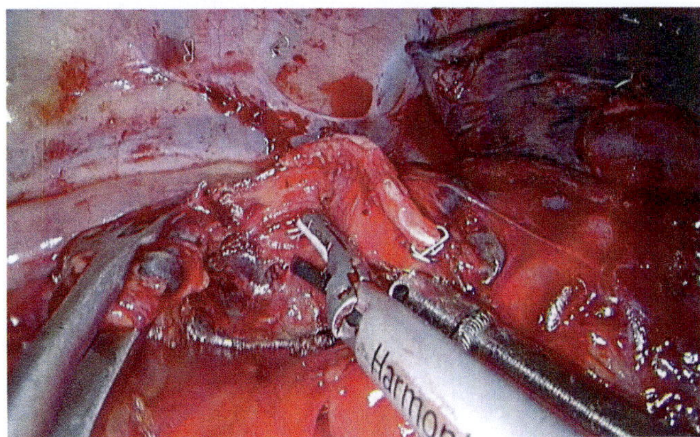

Fig. 3 Right Subcarinal Lymphadenectomy

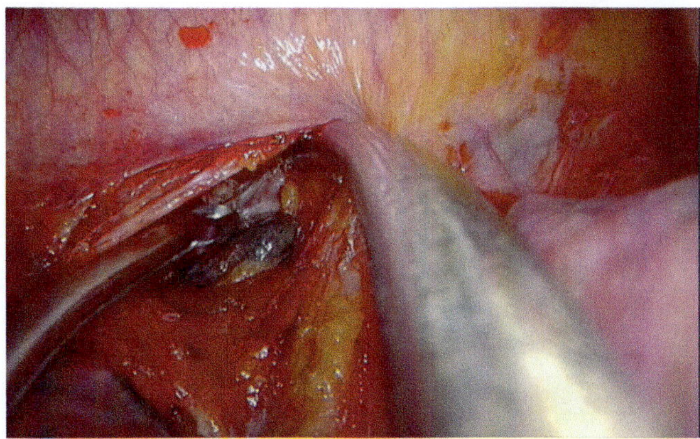

Fig. 5 Left Subcarinal Lymphadenectomy

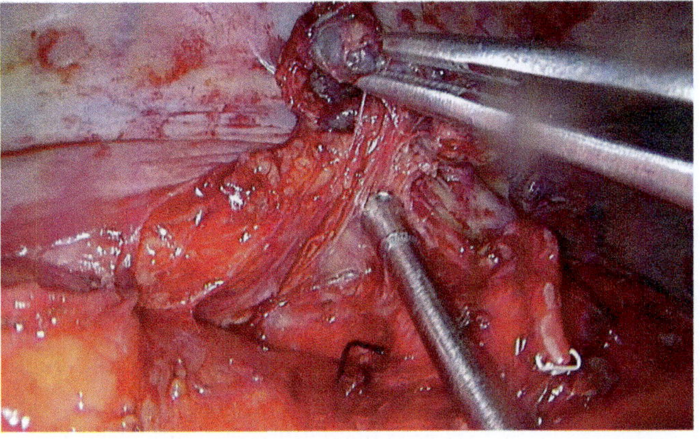

Fig. 4 Right Subcarinal Lymphadenectomy

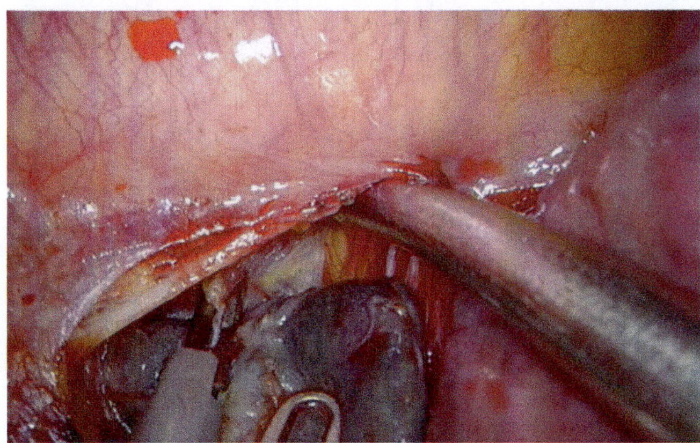

Fig. 6 Left Subcarinal Lymphadenectomy

The mediastinal pleura is opened with a Harmonic scalpel and it is dissected with the grasper or curved suction. Sometimes it is useful to retract the aorta with a sponge stick or with another instrument like a curved suction.

We finish with the harmonic scalpel and remove all the lymph nodes and fat tissues in a bloc (Figs. 5, 6, and 7).

Aortopulmonary Window Space

Five group and six group.

The space above upper left pulmonary vein and between the aorta and the main left pulmonary artery. During the dissection precaution is given to protect the recurrent laryngeal nerve and the phrenic nerve. The first step is to open the anterior mediastinal pleura with the Harmonic scalpel towards the superior left main pulmonary artery. The lymph nodes and fatty tissues are removed with the assistance of a long curve suction or a grasper to avoid bleeding (Figs. 8 and 9).

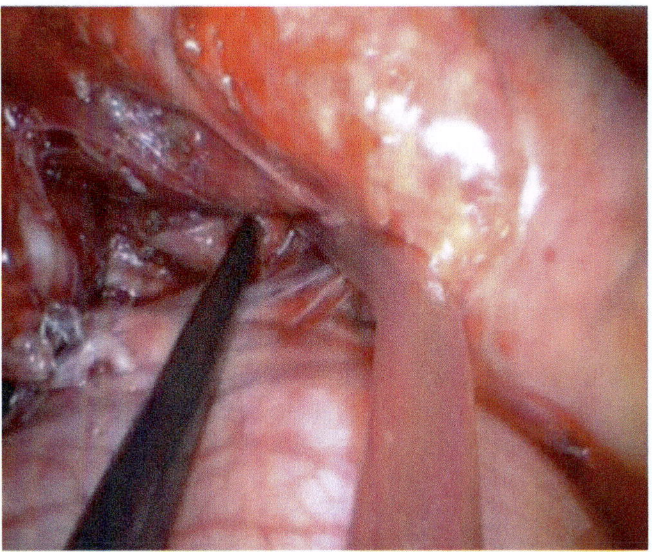

Fig. 7 Left Subcarinal Lymphadenectomy

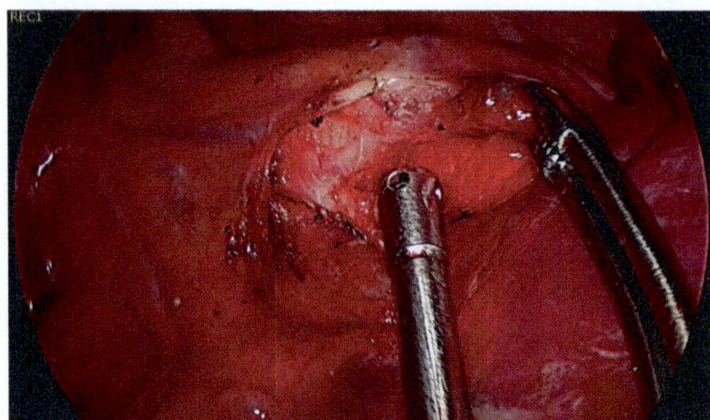

Fig. 8 Aortopulmonary Window Space

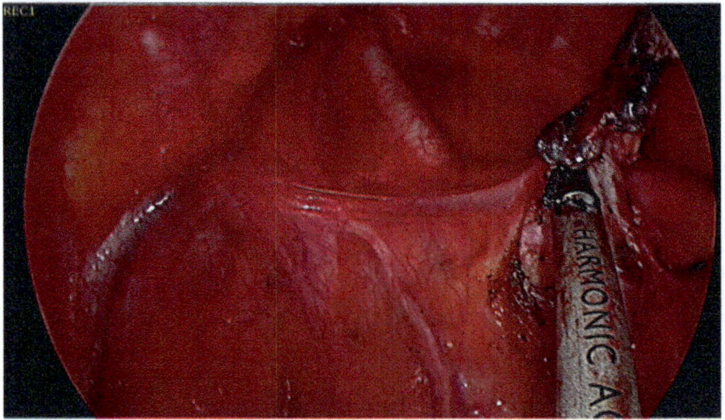

Fig. 9 Aortopulmonary Window Space

Para-oesophageal and Pulmonary Ligament Lymph Nodes

Eight group and nine group.

The lung is pushed cranially with a grasper with a gauze, a curved ring forceps or a endoscopic peanut and the pulmonary ligament and the lymph nodes are dissected with the harmonic scalpel and the curve suction or a grasper.

Hiliar and Interlobar Lymph Nodes

The hiliar lymph nodes are removed usually during the lobectomy. Sometimes the interlobar lymphadenectomy has the difficulty that the nodes frequently are above the pulmonary artery branches. With a grasper and another instrument, like the cautery or the harmonic scalpel a complete dissection of this area it is possible and safe (Video 2).

Comments

Currently, the percentage of lobectomies done by VATS in many hospitals has increased to almost 80% of the lung pulmonary resections [6].

With this volume in VATS for mayor resections by experienced surgeons in the technique, it is possible to perform a complete and radical lymph node dissection by VATS [7], at the same time that VATS is associated with lower morbidity than open approach [8].

The lymphadenectomy with single port, can have even better results than with two or three ports by the direct view and with the experience of the surgeon and easier instrumentation [5].

As more cases are treated with the single-port approach, the number of lymph nodes removed increases—thus reflecting improvement in the surgical technique. Gonzalez Rivas and colleagues [9] analysed the mean number of lymph nodes resected with single port approach and compare that with two and three ports, being the lymph nodes number reported by single port higher than with two or three port VATS (14.5 ± 7 vs. 11.9 ± 6.7). On the other hand more lymph node dissection was performed during the last single port period: 12.2 ± 4.7 versus 16 ± 8 ($p = 0.055$).

In conclusion, lymphadenectomy is an important part of the lung cancer surgery.

To perform a standard lymphadenectomy by single port approach is possible and represents the best view if we compare with three and two ports. Of course, the surgeon's learning curve in VATS lobectomies and the cumulative hospital volume are important factors to consider, in this way it has been associated with improved lymph node dissection.

Disclosures No disclosures.

References

1. D'Amico TA. Videothoracoscopic mediastinal lymphadenectomy. Thorac Surg Clin. 2010;20:207–13.
2. Baisi A, Rizzi A, Raveglia F, Cioffi U. Video-assisted thoracic surgery is effective in systemic lymph node dissection. Eur J Cardiothorac Surg. 2013;44(5):966.
3. Delgado Roel M, Fieira Costa EM, González-Rivas D, Fernández LM, Fernández Prado R, De la Torre M. Uniportal video-assisted thoracoscopic lymph node dissection. J Thorac Dis. 2014;6(Suppl 6):S665–8.
4. Fieira Costa E, Delgado Roel M, Paradela de la Morena M, Gonzalez-Rivas D, Fernandez-Prado R, de la Torre M. Technique of uniportal VATS major pulmonary resections. J Thorac Dis. 2014;6(Suppl 6):S660–4.
5. Gonzalez-Rivas D. VATS lobectomy: surgical evolution from conventional VATS to uniportal approach. ScientificWorldJournal. 2012;2012:780842.

6. Kent M, Wang T, Whyte R, Curran T, Flores R, Gangadharan S. Open, video-assisted thoracic surgery, and robotic lobectomy: review of a national database. Ann Thorac Surg. 2014;97(1): 236–42.
7. Lee PC, Kamel M, Nasar A, Ghaly G, Port JL, Paul S, Stiles BM, Andrews WG, Altorki NK. Lobectomy for non-small cell lung cancer by video-assisted thoracic surgery: effects of cumulative institutional experience on adequacy of lymphadenectomy. Ann Thorac Surg. 2016;101(3):1116–22.
8. Ceppa DP, Kosinski AS, Berry MF, Tong BC, Harpole DH, Mitchell JD, D'Amico TA, Onaitis MW. Thoracoscopic lobectomy has increasing benefit in patients with poor pulmonary function: a society of thoracic surgeons database analysis. Ann Surg. 2012;256(3):487–93.
9. Gonzalez-Rivas D, Paradela M, Fernandez R, Delgado M, Fieira E, Mendez L, Velasco C, De la Torre M. Uniportal video-assisted thoracoscopic lobectomy: two years of experience. Ann Thorac Surg. 2013;95:426–32.

Part V

Advanced Uniportal Techniques

Uniportal Video-Assisted Thoracoscopic Sleeve Resections

Diego Gonzalez-Rivas, Jiang Lei, and Dmitrii Sekhniaidze

Introduction

In 1947 the first bronchoplasty took place to remove a benign tumor [1]. Thereafter, in 1959 the first bronchial carcinoma was removed [2]. A right pneumonectomy with en-bloc resection of the carina was reported in 1950 [3]. Gibbon described in 1959 the first case of a right sleeve pneumonectomy [4] and in the eighties decade, Grillo and coworkers described carinal resections [5]. Pulmonary artery reconstruction for lung cancer was reported in 1950. During the 1970s and 1980s a few groups also described these procedures in a series of cases [6].

Nowadays, as minimally invasive techniques are evolving and are being adopted worldwide, so have the indications. Video-assisted thoracoscopic surgery (VATS), compared to open thoracotomy offers several advantages: decreased postoperative pain [7], shorter removal time of chest tube drainage and shorter length of stay [8], better preservation of pulmonary function [9], and earlier return to regular activities [10]. These results are obtained while respecting the oncologic principles of thoracic surgery. Even more so, there is evidence that thoracoscopic lobectomies may offer fewer complications and better survival rates for early stage tumors [11]. However, there are currently no studies showing survival benefits of VATS in advanced cases of non-small cell lung cancer (NSCLC) over open thoracotomy.

Sleeve procedures allow parenchymal preservation and safe oncologic margins even for patients that can tolerate more extensive resections [12]. Several publications report that sleeve lobectomy is equal to pneumonectomy in terms of survival [13] but are associated to specific complications [14].

Sleeve procedures are contraindicated when pneumonectomy is required due to the extension of the tumor. For example, when the tumor extensively involves the interlobar fissure. The bronchial reconstruction should be carefully assessed at the end of the procedure to determine its likelihood to fail.

The experience gained in VATS throughout the last years, surgical instrument improvements and better high definition cameras are the principal reasons why indications to the most complex procedures have augmented in VATS [15]. Since the approach is less invasive, the uniportal VATS has emerged as an alternative and feasible technique, applicable to all large spectrum of pulmonary resections including sleeve procedures [16, 17].

Preoperative Planning

With preoperative bronchoscopy, CT (Computed Tomography) scan, and PET-CT (Positron emission tomography–computed tomography) scan, (Fig. 1) the indication for a sleeve resection is defined. In the case of uptake on the PET-CT, a mediastinoscopy or endobronchial ultrasound biopsy (EBUS) should be performed prior to the operation. The extension of the tumor should be carefully ascertained and histology should be confirmed with biopsy. A bronchoscopy prior to the surgery can identify the need for a sleeve resection when the tumor is at the entrance of a lobar bronchus, or when the tumor is exophytic and located in a mainstem bronchus. Also when submucosal signs indicate cancer extension. The information obtained through bronchoscopy

Electronic Supplementary Material The online version of this chapter (https://doi.org/10.1007/978-981-13-2604-2_29) contains supplementary material, which is available to authorized users.

D. Gonzalez-Rivas (✉)
Department of Thoracic Surgery, Shanghai Pulmonary Hospital, Tongji University School of Medicine, Shanghai, China

Department of Thoracic Surgery and Minimally Invasive Thoracic Surgery Unit (UCTMI), Coruña University Hospital, Coruña, Spain
e-mail: diego@uniportal.es

J. Lei
Department of Thoracic Surgery, Shanghai Pulmonary Hospital, Tongji University School of Medicine, Shanghai, China

D. Sekhniaidze
Department of Thoracic Surgery, Regional Oncological Center, Tyumen, Russian Federation

D. Gonzalez-Rivas et al. (eds.), *Atlas of Uniportal Video Assisted Thoracic Surgery*,
https://doi.org/10.1007/978-981-13-2604-2_29

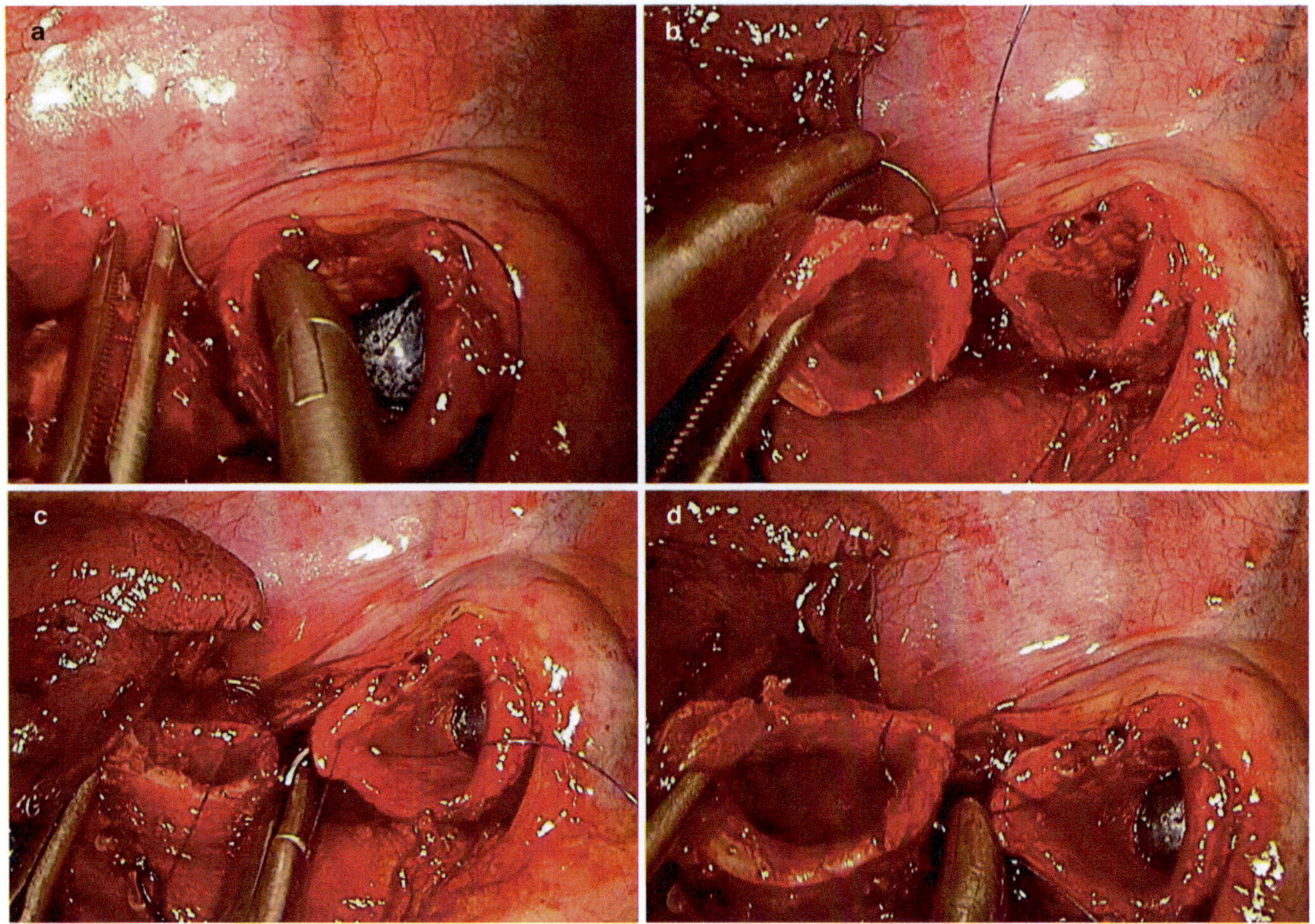

Fig. 1 Running suture for RUL sleeve anastomosis. (**a**) First stitch from inside to outside in the border between cartilaginous and membranous portion. (**b**) With the same needle the stitch is from outside to inside in the intermedius bronchus at the same level. (**c**) With the same needle we continue the running suture from posterior to anterior (from inside to outside in the main bronchus). (**d**) Suture from outside to inside in the intermedius bronchus

is useful at the time of the surgery when the bronchus is incised and divided. A pulmonary function test and perfusion scan to predict postoperative lung function are relevant factors when planning a sleeve resection as well as considering the suitability for surgery.

As part of the postoperative management, patients usually go through physiotherapy, are given mucolitis or humidification and antibiotics. A bronchoscopy should be performed postoperatively to check the integrity of the suture and to clear secretions before discharging the patient home.

Surgical Thoracoscopic Technique

The most convenient location for the incision is in the fourth ICS, between the anterior and middle axillary line (for both sides and also for upper or lower procedures). Based in our experience, the suturing is more complicated if the incision is placed too posterior and perpendicular to the hilum. It is also less ergonomic due to the angle of the needle, this is particularly so when suturing the posterior wall of the bronchus. Placing the incision between the anterior and middle axillary line, always in the fourth intercostal space, facilitates the handling of suture as the needle holder runs parallel to the hilum, making suturing similar to an open anterior thoracotomy.

When performing bronchial suturing using a uniportal VATS approach, it is very important to maintain the camera in the posterior part of the incision and to operate with both hands below the camera. The idea is to reproduce the same principle as in open anterior thoracotomies where the eyes of the surgeon are above his/her hands (Fig. 1). The geometrical explanation of the approach [18] and the ergonomics of the instrumentation [19] are important factors that make a sleeve reconstruction through a uniportal approach less complex. As a result, the anastomosis can be accomplished from a more natural and ergonomic perspective in our opinion. It is recommended to use a wound protector as it prevents fatty tissue from interfering with the suture.

By rotating the table 45° towards the surgeon, the lung exposure improves making it easier to do the posterior bronchial anastomosis, especially the membranous portion.

The uniportal thoracoscopic bronchial sleeve anastomosis should always be performed by a continuous suture. It is less complex and less time consuming compared to interrupted sutures applied by VATS. In our practice we tie the suture extracorporeally, then we wrap one end of the suture around the index and the other end around the pinky finger of the left hand to control tension of the lines and finally with the right hand the knot is pushed down with a thoracoscopic knot pusher [20]. We normally use a continuous absorbable suture with one thread and two needles (Polydioxanone, PDS 3-0) or non-absorbable suture (prolene 3/0). However the anastomosis can also be performed by using an absorbable barbed suture device, the V-Loc™ wound closure device (Medtronic Covidien, US) or Stratafix™ (Johnson & Johnson, US) which avoids knot-tying and provides a secure, strong closure.

Following completion of the anastomosis, it is tested under saline water for evidence of air leaks and we evaluate the anastomosis with a bronchoscopy before extubating. At the end of the operation only one chest tube is normally placed.

Sleeve Bronchoplasty

The end-to-end anastomosis are the most demanding bronchoplastic procedures from all bronchial sleeve resections. The right upper lobe (RUL) bronchoplasty is the most common and use to be the less complex procedure. This is due to the alignment of the main and the intermediate bronchi (Fig. 1). Occasionally, however, the right bronchus is located at the posterior side of the pulmonary artery or the azygos vein, making it less accessible and complicating the anastomosis. The pulmonary ligament should be released to improve lung mobility and reduce tension during and after the anastomosis. Right upper lobe sleeves should begin with the subcarinal lymph node dissection, when required, prior to the anastomosis. In the event of a short stump of the main bronchus, suturing could be difficult and would require the azygos vein to be divided. When this occurs, paratracheal lymphadenectomy should be left for last in order to prevent the proximal bronchi from retracting under the azygos vein into the paratracheal space.

With the use of a long scalpel the bronchus can be initially incised. Then the bronchial circumference section may be completed using a pair of scissors. Anastomosis can be completed in two ways. The first would be to initially fixate with a knot the posterior face and then with a needle perform the running suture from the posterior to the anterior side. After that and next to the first knot, another running suture would be applied on the opposite direction towards the anterior side bringing both suture ends to the anterior face to finally tie both ends (Video 1).

The second and our preferred method would be to use only one thread with two needles. The suturing would start at the posterior side and one of the ends, through a running suture, would be brought to the anterior face. Thereafter, the other end would follow from the posterior to the anterior side, bringing both ends together on the anterior face. This technique allows a faster and even better adjustment of the anastomosis, especially when there is discordance in calibers (Fig. 1, Video 2).

Vascular Reconstruction

A partial resection or total vascular sleeve reconstruction might be required when a tumor invades the pulmonary artery (PA). In these cases it is recommended that a proper dissection and control of the PA (in occasions intrapericardial control might be required) be done prior to the procedure. In order to prevent thrombosis, 5000 IU intravenous heparin must be administered before clamping off the PA. The classic way is to proximally clamp the PA with a large thoracoscopic clamp such as a Chitwood clamp and then distally (or on the inferior pulmonary vein to prevent interference with instruments during anastomosis), to clamp with a bulldog clamp. The pressure of the bulldog clamp should be controlled prior

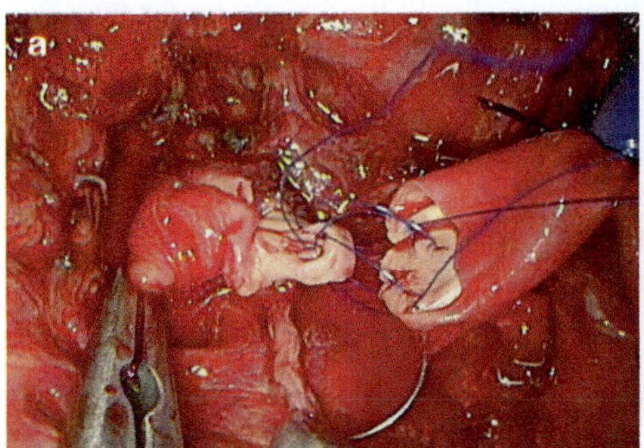

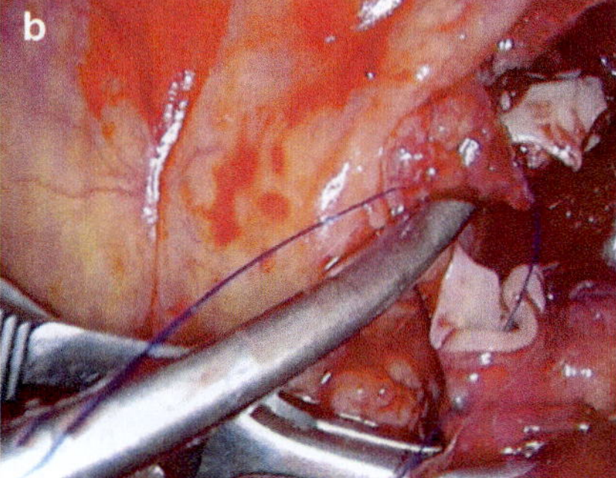

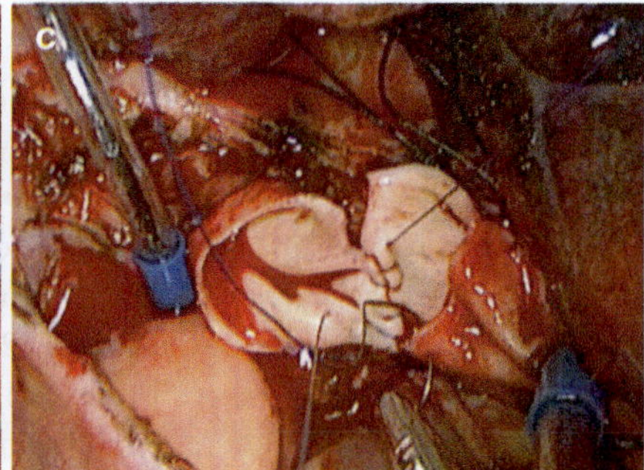

Fig. 2 Different options to clamp the pulmonary artery. (**a**) Proximal clamp and distal torniquet (**b**) proximal clamp and distal bullodog. (**c**) Proximal and distal torniquets

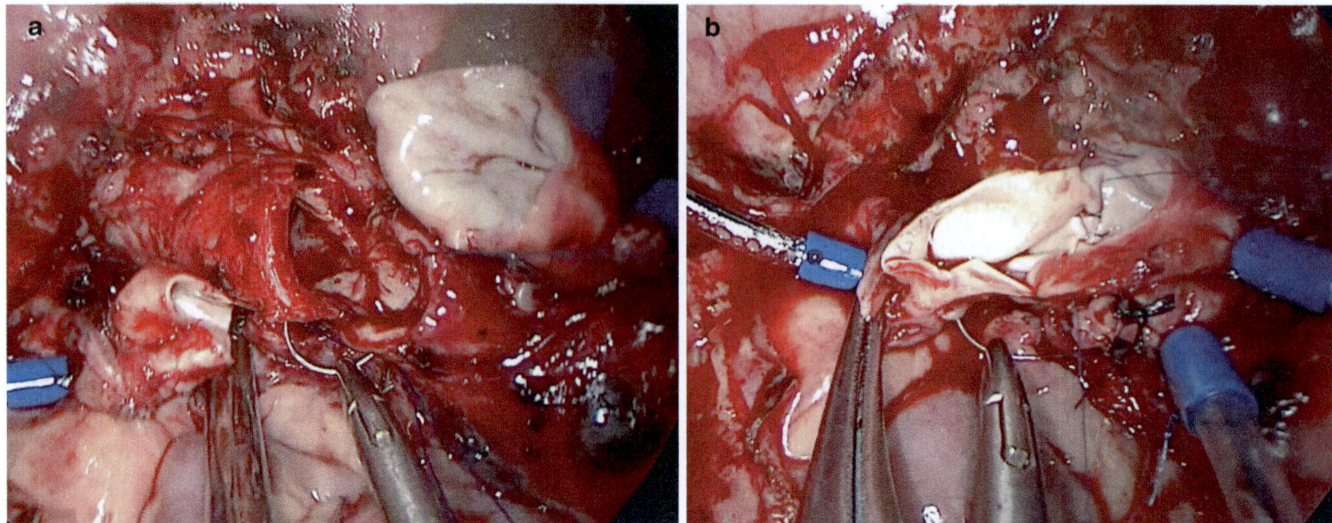

Fig. 3 Double sleeve technique. (**a**) Bronchial anastomosis. (**b**) Vascular reconstruction

to surgery in order to avoid unexpected bleeding. The use of a double vessel loop could suffice as well to clamp the distal part of the artery or inferior pulmonary vein, when performing lateral small angioplastic resections [21].

The pulmonary artery may be alternatively clamped with the use of a vascular tourniquets, both proximally as well as distally by using a triple silk thread system, sling or surg-i-loop. Traction on the tourniquet can be maintained by applying a polymer clip or suture and both tourniquets are placed inside the chest cavity pushed by wet gauzes. This allows more space to work through the incision. On the left side it is advisable to do an intra-pericardial control of the pulmonary artery and to place the tourniquet proximal to the ductus arteriosus. This will avoid any accidental displacement of the tourniquet (Fig. 3). When the involvement of the tumor is too proximal on the PA, the use of the tourniquets is not recommended. The ductus arteriosus should be divided in order to enlarge more than 1 cm on the length of the PA stump, and then use of a thoracoscopic clamp is the safest choice. The clamp must be placed through the incision outside of the wound protector to avoid interference during the anstomosis.

To facilitate vascular reconstructions, the lymphadenectomy, should be done at the beginning of the procedure. First start by dividing the veins, bronchus and then fissure. This provides a larger surgical field to work in as well as a better control of the section of the pulmonary artery involved [22–24].

In an end-to-end anastomosis, it is crucial to carefully align the edges and diameter of both vascular ends in order to avoid stenosis or kinking of the vessel [25]. We recommend to use the same technique we described for bronchus: running 4/0 or 5/0 prolene suture, one thread with two needles.

The suture on the posterior face is placed first and then suturing is done in a postero-anterior direction. Both needle ends meet at the anterior face and are then knotted together.

Before tying completely, the proximal clamp should be released to purge any air and to check the blood flow through the reconstructed section of the artery.

In case of double broncho-vascular sleeve procedures, the bronchus must be sutured first and the vascular anastomosis last in order to avoid traction to the arterial anastomosis (Fig. 3) [26]. The anastomosis should be protected at the end of the procedure with a flap to prevent fistula (Video 3).

RUL Sleeve Lobectomy (Videos 1, 2)

The most frequently described sleeve lobectomy in the literature is the right upper lobe (RUL) [27, 28]. Once the hilar vessels have been divided and the fissure has been opened, the right main bronchus, upper lobe bronchus and intermediate bronchus must be dissected divided with the use of a long scalpel or sharp scissors. The bronchial anastomosis is done with the use of a continuous 3-0 suture (prolene, PDS or barbed suture) as previously described. To compensate for the difference of caliber between both bronchi, the suture intervals on the main bronchus should be slightly larger than the suture intervals on the bronchus intermedius and should be frequently adjusted throughout the anastomosis (Videos 1, 2).

Right Lower Lobe Sleeve Resection (Middle Lobe Bronchus to Intermediate Bronchus Sleeve) (Video 4)

In order to avoid a bilobectomy of the lower and middle lobe, especially in patients with a poor lung function, a reconstruction of the lower lobar bronchus to preserve the middle lobe can be performed by suturing to the bronchus

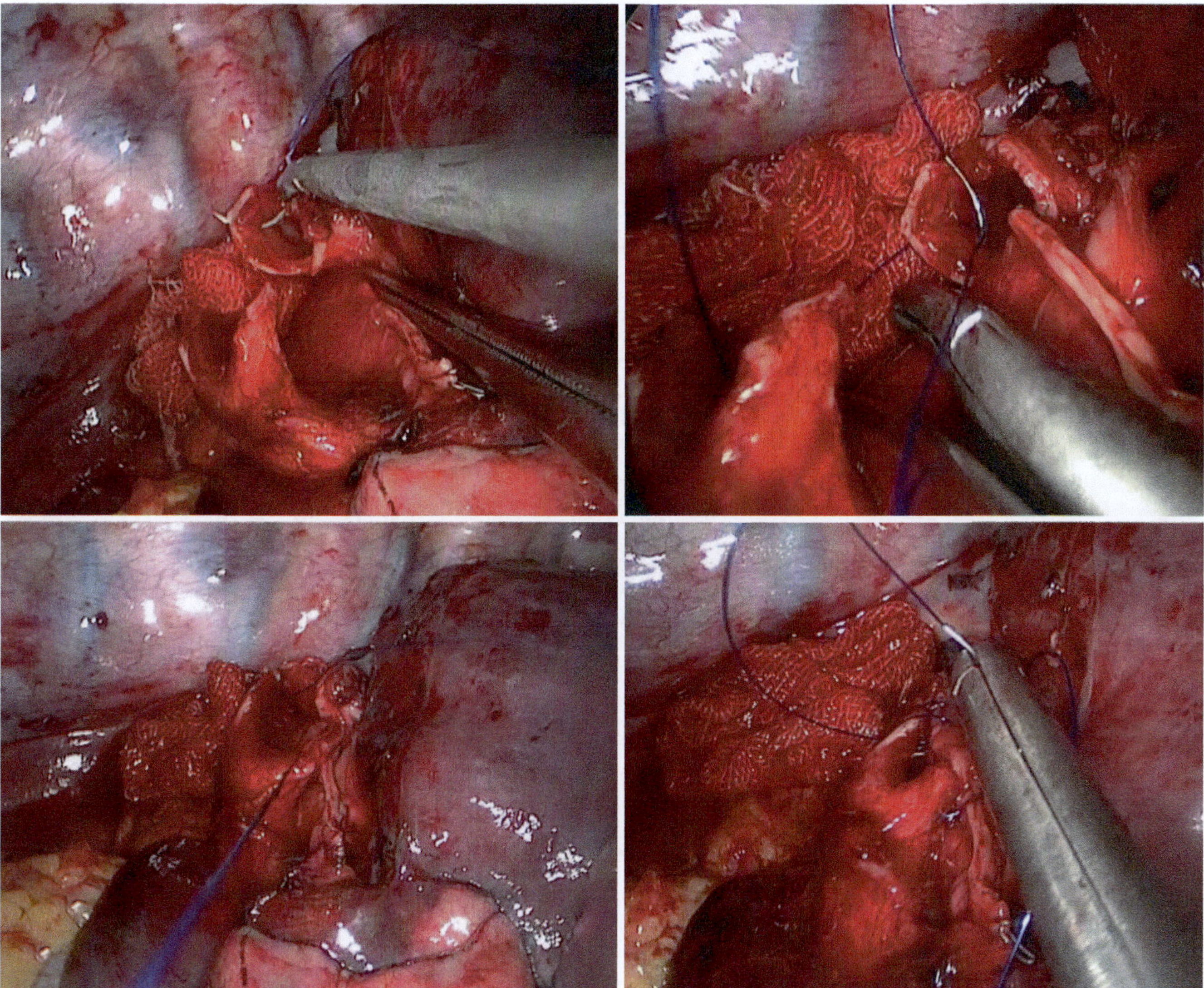

Fig. 4 Surgical technique or running suture for middle lobe anastomosis to bronchus intermedius

intermedius of the middle lobe. Due to the difference in caliber it is essential to perform a tangential cut of the middle bronchus and adjust the caliber of the anastomosis very carefully (Fig. 4).

Right Upper Sleeve Bilobectomy (Video 5)

When there is a tumor that invades the bronchus intermedius to the origin of the superior lobar bronchus, a sleeve bilobectomy that connects the superior bronchus to the main right bronchus via anastomosis can be performed. The anastomosis can be done in the same way as in a RUL sleeve. In this case it is essential to avoid that the lobar bronchus rotates with the suture. The correct subcarinal lymphadenectomy must be performed prior to the anastomosis (Fig. 5).

Left Upper Lobe (LUL) Sleeve Resection (Video 6)

While the longer length of the main left bronchus might seem to make it less complicated to perform left upper sleeve resections, the deeper location of the main stump after bronchial transection, the absence of the intermediate bronchus, the interference with the main PA and the aortic arch, and the short length of upper lobe bronchus, makes the anastomosis more difficult than on the right hemithorax (Fig. 6).

As previously described, anastomosis should be performed using the running suture technique with two needles, for both the anterior and posterior wall (Video 6). The running suture technique can also be performed in two steps: first the posterior 180 degrees of the 360 degree circumference of the bronchus and then the remaining anterior 180 degrees (Fig. 7, Video 6).

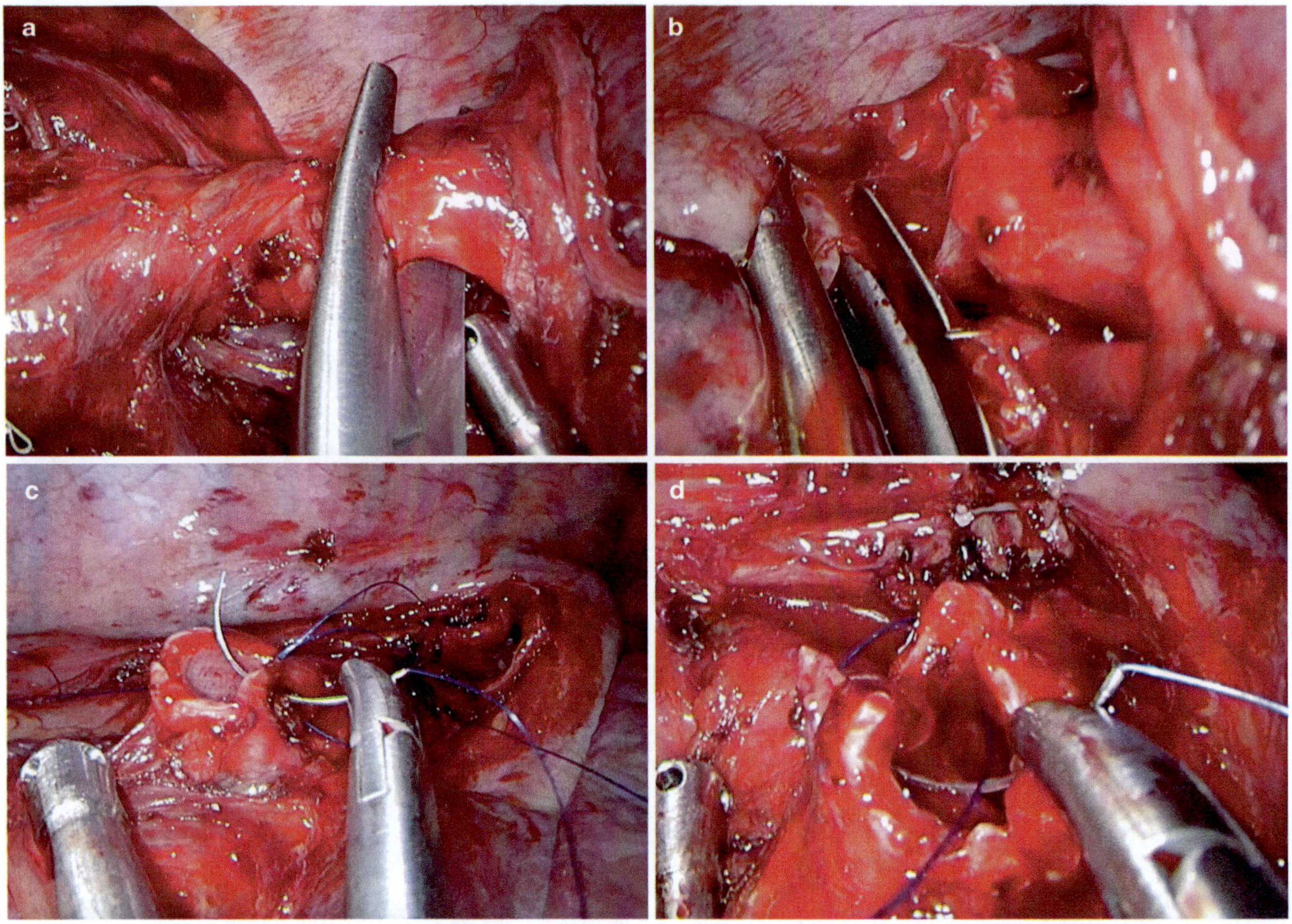

Fig. 5 Surgical technique for RUL sleeve bilobectomy. (**a**) The RUL bronchus is incised. (**b**) The main bronchus is incised. (**c**) A running suture is commenced for the posterior wall. (**d**) The anterior wall is performed to complete the anastomosis from posterior to anterior

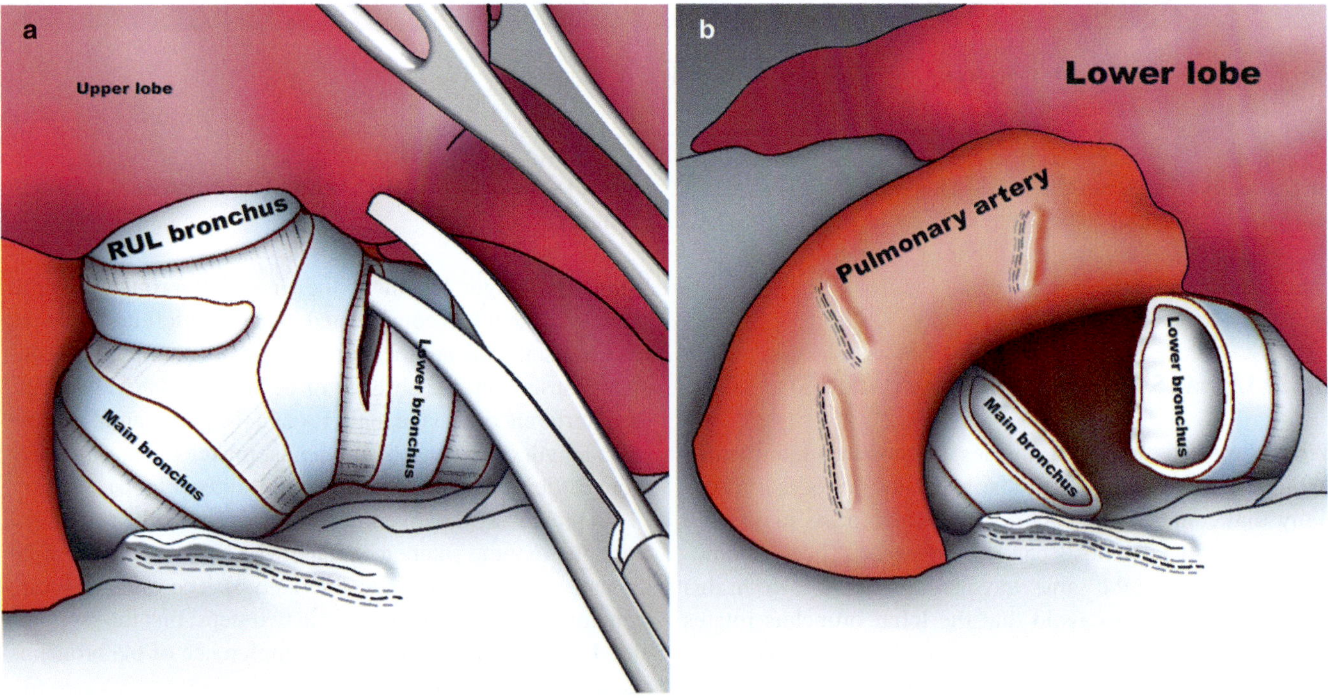

Fig. 6 Left upper lobe sleeve bronchial resection. (**a**) The lower lobe bronchus is transsected by using scissors. (**b**) Bronchial view when the upper lobe is removed

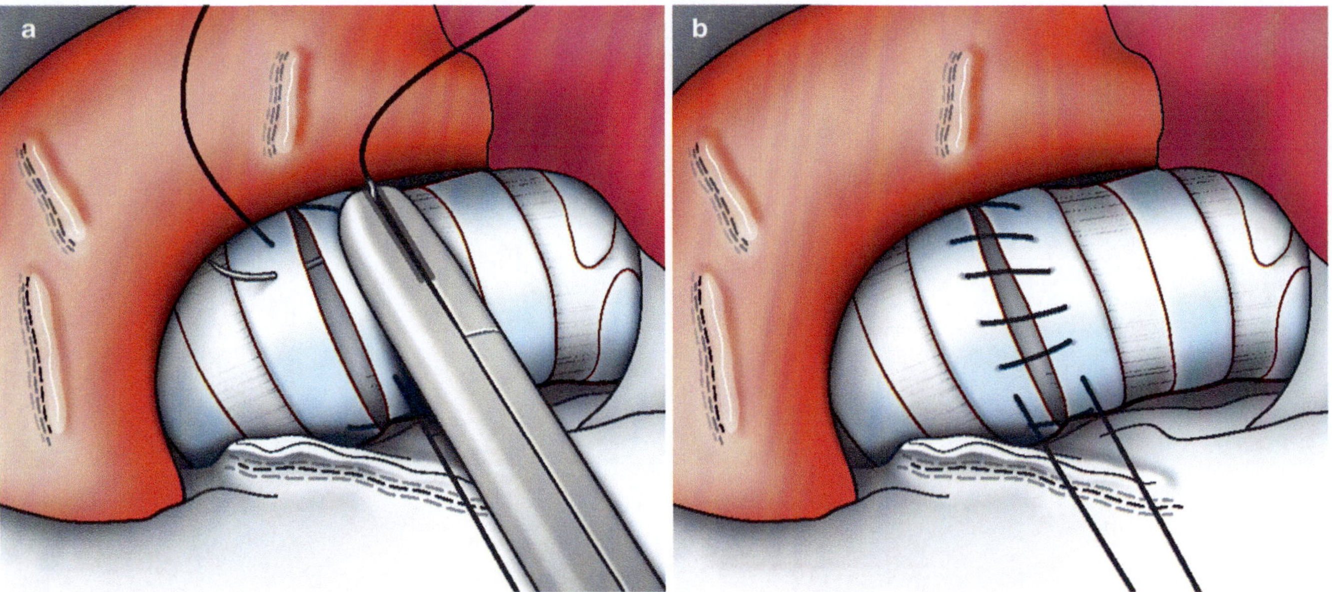

Fig. 7 Left upper lobe sleeve anastomosis. (**a**) Running suture from posterior to anterior. (**b**) Both threads are typed in the anterior part of the anastomosis

Left Lower Sleeve Resection (Video 7)

Due to the presence of the aortic arch, the heart's atrium and pulmonary artery that needs to be retracted in order to perform the anastomosis, the left lower sleeve lobectomy is technically more challenging than the others [17]. The orientation by VATS also makes it more complex to do the anastomosis due to the upper lobe bronchus being reimplanted on the main bronchus from an anterior view position. Next to this, the main bronchus is usually located quite deep, below the descending aorta. The preferred method is a running continuous suture as previously described (Fig. 8).

Sometimes, when the origin of the lingular artery originates from the basal atrial trunk or when it complicates the bronchial dissection, the artery must be sacrificed in order to perform a more secure anastomosis.

Bronchial Sleeve Resection (Lung Sparing)

Whenever possible, bronchoplastic resections that preserve parenchyma, should be attempted. Particularly when treating distal tracheal or centrally located endobronchial tumors. This is especially important for patients with poor pulmonary function [29, 30]. In general terms, the main indications for lung sparing bronchial sleeve resections are in the event of some benign diseases or bronchial low malignant tumors such as mucoepidermoid carcinoma, common carcinoid, and adenoid cystic carcinoma [31, 32]. It is not recommended for pure bronchial resection in the treatment of patients with non-small cell lung cancer because intrapulmonary mediastinal lymph nodes cannot be explored.

Due to the removal of the lobe and the space that is left behind to implement the anastomosis, a standard VAT sleeve lobectomy is technically less challenging than a VATS lung sparing bronchial sleeve resection [29, 30]. The remaining undivided lobar structures limit the exposure of the surgical field for suturing during lung sparing sleeve procedures (Fig. 9).

In the case of endobronchial carcinoid tumors that are located in the bronchus intermedius, the main and the RUL bronchus should be dissected and exposed by removing the subcarinal and peribronchial lymph nodes. After dividing the fissure, the lower lobe's basal artery should be encircled and retracted with a surg-i-loop or tape. The bronchus intermedius must be incised distally above the origin of the right middle bronchus and proximally just below the origin of the RUL bronchus. The anastomosis is initiated by suturing the posterior wall of the bronchus and then is continued from posterior to anterior direction by using a continuous 3-0 PDS or prolene suture. This is done with one of the two needles (one thread with two needle suture). The other needle of the same thread is used to complete the anterior side of the anastomosis and tied together when both ends meet at the anterior aspect (Fig. 9).

If the tumor is located on the right main bronchus, sometimes a double reconstruction of right upper and intermedius bronchus and proximal anastomosis near the carina may be necessary in order to achieve free bronchial margins.

When comparing a thoracoscopic right bronchial sleeve resection with a thoracoscopic reconstruction of a second carina on the left, the anastomosis is usually more complex because of the suturing of the upper and lower lobe bronchus. In addition, the left main bronchus is often hidden behind the left pulmonary artery [33].

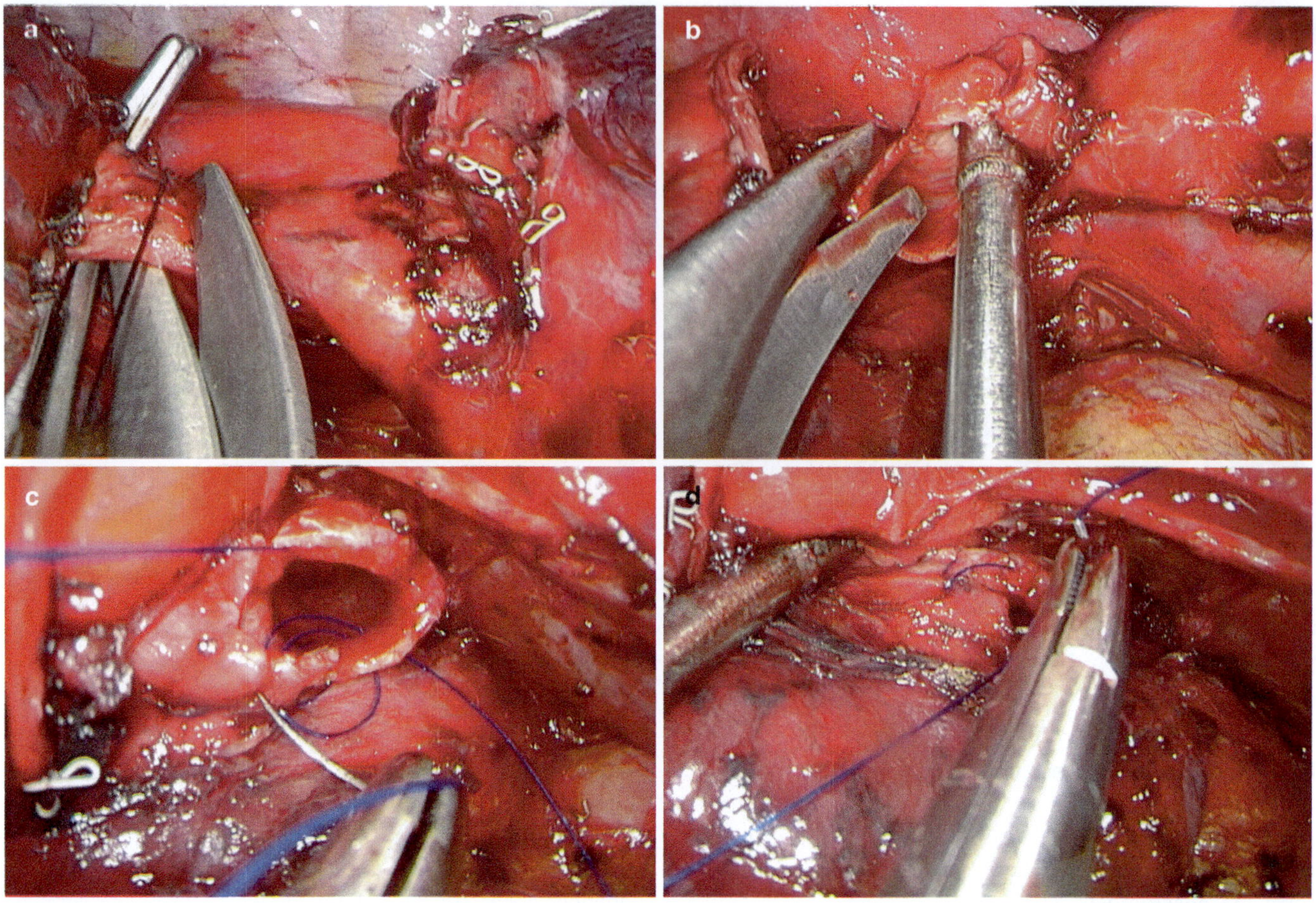

Fig. 8 Left lower sleeve lobectomy. (**a**) The upper lobe bronchus is incised. (**b**) The left main bronchus is incised, (**c**) the anastomosis is commenced in the postero-lateral wall from posterior to anterior, (**d**) finally the anterior wall of the anastomosis is completed in the same direction

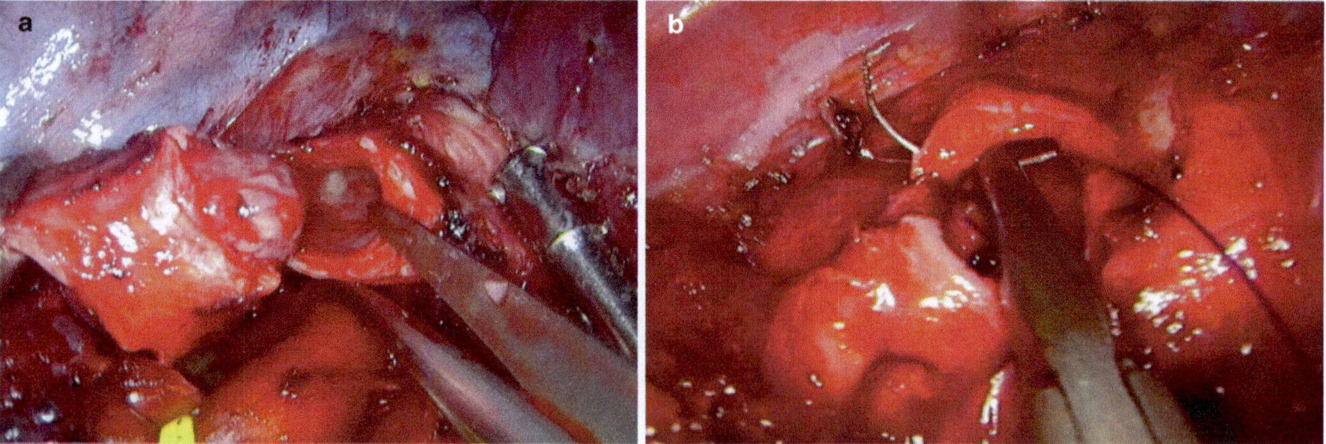

Fig. 9 Bronchus intermedius bronchial resection and anastomosis. (**a**) Proximal resection. (**b**) Completion of posterior wall of the anastomosis. (**c**) Running suture for anterior wall. (**d**) Completion of the procedure

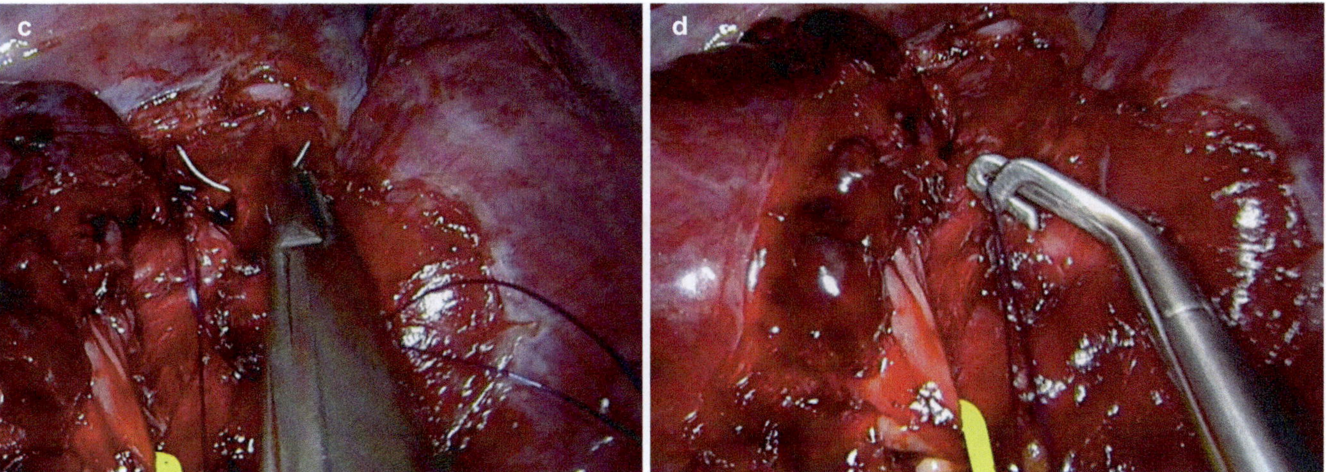

Fig. 9 (continued)

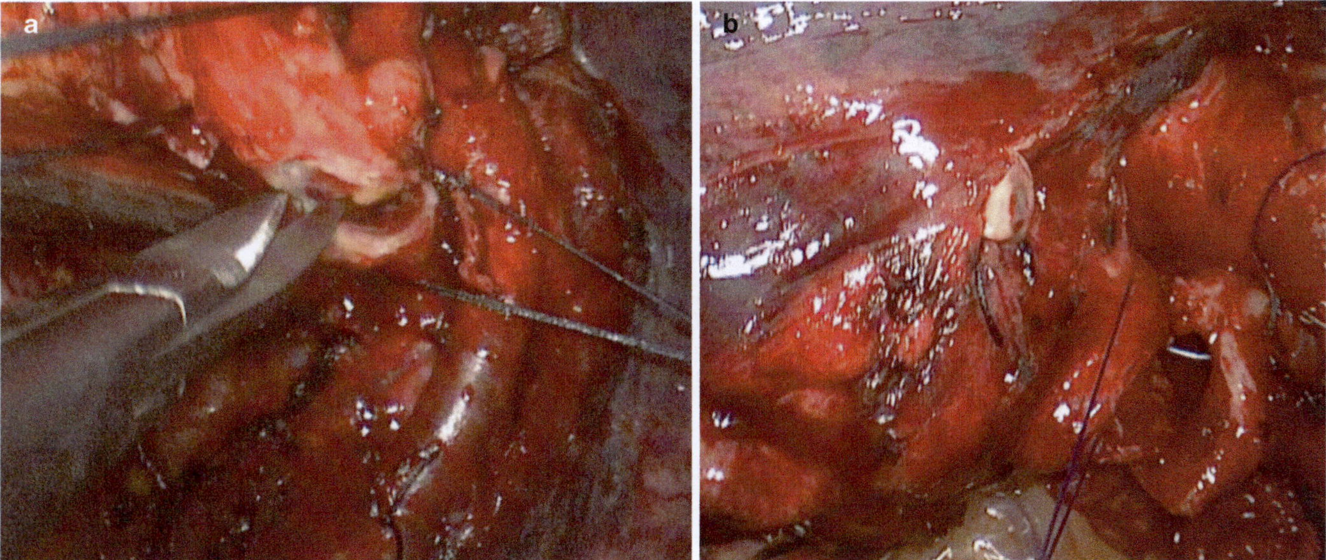

Fig. 10 Left upper lobe lingular sleeve segmentectomy. (**a**) The lingular bronchus is incised with scissors and the lingula is removed. (**b**) The upper lobe bronchus is sutured to the trisegmental bronchus

Sleeve Segmental Procedures (Video 8)

These are very rare procedures and more complicated because the reconstruction is performed on segmental bronchi with lobar bronchus, where the caliber discordance is larger. The objective is generally to avoid a lobectomy in cases that are especially indicated for benign endobronchial pathologies. For example, a benign tumor located at the entrance of the lingular lobe. In this case a resection and anastomosis of the LUL bronchus to the trisegmentary bronchus would be performed (Fig. 10).

Tracheal and Carinal Resection Reconstruction (Video 9)

Tumors invading the distal trachea or carina represent a challenge due to the complexity of airway reconstruction and management [34, 35]. Tracheal or carinal resections, and airway reconstruction on the left side are rather complex due to the limited exposure because of the aortic arch that covers the left main bronchus. It is also a deep operating site due to the natural right deviation of the carina [36]. This complicated procedure has been surgically approached by either

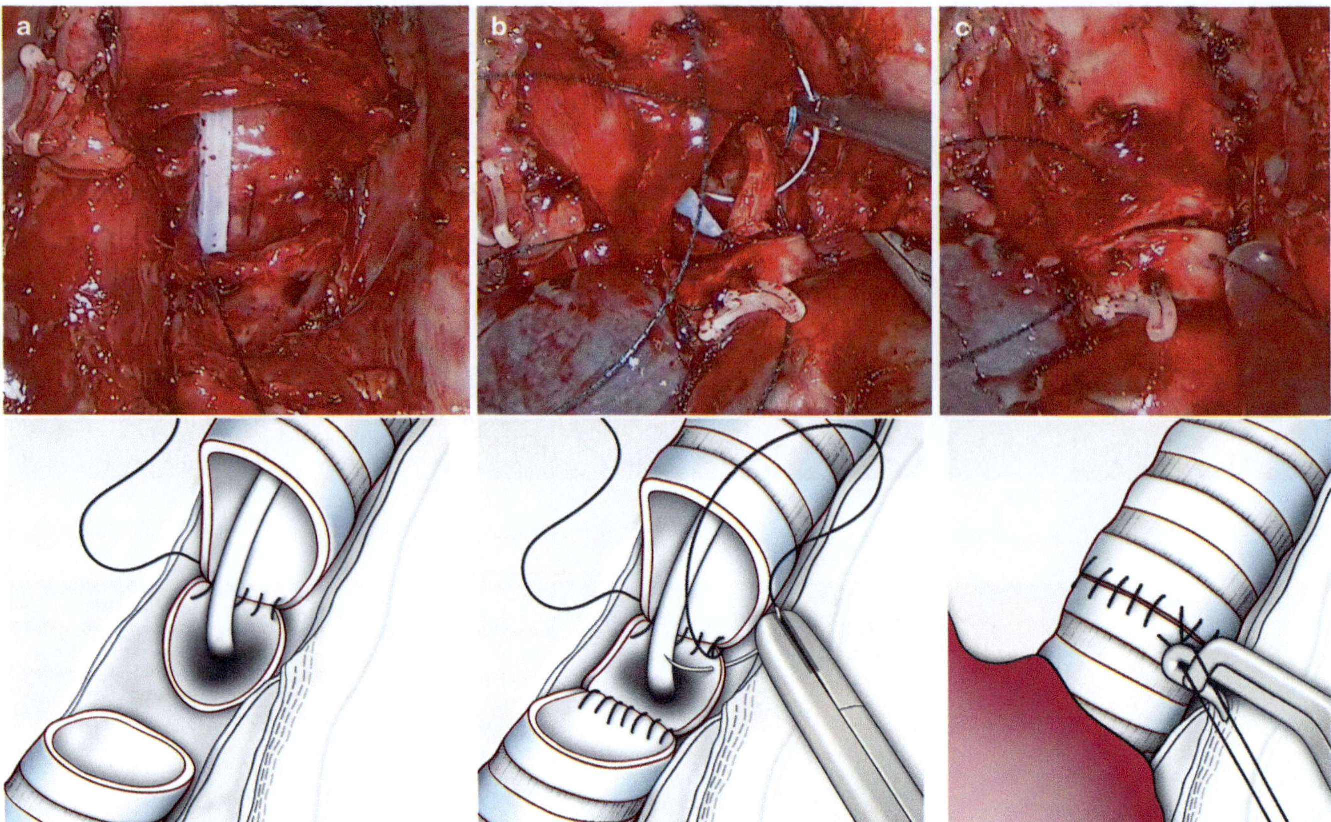

Fig. 11 Carinal sleeve right upper lobectomy with high frequency ventilation jet. (**a**) Running suture is completed between trachea and left main bronchus. (**b**) Lateral anastomosis to suture trachea to left main bronchus. (**c**) Completion of the anastomosis between trachea and bronchus intermedius. Photo With permission of JTD (*Gonzalez-Rivas D, Yang Y, Sekhniaidze D, Stupnik T, Fernandez R, Lei J, Zhu Y, Jiang G. Uniportal video-assisted thoracoscopic bronchoplastic and carinal sleeve procedures. J Thorac Dis 2016;8(Suppl 2):S210-S222*)

right open thoracotomy or median sternotomy [37, 38]. However distal trachea or carinal resections can be performed by uniportal VATS when in expert hands. Tumors that involve the carina or trachea pose several challenges during VATS surgery. They require a total coordination with the anesthesiologist during the airway resection, precise airway management and surgical reconstruction. Next to this, a preoperative plan should be defined in case of emergency.

To perform this procedure through a uniportal thoracoscopic approach, the lung can be ventilated two different ways. One (1) with the use of an intra-surgical field, tracheal tube [39], or two (2) with the use of high frequency jet ventilation (Fig. 11) [40]. The latter can be introduced through the endotracheal tube for ventilation because of the small diameter of the catheter. It also doesn't interfere with the lateral cartilaginous or membranous portion of the anastomosis. Using this approach, intra-field intubation is not needed. In the event that surgical field intubation is required, the tracheal tube could be inserted through the intercoastal incision. A sterile circuit is passed onto the field and prepared to directly ventilate the contralateral single lung using the surgical field tracheal tube.

For a tracheal and carinal resection, a single incision should be performed on the right hemithorax in the third or fourth intercostal space. An adequate dissection of the paratracheal space is required in order to isolate the trachea. A surg-i-loop or tape is passed around the trachea to help with the exposure. It is recommended to do the tracheal incision under bronchoscopic control, based on the location of the tumor. The right main bronchus can usually be transected at the base. When taking the specimen, both surgical margins must be tumor free on an intraoperative frozen-section biopsy. The preservation of continuity of lateral wall of the right and left main stem bronchus allows the re-implantation of the distal trachea to 2/3 of the circumference of the left main bronchus first. Thereafter it is sutured to the 2/3 circumference of the right main bronchus to form the neocarina. The lateral wall of the trachea and left main bronchus are anastomosed in an end-to-end fashion using a running 3-0 PDS suture (Fig. 6b). The patient can be ventilated intermittently through the left main bronchus intubation across an additional 1 cm incision through the surgical field, while doing the anastomosis (Fig. 6a, b). Once anastomosis is finalized, the intrathoracic tracheal tube across the incision is

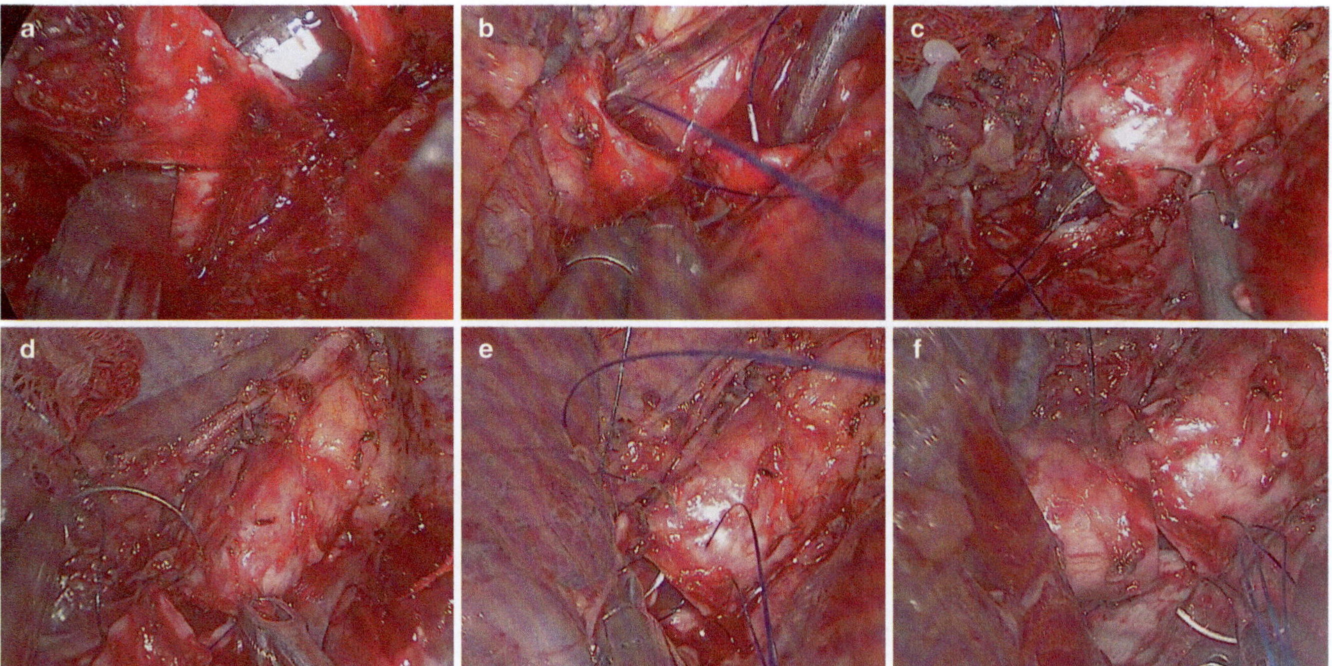

Fig. 12 Carinal sleeve resection without lung resection. (**a**) Incision of left main bronchus (**b**) creation of neocarina between left main and right main bronchus. (**c**) Suture of lateral wall of the trachea and right main bronchus. (**d**) Completion of anastomosis of membranous portion between trachea and right main bronchus. (**e**) Running suture for lateral cartilaginous portion, (**f**) completion of anastomosis with interrupted sutures

removed and the endotracheal tube is carefully advanced across the anastomosis for single lung ventilation. An end-to-side anastomosis should be performed to re-implant the right bronchus to the airway at the joint created from the distal trachea and left main stem bronchus (LMB). While adjusting the caliber in a tension-free manner (Video 9).

For RUL tumors that involve the carina, the complex part of the operation is to make an optimal reconstruction due to the mismatch between the distal trachea, LMB and bronchus intermedius (BI). To avoid mismatch, a neo-carina is created with an end-to-end anastomosis of distal trachea to the lateral wall of the LMB (LMB to BI) and re-implantation of the neo-carina to the trachea can be performed (Fig. 11). The high frequency ventilation jet is quite useful. It facilitates the anastomosis of the distal trachea to the main stem bronchus avoiding the insertion of a tracheal tube through the incision and maintains oxygenation [40]. Alternatively, while preserving parenchyma, the carina can also be resected and then a total end-to-end anastomosis performed between the trachea and the left main bronchus, followed by the anastomosis of the lateral, cartilaginous wall of the trachea to the right main bronchus (Fig. 12, Video 9). For a better exposure to perform the carinal resection, the azygos vein should be divided. To ventilate the left lung, through a 2 mm endotracheal catheter, a high-frequency jet ventilation is inserted. As previously described, a running suture facilitates the reconstruction. The left side wall is first formed between the trachea and left main bronchus, thereafter the sutured membranous trachea and then left main bronchus. After that the neo-carina of lateral wall of left main bronchus and right main bronchus is created. Lastly, all three (left main bronchus, front wall of the trachea and right main bronchus) are anastomosed.

When a tumor involves the hilum of the lung up to the carinal division we can perform a carinal pneumonectomy following the same technique with anastomosis of trachea to the main bronchus (Fig. 13).

Literature Review and Discussion

During the last decade, VATS has evolved from the conventional three-port technique to the uniportal approach [41–43]. Minimally invasive surgery compared to conventional open surgery for cancer has proven to offer many benefits over traditional open surgery. It reduces postoperative pain and offers faster patient recovery without compromising oncologic results [6–10]. On the other hand, VATS procedures are initially more technically challenging due to the steep learning curve, no direct vision, lack of palpation, and the surgeon adapting to a 2D or 3D monitor view [44].

As surgeons gain more experience with thoracoscopic suturing and tying techniques, along with the development of new dedicated thoracoscopic instruments, bronchoplastic procedures are now being performed thoracoscopically by expert surgeons [28, 45]. Several publications report that an open sleeve lobectomy results in a better survival rate

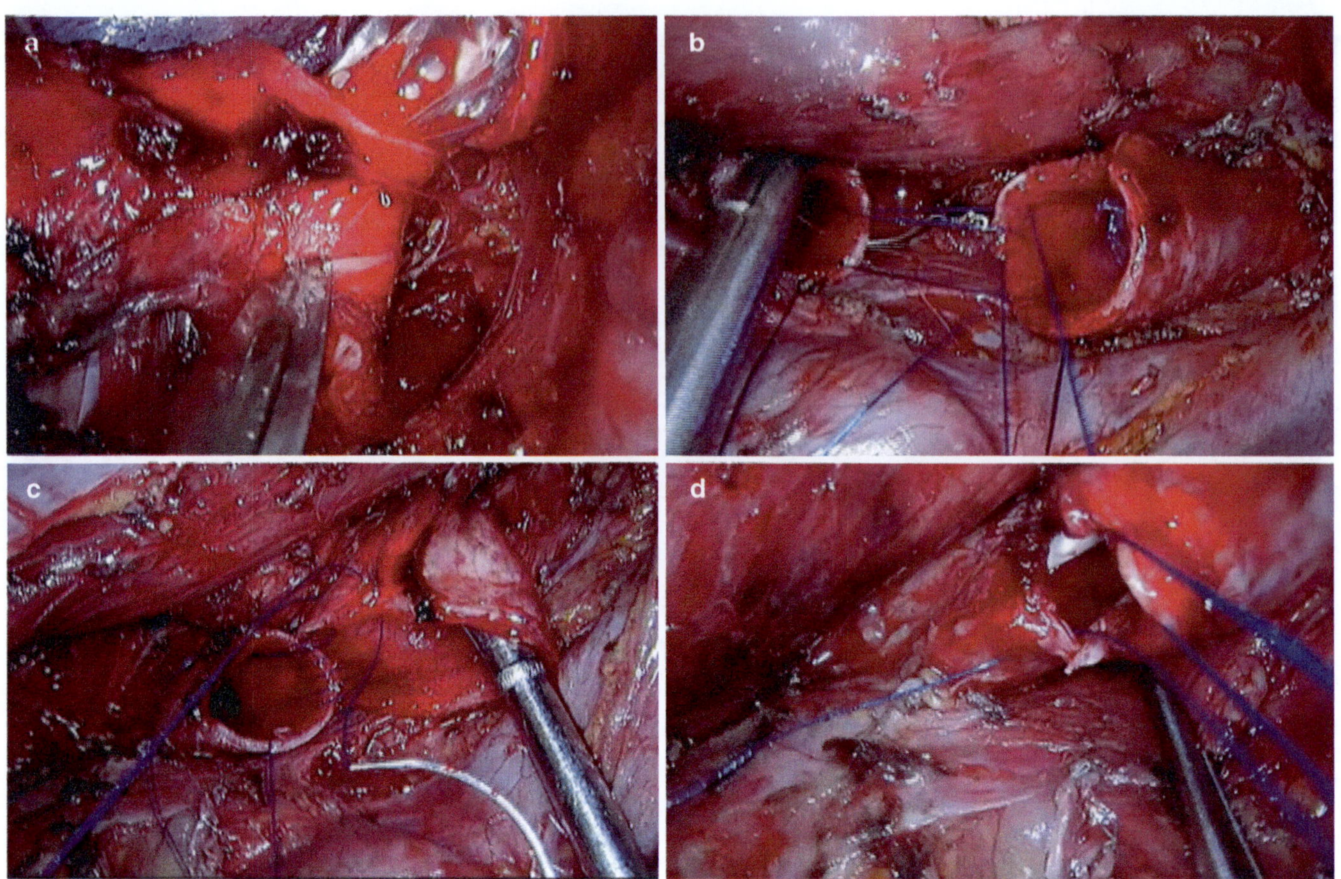

Fig. 13 Carinal sleeve pneumonectomy. (**a**) Trachea is incised and the left main bronchus is cut. (**b** and **c**) Running suture of posterior wall between trachea and left main bronchus. (**d**) Running suture for anterior wall

compared to pneumonectomy. Sleeve resections avoid loss in lung function, and reduce perioperative mortality [46, 47]. In contrast, there aren't many articles reporting series of VATS sleeve resections. These are slowly increasing in number over the last decade [28]. The first article reporting conventional multi-port VATS sleeves was published 16 years ago [48] and only 5 years ago the first were reported by the uniportal approach [16]. The concerns of performing a radical resection and a correct sleeve anastomosis is one of the main reasons for the slow adoption of the thoracoscopic technique. Some authors consider that a surgeon should perform a minimum number of 25–30 VATS cases to overcome the learning curve and safely perform, advanced cases by a VATS approach [49]. Other publications describe hybrid VATS sleeve resections, with direct visualization through the utility incision to avoid a conventional thoracotomy [50].

As with any other surgical procedure, sleeve lobectomies by VATS has its natural learning curve. Based on our own experience, surgeons should have done at least 200 VATS lobectomies or more and at least 20 cases of open sleeve procedures in order to lay the anatomical and operative technical foundation required for a surgeon to be sufficiently experienced to perform a thoracoscopic sleeve resection [51].

The same principles of open surgery apply to VATS bronchoplasties. Using monofilament absorbable sutures for smooth placement and sliding of the knots is recommended. The manipulation of instruments and sutures in VATS is more crucial than in open an open thoracotomy approach. The tension of the suture line can be carefully adjusted with a knot pusher instrument.

Some publications have reported that the use of interrupted sutures is recommended to allow better size matching, less anastomotic-site ischemia and to prevent loosening and entanglement of the sutures [28, 52].

Other publications describe an improved suturing technique by using both continuous suturing for the membranous portion of the bronchus and interrupted suturing for the cartilaginous portions [53]. Based on our experience, the use of a continuous suture performed in two steps for the posterior and the anterior bronchial wall, results in less suture tangling and is faster [45, 54]. A new absorbable barbed suture, the V-Loc™ wound closure device can be used to avoid knot-tying [20].

Unless the tumor had received previous radiation therapy or the patient presented signs of infection, we do not buttress the anastomosis [55]. If needed though, mediastinal fat, thymus, pericardial pedicle, or an intercostal muscle flap may be used.

In the literature there aren't many articles that report vascular, bronchial or combined broncho-vascular sleeve procedures. Most of them are related to an open thoracotomy approach and even less are performed by VATS [52, 54, 56]. As our single incision VATS approach experience has grown over the years [57], so has the rate of our reconstruction procedures by uniportal approach, in this way reducing the incidence of pneumonectomies [21, 22, 26, 58].

Going through the literature, we have found a number of publications describing sleeve procedures of the right upper lobe for NSCLC using four ports [59], three ports [60, 61] or two ports [62]. A few other publications describe partial removal of the PA [63], as well as double sleeve procedures on the left side [64].

Mahtabifard et al., reported one of the earlier series of 13 sleeve resections, that described a relatively short median operative time of 167 min (range, 90–300) and a chest tube duration of 3 days (range 2–6). However, the post-operative morbidity was 31% [52].

In the recent years, some of the larger series describing VATS bronchoplasties came from Asia. Particularly Agastian et al., described 21 VATS bronchoplastic procedures (representing 9.1% of all of his VATS procedures in his series). Most of them for NSCLC resections which included wedge, sleeve bronchoplasty and other extended bronchoplasties. The authors, in these series, used an interrupted suture technique for the anastomosis with mean surgical time 287 min (range 135–540) and mean hospital stay of 5.2 days [28].

As experience with the VATS approach increases, more advanced procedures such as carinal or tracheal resections can be successfully performed through a Uniportal VATS [45, 58]. However, VATS for these types of cases could represent a challenge even for the experienced thoracic surgeon. The reasons include intraoperative airway management and the inherent technical difficulties with the anatomic reconstruction.

The surgical technique as well as the airway management for carinal resections are traditionally described with the use of an open surgery approach [36, 37, 39]. The common approaches for this are either by median sternotomy of right thoracotomy [39]. The uniportal VATS approach for tracheal or carinal resections is an emergent procedure and should be performed through the right side of the patient. The Ventilation, after a uniportal VATS tracheal or carinal resection, can be maintained by using an intrafield single-lumen tune or a high ventilation jet [45, 58]. It is also possible to perform these procedures with no intubation, under spontaneous ventilation [65].

One of the most active group for sleeve resections and complex reconstructions is He's group from China. Within their series, they include broncho-vascular reconstructions, tracheal and carinal resections in intubated and a non-intubated patients with excellent postoperative outcomes [65]. In a multicenter study including 3 centers in China, a series of 12 carinal and tracheal resections are reported. In these series they describe five different types of VATS airway reconstructions while sparring parenchyma or with lobectomy. The first (1) reconstruction includes right bronchial resection with a partial carinal reconstruction; second (2), left bronchial resection with carinal reconstruction; third (3), tracheal resection and reconstruction; fourth (4), tracheal or right bronchial resection with carinal reconstruction, and fifth (5), right pneumonectomy with carinal reconstruction. The mean operative time was 224 ± 78 min and the mean hospital stay was 12.5 days. No postoperative major morbidity or mortality was reported [66].

There are even less publications describing double sleeve procedures by VATS [64]. Our group published several case reports of uniportal broncho plastic procedures which included combined broncho—vascular sleeve resections [26, 45, 58, 67], and vascular reconstruction [22].

Hung et al., described a retrospective multi-center study with 13 thoracoscopic double sleeve resections for NSCLC patients. The median operative time was 263 min, and the median LOS was 10 days [67]. A Russian group recently reported a series of four double sleeve (LUL) and two carinal resections through uniportal VATS. In one case a right upper sleeve carinal lobectomy, and in the other a right sleeve carinal pneumonectomy. The mean operation time was 280 ± 13 min and no conversion occurred. The mean LOS was 10.8 ± 0.8 days and no postoperative mortality [68].

Recently, the group of He Jianxing published an important study of 32 tracheal and carinal resections performed by VATS comparing 18 cases under spontaneous ventilation with 14 cases with endotracheal intubation. The non intubated group showed faster recovery and shorter hospital length of stay [69].

Conclusions

The approach for sleeve resections has evolved from open techniques, to hybrid mini-thoracotomy procedures with video-assistance, and currently to a single incision (Uniportal) approach. These procedures should be performed as an alternative to pneumonectomy provided that complete tumor resection can be achieved. The preservation of parenchyma should improve lung functional capacity and so possibly improves quality of life as well as reduces the risk of operative mortality. The experience acquired with established minimally invasive techniques such as the uniportal VATS approach, allows expert surgeons to perform advanced procedures that include both, VATS vascular & bronchial sleeves, and carinal & tracheal resections, with good postoperative outcomes. Long term follow-up results and evaluation of series of patients will need to be studied for these complicated cases, performed with the uniportal VATS approach.

References

1. Price-Thomas C. Conservative resection of the bronchial tree. J R Coll Surg Edinb. 1956;1:169.
2. Allison PR. Course of thoracic surgery in Groningen. Quoted by Jones PH. Lobectomy and bronchial anastomosis in the surgery of bronchial carcinoma. Ann R Coll Surg Engl. 1959;25:20–38.
3. Abbott OA. Experiences with the surgical resection of the human carina, tracheal wall, and contralateral bronchial wall in cases of right total pneumonectomy. J Thorac Surg. 1950;19:906–22.
4. Gibbon JH, in discussion to Chamberlain M, et al. Bronchogenic carcinoma: an aggressive surgical attitude. J Thorac Cardiovasc Surg. 1959;38:727.
5. Grillo HC. Carinal reconstruction. Ann Thorac Surg. 1982;34:356–73.
6. Vogt-Moykopf I, Fritz T, Meyer G, Bülzerbruck H, Daskos G. Bronchoplastic and angioplastic operation in bronchial carcinoma: long-term results of a retrospective analysis from 1973 to 1983. Int Surg. 1986;71:211–20.
7. Yan TD, Black D, Bannon PG, McCaughan BC. Systematic review and meta-analysis of randomized and nonrandomized trials on safety and efficacy of video-assisted thoracic surgery lobectomy for early-stage non-small-cell lung cancer. J Clin Oncol. 2009;27:2553–62.
8. Onaitis MW, Petersen RP, Balderson SS, Toloza E, Burfeind WR, Harpole DH Jr, et al. Thoracoscopic lobectomy is a safe and versatile procedure: experience with 500 consecutive patients. Ann Surg. 2006;244:420–5.
9. Kaseda S, Aoki T, Hangai N, Shimizu K. Better pulmonary function and prognosis with video-assisted thoracic surgery than with thoracotomy. Ann Thorac Surg. 2000;70:1644–6.
10. Yang X, Wang S, Qu J. Video-assisted thoracic surgery (VATS) compares favorably with thoracotomy for the treatment of lung cancer: a five-year outcome comparison. World J Surg. 2009;33:1857–61.
11. Ng CS, Wan S, Hui CW, Lee TW, Underwood MJ, Yim AP. Video-assisted thoracic surgery for early stage lung cancer – can short-term immunological advantages improve long-term survival? Ann Thorac Cardiovasc Surg. 2006;12:308–12.
12. Maurizi G, D'Andrilli A, Anile M, Ciccone AM, Ibrahim M, Venuta F, et al. Sleeve lobectomy compared with pneumonectomy after induction therapy for non-small-cell lung cancer. J Thorac Oncol. 2013;8:637–43.
13. De Leyn P, Rots W, Deneffe G, Nafteux P, Coosemans W, Van Raemdonck D, et al. Sleeve lobectomy for non-small cell lung cancer. Acta Chir Belg. 2003;103:570–6.
14. Krüger M, Uschinsky K, Hässler K, Engelmann C. Postoperative complications after bronchoplastic procedures in the treatment of bronchial malignancies. Eur J Cardiothorac Surg. 1998;14:46–52.
15. Ng CS. Thoracoscopic sleeve resection-the better approach? J Thorac Dis. 2014;6:1164–6.
16. Gonzalez-Rivas D, Fernandez R, Fieira E, Rellan L. Uniportal video-assisted thoracoscopic bronchial sleeve lobectomy: first report. J Thorac Cardiovasc Surg. 2013;145:1676–7.
17. Gonzalez-Rivas D, Delgado M, Fieira E, Pato O. Left lower sleeve lobectomy by uniportal video-assisted thoracoscopic approach. Interact Cardiovasc Thorac Surg. 2014;18:237–9.
18. Bertolaccini L, Rocco G, Viti A, Terzi A. Geometrical characteristics of uniportal VATS. J Thorac Dis. 2013;5:214–6.
19. Bertolaccini L, Viti A, Terzi A. Ergon-trial: ergonomic evaluation of single-port access versus three-port access video-assisted thoracic surgery. Surg Endosc. 2015;29:2934–40.
20. Nakagawa T, Chiba N, Ueda Y, Saito M, Sakaguchi Y, Ishikawa S. Clinical experience of sleeve lobectomy with bronchoplasty using a continuous absorbable barbed suture. Gen Thorac Cardiovasc Surg. 2015;63(11):640–3.
21. Gonzalez-Rivas D, Fieira E, De la Torre M, Delgado M. Bronchovascular right upper lobe reconstruction by uniportal video-assisted thoracoscopic surgery. J Thorac Dis. 2014;6:861–3.
22. Gonzalez-Rivas D, Delgado M, Fieira E, Mendez L. Single-port video-assisted thoracoscopic lobectomy with pulmonary artery reconstruction. Interact Cardiovasc Thorac Surg. 2013;17:889–91.
23. Yu DP, Han Y, Zhao QY, Liu ZD. Pulmonary lobectomy combined with pulmonary arterioplasty by complete video-assisted thoracic surgery in patients with lung cancer. Asian Pac J Cancer Prev. 2013;14:6061–4.
24. Nakanishi R, Yamashita T, Oka S. Initial experience of video-assisted thoracic surgery lobectomy with partial removal of the pulmonary artery. Interact Cardiovasc Thorac Surg. 2008;7:996–1000.
25. Xu X, Huang J, Pan H, Chen H, He J. Video-assisted thoracoscopic bronchoplasty/pulmonary arterial angioplasty. J Thorac Dis. 2016;8(3):544–52.
26. Gonzalez-Rivas D, Delgado M, Fieira E, Fernandez R. Double sleeve uniportal video-assisted thoracoscopic lobectomy for non-small cell lung cancer. Ann Cardiothorac Surg. 2014;3(2):E2.
27. Yang R, Shao F, Cao H, Liu Z. Bronchial anastomosis using complete continuous suture in video-assisted thoracic surgery sleeve lobectomy. J Thorac Dis. 2013;5:321–2.
28. Agasthian T. Initial experience with video-assisted thoracoscopic bronchoplasty. Eur J Cardiothorac Surg. 2013;44:616–23.
29. Bagan P, Le Pimpec-Barthes F, Badia A, Crockett F, Dujon A, Riquet M. Bronchial sleeve resections: lung function resurrecting procedure. Eur J Cardiothorac Surg. 2008;34:484–7.
30. Cerfolio RJ, Deschamps C, Allen MS, Trastek VF, Pairolero PC. Mainstem bronchial sleeve resection with pulmonary preservation. Ann Thorac Surg. 1996;61:1458–62.
31. Bölükbas S, Schirren J. Parenchyma-sparing bronchial sleeve resections in trauma, benign and malign diseases. Thorac Cardiovasc Surg. 2010;58:32–7.
32. Ragusa M, Vannucci J, Cagini L, Daddi N, Pecoriello R, Puma F. Left main bronchus resection and reconstruction: a single institution experience. J Cardiothorac Surg. 2012;7:29.
33. Tang J, Cao M, Qian L, Fu Y, Tang J, Zhao X. The pure distal left main bronchial sleeve resection with total lung parenchymal preservation: report of two cases and literature review. J Thorac Dis. 2014;6:294–8.
34. Regnard JF, Fourquier P, Levasseur P. Results and prognostic factors in resections of primary tracheal tumors: a multicenter retrospective study. J Thorac Cardiovasc Surg. 1996;111:808–13.
35. Maziak DE, Todd TR, Keshavjee SH, Winton TL, Van Nostrand P, Pearson FG. Adenoid cystic carcinoma of the airway: thirty-two-year experience. J Thorac Cardiovasc Surg. 1996;112:1522–31.
36. Maeda M, Nakamoto K, Tsubota N, Okada T, Katsura H. Operative approaches for left-sided carinoplasty. Ann Thorac Surg. 1993;56:441–5.
37. Porhanov VA, Poliakov IS, Selvaschuk AP, Grechishkin AI, Sitnik SD, Nikolaev IF, et al. Indications and results of sleeve carinal resection. Eur J Cardiothorac Surg. 2002;22:685–94.
38. Shao F, Yang R, Xu D, Zou W, Ma G, Cao H, et al. Bronchial sleeve lobectomy and carinal resection in the treatment of central lung cancer: a report of 92 cases. Zhongguo Fei Ai Za Zhi. 2010;13:1056–8.
39. Weder W, Inci I. Carinal resection and sleeve pneumonectomy. Thorac Surg Clin. 2014;24:77–83.
40. Watanabe Y, Murakami S, Iwa T, Murakami S. The clinical value of high-frequency jet ventilation in major airway reconstructive surgery. Scand J Thorac Cardiovasc Surg. 1988;22:227–33.
41. Ng CS, Rocco G, Wong RH, Lau RW, Yu SC, Yim AP. Uniportal and single-incision video-assisted thoracic surgery: the state of the art. Interact Cardiovasc Thorac Surg. 2014;19:661–6.
42. Rocco G. One-port (uniportal) video-assisted thoracic surgical resections-A clear advance. J Thorac Cardiovasc Surg. 2012;144:27–31.

43. Ng CS, Lau KK, González-Rivas D, Rocco G. Evolution in surgical approach and techniques for lung cancer. Thorax. 2013;68:681.
44. Petersen R, Hansen H. Learning thoracoscopic lobectomy. Eur J Cardiothorac Surg. 2010;37:516–52.
45. Gonzalez-Rivas D, Yang Y, Sekhniaidze D, Stupnik T, Fernandez R, Lei J, Zhu Y, Jiang G. Uniportal video-assisted thoracoscopic bronchoplastic and carinal sleeve procedures. J Thorac Dis. 2016;8(Suppl 2):S210–22.
46. Rendina E, De Giacomo T, Venuta F, Ciccone A, Coloni G. Lung conservation techniques: bronchial sleeve resection and reconstruction of the pulmonary artery. Semin Surg Oncol. 2000;18: 165–72.
47. Burfeind WR Jr, D'Amico TA, Toloza EM, Wolfe WG, Harpole DH. Low morbidity and mortality for bronchoplastic procedures with and without induction therapy. Ann Thorac Surg. 2005;80:418–21.
48. Santambrogio L, Cioffi U, De Simone M, Rosso L, Ferrero S, Giunta A. Video-assisted sleeve lobectomy for mucoepidermoid carcinoma of the left lower lobar bronchus: a case report. Chest. 2002;121:635–6.
49. Nakanishi R, Fujino Y, Yamashita T, Shinohara S, Oyama T. Thoracoscopic anatomic pulmonary resection for locally advanced non-small cell lung cancer. Ann Thorac Surg. 2014;97:980–6.
50. Shao WL, Liu LX, He JX, Yang YY, Chen HZ, Wu ZF, et al. Bronchial sleeve resection and reconstruction of pulmonary artery by video-assisted thoracic small incision surgery for central lung cancer: a report of 139 cases. Zhonghua Wai Ke Za Zhi. 2007;45:1530–2.
51. Gonzalez D, De la Torre M, Paradela M, Fernandez R, Delgado M, Garcia J, et al. Video-assisted thoracic surgery lobectomy: 3-year initial experience with 200 cases. Eur J Cardiothorac Surg. 2011;40:e21–8.
52. Mahtabifard A, Fuller CB, McKenna RJ Jr. Video-assisted thoracic surgery sleeve lobectomy: a case series. Ann Thorac Surg. 2008;85:729–32.
53. Li Y, Wang J. Video-assisted thoracoscopic surgery sleeve lobectomy with bronchoplasty: an improved operative technique. Eur J Cardiothorac Surg. 2013;44:1108–12.
54. Gonzalez-Rivas D, Marin JC, Granados JP, Llano JD, Cañas SR, Arqueta AO, de la Torre M. Uniportal video-assisted thoracoscopic right upper sleeve lobectomy and tracheoplasty in a 10-year-old patient. J Thorac Dis. 2016;8(9):E966–9. https://doi.org/10.21037/jtd.2016.08.06.
55. Tsuchiya R. Bronchoplastic techniques. In: Pearson FG, Cooper JD, Deslauriers J, editors. Thoracic surgery. 2nd ed. Philadelphia: Churchill Livingstone; 2002. p. 1005–13.
56. Kara HV, Balderson SS, D'Amico TA. Challenging cases: thoracoscopic lobectomy with chest wall resection and sleeve lobectomy-Duke experience. J Thorac Dis. 2014;6:637–40.
57. Gonzalez-rivas D, Fieira E, Delgado M, Mendez L, Fernandez R, De la Torre M. Uniportal video-assisted thoracoscopic lobectomy. J Thorac Dis. 2013;5:234–45.
58. Gonzalez-Rivas D, Yang Y, Stupnik T, Sekhniaidze D, Fernandez R, Velasco C, Zhu Y, Giang G. Uniportal video-assisted thoracoscopic bronchovascular, tracheal and carinal resections. Eur J Cardiothorac Surg. 2015;49:i6–i16. https://doi.org/10.1093/ejcts/ezv410.
59. Li X, Pan X, Zhang C, Zhu D, Zhao J. Video-assisted thoracoscopic sleeve lobectomy. J Thorac Dis. 2014;6:1351–3.
60. Liu K, Jin C, Tian H, Shen W. Total video-assisted thoracic surgery sleeve lobectomy: suture by both hands. Thorac Cardiovasc Surg Rep. 2013;2:43–5.
61. Lu H, Zhang Z, Li W, Hu D. Video-assisted thoracic surgery right sleeve lobectomy. J Thorac Dis. 2013;5:323–4.
62. Jiao W, Zhao Y, Huang T, Shen Y. Two-port approach for fully thoracoscopic right upper lobe sleeve lobectomy. J Cardiothorac Surg. 2013;8:99.
63. Han Y, Zhou S, Yu D, Song X, Liu Z. Video-assisted thoracic surgery (VATS) left upper sleeve lobectomy with partial pulmonary artery resection. J Thorac Dis. 2013;5:301–3.
64. Liu L, Mei J, Pu Q, Ma L. Thoracoscopic bronchovascular double sleeve lobectomy for non-small-cell lung cancer. Eur J Cardiothorac Surg. 2014;46:493–5.
65. Peng G, Cui F, Ang KL, Zhang X, Yin W, Shao W, Dong Q, Liang L, He J. Non-intubated combined with video-assisted thoracoscopic in carinal reconstruction. J Thorac Dis. 2016;8(3):586–93. https://doi.org/10.21037/jtd.2016.01.58.
66. Li J, Wang W, Jiang L, Yin W, Liu J, Shao W, Chen H, Ang KL, Jiao W, Kang M, He J. Video-assisted thoracic surgery resection and reconstruction of carina and trachea for malignant or benign disease in 12 patients: three centers' experience in China. Ann Thorac Surg. 2016;102(1):295–303.
67. Huang J, Li J, Qiu Y, Xu X, Sekhniaidze D, Chen H, et al. Thoracoscopic double sleeve lobectomy in 13 patients: a series report from multi-centers. J Thorac Dis. 2015;7:834–42.
68. Lyscov A, Obukhova T, Ryabova V, Sekhniaidze D, Zuiev V, Gonzalez-Rivas D. Double-sleeve and carinal resections using the uniportal VATS technique: a single centre experience. J Thorac Dis. 2016;8(Suppl 3):S235–41.
69. Jiang L, Liu J, Gonzalez-Rivas D, Shargall Y, Kolb M, Shao W, Dong Q, Liang L, He J. Thoracoscopic surgery for tracheal and carinal resection and reconstruction under spontaneous ventilation. J Thorac Cardiovasc Surg. 2018;155(6):2746–54.

Sleeve Resection

Hyun Koo Kim and Kook Nam Han

Abstract

The uniportal approach to video-assisted thoracoscopic surgery (VATS) sleeve resection may be considered for patients undergoing conventional VATS sleeve resection. In this chapter, we describe the technical details of the uniportal VATS approach for bronchial sleeve resection. Further study is needed to address the long-term outcomes and the ability of thoracic surgeons to carry out these crowded surgical techniques.

Introduction

Sleeve resection was conceived as an alternative to pneumonectomy for patients with central lung lesions and limited pulmonary function [1–3]. Knowledge of planned and unplanned options for bronchoplastic technique during lung resection is essential for the general thoracic surgeon [4–6]. The major goal of this procedure is the preservation of normal lung function to improve postoperative pulmonary function [1, 2, 7–12]. The first report of video-assisted thoracoscopic surgery (VATS) sleeve lobectomy in 2002 suggested that the procedure should only be performed by an experienced VATS surgeon [13–17]. Since then, VATS sleeve resection has become a feasible option for some patients, and has consistent postoperative outcomes [18, 19]. Recently, some groups have reported their experiences with uniportal VATS bronchial and vascular sleeve resection [15, 20, 21]. The uniportal VATS approach has also been a challenging option for sleeve resection, and thus is not widely used. The potential advantages of the uniportal VATS approach in sleeve resection are a direct view and geometry similar to that of a thoracotomy. Technically, uniportal VATS sleeve resection can be performed in selected patients if the thoracic surgeon is experienced in uniportal VATS procedures for major lung resection. Specifically, thoracic surgeons should be thoroughly experienced in the suturing technique through a uniportal VATS field because bronchoplastic anastomosis is critical to prevent a postoperative bronchopleural fistula, and there can be technical difficulty in handling the suture material and instruments through a single, small (2–4 cm) incision. Newly introduced three-dimensional (3D) or high definition (HD) video surgery systems could be useful options for complex VATS procedures, with better visual performance and improved depth perception (Fig. 1).

Operative Technique

The position and port required for the uniportal approach in sleeve resection are the same as those used for upper or lower lobe resection. Performance of a bronchoplastic technique through a uniportal approach requires mobilization of the vascular and bronchial structures, thus enabling accurate suturing technique through a uniportal VATS view (Fig. 2). Once full mobilization of the bronchus and transection of the vascular structures are achieved and the target lobe fissure and complete systemic lymph node dissection are completed, the remnant vascular structures are encircled and retracted with rubber or umbilical tape to expose the bronchial structure. After careful inspection of the location of the tumor, assisted by a pediatric fiberoptic bronchoscope, a blade or endoscopic scissors are used to open the bronchus away from the bronchial lesion. Too close a resection margin, or opening too close to positive malignant cells in the frozen examination section might lead to conversion to bilobectomy or pneumonectomy. Hilar and mediastinal

Electronic Supplementary Material The online version of this chapter (https://doi.org/10.1007/978-981-13-2604-2_30) contains supplementary material, which is available to authorized users.

H. K. Kim (✉) · K. N. Han
Department of Thoracic and Cardiovascular Surgery,
Korea University Guro Hospital, Seoul, Republic of Korea
e-mail: kimhyunkoo@korea.ac.kr

D. Gonzalez-Rivas et al. (eds.), *Atlas of Uniportal Video Assisted Thoracic Surgery*,
https://doi.org/10.1007/978-981-13-2604-2_30

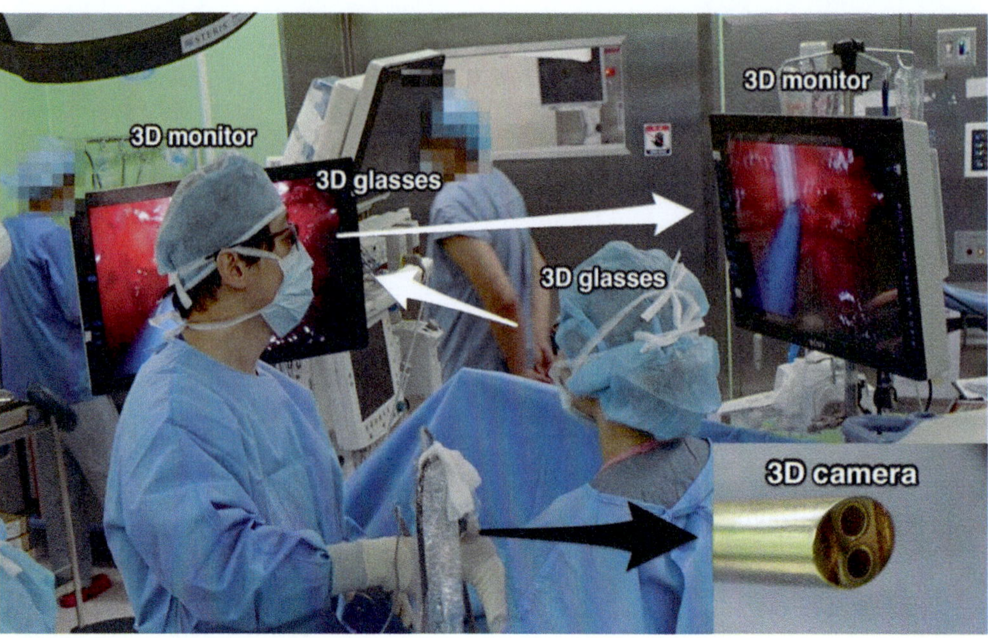

Fig. 1 Uniportal thoracoscopic surgery using a three-dimensional video system

release procedures are helpful to approximate the proximal and distal bronchus. If there is a size discrepancy between two bronchi, trimming of the distal bronchus is needed to prevent stenosis and distal lobe atelectasis. In our experience, suturing in a uniportal field through a small incision is not a simple procedure, and there is often conflict between the inserted instruments. Curved and flexible endoscopic instruments are useful for suturing. Additionally, an endoscopic needle holder such as the Scanlan VATS/MIS (Scanlan International, MN, USA) enables precise suturing in a uniportal VATS approach. We prefer polydioxanone monofilament suture (PDS; Ethicon, USA) as the material for anastomosis of the bronchus, in particular in cases of complete end-to-end anastomosis requiring continuous suturing at the membranous portion and interrupted sutures at the anterior bronchus wall (Fig. 3). Wedge bronchoplasty can be completed with interrupted sutures. Knot ties lie outside of the bronchus wall and are advanced with a knot pusher or sometimes by the second finger. After closure or anastomosis of the bronchus is completed, lung inflation under water submersion to evaluate dehiscence is important to prevent a postoperative fistula. Reinforcement of muscle or the intercostal flap is helpful in cases of preoperative radiation therapy. Fiberoptic bronchoscopy is used to evaluate an anastomotic stenosis or dehiscence, and for removal of secretions (Video 1).

Results

There are no published results of uniportal VATS sleeve resection being carried out in large series or randomized trials, compared with conventional VATS or open thoracotomy. However, several case reports and a series by a uniportal VATS expert have demonstrated acceptable operative results and potential benefits in selected patients [20, 22–24]. New developments in thoracoscopic instruments and display devices promise the expanded application of the uniportal VATS approach to complex thoracic procedures including bronchovascular, tracheal, and carinal reconstruction [25, 26]. Future study is necessary to discuss the oncologic outcomes of uniportal sleeve resection, which is not available currently.

Conclusions

Sleeve resection by a uniportal VATS approach is a feasible option for patients requiring sleeve resection. However, this technique is still a demanding procedure, even for experts in uniportal VATS, and there are few reports regarding postoperative outcomes and safety in a large population. Future studies are needed to achieve an oncologically acceptable procedure with comparable operative risk to sleeve resection via open thoracotomy or conventional VATS.

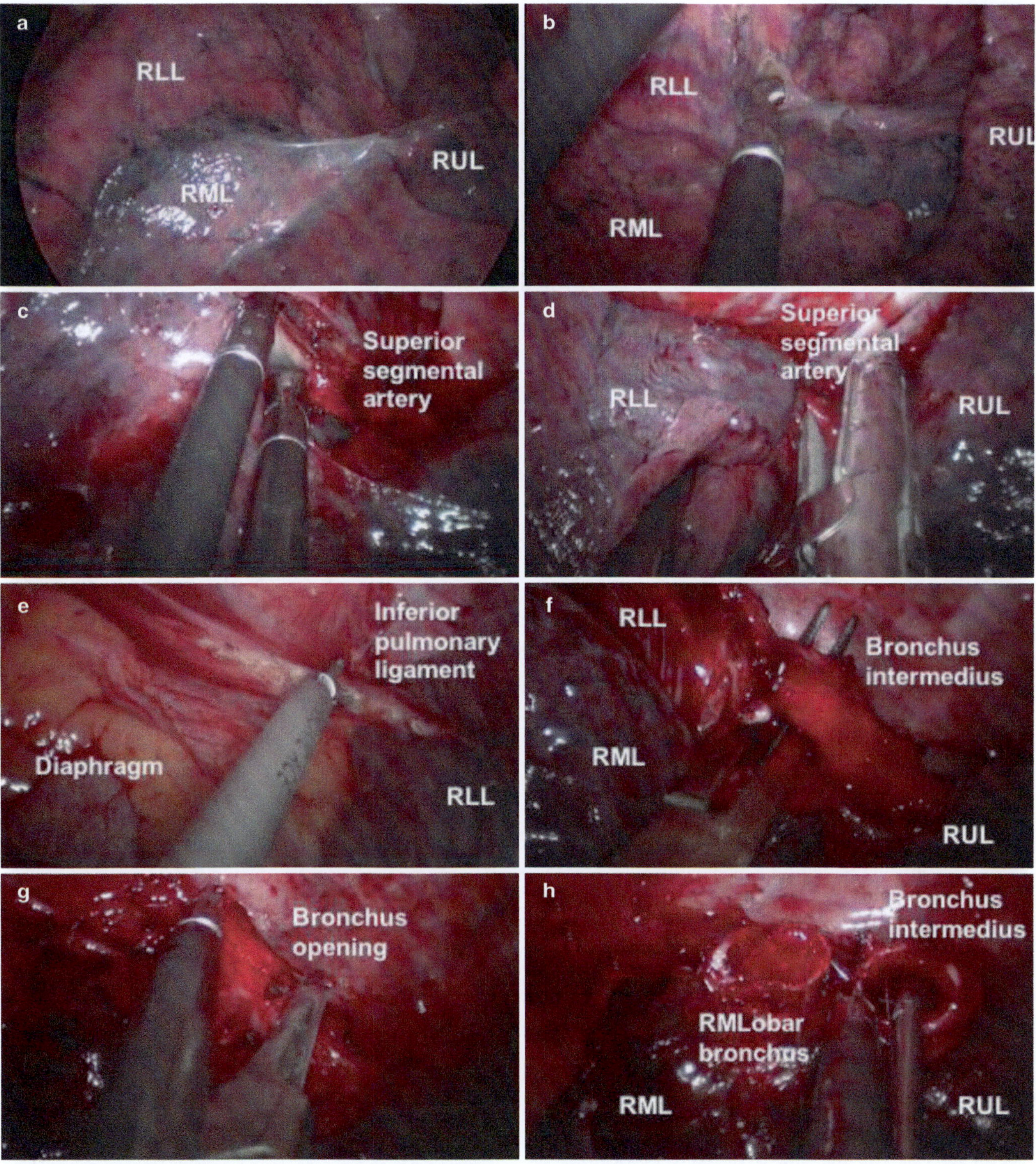

Fig. 2 Uniportal VATS for right lower lobe sleeve resection; (**a**) surgical view from the uniportal approach, (**b**) dissection of the interlobar plane, (**c**) identification of the lower lobar vessel, (**d**) transection of the superior segmental artery, (**e**) division of the inferior pulmonary ligament, (**f**) isolation of the bronchus intermedius, (**g**) opening of the bronchus intermedius with a blade, (**h**) posterior wall anastomosis between the middle lobar bronchus and bronchus intermedius, (**i**) anterior wall anastomosis by interrupted suture, (**j**) completed anastomosis

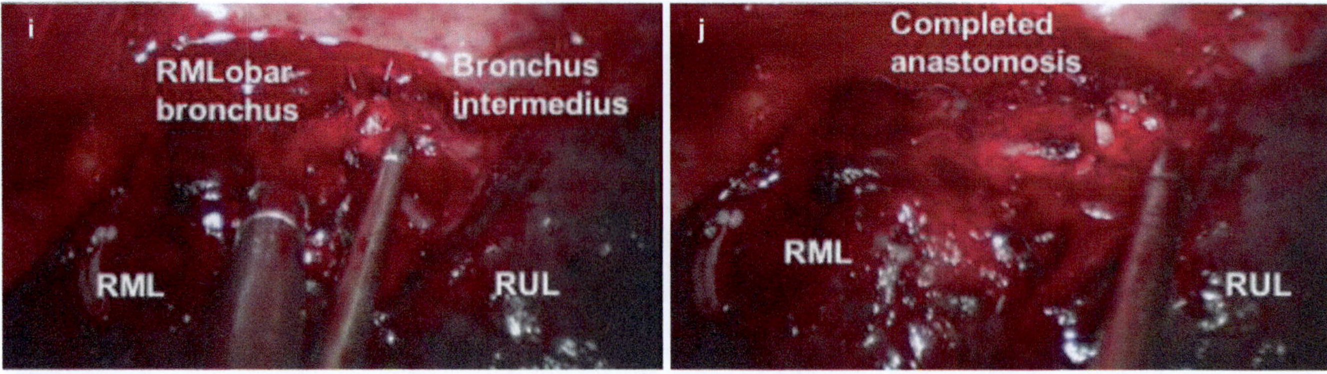

Fig. 2 (continued)

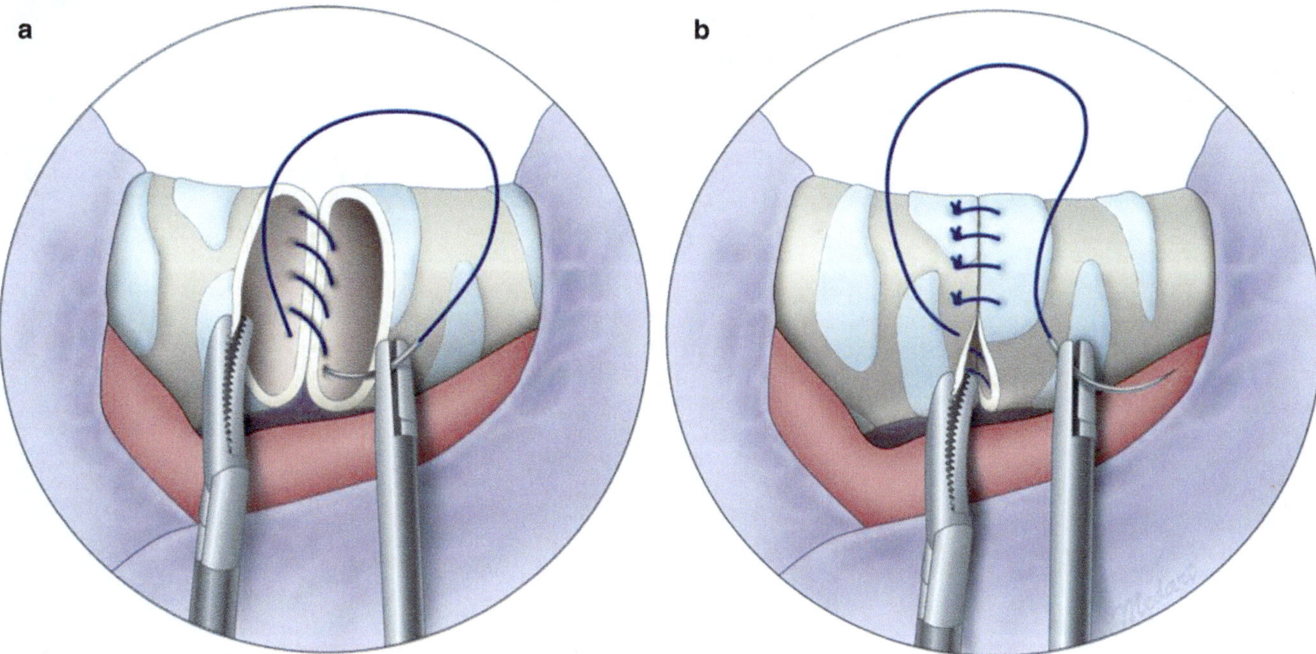

Fig. 3 Bronchial anastomosis with the uniportal approach; (**a**) continuous suturing of the posterior wall, (**b**) suturing the anterior wall by the single-stitch technique

References

1. Deslauriers J, Gregoire J, Jacques LF, et al. Sleeve lobectomy versus pneumonectomy for lung cancer: a comparative analysis of survival and sites or recurrences. Ann Thorac Surg. 2004;77:1152–6;discussion 1156.
2. Park JS, Yang HC, Kim HK, et al. Sleeve lobectomy as an alternative procedure to pneumonectomy for non-small cell lung cancer. J Thorac Oncol. 2010;5:517–20.
3. D'Andrilli A, Maurizi G, Andreetti C, et al. Sleeve lobectomy versus standard lobectomy for lung cancer: functional and oncologic evaluation. Ann Thorac Surg. 2016;101:1936–42.
4. Yamamoto K, Miyamoto Y, Ohsumi A, et al. Sleeve lung resection for lung cancer: analysis according to the type of procedure. J Thorac Cardiovasc Surg. 2008;136:1349–56.
5. Fréchette É, Deslauriers J. Surgical anatomy of the bronchial tree and pulmonary artery. Semin Thorac Cardiovasc Surg. 2006;18:77–84.
6. Ashiku S, MM DC Jr. Parenchymal-sparing procedures in lung cancer: sleeve resection of the lung for proximal lesions. Oper Tech Thorac Cardiovasc Surg. 2006;11:295–309.
7. Takeda S, Maeda H, Koma M, et al. Comparison of surgical results after pneumonectomy and sleeve lobectomy for non-small cell lung cancer: trends over time and 20-year institutional experience. Eur J Cardiothorac Surg. 2006;29:276–80.
8. Yildizeli B, Fadel E, Mussot S, et al. Morbidity, mortality, and long-term survival after sleeve lobectomy for non-small cell lung cancer. Eur J Cardiothorac Surg. 2007;31:95–102.
9. Ferguson MK, Lehman AG. Sleeve lobectomy or pneumonectomy: optimal management strategy using decision analysis techniques. Ann Thorac Surg. 2003;76:1782–8.

10. Bagan P, Berna P, Pereira JC, et al. Sleeve lobectomy versus pneumonectomy: tumor characteristics and comparative analysis of feasibility and results. Ann Thorac Surg. 2005;80:2046–50.
11. Balduyck B, Hendriks J, Lauwers P, Van Schil P. Quality of life after lung cancer surgery: a prospective pilot study comparing bronchial sleeve lobectomy with pneumonectomy. J Thorac Oncol. 2008;3:604–8.
12. Khargi K, Duurkens VA, Verzijlbergen FF, et al. Pulmonary function after sleeve lobectomy. Ann Thorac Surg. 1994;57:1302–4.
13. Sekhniaidze D, Gonzalez-Rivas D. Uniportal video-assisted thoracoscopic sleeve resection. Ann Cardiothorac Surg. 2016;5:145–6.
14. Xie D, Wang H, Fei K, et al. Single-port video-assisted thoracic surgery in 1063 cases: a single-institution experiencedagger. Eur J Cardiothorac Surg. 2016;49(Suppl 1):i31–6.
15. Gonzalez-Rivas D, Yang Y, Stupnik T, et al. Uniportal video-assisted thoracoscopic bronchovascular, tracheal and carinal sleeve resectionsdagger. Eur J Cardiothorac Surg. 2016;49(Suppl 1):i6–16.
16. Agasthian T. Initial experience with video-assisted thoracoscopic bronchoplasty. Eur J Cardiothorac Surg. 2013;44:616–23.
17. Santambrogio L, Cioffi U, De Simone M, et al. Video-assisted sleeve lobectomy for mucoepidermoid carcinoma of the left lower lobar bronchus: a case report. Chest. 2002;121:635–6.
18. Li Y, Wang J. Video-assisted thoracoscopic surgery sleeve lobectomy with bronchoplasty: an improved operative technique. Eur J Cardiothorac Surg. 2013;44:1108–12.
19. Zhou S, Pei G, Han Y, et al. Sleeve lobectomy by video-assisted thoracic surgery versus thoracotomy for non-small cell lung cancer. J Cardiothorac Surg. 2015;10:116.
20. Andrade H, Joubert P, Vieira A, Ugalde Figueroa P. Single-port right upper lobe sleeve lobectomy for a typical carcinoid tumour. Interact Cardiovasc Thorac Surg. 2017;24(2):315–6.
21. Gonzalez-Rivas D, Fernandez R, Fieira E, Rellan L. Uniportal video-assisted thoracoscopic bronchial sleeve lobectomy: first report. J Thorac Cardiovasc Surg. 2013;145:1676–7.
22. Gonzalez-Rivas D, Fieira E, Delgado M, et al. Uniportal video-assisted thoracoscopic sleeve lobectomy and other complex resections. J Thorac Dis. 2014;6:S674–81.
23. Lyscov A, Obukhova T, Ryabova V, et al. Double-sleeve and carinal resections using the uniportal VATS technique: a single centre experience. J Thorac Dis. 2016;8:S235–41.
24. Gonzalez-Rivas D, Delgado M, Fieira E, Pato O. Left lower sleeve lobectomy by uniportal video-assisted thoracoscopic approach. Interact Cardiovasc Thorac Surg. 2014;18:237–9.
25. Ng CS, Rocco G, Wong RH, et al. Uniportal and single-incision video-assisted thoracic surgery: the state of the art. Interact Cardiovasc Thorac Surg. 2014;19:661–6.
26. Ng CS, Wong RH, Lau RW, Yim AP. Single port video-assisted thoracic surgery: advancing scope technology. Eur J Cardiothorac Surg. 2015;47:751.

Tracheal and Carina Resection/ Reconstruction

Guilin Peng, Wei Wang, Minzhang Guo, Hui Pan, and Jianxing He

Abstract

Trachea and carina resection and reconstruction is a difficult surgical technique. In the past, such procedures were completed via large incisions (Pearson FG, Thompson DW, Weissberg D, Simpson WJ, Kergin FG, Ann Thorac Surg 18:16–29, 1974) and, consequently, patients' time to make a full recovery was much longer. In addition, the high potential for postoperative complications have led to many thoracic surgeons avoiding performing these procedures. With the advances of surgical techniques and equipment (Jiao W, Zhu D, Cheng Z, Zhao Y, Ann Thorac Surg 99:e15–7, 2015), including advances in the management of anesthesia, the implementation of tracheal and carina resection/reconstruction is now feasible under complete video-assisted thoracoscopic surgery (c-VATS). For surgeons with extensive VATS experience, the uniportal technique is also a feasible and safe choice that further reduces surgical injury and may accelerate postoperative recovery. Here we introduce two cases: one tracheal and one carinal resection/reconstruction performed under the uniportal VATS technique.

Electronic Supplementary Material The online version of this chapter (https://doi.org/10.1007/978-981-13-2604-2_31) contains supplementary material, which is available to authorized users.

G. Peng · W. Wang · M. Guo · H. Pan · J. He (✉)
Department of Thoracic Surgery, The First Affiliated Hospital of Guangzhou Medical University, Guangzhou, China

Guangzhou Institute of Respiratory Disease & China State Key Laboratory of Respiratory Disease, Guangzhou, China

National Clinical Research Center for Respiratory Disease, Guangzhou, China

Introduction

Tracheal resection was first described by Mathey in 1957 [1]. Thereafter, these procedures became more common and different approaches were developed for the different lesion positions within the trachea and carina, including the right thoracic approach, the median sternotomy approach (even under the extracorporeal circulation) and the cervical approach. In recent years, for large medical centers with extensive VATS experience, this has extended to include complete video assisted thoracic surgery (c-VATS) trachea and carina resections and reconstructions [2].

Developments in the field of surgery have led to a significant increase in the complexity of surgical procedures while simultaneously reducing the length and number of incisions required to complete procedures. Most recently this means uniportal procedures [3]. Uniportal VATS has been gaining popularity, particularly within this past year. Current publications using this procedure range from wedge resection to bronchial sleeve and other complex resections. It offers a directly visual field similar to open surgery and reduces postoperative pain [3].

In cases of tracheal or carinal tumors, obtaining satisfactory oxygenation i.e. intra-operative ventilatory support, is a very important procedure, and requires significant consideration when selecting the method. Choices can include small size (4.5 F reinforced endotracheal tube well lead) tracheal intubation or high-frequency cross field ventilation [2]. In the following cases spontaneous respiration anesthesia is used; as a result, these methods are used only as short-term extra support and are not a primary ventilation method.

Preoperative Preparation

Bronchoscopy is a very important preoperative method used in the measurement of the distance of the tumor from the carina or glottis. In addition, we often acquire pathology

D. Gonzalez-Rivas et al. (eds.), *Atlas of Uniportal Video Assisted Thoracic Surgery*,
https://doi.org/10.1007/978-981-13-2604-2_31

through bronchoscopic exam. When under submucosa growth may be present, characteristic of adenoid cystic carcinoma for example, we perform bronchoscopic multiple punch biopsy to confirm negative margins. Performing this procedure preoperatively allows better operative planning and increases the perioperative negative margin rates of the resection area.

Cough and dyspnea are the main symptoms presented in patients with tracheal tumors. Some preoperative therapeutic options performed under bronchoscopy can reduce symptoms and increase the safety of the operation. Galvanocautery and argon plasma coagulation (APC) are all suitable methods for preoperative therapy in patients with obstructing tumors.

Advances in CT imaging technology and data processing have given us refactoring technology which can help us distinguish individuals' anatomic features in relation to the tumor such as the esophagus, arteries, and veins.

Induction of Anesthesia

Our extensive experience with spontaneous ventilation procedures under non-intubated anesthesia since the concept was first introduced by Pompeo et al. in 2004 [4], has allowed us to apply this method in complex procedures. In this case we have found that the use of spontaneous breathing anesthesia in tracheal and carinal resections and reconstructions has simplified oxygen support as it avoids the need of switching ventilation approaches during conventional cross-field ventilation [5]. Furthermore, it provides better operative exposure and visualization. Therefore, we have used the same spontaneous ventilation technique in both of the herein reported cases.

Midazolam (0.06 mg/kg) and atropine (0.01 mg/kg) were injected intramuscularly 30 min before the anesthesia. Intra-operative thoracic epidural analgesia was administered at the level of T6–7 using 0.25% ropivacaine (12 mL bolus initially, followed by 5 mL bolus every 30 min). Anesthesia was achieved by intravenous injection of remifentanil (0.05 mg/kg/min), dexmedetomidine (0.5–1.0 μg/kg/h) and propofol (1.5–2.5 μg/mL). Patients were allowed to breathe spontaneously with supplementary oxygen through a laryngeal mask, aiming for a respiration rate of 12–20 breaths/min and oxygenation saturation of more than 90%. High-frequency jet ventilation and/or bronchus intubation are used only in the event that a patient's oxygen saturation falls below 90% to ensure sufficient, stable oxygenation particularly during resection of the trachea. The patient's vital signs, arterial blood gases, electrocardiogram, and bispectral index (BIS) were monitored throughout the operation.

Position and Incision Selection

The length of the trachea is about 11–13 cm in normal patients and tumors may be located at any position including the carina. We divide the incision selection for these patients into three options:

1. Cervical approach: Patients with a tumor located under the glottis and above the sternal notch should be placed in a supine position with cervical extension. Particular attention must be given when patients have a tumor located close to the glottis. Removal of such tumors can result in destruction of the structure around the glottis. In these patients, the recurrent laryngeal nerve should be explored before the operation. In the event that the laryngeal nerve or glottis is destroyed by the tumor, tracheostomy or tracheal stent implantation can be considered for unresectable tumors.
2. Median sternotomy approach: In the event that exposure of the tumor is difficult and invasion of surrounding tissues is found, thoracic surgeons may consider a median sternotomy approach, this is also a safer approach when preparation for extracorporeal circulation is required.
3. Right thoracic approach: When a tumor is located at the lower portion of the trachea or the carina, a right thoracic approach can offer good exposure assisted by the thoracoscope. Using the right thoracic approach the aorta and other large arteries can be avoided which reduces the risk for major bleeds. The operating port at third intercostal space between the anterior and mid-axillary line is suitable for exposure and anastomosis.

Surgical Technique

We report two cases with different tumor locations resected under uniportal VATS. Both were completed using the right thoracic approach. As both patients had a BMI < 25 and an ASA grade < II and no other anesthetic contraindications were found, spontaneous ventilation was selected as the anesthetic approach.

Case 1

A 46 year old male patient with distal tracheal keratotic squamous cell carcinoma (tumor diameter of approximately 29 mm) was admitted to the hospital. The CT scan and bronchoscopic image of the tumor are shown below (Fig. 1a–c). Five days before the operation, argon plasma coagulation (APC) was applied through the bronchoscope to relieve the tracheal obstruction and increase the safety of the operation.

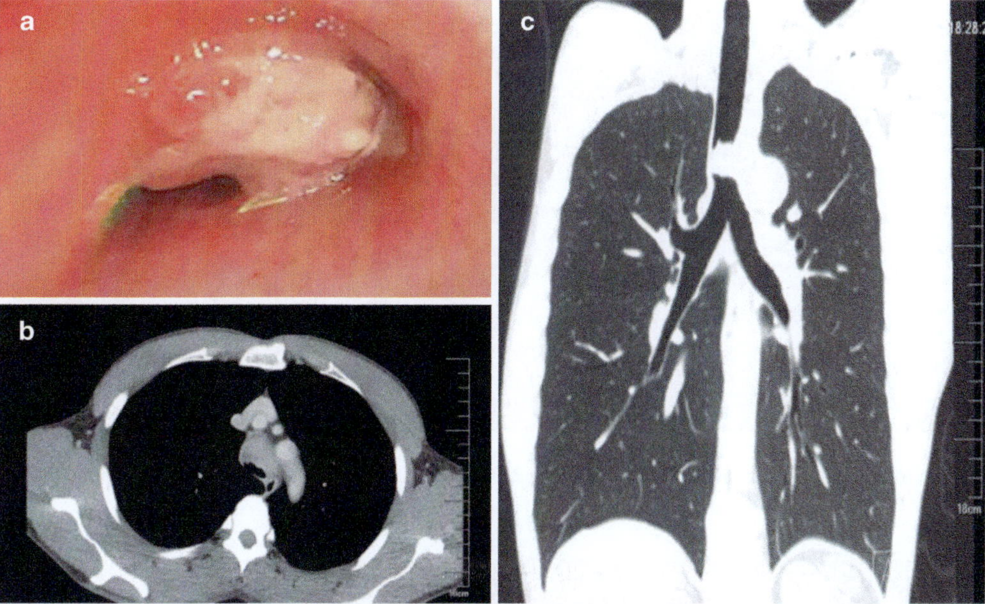

Fig. 1 (**a**) The tracheal view under the bronchoscope; (**b** and **c**) the chest computed tomography (CT) showed a nodule located at the lower trachea, 17 mm away from the carina

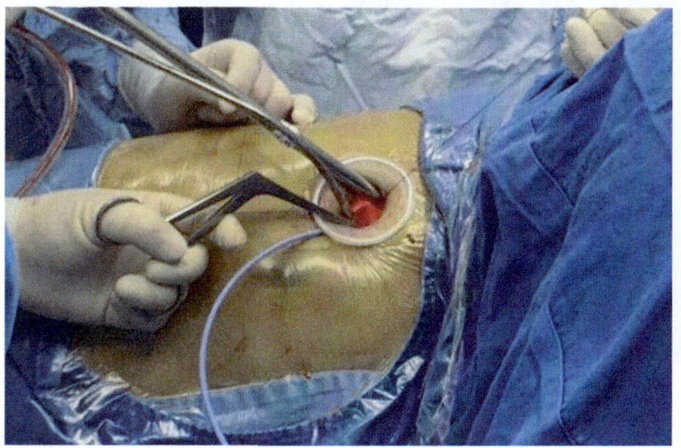

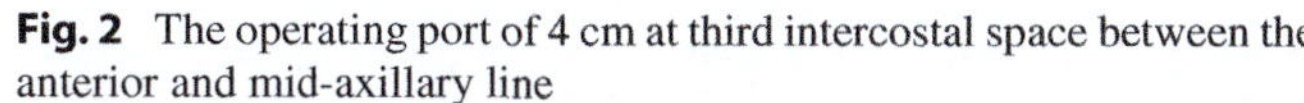

Fig. 2 The operating port of 4 cm at third intercostal space between the anterior and mid-axillary line

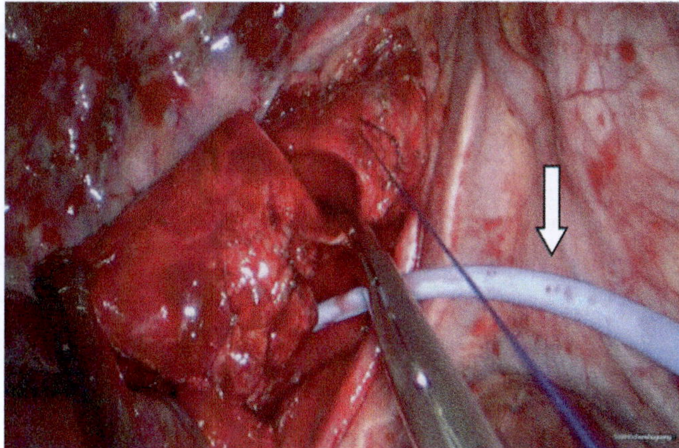

Fig. 3 The diseased trachea with tumor and the blue high-frequency oxygen tube

One port was created at the third intercostal space between the anterior and mid-axillary line with a length of 4 cm (Fig. 2). The azygos vein was cut for a better exposure of the tumor. About 4 cm of the trachea was resected in total. During resection of the trachea, the patients' SpO_2 fell below 90%, as a result a high frequency oxygenation tube was inserted to the lower trachea until satisfactory oxygenation was assured (Fig. 3). End-to-end anastomosis of the trachea using 2-0 Prolene continuous suture was used starting from the membranous section of the trachea (Fig. 4). Separation of the surrounding tissues from the trachea can reduce the tension of the trachea and benefit surgeons when performing end-to-end anastomosis. Continuous suture is selected in our center for most surgical procedures to avoid wire wrapping and reduce the suture time (Fig. 5). Reinforcement sutures are very important for reducing the tension on the anastomosis (Fig. 6). The postoperative CT scan and bronchoscopy show the new carina (Fig. 7).

Case 2

A 40 year old female with lymphoepithelioma-like carcinoma (40 mm) located in the lower trachea and the initial opening of the right main bronchus underwent tracheal resection using the non-intubated technique described above. Diagnostic CT scan and bronchoscopic images are shown below (Fig. 8a–c). Bronchoscopic multiple punch biopsy was performed to confirm the negative margins around the tumor for preoperative planning.

One 5 cm port was made in the third intercostal space between the anterior and mid-axillary line (Fig. 9). About 3.5 cm trachea and part of the right main bronchus were resected. A high frequency oxygenation tube was inserted to the left main bronchus for a short period of time when the patients' SpO_2 fell below 90% (Fig. 10). Reconstruction included two sets of anastomosis completed using 2-0 Prolene continuous suture. The first was between the left side

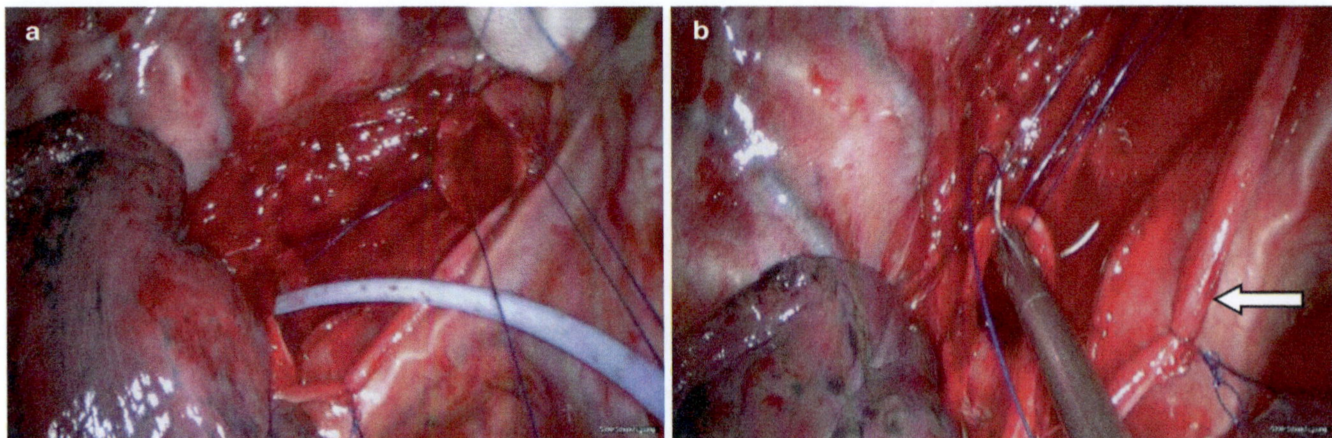

Fig. 4 (**a**) The convolution of the both ends, using 2-0 Prolene stitches. (**b**) The white arrow points out the suspension of the vagus nerve

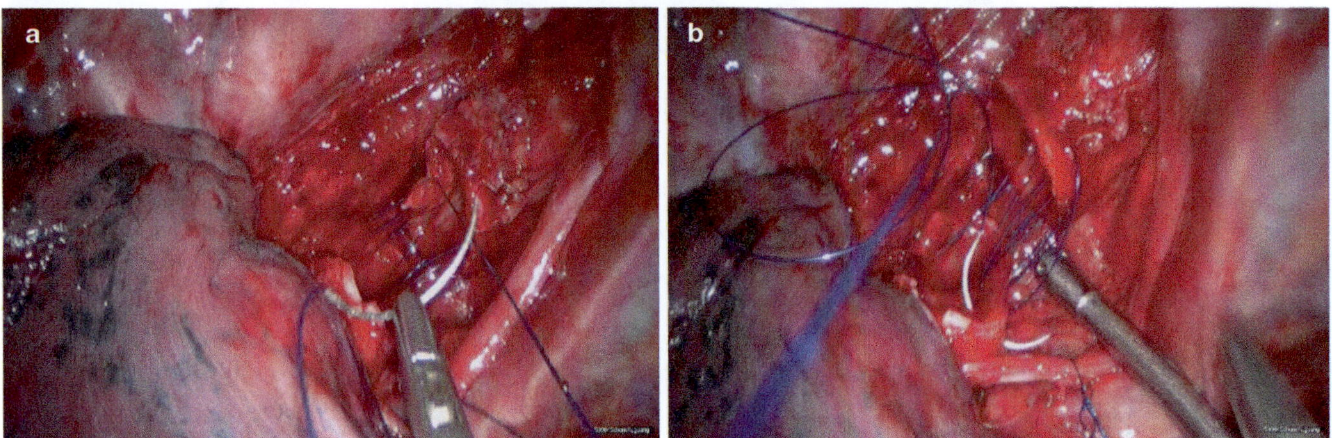

Fig. 5 (**a**) The anastomosis process of the tracheal stump. (**b**) Avoiding wire wrapping during the anastomosis process

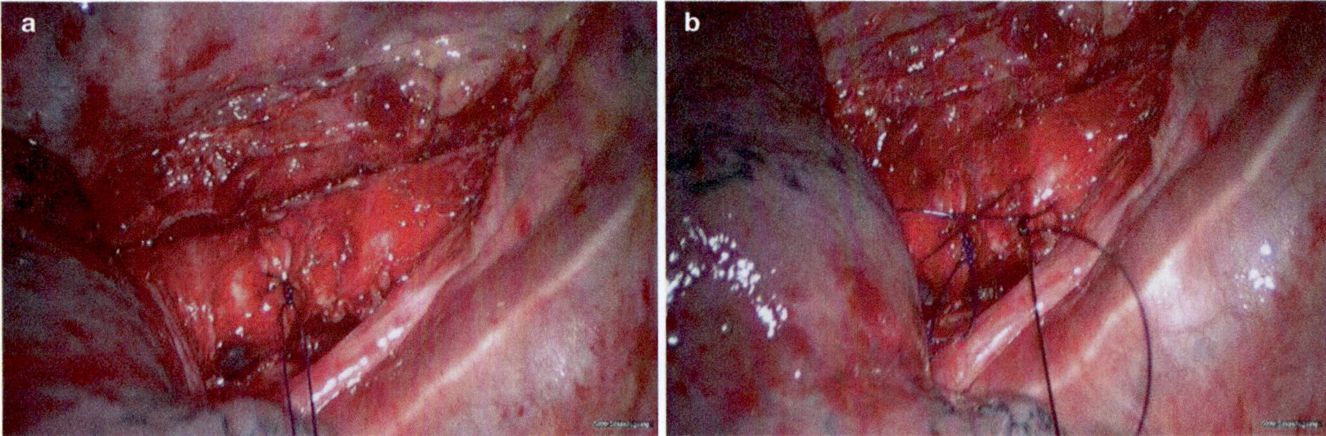

Fig. 6 (**a**) The completed anastomosis of the trachea. (**b**) Reinforcing sutures of the anastomotic stoma

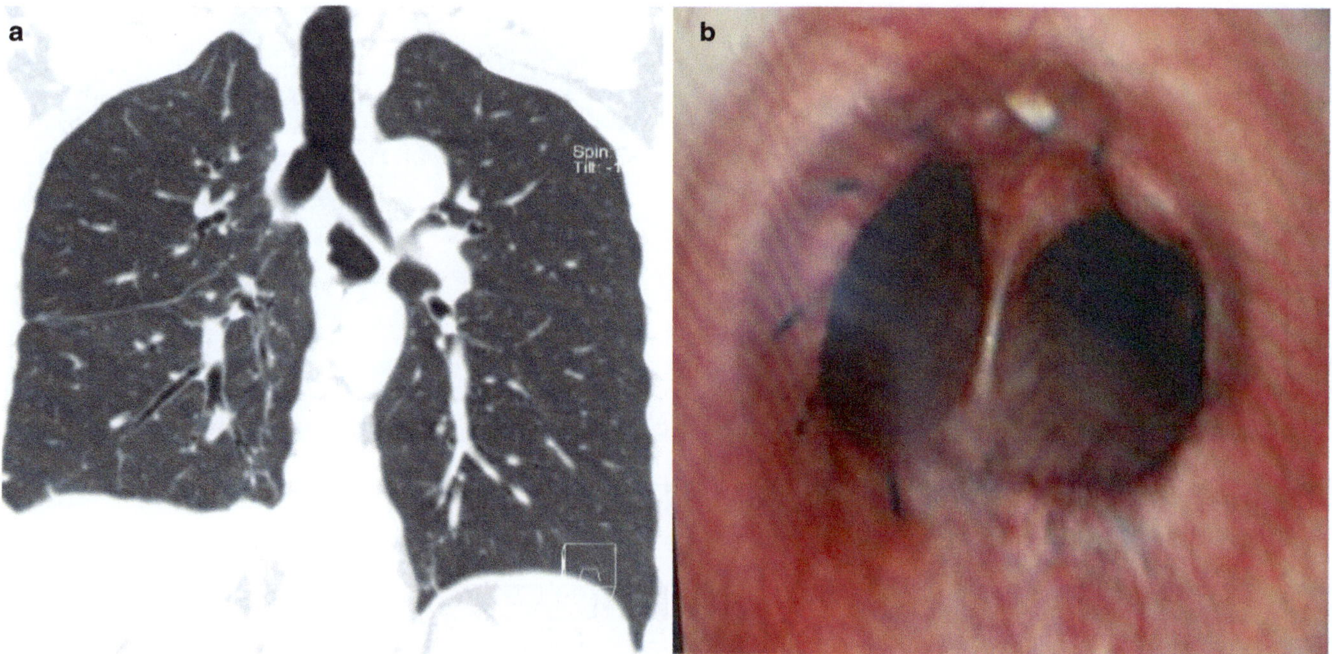

Fig. 7 (**a**) Postoperative CT Scan. (**b**) Postoperative bronchoscope view of the anastomotic stoma

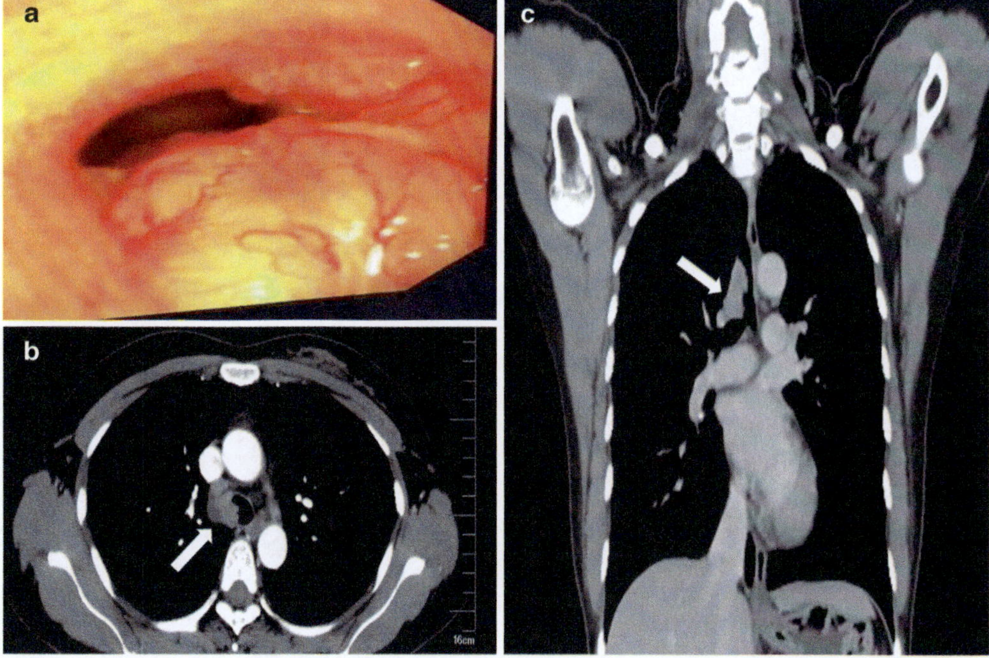

Fig. 8 (**a**) The endotracheal view under the bronchoscope; (**b** and **c**) the chest computed tomography (CT) showed the tumor located at the lower tracheal and the initial part of the right main bronchus, with the diameter of about 40 mm

of the trachea and the left main bronchus beginning from the membranous section of the trachea (Fig. 11). The second was between the newly constructed half of the carina and the right main bronchus, creating a new carina (Fig. 12). After reconstruction of the carina two reinforcement sutures were placed (Fig. 13).

The time of operation was 5 h and the process of the anastomosis was about 120 min, the intra-operative blood loss was about 50 mL. The patient returned to our hospital 1 month postoperatively for follow-up. CT scan and the bronchoscopic exams revealed no stenosis nor signs of recurrence (Fig. 14).

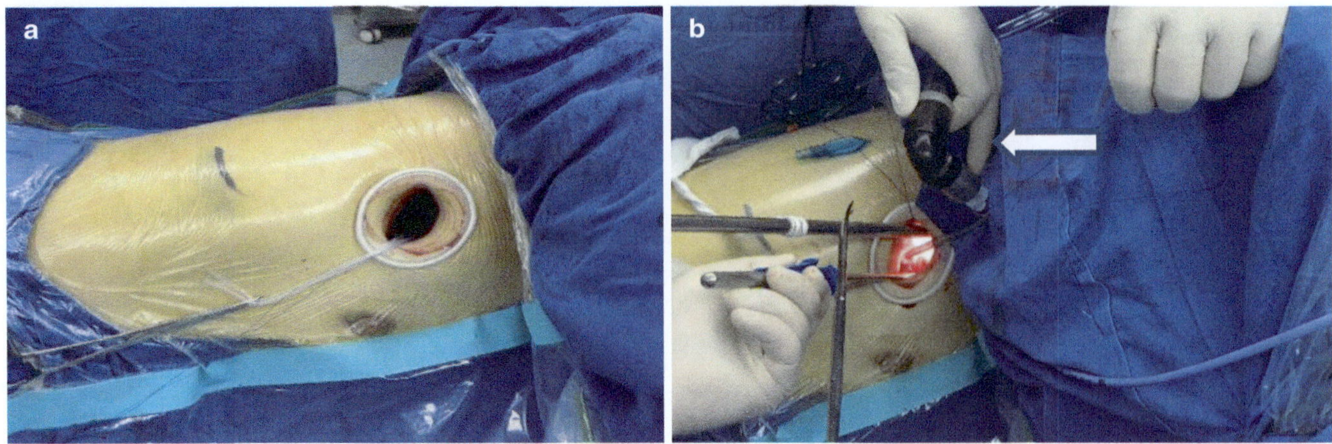

Fig. 9 (**a**) The 5 cm operating port at third intercostal space between the anterior and mid-axillary line. (**b**) The tracheal intubation connected to the ventilator

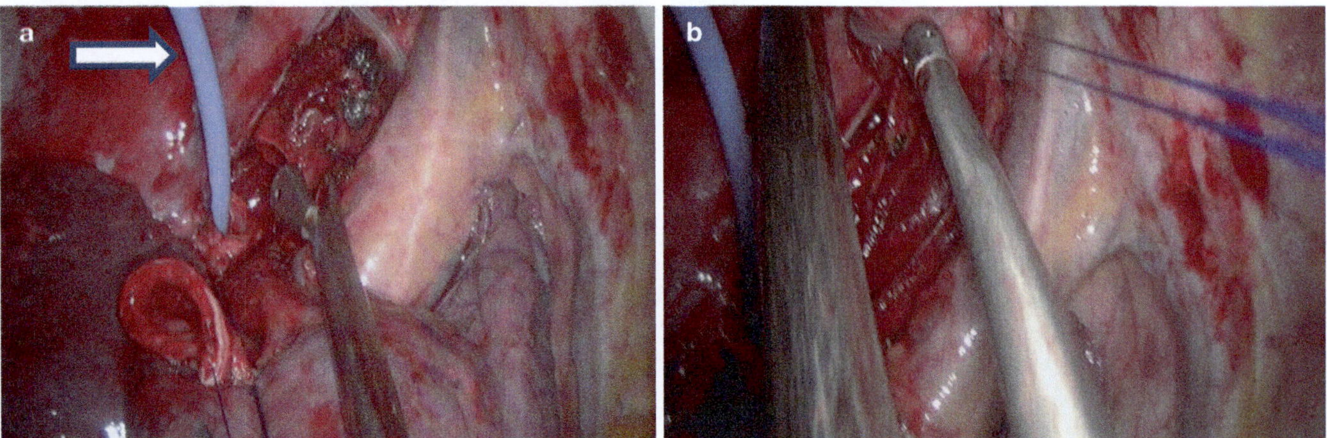

Fig. 10 (**a** and **b**) Anatomy of the trachea with tumor, the blue high-frequency oxygen tube

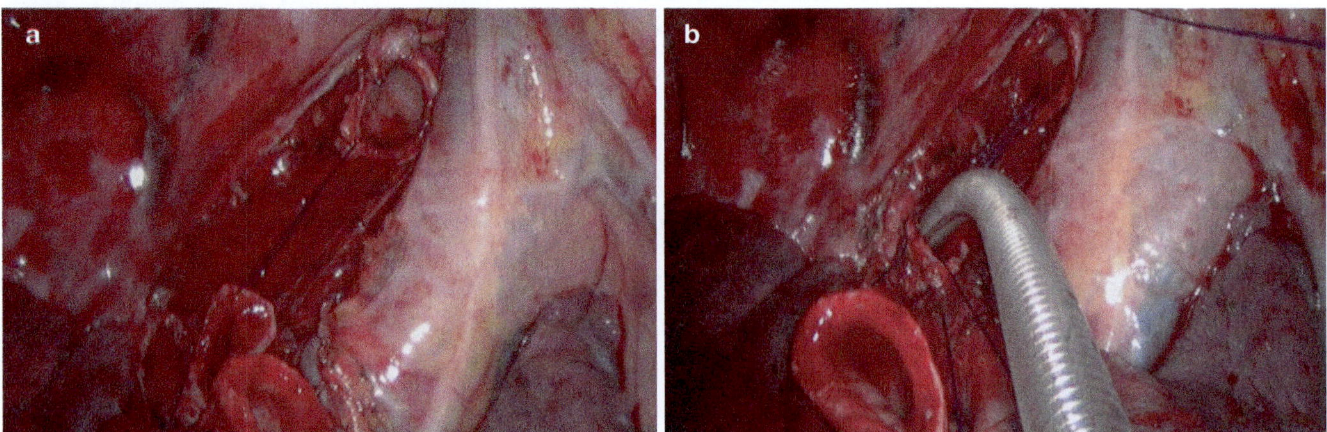

Fig. 11 (**a**) The convolution of the trachea and the left main bronchus, using 2-0 Prolene. (**b**) The tracheal intubation inserted to the left main bronchus for better oxygenation

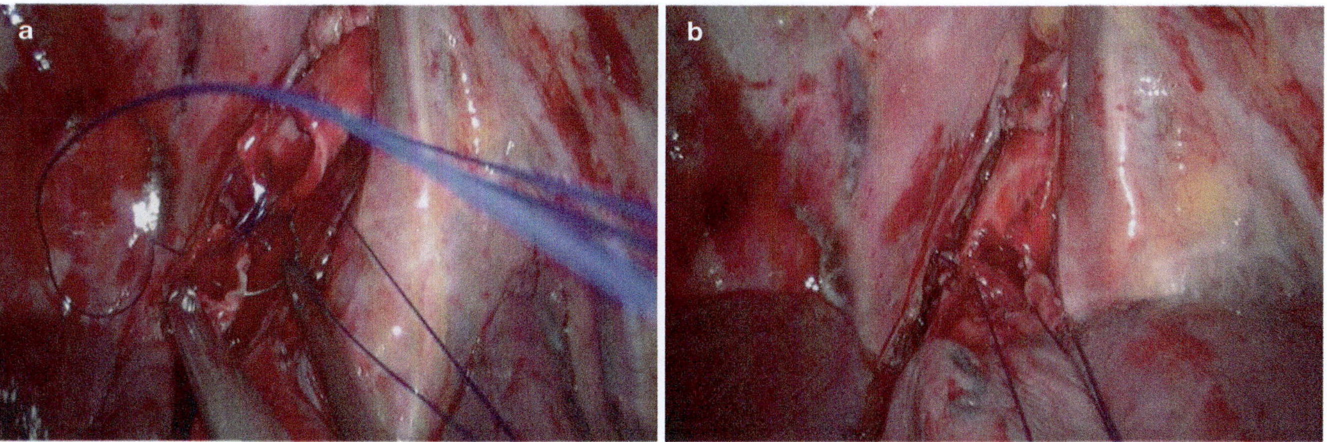

Fig. 12 (**a**) The anastomosis of the left main bronchus and trachea; (**b**) the anastomosis of the right main bronchus and the artificial gap

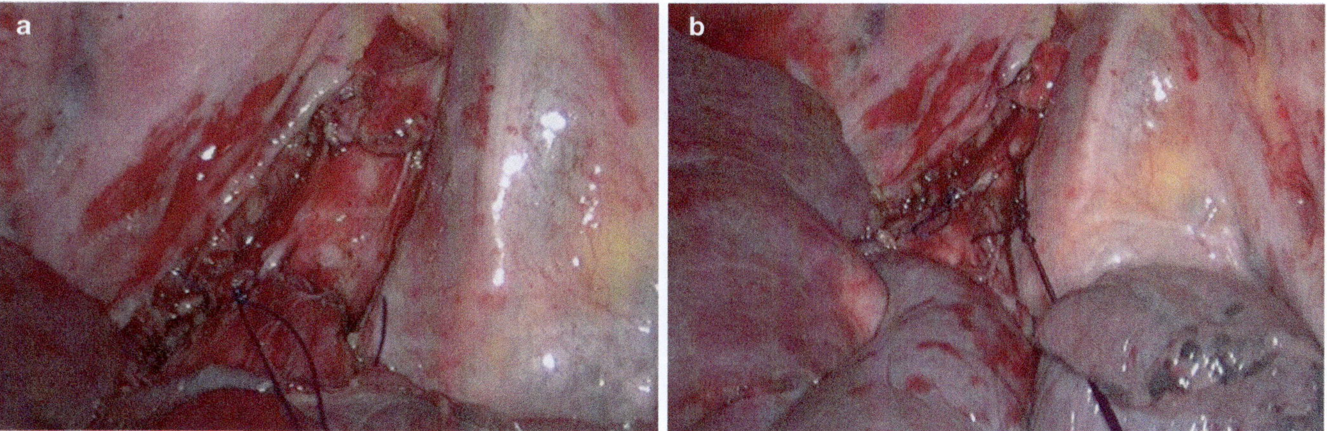

Fig. 13 (**a**) Completed anastomosis of the trachea. (**b**) Reinforcement suture of the anastomotic stoma

Post-operative Care

Two prophylactic chin sutures were placed at the end of the procedure to protect the anastomosis from excessive neck extension. Patients were discharged after the chin sutures were removed (about 2 weeks postoperatively to assure proper healing). We suggest that the patient keep the head leaned forward for about 1 month to lower tension and protect the anastomosis.

Mechanical assisted expectoration is very important for patients whose cervical movement is limited postoperation. Out of bed activity is also very important to reduce postoperative complications such as pulmonary embolism and venous thromboembolism and to speed up patient recovery.

Both patients returned to the hospital for follow up observation 1 month postoperation. Follow-up included CT scan and the bronchoscopic exam and confirmed no stenosis or signs of recurrence.

Conclusion

Tracheal and carinal resection/reconstruction is a challenging procedure, both because of the complex technique involved in the completion of these procedures and the possibilities of severe postoperative complications. The question of how to reduce trauma and increase peri-operative safety is of critical concern to surgeons with enough experience to perform these procedures.

In the past, surgical procedures were completed using large incisions (even extracorporeal circulation) first for lack of the technology and anatomical knowledge necessary to complete procedures through smaller incisions, and later for safety. In recent years, we have been able to reduce trauma via multiport video assisted thoracic surgery (VATS). Now, with the advances of surgical technique and imaging equipment, uniportal VATS is making an impact in the thoracic surgery world. Uniportal VATS is a good choice for patients requiring

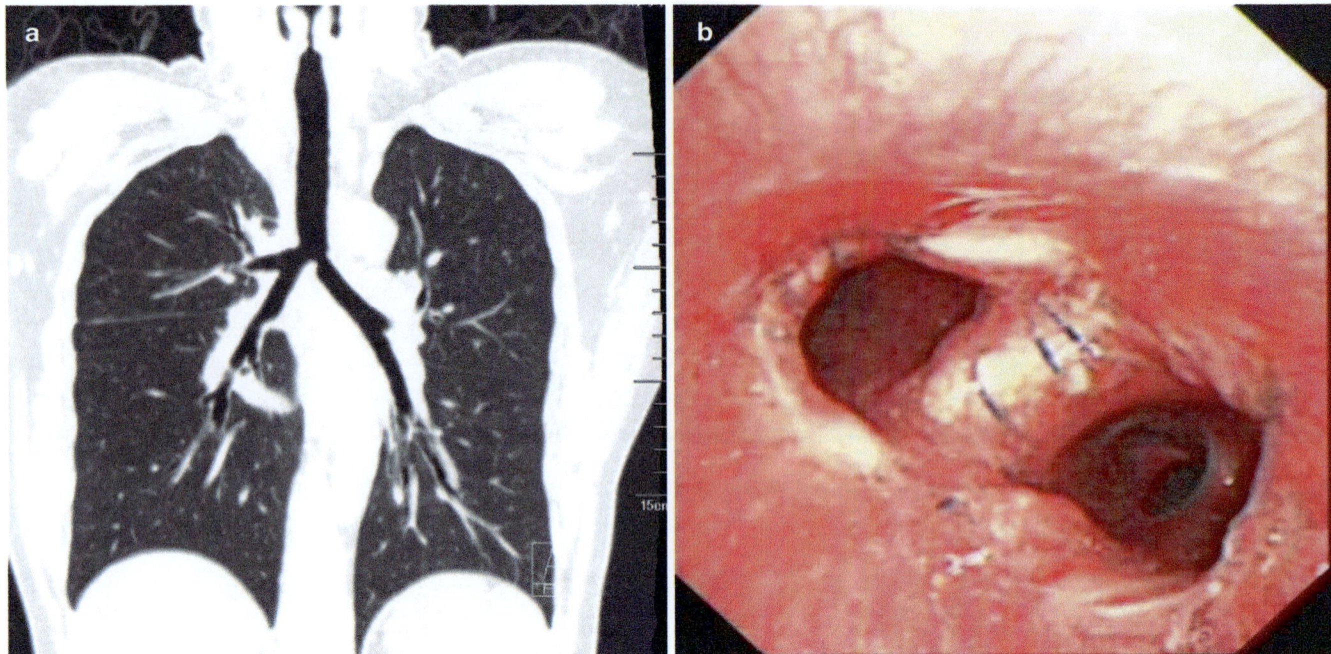

Fig. 14 (**a**) The postoperative CT Scan. (**b**) The postoperative bronchoscopic view of the anastomotic stoma

tracheal or carinal tumor resection and reconstruction, as it may offer potential advantages such as less surgical trauma, less postoperative pain, faster recovery, and better cosmetic results. In general, uniport procedures have the advantage of a direct visual field, for beginners this is a significant advantage as it makes manipulation easier by providing a view similar to thoracotomy. In regards to thoracic surgeons with extensive experience minimally invasive procedures, advantages are the same and switching from multiport to uniportal VATS requires only some special uniportal equipment and good coordination with assistants. For patients with tracheal disease, uniportal VATS is a good option, because of the potential advantages of reduced access trauma, less postoperative pain and better cosmetic results [6]. For surgical centers with vast experience in advanced VATS procedures, the uniportal technique may offer a less invasive alternative option even for complex operative procedures. In our opinion uniportal tracheal and carina resection/reconstruction procedures could be implemented in centers with full surgical experience.

During both multiport and uniportal tracheal procedures the presence of a tracheal tube during anastomosis results in poor surgical field and high anastomotic tension, which directly increases the surgical difficulty and prolongs the operative time. Thus, in this article we also describe the application of a novel spontaneous breathing c-VATS surgery. This use of this technique provides good exposure of the resection area and greater flexibility of the trachea during the anastomotic process [7]. During this spontaneous ventilation procedure, if the SpO_2 falls below 90% or the CO_2 increases to 80 mmHg or more, high frequency ventilation or bronchus intubation can be used to improve the situation. However, if these methods are unsuccessful, conversion of anesthetic procedure to traditional tracheal intubation should be performed without hesitation.

References

1. Mathey J, Binet JP, Galey JJ, et al. Tracheal and tracheobronchial resections: technique and results in 20 cases. J Thorac Cardiovasc Surg. 1966;51:1–13.
2. Xu X, Chen H, Yin W, et al. Thoracoscopic half carina resection and bronchial sleeve resection for central lung cancer. Surg Innov. 2014;21:481–6.
3. Anile M, et al. Uniportal video assisted thoracoscopic lobectomy: going directly from open surgery to a single port approach. J Thorac Dis. 2014;6:641–3.
4. Pompeo E, Mineo D, Rogliani P, Sabato AF, Mineo TC. Feasibility and results of awake thoracoscopic resection of solitary pulmonary nodules. Ann Thorac Surg. 2004;78:1761–8.
5. Blasberg JD, Wright CD. Surgical considerations in tracheal and carinal resection. Semin Cardiothorac Vasc Anesth. 2012;16:190–5.
6. Gonzalez-Rivas D. Recent advances in uniportal video-assisted thoracoscopic surgery. Chin J Cancer Res. 2015;27(1):90–3. https://doi.org/10.3978/j.issn.1000-9604.2015.02.03.
7. Peng G, Cui F, et al. Spontaneous breathing combined with video-assisted thoracoscopic in carinal reconstruction. J Thorac Dis. 2016;8(3):586–93.

Uniportal VATS Chest Wall and Diaphragm Resection and Reconstruction

Firas Abu Akar and Diego Gonzalez-Rivas

Introduction

Lung cancer is one of the leading causes of death around the world. Only a small percentage (5%) of cases of pulmonary tumors that are subjected to resection is needed to be removed en bloc with a part from the chest wall due to its involvement by the tumor. These patients are divided into two groups for historical and anatomical reasons, tumors involving and/or superior to the second rib (Pancoast), and tumors located inferior to the second rib. The issue of post-thoracotomy pain is increased after chest wall resection, especially after resections involving the paravertebral area, en bloc resection of the chest wall together with the lobe is the procedure of choice to achieve complete resection in lung cancer invading the chest wall relying on most of the series advocated that [1–3]. Surgical treatment of non-small cell lung cancer (NSCLC) invading the chest wall by extrapleural or "en bloc" resection is widely adopted and justified by the good results, in terms of morbidity and relief of pain. Survival always depends on the nodal status.

Diaphragmatic involvement by NSCLC is rarer than the chest wall with only 0.5% of the cases of resectable locally advanced lung tumors. However, because of the paucity of these cases, there are also few reports and publication concerning of the results in this entity. VATS resection of the affected lung lobe en-bloc with the chest wall or the diaphragm is a relatively new technique, which gained popularity due to improved visual field provided in addition to the benefit of reducing the surgical trauma and providing less painful and faster recovery to the patients. As the experience has increased, surgeons have been able to perform more radical and complex resections. To date Uniportal VATS is the least invasive technique used for performing thoracic operations, few publications have been released describing en-bloc resection of lung tumors involving the chest wall or the diaphragm.

Electronic Supplementary Material The online version of this chapter (https://doi.org/10.1007/978-981-13-2604-2_32) contains supplementary material, which is available to authorized users.

F. A. Akar
Department of Cardiothoracic surgery, Makassed Charitable Society Hospital, East Jerusalem, Israel

Department of Cardiothoracic Surgery, Shaare Zedek Medical Center (SZMC), Jerusalem, Israel

D. Gonzalez-Rivas (✉)
Department of Thoracic Surgery, Shanghai Pulmonary Hospital, Tongji University School of Medicine, Shanghai, China

Department of Thoracic Surgery and Minimally Invasive Thoracic Surgery Unit (UCTMI), Coruña University Hospital, Coruña, Spain
e-mail: diego@uniportal.es

Discussion

Incidence

The vast majority of chest wall lesions is caused by the direct invasion of adjacent malignancies or metastatic lesions with about 40% of cases due to direct invasion of lung cancer [4–6]. A series of 4688 patients with non-small cell lung cancer (NSCLC) undergoing tumor resection was reported by Weksler et al. [7], They found diaphragmatic involvement in eight (0.17%), outcomes of these patients were unfavorable. Yokoi et al. found the diaphragm was involved in 36/16771 (0.38%) of patients with NSCLC.

Staging and Prognosis

According to the last International Association for the Study of Lung Cancer (IASLC) TNM staging [8], NSCLC involving the diaphragm or the chest wall is considered to be a T3 disease. Although surgery is indicated in T3 disease, contraindications to surgery are based on the histopathological type, the extension of the tumor, and the patient's overall general condition [9]. Five-year survival in NSCLC involving the chest wall approximates 50% for T3N0M0 patients. However, patients with N1 and N2 disease, have less than 10% 5-year survival, and adjuvant radiotherapy appears to

D. Gonzalez-Rivas et al. (eds.), *Atlas of Uniportal Video Assisted Thoracic Surgery*,
https://doi.org/10.1007/978-981-13-2604-2_32

have no effect on survival [9]. Yokoi et al. [10] noticed that patients with T3 NSCLC involving the diaphragm have a 5-year survival of 22.6% with complete resection, but patients with incomplete resection did not achieve 4-year survival (P = 0.024). Patients with completely resected T3N0M0 and T3N1-2M0 tumors had a survival of 28.3% and 18.1%, respectively (P = 0.013). Diaphragmatic invasion depth has its significant effect on the prognosis. Patients with superficial invasion (involvement of subpleural, pleural or parietal layers) have a 5-year survival of 33.0%, whereas in patients who had a deep invasion (peritoneal or muscle infiltration) was 14.3% (P = 0.036), and these results were confirmed by Galetta et al. [11]. The 5-year survival rate for T3N0 patients with superficial invasion tumors was 43%, whereas that of patients with T3N+ or deep invasion was worse. Possibly due to their rarity, we have only a few reports have been published concerning the surgical results of patients with primary lung tumors invading the diaphragm [7, 10–15]. Cure with acceptable mortality was offered by en bloc resection of the lung and diaphragm [10]. It has been suggested that lesion invading the muscular layer or deeper to it, warrant a higher degree of staging than T3, in that although these cancers are generally technically resectable, oncologically they are almost incurable [10, 14]. Five other cases were reported by Inoue et al. and there were no 3-year survivors among these patients. They suggested that such NSCLC invading the diaphragm may consider a T4 disease [12]. According to Doyle and Ainser [16] this poor prognosis attributed to the extensive lymphatic and venous drainage of the diaphragm which could be responsible for early systemic dissemination of the disease. Further explaining that "once the tumor cells have reached into the diaphragmatic muscle, there is almost always a liver involvement or retroperitoneal lymph nodes metastases or both". Surgical resection is still the only reliable curative method. Downey et al. [17] concluded that no difference was observed between en bloc and extrapleural resection in terms of local recurrence or survival. They found no difference in survival based on the invasion depth of chest wall. Long-term survival in patients with chest wall involvement undergoing surgical resection is strongly related to regional lymph node involvement and achieving R0 resection. They also concluded that 5-year survival in patients undergoing incomplete resection was only 4%, results similar to those who did not undergo surgery.

The Role of VATS

The introduction of video-assisted thoracoscopic surgery (VATS) for lobectomy was at the beginning of the1990s [18], and within few years it has become a standard for selected cases of pulmonary resections, especially for early stage NSCLC [19–21]. With gaining experience in VATS and with technological advances in equipment, VATS was applied to more complex conditions. Even though there have been no prospective "RCTs", comparing open thoracotomy to VATS approaches, a number of propensity-matched studies have demonstrated some advantages of VATS over open procedures reduction of post-operative pain, quicker return to normal life activities, preferable conserved lung function, shorter chest drainage time, shorter length of hospital stay, reduced inflammatory reaction and a lower incidence of arrhythmia [19–22]. At the beginning of the new millennium, Widmann and colleagues reported the feasibility of VATS en bloc resection of the chest wall for lung cancer [23]. And since then only a few reports were published concerning the feasibility of pure VATS or "hybrid" thoracoscopic lobectomy en-bloc with chest wall resections [22, 24, 25]. The hybrid approach has been shown to be feasible and effective in selected patients, the use of a limited incision without rib spreading allowed complete R0 resections in all cases without increased morbidity compared to conventional thoracotomy according to a study reported by Berry MF and colleagues [26]. Nonetheless, patients seem to benefit when rib spreading is avoided even for chest wall resection. This is due to less postoperative pain and better postoperative pulmonary functions [22, 24, 26], especially since respiratory insufficiency is the leading cause of mortality after combined resection [27]. VATS is somewhat limited in cases of large tumors (>7 cm) that require the resection of the first rib (Pancoast). This is explained by the need for dissection close to the thoracic outlet, as well as the visual limitation at the apical area of the thorax. When the transverse processes are involved by the tumor, also not ideally suited for thoracoscopy [22, 26]. Uniportal VATS is an emerging technique was introduced in the beginnings of the new millennium [28–30]. This new approach was taken forward and evolved to major lung resections by Gonzalez-Rivas and his group [31–34]. Since the report of uniportal VATS lobectomy in 2011 [31] this technique was expanded to complex procedures such as segmental resections, sleeve resections and pneumonectomies [32–34]. Uniportal VATS surgery has since acquired wide popularity with more surgeons espoused this approach over the conventional multi-portal VATS approach. In addition, one notable advantage of uniportal VATS is the more "intuitive" visualization and instrument deployment afforded by the system. The technique enables inserting both camera and instruments in parallel, thus no different view than the way in open surgery [35]. In 2013 Gonzalez Rivas and his group reported a case of uniportal VATS right upper lobectomy with chest wall resection by posterior approach [36], and they further described the hybrid uniportal technique with a number of videos in the web [37–39]. Although hybrid or pure uniportal VATS approach for resecting tumors involving the chest wall seems to be feasible and safe, more studies are needed to prove the superiority of uniportal VATS over other conventional techniques. Multiple reports have been published describing VATS plication of the diaphragm for paralyzed diaphragm or diaphragmatic reconstruction after repair of eventration [40–47]. To date, there are not any reports describing uniportal VATS resection and reconstruction of the diaphragm in NSCLC tumors involving the diaphragm.

Surgery

Anesthesia

General anesthesia is usually utilized. Separated-lung ventilation achieved by employing a double-lumened tube or bronchial blocker device under the guidance of the fiberoptic bronchoscope. The authors prefer to use the double-lumened tube for right-sided lung resections as we believe that it gives a superior lung deflation during the surgery. Arterial line employed for hemodynamic and monitoring of the ABGs. Peripheral IV accesses are usually utilized for injecting fluids and intravenous medications. A urinary catheter is routinely inserted. Paravertebral anesthesia could be applied before to the beginning of the surgery; alternatively, intercostal nerve blockage can be done by the surgeon at the end of the procedure. The epidural catheter could be used in cases of extensive chest wall resection.

Positioning

The patient is laid in a lateral decubitus position, both arms along the body (Prayer's position) (Fig. 1a, b). Breaking the table at a point superior to the iliac crest can enhance the widening of the intercostal spaces. In middle and lower lobe operations, the main operator and the assistant stands to face the patient. This will give similar thoracoscopic dimensions and harmonious movements for both of them during the surgery (Fig. 2a). In upper lobe procedures, the main operator stands anterior to the patient while the helper can stand posterior to the patient, this can provide more comfortable space to the surgeon during the surgery (Fig. 2b). The scrub nurse usually placed in the back of the patient [45].

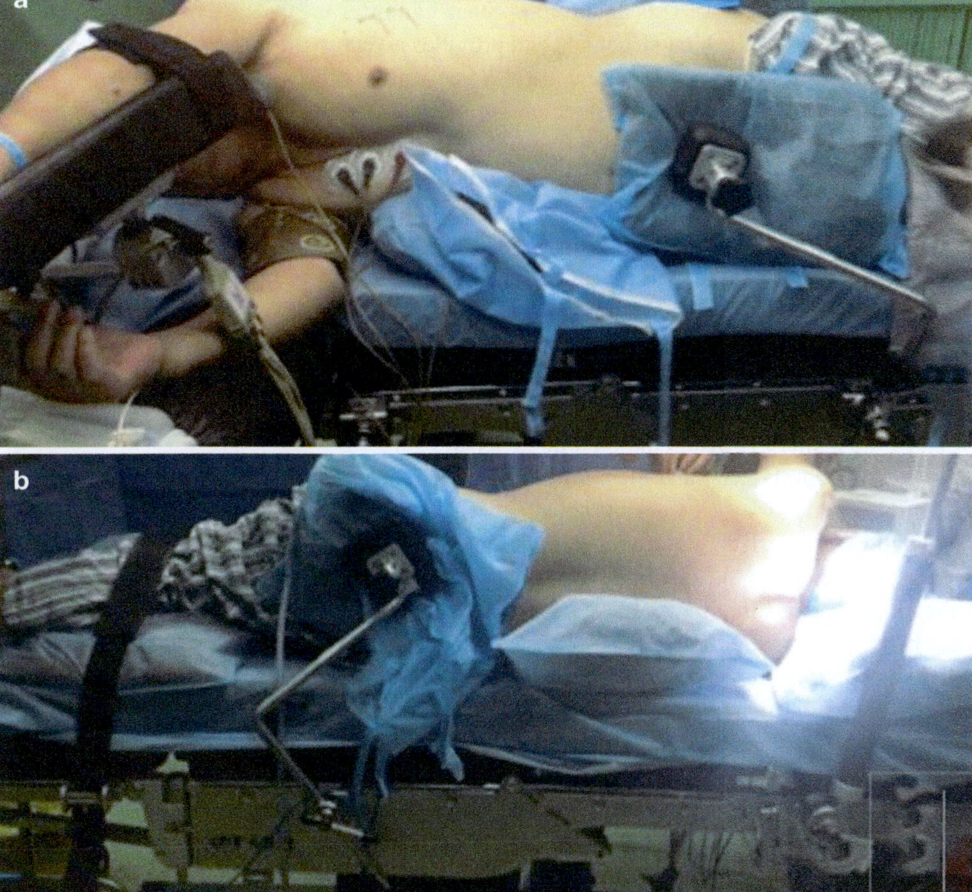

Fig. 1 Patient positioning during the surgery "Prayer's position", **(a)** anterior view **(b)** posterior view

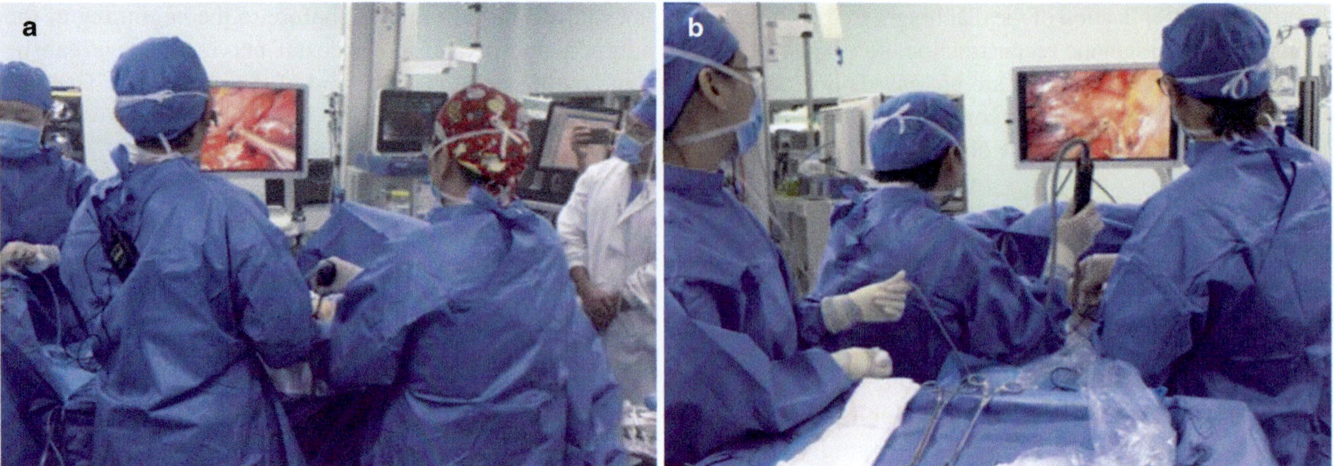

Fig. 2 Different position of the surgeons according to the type of surgery, **(a)** during lower and middle lobe surgery **(b)** during an upper lobe surgery

Technique

Lobectomy with Chest Wall Resection

As a standard, the authors prefer to create an anterior axillary line incision at the level of the fifth intercostal space with a length of 2.5–5 cm (Fig. 3). This anterior approach can offer a very good access to the hilar structures and provides a very good angle for introducing the staplers [48]. We never use a rib retractor or trocar in the uniportal technique, but we routinely use the wound protector (Fig. 4a), especially in obese patients. This can protect the wound tissue from contamination with the tumor cells and also minimize frequent camera contamination during the surgery. If the wound protector is unavailable, retracting the wound with two stitches "one from each side" could be also helpful for keeping the wound open and avoiding the taint of the camera (Fig. 4b). The thoracoscope (preferably 10 mm 30°) should be placed and maintained in the posterior angle of the wound (Figs. 5 and 6). Once the camera is inside the pleural cavity the surgeon explores the pleural cavity and makes a decision, whether to do the lobectomy first or to resect the affected area of the chest wall before performing the lobectomy, this decision is taken according to the location of the tumor and the situation of the inter-lobar fissure, we usually start with the easier part. After breaking of the adhesions, dissection of the chest wall tissue surrounding the tumor, with an identification of the involved ribs (Fig. 6), anterior and posterior dissection of the subperiosteal part of the ribs, and dividing the intercostal muscles. This dissection is enhanced with magnified visualization provided by HD camera. The attachment between the lung and the chest wall could be somehow helpful by retracting the affected lobe and facilitating the exposure of the

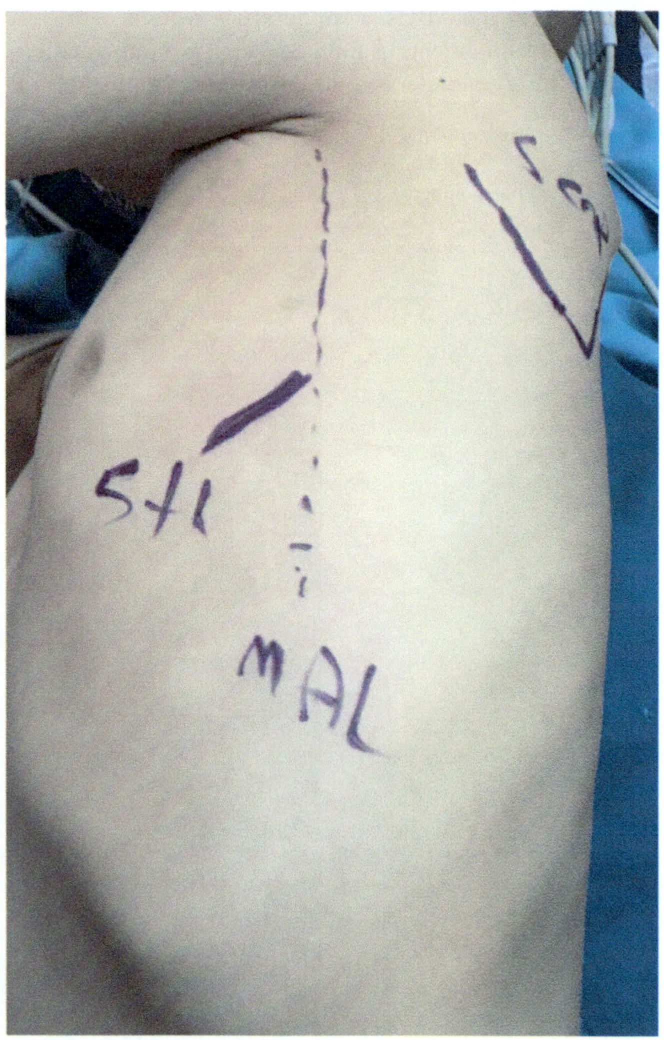

Fig. 3 Location of the incision "anterior axillary line"

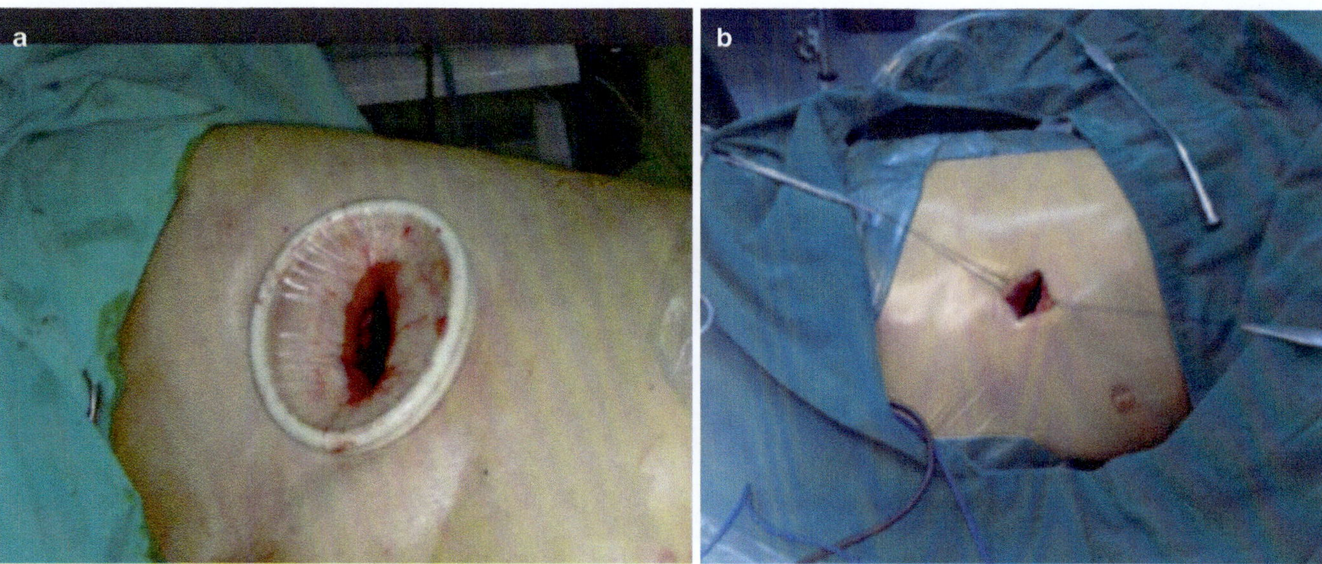

Fig. 4 (**a**) Wound soft tissue protector. (**b**) Two stitches technique

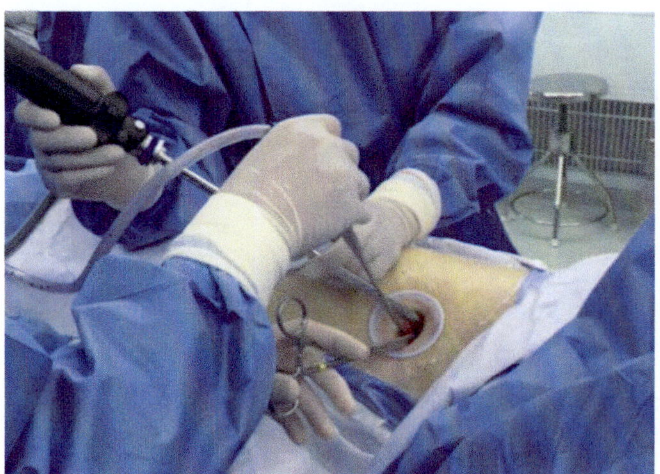

Fig. 5 The location of the thoracoscope during the surgery "at the posterior part of the incision"

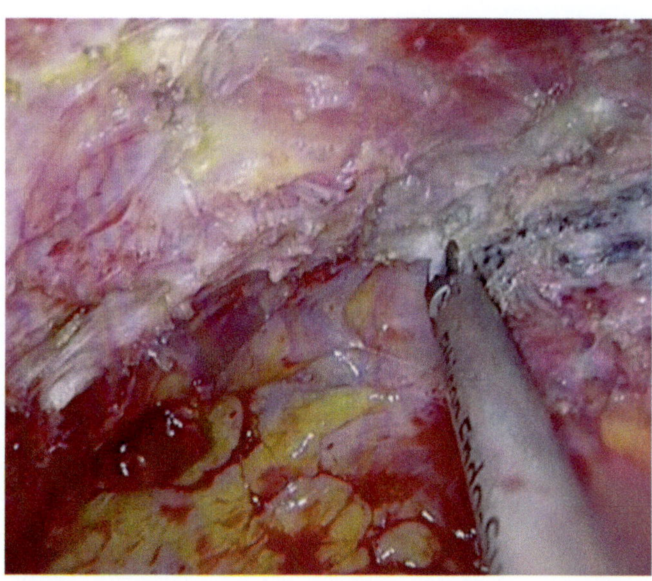

Fig. 6 Dissecting and marking the boundaries of the resection from inside the cavity

hilum (Fig. 7). Dissecting the hilar structures could be done before excising the chest wall and the ribs, as shown in the video (Video 1). Left upper lobectomy was performed first by dissecting encircling and stapling the vascular and bronchial branches to the upper lobe, while the left upper lobe is still attached to the chest wall completing the lobectomy is done by dividing the interloper fissure (Fig. 8). A longitudinal posterior incision then performed (Fig. 9). The tumor borders marked under thoracoscopic guidance after digital palpation (Fig. 10). The involved ribs excised around the tumor using a rib cutter with respecting the safety margins so as to achieve R0 resection (one rib and intercostal tissue above and below the tumor should also be included in the resection) (Fig. 11a–b) [49]. After resecting the involved part of the chest wall, the specimen fall inside the pleural cavity and retrieved later using a protective bag. The location of the chest wall invasion is a point of a great importance. Posterior invasion is usually an easier procedure to perform through

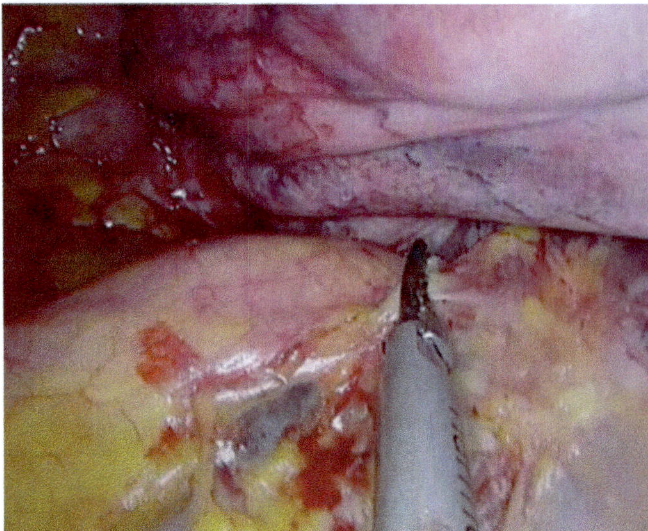

Fig. 7 Attachment between the lung and the chest wall facilitating the retraction of the lobe and the exposure of the hilum

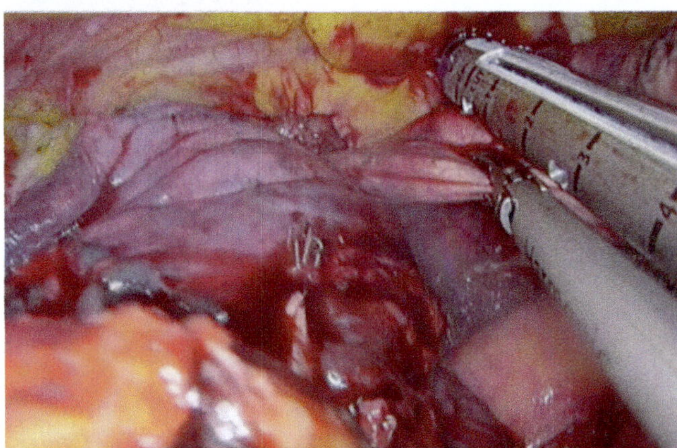

Fig. 8 Dividing the interlobar fissure

uniportal VATS, while in case of anterior invasion of the chest wall the procedure is more complex due to the proximity to the utility incision and the difficulty to find the comfortable angles for a good view and use of rib cutter. Using the endoscopic rib cutter (Fig. 12) makes total thoracoscopic rib resection (rather than the hybrid) feasible and safe through a single incision with no need for additional incision over the resected chest wall area [50].

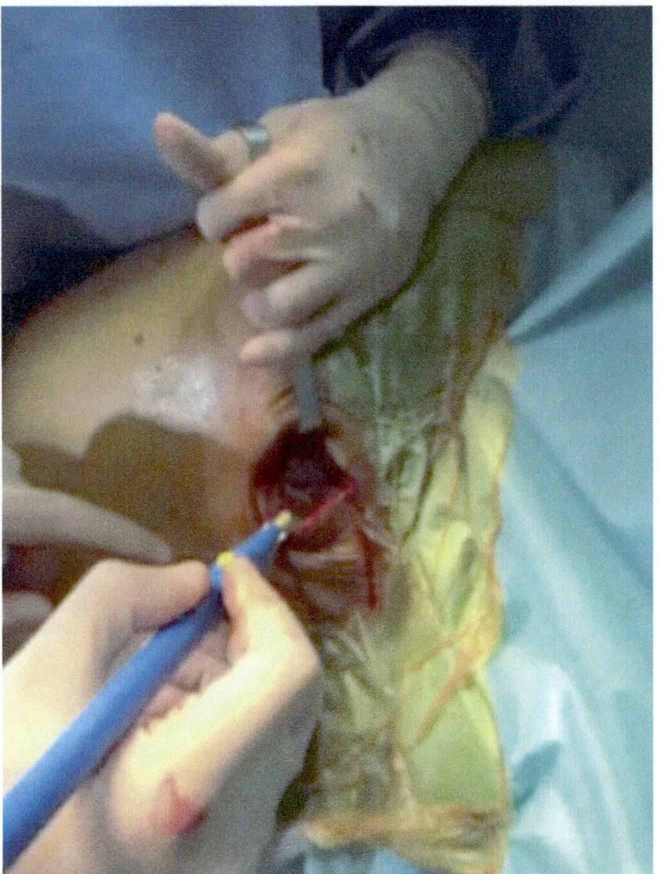

Fig. 9 Posterior longitudinal incision

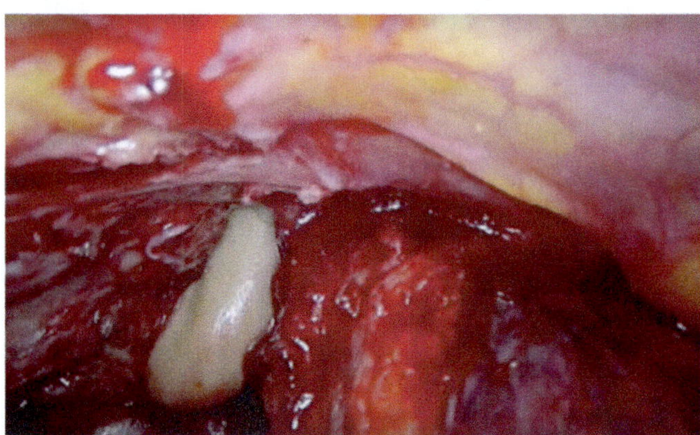

Fig. 10 Digital palpation marking of the tumor borders

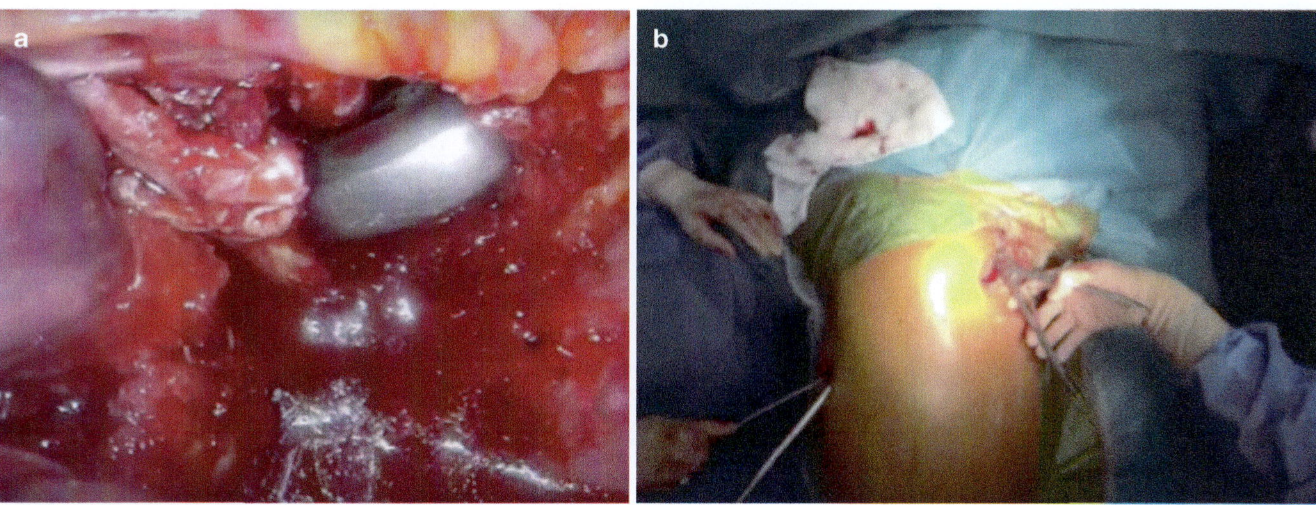

Fig. 11 (**a, b**) Using rib cutter to resect the involved chest wall segment

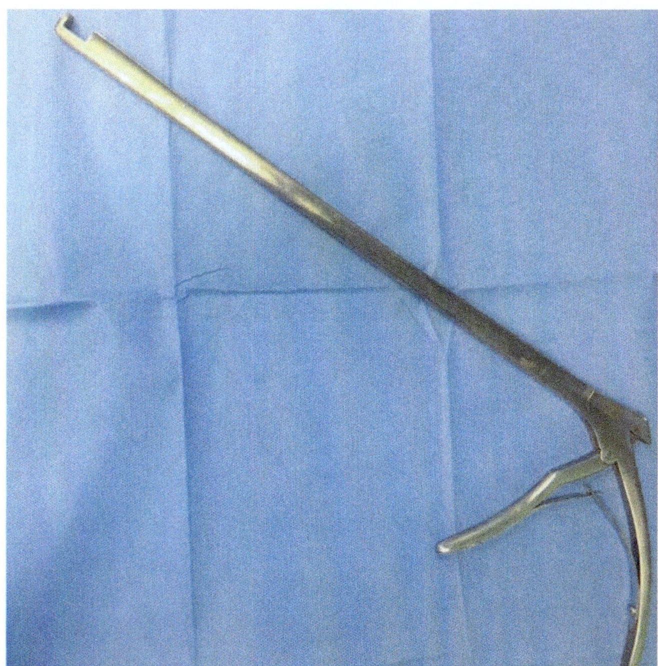

Fig. 12 Thoracoscopic rib cutter

Thoracoscopic rib resection using the Gigli saw (Fig. 13a, b) is useful in some situations as in the case of deep ribs resection [50, 51]. After completing lymph nodes dissection or sampling, thoracoscopic hemostasis and pneumostasis are done a chest tube inserted through the anterior incision which then all the incisions are closed in layers (Figs. 14a and 14b). Depending on its size and location the posterior incision could be closed with or without using prosthetic materials, chest wall reconstruction is carried out as needed to prevent physiological impairment due to paradoxical chest wall movement, scapular tip entrapment, or for cosmetics reasons. For posterior chest wall remaining defects, the scapula and the remaining chest wall muscles are usually sufficient to cover and support the defect whereas anterior and lateral defects more often require reconstruction using a prosthetic graft (Marlex mesh, Vicryl or Gore-Tex patch, etc.) especially when a large defect is present [49, 52]. Before closure of the skin, additional tissue may be brought over the site of the original defect to support the closure if necessary.

Lobectomy with Diaphragm Resection and Reconstruction

Three to five centimeter incision, at the fifth intercostal space in the anterior axillary line area, without using a rib-spreaders or thoracoscopic trocar. Ten millimeter 30° thoracoscope used and remains in the posterior part of the incision during the surgery (Fig. 5). Resection of the involved part of the diaphragm could be done at the beginning or at the end of surgery depending on the situation, with respect to the safety margins so as to achieve R0 resection. Bimanual instrumentation has a major role in uniportal VATS surgeries, during diaphragmatic resection done applying traction on the diaphragm to avoid injuring abdominal structures and to facilitate the resection is done using the suction device or lung grasper then the involved part of the diaphragm resected using an energy device (Fig. 15, Video 2). The remaining diaphragmatic defect then closed primarily with continuous non-absorbable sutures (Fig. 16), and the knots are tied pushed using the knot pusher, large defects should be closed using synthetic materials such as a Gore-Tex patch (W. L. Gore and Associates, Flagstaff, AZ) or Prolene mesh (Ethicon, Somerville, NJ) and the operation continued as usual.

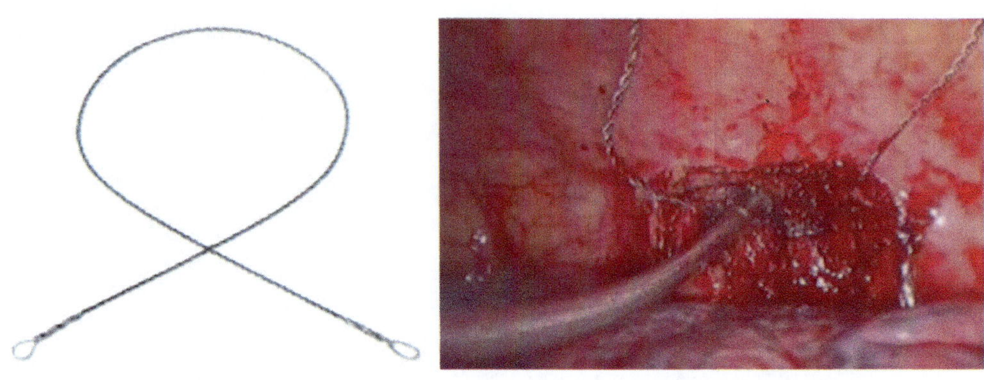

Fig. 13 (**a, b**) Thoracoscopic Gigli Saw

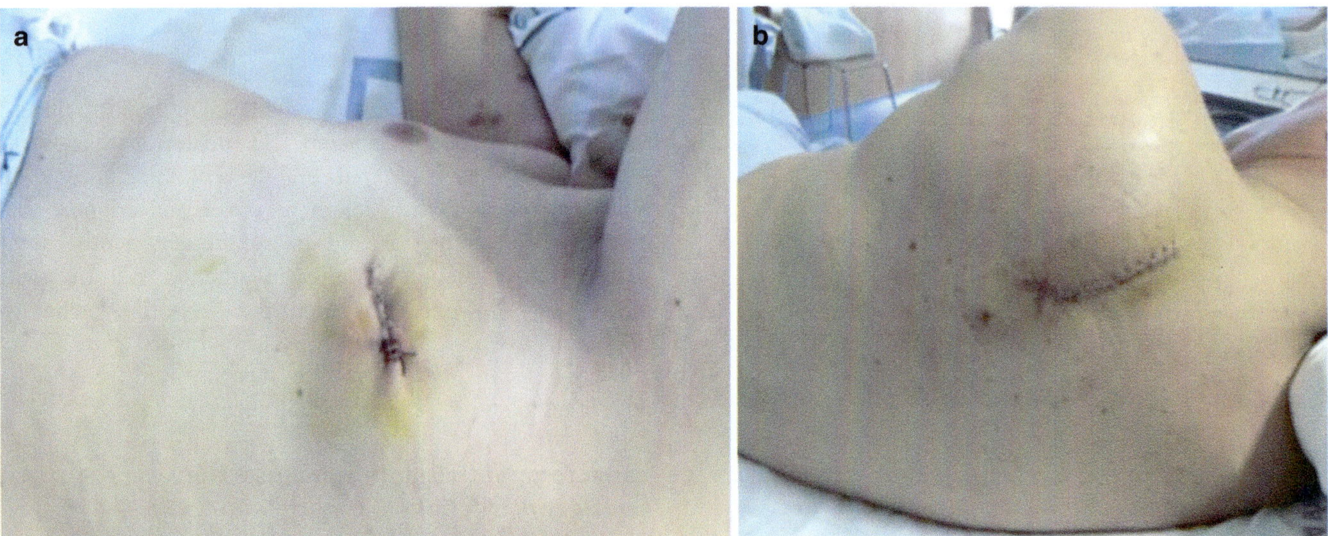

Fig. 14 (**a, b**) Closure of the wounds

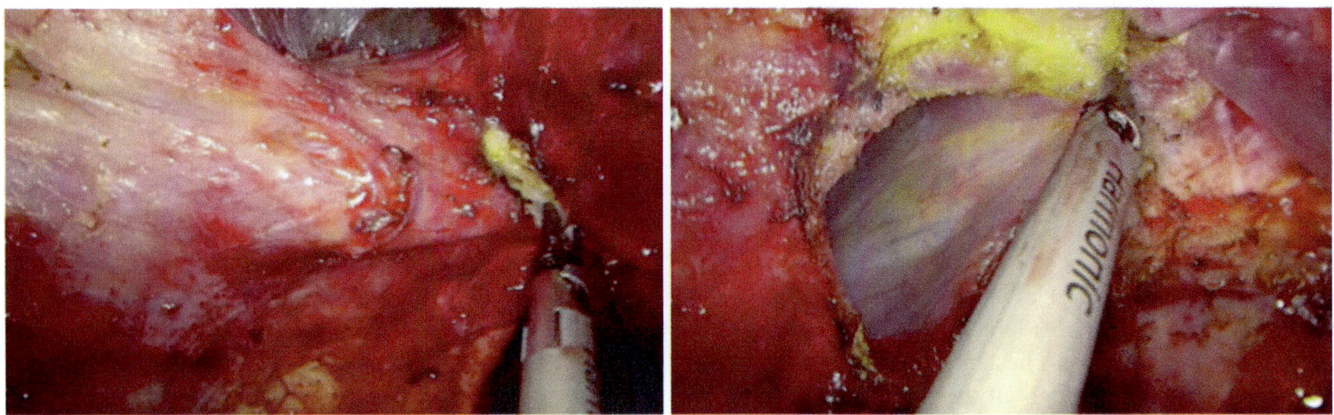

Fig. 15 Retracting and opening the diaphragm using an energy device

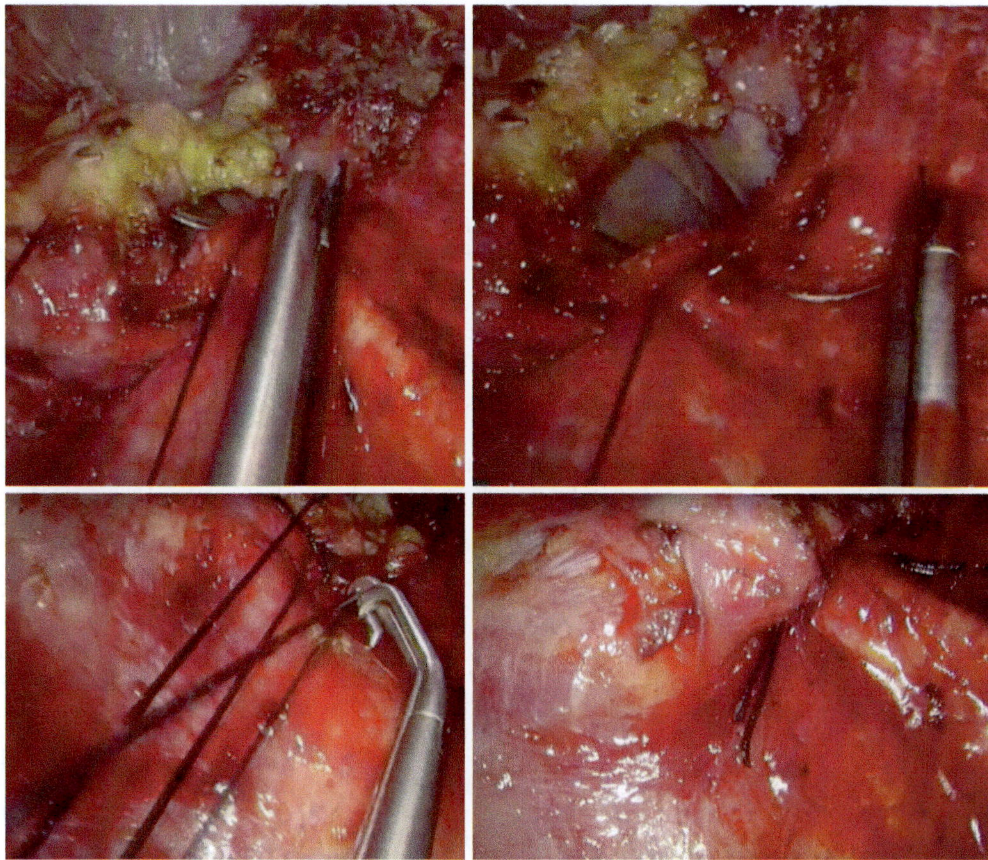

Fig. 16 Closure of the diaphragm with non-absorbable sutures

References

1. Ramsey HE, Cliffion EE. Chest wall resection for primary carcinoma of the lung. Ann Surg. 1968;167:342–51.
2. Albertucci M, DeMeester TR, Rothberg M, Hagen JA, Santoscoy R, Smyrk TC. Surgery and the management of peripheral lung tumors adherent to the parietal pleura. J Thorac Cardiovasc Surg. 1992;103:8–13.
3. Facciolo F, Cardillo G, Lopergolo M, Pallone G, Sera F, Martelli M. Chest wall invasion in non-small cell lung caricinoma: a rationale for en bloc resection. J Thorac Cardiovasc Surg. 2001; 121:649–56.
4. Martini N, McCormack PM, Bains MS. Chest wall tumors: clinical results of treatment. In: Grillo HC, Eschapasse H, editors. International trends in general thoracic surgery. Volume 2. Major challenges. Philadelphia: Saunders; 1987. p. 285.
5. Mansour KA, Thourani VH, Losken A, Reeves JG, Miller JI Jr, Carlson GW, Jones GE. Chest wall resections and reconstruction: a 25-year experience. Ann Thorac Surg. 2002;73(6):1720–5;discussion 1725–6.
6. Weyant MJ, Bains MS, Venkatraman E, Downey RJ, Park BJ, Flores RM, Rizk N, Rusch VW. Results of chest wall resection and reconstruction with and without rigid prosthesis. Ann Thorac Surg. 2006;81(1):279–85.
7. Weksler B, Bains M, Burt M, Downey R, Martini N, Rusch V, Ginsberg R. Resection of lung cancer invading the diaphragm. J Thorac Cardiovasc Surg. 1997;114(3):500–1.
8. Goldstraw P, Crowley J, Chansky K, Giroux DJ, Groome PA, Rami-Porta R, et al. The IASLC lung cancer staging project: proposals for the revision of the TNM stage groupings in the forthcoming (seventh) edition of the TNM classification of malignant tumors. J Thorac Oncol. 2007;2:706–14.
9. Pairolero PC. Extended resections for lung cancer. How far is too far? Eur J Cardiothorac Surg. 1999;16(Suppl 1):S48–50.
10. Yokoi K, Tsuchiya R, Mori T, Nagai K, Furukawa T, Fujimura S, Nakagawa K, Ichinose Y. Results of surgical treatment of lung cancer involving the diaphragm. J Thorac Cardiovasc Surg. 2000;120(4):799–805.
11. Galetta D, Borri A, Casiraghi M, Gasparri R, Petrella F, Tessitore A, Serra M, Guarize J, Spaggiari L. Outcome and prognostic factors of resected non-small-cell lung cancer invading the diaphragm. Interact Cardiovasc Thorac Surg. 2014;19(4):632–6;discussion 636.
12. Inoue K, Sato M, Fujimura S, Sakurada A, Takahashi S, Usuda K, Kondo T, Tanita T, Handa M, Saito Y, Sagawa M. Prognostic assessment of 1310 patients with non-small-cell lung cancer who underwent complete resection from 1980 to 1993. J Thorac Cardiovasc Surg. 1998;116(3):407–11.
13. Adebonojo SA, Bowser AN, Moritz DM, Corcoran PC. Impact of revised stage classification of lung cancer on survival: a military experience. Chest. 1999;115(6):1507–13.
14. Rocco G, Rendina EA, Meroni A, Venuta F, Della Pona C, De Giacomo T, Robustellini M, Rossi G, Massera F, Vertemati G, Rizzi A, Coloni GF. Prognostic factors after surgical treatment of lung cancer invading the diaphragm. Ann Thorac Surg. 1999;68(6):2065–8.

15. Riquet M, Porte H, Chapelier A, Brichon PY, Bernard A, Dujon A, Dahan M, Bonette P, Guidicelli R, Jancovici R, Monteau M, Moreau JL, Moreau JM, Peillon C, Bellenot F, Faillon JM, Mouroux J. Resection of lung cancer invading the diaphragm. J Thorac Cardiovasc Surg. 2000;120(2):417–8.
16. Doyle LA, Aisner J. Clinical presentation and staging. In: Roth JA, Ruckdeschel JC, Weinsenburger TH, editors. Thoracic oncology. 2nd ed. Philadelphia: WB Saunders; 1995. p. 26–48.
17. Downey RJ, Martini N, Rusch VW, Bains MS, Korst RJ, Ginsberg RJ. Extent of chest wall invasion and survival in patients with lung cancer. Ann Thorac Surg. 1999;68(1):188–93.
18. Roviaro G, Rebuffat C, Varoli F, Vergani C, Mariani C, Maciocco M. Videoendoscopic pulmonary lobectomy for cancer. Surg Laparosc Endosc. 1992;2(3):244–7.
19. McKenna RJ Jr, Houck W, Fuller CB. Video-assisted thoracic surgery lobectomy: experience with 1,100 cases. Ann Thorac Surg. 2006;81(2):421–5.
20. Daniels LJ, Balderson SS, Onaitis MW, D'Amico TA. Thoracoscopic lobectomy: a safe and effective strategy for patients with stage I lung cancer. Ann Thorac Surg. 2002;74(3):860–4.
21. Balderson SS, D'Amico TA. Thoracoscopic lobectomy for the management of non-small cell lung cancer. Curr Oncol Rep. 2008;10(4):283–6.
22. Kara HV, Balderson SS, D'Amico TA. Challenging cases: thoracoscopic lobectomy with chest wall resection and sleeve lobectomy-Duke experience. J Thorac Dis. 2014;6(Suppl 6):S637–40.
23. Widmann MD, Caccavale RJ, Bocage JP, Lewis RJ. Video-assisted thoracic surgery resection of chest wall en bloc for lung carcinoma. Ann Thorac Surg. 2000;70(6):2138–40.
24. Demmy TL, Nwogu CE, Yendamuri S. Thoracoscopic chest wall resection: what is its role? Ann Thorac Surg. 2010;89(6):S2142–5.
25. Caronia FP, Ruffini E, Lo Monte AI. The use of video-assisted thoracic surgery in the management of Pancoast tumors. Interact Cardiovasc Thorac Surg. 2010;11(6):721–6.
26. Berry MF, Onaitis MW, Tong BC, Balderson SS, Harpole DH, D'Amico TA. Feasibility of hybrid thoracoscopic lobectomy and en-bloc chest wall resection. Eur J Cardiothorac Surg. 2012;41(4):888–92.
27. Stoelben E, Ludwig C. Chest wall resection for lung cancer: indications and techniques. Eur J Cardiothorac Surg. 2009;35(3):450–6.
28. Nesher N, Galili R, Sharony R, Uretzky G, Saute M, et al. Videothorascopic sympathectomy (VATS) for palmar hyperhidriosis: summary of a clinical trial and surgical results. Harefuah. 2000;138(11):913–6.
29. Rocco G, Martin-Ucar A, Passera E, et al. Uniportal VATS wedge pulmonary resections. Ann Thorac Surg. 2004;77(2):726–8.
30. Rocco G, Martucci N, La Manna C, Jones DR, De Luca G, La Rocca A, Cuomo A, Accardo R, et al. Ten-year experience on 644 patients undergoing single-port (uniportal) video-assisted thoracoscopic surgery. Ann Thorac Surg. 2013;96(2):434–8.
31. Gonzalez-Rivas D, Paradela M, Garcia J, Dela Torre M, et al. Single-port video-assisted thoracoscopic lobectomy. Interact Cardiovasc Thorac Surg. 2011;13(5):539–41.
32. Gonzalez-Rivas D, Mendez L, Delgado M, Fieira E, Fernandez R, de la Torre M. Uniportal video-assisted thoracoscopic anatomic segmentectomy. J Thorac Dis. 2013;5(Suppl 3):S226–33.
33. Gonzalez-Rivas D, Yang Y, Stupnik T, Sekhniaidze D, Fernandez R, Velasco C, Zhu Y, Jiang G. Uniportal video-assisted thoracoscopic bronchovascular, tracheal and carinal sleeve resections. Eur J Cardiothorac Surg. 2016;49(Suppl 1):i6–i16.
34. Gonzalez-Rivas D, Stupnik T, Fernandez R, de la Torre M, Velasco C, Yang Y, Lee W, et al. Intraoperative bleeding control by uniportal videoassisted thoracoscopic surgery. Eur J Cardiothorac Surg. 2016;49(Suppl 1):i17–24.
35. Bertolaccini L, Rocco G, Viti A, Terzi A. Geometrical characteristics of uniportal VATS. J Thorac Dis. 2013;5(Suppl 3): S214–6.
36. Gonzalez-Rivas D, Fernandez R, Fieira E, Mendez L. Single-incision thoracoscopic right upper lobectomy with chest wall resection by posterior approach. Innovations (Phila). 2013;8(1):70–2.
37. Gonzalez-Rivas D, Fieira E, Delgado M, et al. Lower lobectomy with chest wall resection. Asvide 2014;1:347. Available http://www.asvide.com/articles/360.
38. Gonzalez-Rivas D, Fieira E, Delgado M, et al. Superior sulcus tumor. Asvide 2014;1:346. Available http://www.asvide.com/articles/359.
39. Gonzalez-Rivas D, Fieira E, Delgado M, de la Torre M, Mendez L, Fernandez R. Uniportal video-assisted thoracoscopic sleeve lobectomy and other complex resections. J Thorac Dis. 2014;6(Suppl 6): S674–81.
40. Moon SW, Wang YP, Kim YW, Shim SB, Jin W. Thoracoscopic plication of diaphragmatic eventration using endostaplers. Ann Thorac Surg. 2000;70(1):299–300.
41. Shary TM, Hebra A. A simple technique for thoracoscopic treatment of diaphragmatic eventration. Am Surg. 2013; 79(9):893–5.
42. Matsubara H, Miyauchi Y, Ichihara T, Matsuoka H, Kunimitsu T, Uchida T, Onuki Y, Hasuda N, Oyachi N, Takano K, Suzuki S. Thoracoscopic diaphragmatic plication for eventration of diaphragm in children using no-knife automatic suturing device. Kyobu Geka. 2014;67(11):976–9;Japanese.
43. Ikeda M, Sonobe M, Bando T, Date H. Reconstruction of recurrent diaphragmatic eventration with an elongated polytetrafluoroethylene sheet. Interact Cardiovasc Thorac Surg. 2013;17(2):433–5.
44. Kara HV, Roach MJ, Balderson SS, D'Amico TA. Thoracoscopic diaphragm plication. Ann Cardiothorac Surg. 2015;4(6):573–5.
45. Dunning J. Thoracoscopic diaphragm plication. Interact Cardiovasc Thorac Surg. 2015;20(5):689–90.
46. Wu HH, Chen CH, Chang H, Liu HC, Hung TT, Lee SY. A preliminary report on the feasibility of single-port thoracoscopic surgery for diaphragm plication in the treatment of diaphragm eventration. J Cardiothorac Surg. 2013;8:224.
47. Ahn JH, Suh JH, Jeong JY. Robot-assisted thoracoscopic surgery with simple laparoscopy for diaphragm eventration. Thorac Cardiovasc Surg. 2013;61(6):499–501.
48. Gonzalez-Rivas D, Fieira E, Delgado M, Mendez L, Fernandez R, de la Torre M. Uniportal video-assisted thoracoscopic lobectomy. J Thorac Dis. 2013;5(Suppl 3):S234–45.
49. Shields TW, editor. General thoracic surgery. 7th ed. Philadelphia: Lippincott Williams & Wilkins; 2009. p. 1420–2616.
50. Hennon MW, Demmy TL. Thoracoscopic resection and re-resection of an anterior chest wall chondrosarcoma. Innovations (Phila). 2012;7(6):445–7.
51. Huang CL, Cheng CY, Lin CH, Wang BY. Single-port thoracoscopic rib resection: a case report. J Cardiothorac Surg. 2014; 9:49.
52. Shields TW, editor. General thoracic surgery. 7th ed. Philadelphia: Lippincott Williams & Wilkins; 2009. p. 654–2616.

Troubleshooting: Management of Bleeding

Ricardo Fernandez Prado, Juan Pablo Ovalle Granados, Luis Fernandez Vago, Eva Maria Fieira Costa, Marina Paradela De La Morena, Maria Delgado Roel, Diego Gonzalez-Rivas, and Mercedes De La Torre Bravos

Abstract

The first video-assisted thoracic surgery (VATS) anatomic lobectomy for lung cancer was described two decades ago. During this time VATS has become a safe and effective approach for the treatment of lung cancer with a low level of morbidity and mortality.

Nowadays, thanks to advances in VATS and the experience gained, most pulmonary resections can be performed by video-assisted thoracoscopy in a safe way.

By gaining experience, more complex or advanced cases are approached using the VATS technique. However, as VATS lobectomy is applied to more advanced cases, the conversion rate to open thoracotomy can increase, especially during the learning curve, mostly because of the occurrence of intraoperative complications.

The best plan to solve complications during VATS lobectomy is to avoid them. Perform a pulmonary resection as safe as possible by VATS depends on the patient selection, the patient's characteristics and the anticipated technical aspects of the case as well as a careful pulmonary dissection. Regardless of all the prevention of intraoperative complications, these can occur, so we must develop plans or strategies to minimize them if they occur.

The correct assessment of any bleeding is paramount during thoracoscopic major procedures. Major vessel injury may cause massive bleeding in case of an inadequate management of the defect. If bleeding occurs, a sponge stick should be available to apply pressure immediately to control the haemorrhage. Then a decision must be made promptly as to whether thoracotomy is needed or if it can be solved through the VATS approach. This will depend mostly on the surgeon's experience.

What should be clear is that an intraoperative complication should not become an intraoperative catastrophe.

Introduction

The VATS (Video Assisted Thoracic Surgery) approach for lobectomy was first introduced in 1992 [1]. We know that the vats approach offer many advantages over the thoracotomy. Less pain, shorter hospital stay, faster recovery to full activity, less amount of perioperative complications, more effective administration of adjuvant chemotherapy and even better survival rate [2–4].

VATS lobectomy represents a technical challenge, particularly early in the surgeon's learning curve, when compared to the more conventional open approach and because of the intraoperative complications.

The learning curve of the thoracoscopic approach carries along an increase in the number of intraoperative complications [5]. The major intraoperative complication which worries any surgeon is the bleeding. It is the most frequent reason for an emergent conversion to a thoracotomy during the learning curve [6].

The best plan to solve complications during VATS lobectomy is to avoid them.

Perform a pulmonary resection as safe as possible by VATS depends on the patient selection, the patient's characteristics and, the anticipated technical aspects of the case, the radiographic appearance of the target area as well as a careful pulmonary dissection [7].

Electronic Supplementary Material The online version of this chapter (https://doi.org/10.1007/978-981-13-2604-2_33) contains supplementary material, which is available to authorized users.

R. F. Prado (✉) · J. P. O. Granados · L. F. Vago · E. M. F. Costa
M. P. De La Morena · M. D. Roel · M. De La Torre Bravos
Department of Thoracic Surgery, Coruña University Hospital, A Coruña, Spain

D. Gonzalez-Rivas
Department of Thoracic Surgery, Shanghai Pulmonary Hospital, Tongji University School of Medicine, Shanghai, China

Department of Thoracic Surgery and Minimally Invasive Thoracic Surgery Unit (UCTMI), Coruña University Hospital, Coruña, Spain
e-mail: diego@uniportal.es

D. Gonzalez-Rivas et al. (eds.), *Atlas of Uniportal Video Assisted Thoracic Surgery*,
https://doi.org/10.1007/978-981-13-2604-2_33

Our purpose is to describe how to face intraoperative complications and avoiding catastrophic complications. Flores RM et al. define catastrophic complication is defined as an event that results in an additional unplanned major surgical procedure other than the intended lobectomy [8].

We describe the reasons and different types of intraoperative bleedings and the steps to manage them through uniportal VATS.

Bleeding During VATS Lobectomies

The most dangerous intraoperative complication is major bleeding. Our experience is that as the surgeons experience in VATS grows, the rate of intraoperative complications decreases while the rate of bleeding does not decrease to a very low rate. The reason is that more complex cases are done which imply more risk of intraoperative bleedings.

The uniportal VATS approach usually offers excellent visibility of the operative field, thus intrathoracic hemorrhage is rare.

Diego Gonzalez-Rivas et al. [9] classify the main causes of thoracoscopic bleeding into:

- Inexperience of the surgeon
- Difficult vascular dissection: fused artery or vein
- Calcified or malignant hilar lymph nodes
- Vascular injury with cautery or energy devices
- Vascular laceration by the endostapler (limited angle or forced insertion)
- Vascular injury on the posterior wall with a right-angled clamp or scissors
- Failure of staplers (especially when dealing with a thick fissure)
- Laceration during blunt dissection
- Metal or polymer vascular clip loosening or misplacement
- Excessive traction of fragile vessels (after chemotherapy, corticoid treatment or in elderly patients).

If bleeding occurs, do not forget the first and main step: press on the bleeding area with a sponge stick to control the hemorrhage. We must always have a sponge stick ready to press immediately to control the bleeding (Fig. 1); once the bleeding is temporarily controlled we must decide if we can control the hemorrhage by VATS or if on the contrary we must convert to thoracotomy [10]. This decision will depend mainly on the experience and confidence of the surgeon. A very good knowledge of the anatomy, precaution in the dissection and the quick conversion to a thoracotomy must be factors that prevent irreversible situations.

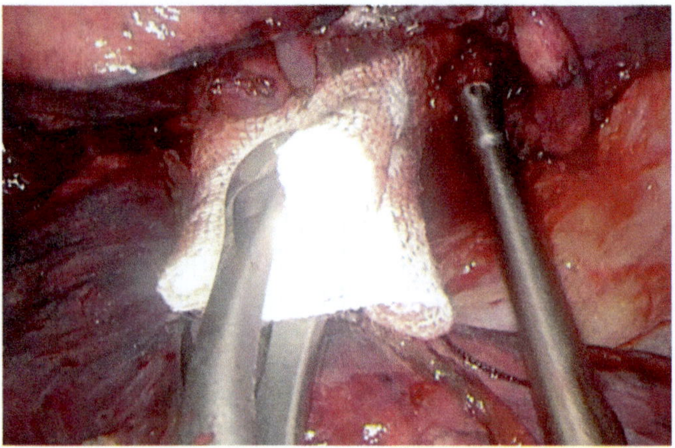

Fig. 1 Sponge stick pressing to control the bleeding

In relation to bleeding from the pulmonary artery, a very careful vascular dissection is essential, in addition to preventing excessive traction of the vessels, especially in the case of central tumors (Videos 1 and 2). Some authors recommend avoiding the use of monopolar scissors or energy devices near vascular structures to prevent thermal injuries from ultrasonic coagulation shears [11] (Video 3). However, in our experience, energy devices are very safe in expert hands and can be used even for anatomic hilar dissection.

Demmy published a trouble shooting guide showing tips and tricks to solve complications during VATS lobectomies [12]. The author describes different methods to control intraoperative bleeding such as by using thrombostatic material, biological sealants or the discrete use of energy devices. They do not recommended to use clips on delicate pulmonary arteries due to the risk of vascular injuries, traction or even the accidental displacement of the clip during manipulation of the lobe. Effectively the use of clips can cause bleeding when the lobe is manipulated, but in our experience if we take into account when mobilizing the lobe we should not have problems. The use of clips is safe when a careful posterior manipulation of the lobe is performed [13].

To make a VATS lobectomy as safe as possible we must consider the characteristics of the patient and previously identify the technical difficulties or anatomical anomalies that may cause intraoperative complications. Care must be taken to avoid injuring unexpected small branches (Video 4).

The right instruments are basic to perform a safe VATS and to be able to solve an intraoperative bleeding. High definition thoracoscopic view is essential in addition to long quality instruments with double articulation (Scanlan International Inc.).

In addition to the above, the experience, as D'Amico describes [5], is a determining factor to solve an intraoperative complication through VATS approach.

We can classify intraoperative bleedings in three categories: oozing, minor and major bleeding.

Usually oozing bleeding type is produced after releasing adhesions (Video 5). The release of adhesions often creates pleural bleeding. Normally this type of bleeding is self-limiting or is solved by compression or direct coagulation on the bleeding surface. We can also use haemostatic material.

Minor bleeding is originated from injuries in small branches (smaller than 5 mm), is usually caused by excessive traction or small pulmonary tears in distal lobar arteries. Normally it is solved after releasing traction and compressing. We can also cause minor bleeding during lymphadenectomy by injuring small lymphatic vessels. Minor bleeding is usually controlled by applying pressure, using energy devices, sealants or metallic or polymer clips (Click aV, Grena®). Minor bleeding must be carefully managed. It must be avoided that a minor bleeding becomes a major bleeding.

If the bleeding is important, we consider it major bleeding. Normally originating on the lobar branches or on the main pulmonary artery or vein. If it is not properly managed it will put the patient's security at risk. It is common that major bleeding is a cause of conversion to a thoracotomy. However with enough experience most of the bleeding that occurs during the vats approach can be solved thoracoscopically (Video 6).

There are different methods to control major bleeding. Direct compression on the bleeding origin, use of sealants, use of clips or control through a direct suture.

Compression on the bleeding origin is the first step to be taken when a bleeding occurs. At the same time it is important to suck up the blood around in order to have a good view of the bleeding point. Once we check that the bleeding is controlled we can decide if it is necessary to convert [10] or if it can be solved through the VATS approach. This will depend mostly on the surgeon's experience. While compression, the main trunk of the artery can be dissected in order to clamp it if it is necessary. After initial compression the use of topic sealants can be useful in selected cases if there is a small tear and the bleeding is controllable.

The use of metal or polymer clips is a safe option to divide small pulmonary vessels. We recommend using two proximal clips to control the proximal end of small arteries and energy device to divide the distal end of the vessel. In this way we avoid the accidental displacement of the distal clip while manipulating the lobe, as well as, we guarantee an additional vascular sealing. When we apply a clip over a bleeding zone we must be sure that there is sufficient surface to secure the clip at the base of the vessel. For a right placing, bimanual instrumentation and lung traction are essential (Video 7).

Sometimes the bleeding is not controlled with the previous measures then must be repaired by means of direct suture. The first step must always be to compress the bleeding point, suck up the blood around in order to have a good exposure. In the event of an important defect it is highly recommended to dissect and control the main pulmonary artery and use a clamp or a vessel loop to suppress the afferent vascular flow. This way we can better assess the defect and apply the suture with more precision and safety. Bimanual instrumentation is crucial keeping the camera at the posterior position and the instruments at the anterior. This way we get a direct vision of the target area and we can mimic the same manoeuvres as in open surgery (Video 8).

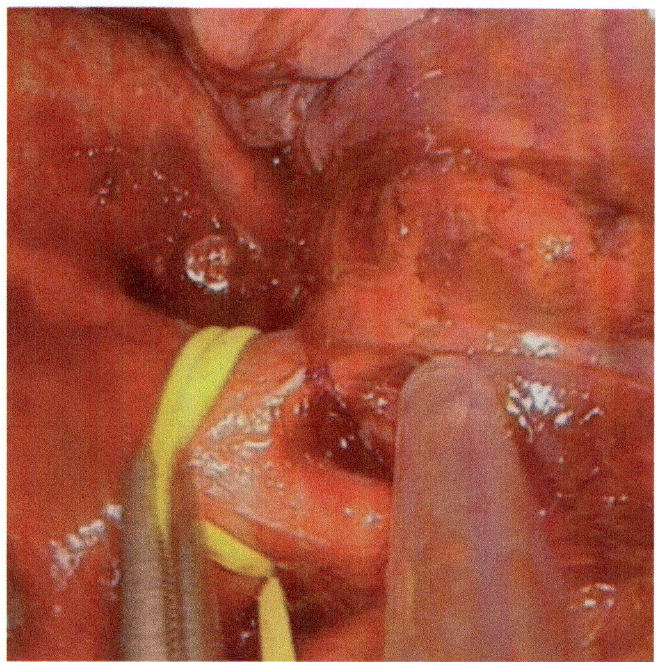

Fig. 2 Control of the pulmonary artery with a vessel loop

Mei J et al. described a "Suction-Compression Angiorrhaphy Technique" to overcome a serious bleeding [14]. They describe the control of the bleeding with an initial phase of compression with endoscopic suction and then the performance of an angiorrhaphy with suture.

Others authors have described preventive control techniques and pulmonary artery clamping during the dissection in complex cases such as proximal hilar tumors or calcified adenopathies involving arteries [15, 16].

We recommend in complex cases the control of the main pulmonary artery with a vessel loop (Fig. 2). In the event of a bleeding, by exercising traction on the vessel loop the artery can be temporarily occluded or we can use a clamp but the artery needs to be dissected at that time.

What should be clear is that an intraoperative complication should not become an intraoperative catastrophe.

References

1. Roviaro G, Rebuffat C, Varoli F, Vergani C, Mariani C, Maciocco M. Videoendoscopic pulmonary lobectomy for cáncer. Surg Laparosc Endosc. 1992;2:244–7.
2. Yan TD, Black D, Bannon PG, McCaughan BC. Systematic review and meta-analysis of randomized and nonrandomized trial son safety and efficacy of video assisted thoracic surgery lobectomy for early-stage non-small-cell lung cáncer. J Clin Oncol. 2009;27:2553–62.
3. Mc Kenna RJ Jr, Houck W, Fuller CB. Video assisted thoracic surgery lobectomy: experience with 1,100 cases. Ann Thorac Surg. 2006;81:421–6.
4. Daniels LJ, Balderson SS, Onaitis MW, et al. Thoracoscopic lobectomy: a safe and effective strategy for patients with stage I lung cancer. Ann Thorac Surg. 2002;74(3):860–4.
5. Berry F, D'Amico T. Complications of thoracoscopic pulmonary resection. Semin Thorac Cardiovasc Surg. 2007;19:350–4.
6. Swada S, Komori E, Yamashita M. Evaluation of video-assisted thoracoscopic surgery requiring emergency conversion to thoracotomy. Eur J Cardiothorac Surg. 2009;36(3):487–90.
7. Hanna J, Berry M, D'Amico T. Contraindications of video-assisted thoracoscopic surgical lobectomy and determinants of conversion to open. J Thorac Dis. 2013;5(Suppl 3):S182–9.
8. Flores RM, Ihekweazu U, Dycoco J, et al. Video-assisted thoracoscopic surgery (VATS) lobectomy: catastrophic intraoperative complications. J Thorac Cardiovasc Surg. 2011;142:142–7.
9. Gonzalez-Rivas D, Stupnik T, Fernandez R. Intraoperative bleeding control by uniportal video-assisted thoracoscopic surgery. Eur J Cardiothorac Surg. 2016;49(Suppl 1):i17–24.
10. Imperatori A, Rotolo N, Gatti M, et al. Peri-operative complications of video-assisted thoracoscopic surgery (VATS). Int J Surg. 2008;6(Suppl 1):S78–81.
11. Cormier B, Nezhat F, Sternchos J, Sonoda Y, Leitao MM Jr. Electrocautery-associated vascular injury during robotic-assisted surgery. Obstet Gynecol. 2012;120:491–3.
12. Demmy TL, James TA, Swanson SJ, McKenna RJ Jr, D'Amico TA. Troubleshooting video-assisted thoracic surgery lobectomy. Ann Thorac Surg. 2005;79:1744–52.
13. Fernandez Prado R, Fieira Costa E, Delgado Roel M, Fernandez LM, de la Morena P, de la Torre M, Gonzalez-Rivas D. Management of complications by uniportal video-assisted thoracoscopic surgery. J Thorac Dis. 2014;6(S6):S669–73.
14. Mei J, Pu Q, Liao H, et al. A novel method for troubleshooting vascular injury during anatomic thoracoscopic pulmonary resection without conversion to thoracotomy. Surg Endosc. 2013;27:530–7.
15. Nakanishi R, Oka S, Odate S. Video-assisted thoracic surgery major pulmonary resection requiring control of the main pulmonary artery. Interact Cardiovasc Thorac Surg. 2009;9:618–22.
16. Kamiyoshihara M, Nagashima T, Ibe T, Takeyoshi I. A tip for controlling the main pulmonary artery during video-assisted thoracic major pulmonary resection: the outside-field vascular clamping technique. Interact Cardiovasc Thorac Surg. 2010;11: 693–5.

Uniportal Minimally Invasive Esophagectomy

Sun-Moa Yang and Jang-Ming Lee

Abstract

There is growing evidence that minimally invasive esophagectomy (MIE) combining various procedures including VATS and laparoscopy is helpful in lowering postoperative complications while providing similar oncological outcomes. Traditionally, all of the procedures including esophagectomy and esophageal reconstruction are performed with multi-port approaches. In current chapter, we described how these procedures can be performed with single-incision both in the laparoscopic and thoracoscopic phases. With patient and meticulous tissue dissection this complex surgical procedure can be safely and efficiently performed, providing equivalent perioperative outcomes and less postoperative pain.

Introduction

Surgery, as the main stay for treating esophageal cancer, is still plagued by substantial perioperative morbidity and mortality. Minimally invasive esophagectomy (MIE) combining laparoscopic and thoracosopic procedures is gradually accepted as a feasible approach in treating esophageal cancer, [1–10]. The single-incision approach has gradually been adopted in performing various thoracoscopic and laparoscopic procedures including pulmonary lobectomy, gastrectomy and colectomy [11–16]. Here, we describe our experience using a single-incision thoracosopic and laparoscopic approach for treating esophageal cancer which has been published for the first time in literature before [17].

Electronic Supplementary Material The online version of this chapter (https://doi.org/10.1007/978-981-13-2604-2_34) contains supplementary material, which is available to authorized users.

S.-M. Yang · J.-M. Lee (✉)
Department of Surgery, National Taiwan University Hospital, Taipei City, Taiwan
e-mail: Jangming@ntuh.gov.tw

Patient Selection

The selection criteria for single incision minimally invasive esophagectomy (SIMIE) included: (1) no evidence of tumor invasion to the adjacent organs in imaging studies (excluding T4 disease); (2) no previous history of abdominal or thoracic surgery; (3) patient's tolerance to one-lung ventilation during surgery.

Surgical Anatomy for Esophagus and Regional Lymph Nodes

The esophagus is a part of the alimentary tract, extending from the pharynx to the stomach with approximately 25 cm in length. It begins at the lower margin of the cricoid cartilage opposite the C6 vertebra and enters the gastric orifice at the level of the T12 vertebra. The esophagus can be divided into a cervical, thoracic and abdominal segment. The cervical part lies between the deep and the middle cervical fascia and anteriorly attached to the trachea, with deviation slightly to the left. Dissection of the thoracic and abdominal part of the esophagus is mandatory for most esophagectomy procedures. The cervical part can remain intact during subtotal esophagectomy with intrathoracic anastomosis. The thoracic esophagus descends through the mediastinum and turns slightly to the right of the spine. The ventral thoracic esophagus is covered by the trachea and the left main stem bronchus. The thoracic aorta descends on the left side of the esophagus in the lower dorsal mediastinum. On the right side there is the mediastinal pleura and the azygos vein. The vertebral column, the thoracic duct, and the intercostal arteries are located dorsally. The abdominal part enters the diaphragm from the esophageal hiatus to enter the cardiac part of the stomach.

For the surgery of esophageal cancer, knowledge of the lymphatic drainage and the location of regional lymph nodes is essential. The lymphatic capillary vessels form a plexus in the submucosal layer, and the flow of lymph runs mainly in a

D. Gonzalez-Rivas et al. (eds.), *Atlas of Uniportal Video Assisted Thoracic Surgery*,
https://doi.org/10.1007/978-981-13-2604-2_34

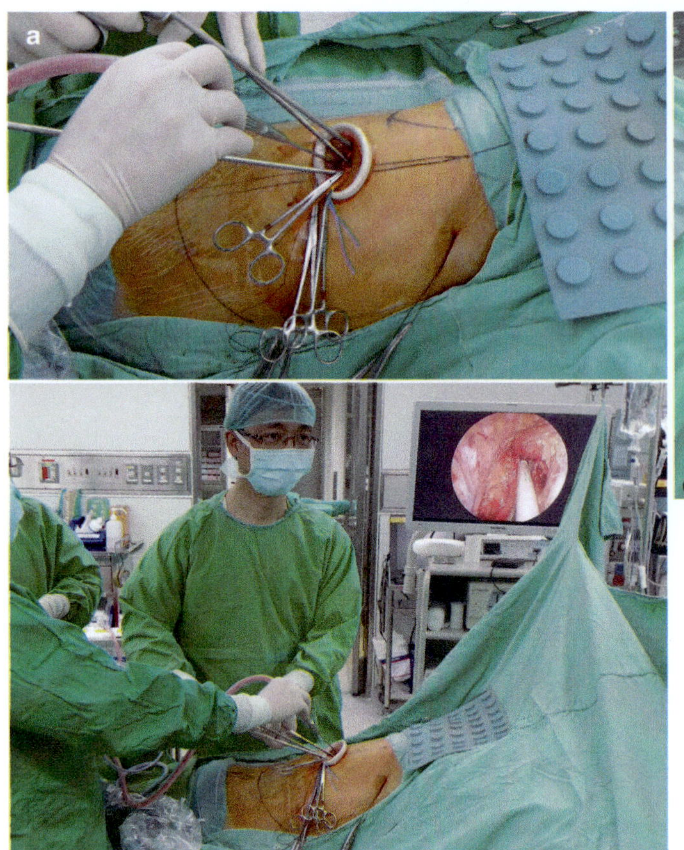

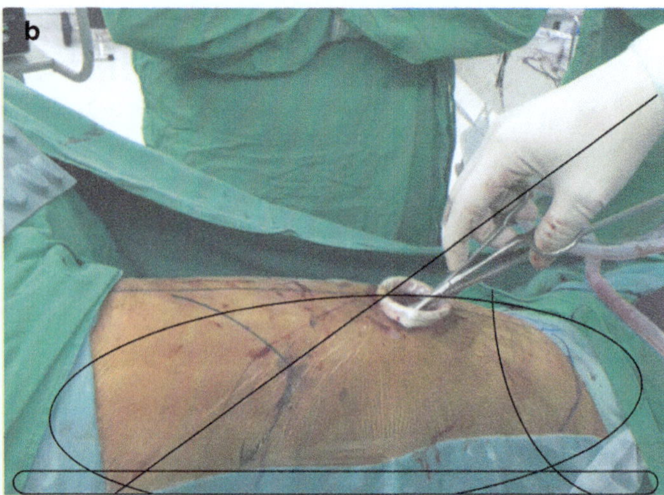

Fig. 1 The incision of single-port VATS in the chest. The angle between the axes of the oesophagus and surgical instrumentation must be kept in excess of 30° to facilitate a smooth dissection for the area near the right recurrent laryngeal nerve area

longitudinal direction. Lymph flow from the upper mediastinum enters the superior paraesophageal lymph nodes which are laterally attached to the esophagus, and the prevertebral lymph nodes, located caudally. Lymphatic drainage of the middle mediastinum courses into the medial paraesophageal lymph nodes and into the paratracheal, tracheobronchial and bronchopulmonary lymph nodes. The lower mediastinal lymphatics runs into the inferior paraesophageal and prevertebral lymph nodes. The superior diaphragmatic lymph nodes rest on the diaphragm along the dorsal connection between the pericardium and the diaphragm.

Operative Methods

Esophagectomy through right side transthoracic approach is widely adopted in treating esophageal cancer because of its superiority in paraesophageal and mediastinal lymph node exposure.

Incision and Access

With the patients in a lateral position, we usually make a right sided 3–4 cm incision through the sixth or seventh intercostal space on the mid-axillary line. The angle between the axis of the oesophagus and surgical instrumentation must be kept in excess of 30° to facilitate a smooth dissection for the area near the right recurrent laryngeal nerve area (Fig. 1a, b).

Surgical Exposure Under Uniportal Thoracoscopy

When patient in lateral decubitus position, the posterior mediastinum and its underlying esophagus would be covered by posterior aspect of right upper lobe and right lower lobe, which makes them unable to be approached directly, especially when lung collapse is not optimal. Under multiportal VATS setting, we usually use endoscopic retractor to move pulmonary lobe laterally and provide enough tension for tissue dissection (Fig. 2). To reduce the collision of the instrument when doing uniportal VATS, we replaced the retractor with the serial retention sutures at posterior mediastinum pleura then pull out anteriorly through endoscopic closure device (Fig. 3). After mediastinal pleural opening, we can keep the tension over dissection plain by pulling and fixation of the suture lines from outside (Fig. 4).

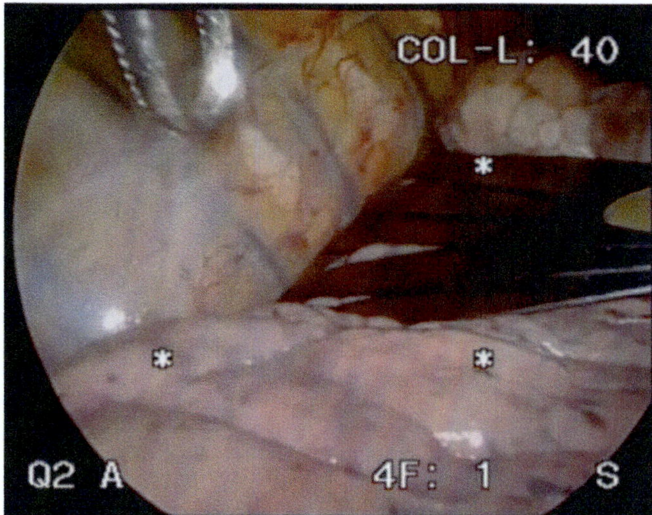

Fig. 2 Under multiportal VATS setting, an endoscopic retractor is used to keep pulmonary lobe laterally and provide enough tension for tissue dissection

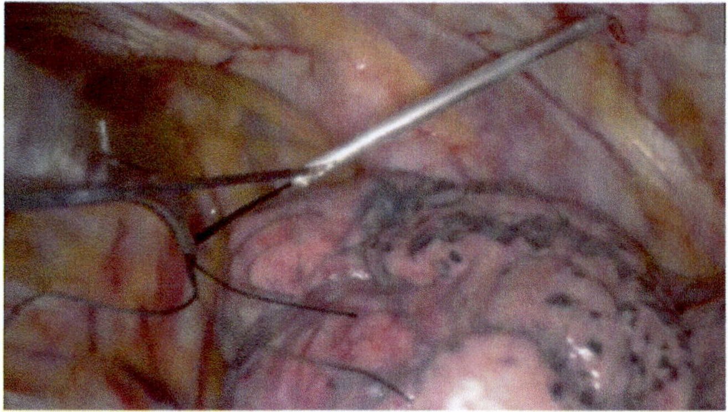

Fig. 3 Under uniportal VATS, a serial retention sutures are fixed at posterior mediastinum pleura then pull out anteriorly through endoscopic closure device to reduce the collision of the instrument

Mobilization and Dissection of Esophagus

After adequate exposure of posterior mediastinum using retention sutures (Fig. 5), the mobilization of the esophagus begin with azygos vein division and opening of the posterior mediastinum pleura. During dissection around the esophagus, care should be taken to the arterial blood supply from thoracic aorta and the inadvertent injury to the thoracic duct if ligation is not routinely performed, besides, using of energy device would be helpful both in better hemostasis and sealing of lymphatics (Fig. 6). Looping of the esophagus using ribbon was routinely performed in tri-incision procedure at our institute to facilitate the dissection of the esophagus (Fig. 7). When doing Ivor-Lewis procedure, the distal esophagus end can be grasped and pulled upward to enhance mobilization of the esophagus after division of the gastric tube, and looping of the esophagus is not recommended (Fig. 8).

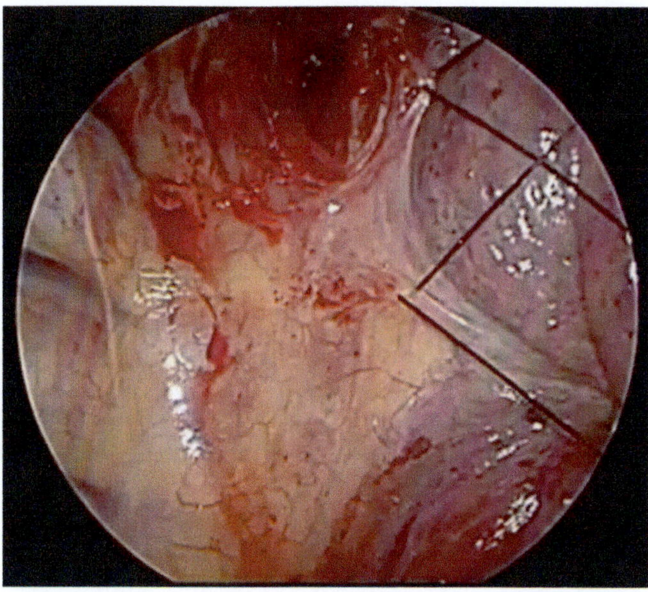

Fig. 4 After mediastinal pleural opening, we can keep the tension over dissection plain by pulling and fixation the suture line from outside

Mediastinal Lymphadenectomy

Pretracheal and right side recurrent laryngeal lymph node dissection can be performed prior to the mobilization of the esophagus. Before the lymphadenectomy of this area, the vagus nerve should be identified, and along its proximal insertion the right recurrent laryngeal nerve can be found with the underlying right subclavian artery, which presented with pulsation. With preserving the right recurrent laryngeal nerve, the lymph nodes in this area (Node zone, 106recR, UICC system) can be removed with branches from vagus nerve. Use of curved long-shaft scissor can be helpful during dissection of this area (Fig. 9). The pretracheal area can be approached easily after dividing the azygous vein, and the pretracheal lymph nodes (Node 106R) are removed with precaution of SVC injury (Fig. 10). The adequate exposure of the subcarinal area (Node 107) can be made by traction suture and even better after esophagus mobilization (Fig. 11). Inadvertent injury of the thoracic duct should be avoided during the dissection of this area. Left recurrent laryngeal area (Node 106recL) (Fig. 12) is deeply located using right side thoracoscopic approach, hence we usually perform the lymph node dissection in this area after fully mobilizing the esophagus in tri-incision procedure and after esophagectomy in Ivor-Lewis procedure. In addition to traction suture, using one instrument to push trachea laterally is usually mandatory for better exposure of the left recurrent laryngeal area (Fig. 13).

Fig. 5 Exposure of posterior mediastinum provided by using retension sutures

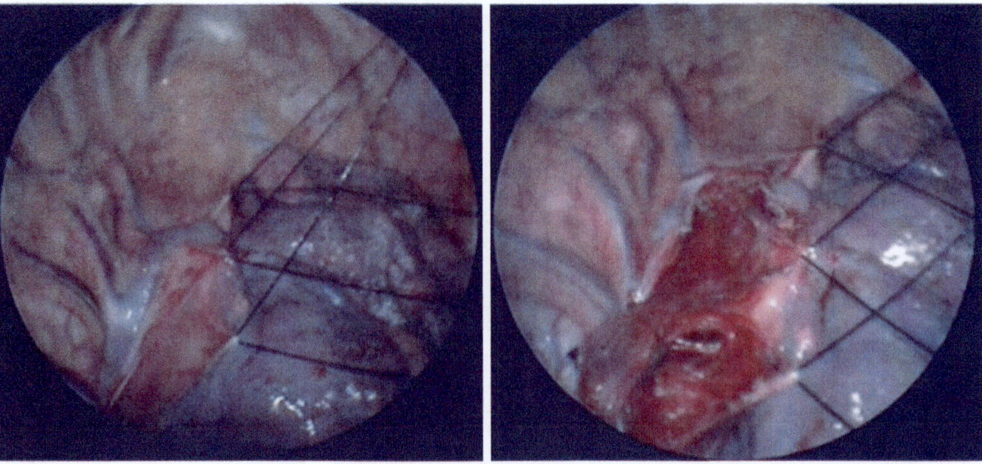

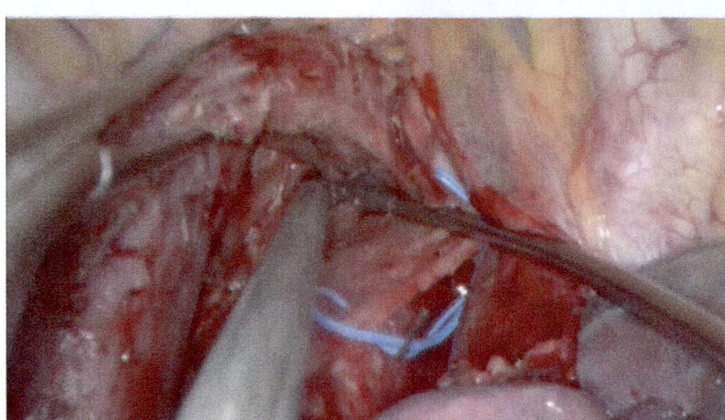

Fig. 6 Dissection around the esophagus by using the energy device

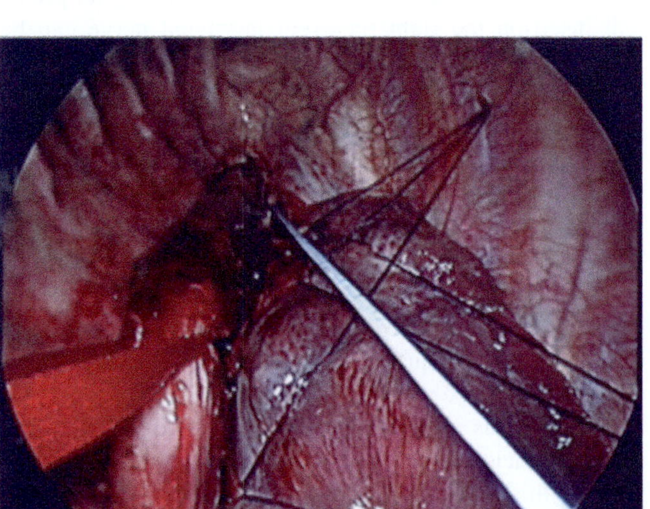

Fig. 7 Looping of the esophagus using ribbon in tri-incision esopahectomy in the chest

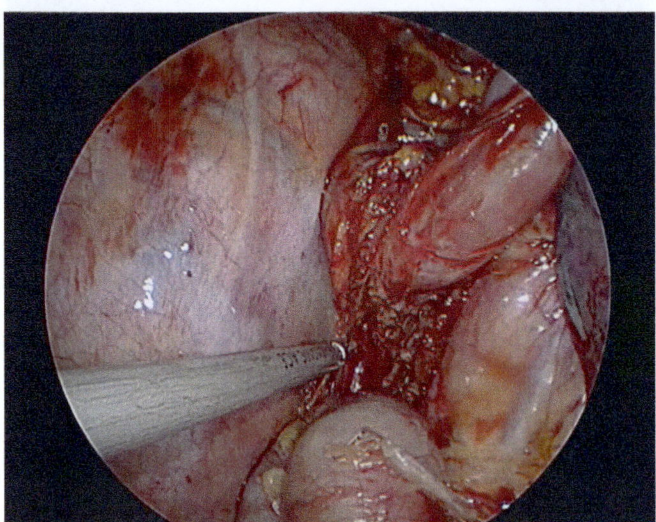

Fig. 8 In Ivor-Lewis procedure, distal esophagus end can be grasped and pulled upward to enhance mobilization of the esophagus after division of the gastric tube

Gastric Mobilization Under Uniportal Laparoscopy

For the single-incision laparoscopic gastric mobilization, a 3-cm incision is made along the umbilicus and a surgical wound-protector (GelPoint, Applied Medical, CA, USA) is applied, through which the two or three surgical instruments and a 5 or 10-mm camera used in the laparoscopic procedure are inserted (Fig. 14). The liver is retracted with a self-retaining fixing stitch passed through the diaphragmatic hiatus and tightened extra-corporally (Fig. 15a, b). The stomach is mobilized via opening the greater and lesser sac

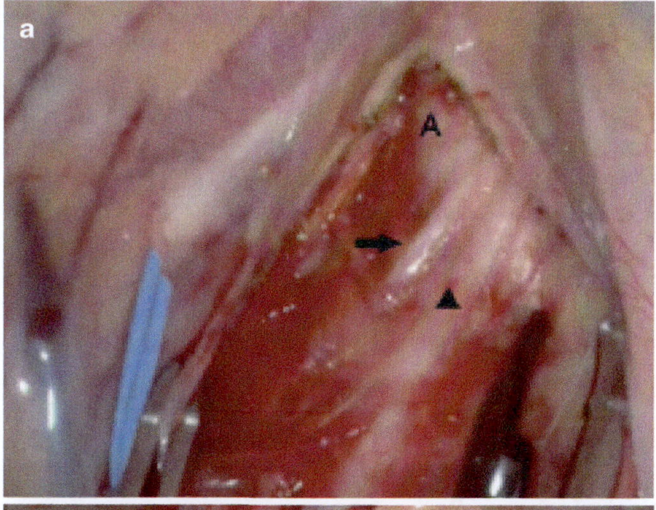

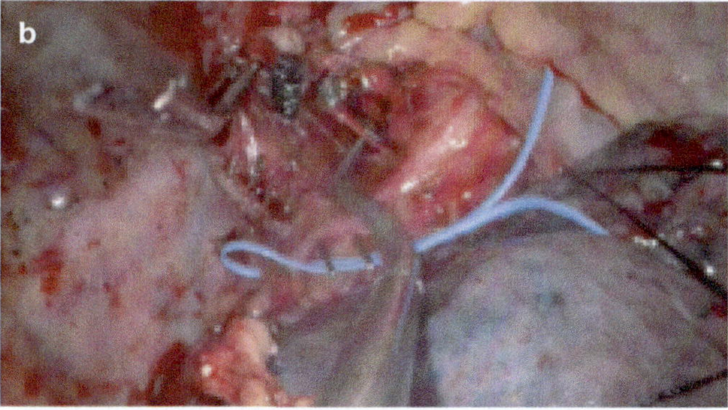

Fig. 9 With preserving the right side recurrent laryngeal nerve (arrow) near the right subclavian artery (A), the lymph nodes in this area (106recR, UICC system) can be removed with branches from vagus nerve (triangle)

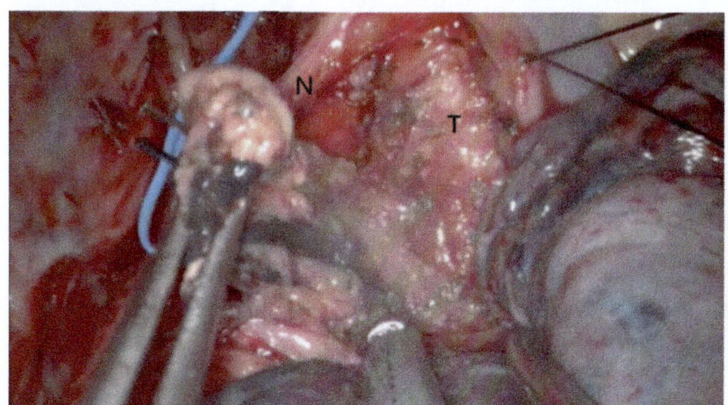

Fig. 10 Lymph node dissection in the pretracheal region (106R) between the trachea (T) and vagus nerve (N) with precaution to prevent SVC injury

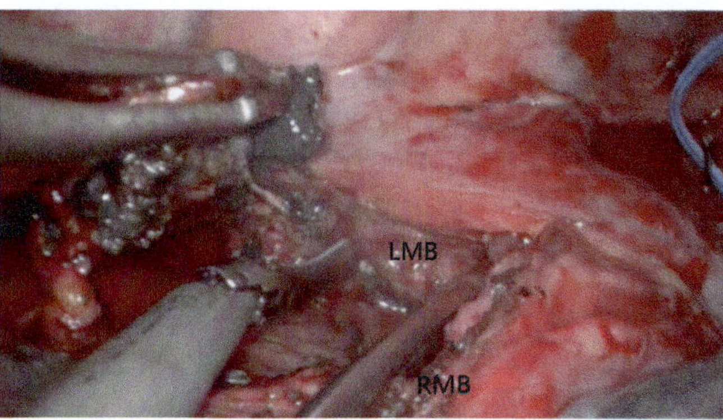

Fig. 11 The exposure of the subcarinal area (107) between the left (LMB) and right main bronchus (RMB)

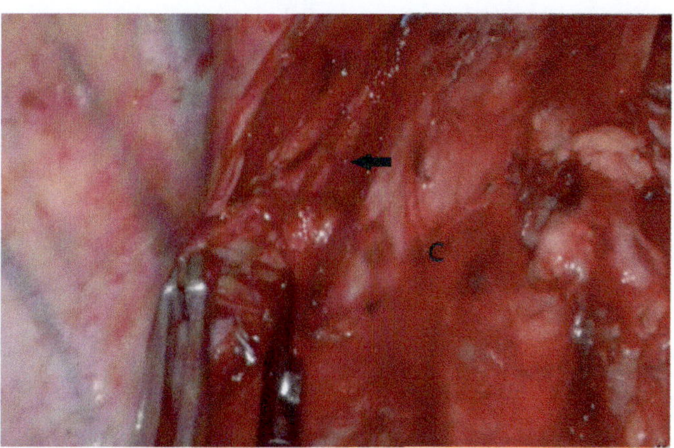

Fig. 12 Exposure for lymph node dissection along the left side recurrent laryngeal area (106recL)

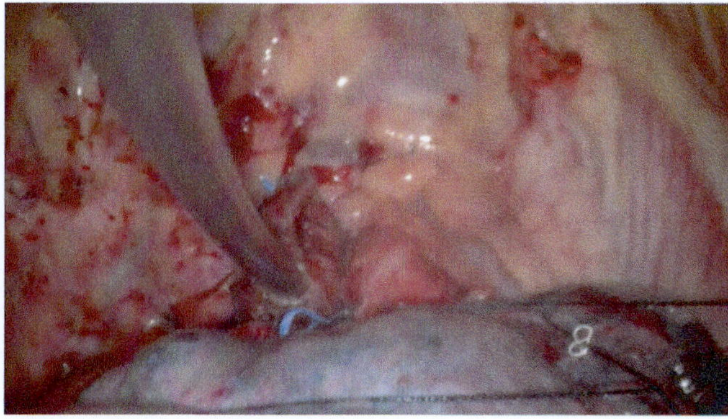

Fig. 13 Using one instrument to push trachea laterally for better exposure of the left side recurrent laryngeal area

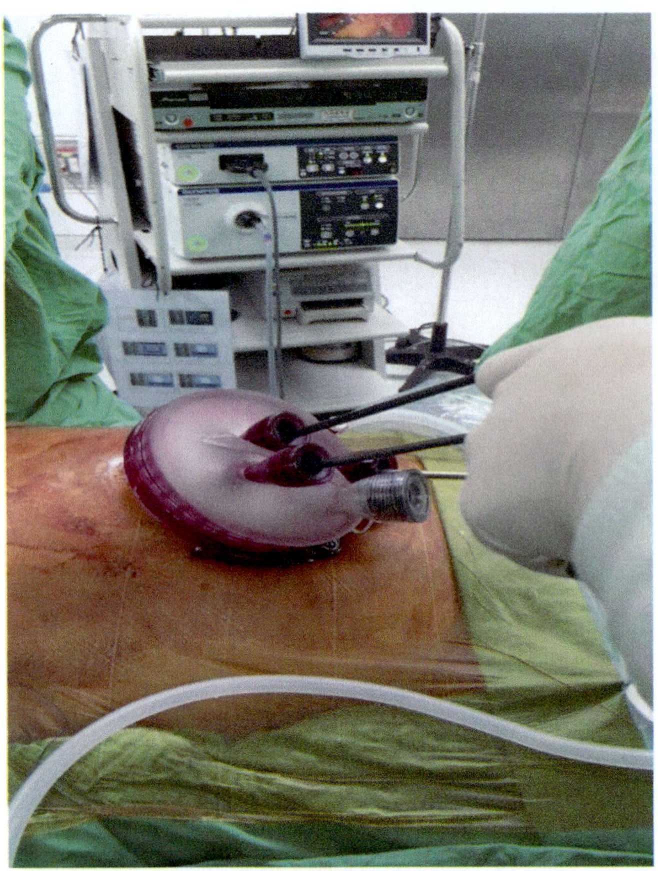

Fig. 14 During single-port laparoscopic procedures, a 3-cm incision is made along the umbilicus and a surgical wound-protector (GelPoint, Applied Medical, CA, USA) is applied

along the greater and lesser curvature respectively. The short and left gastric arteries are divided with ultrasonic or bi-polar scissors while preserving the right gastric and gastroepiploic arteries during the procedure of gastric mobilization. Lymph nodes dissection in the hiatus, lesser curvature, left gastric and celiac trifurcation are performed (Fig. 16). A feeding jejunostomy is performed on the jejunum 40 cm from the Treitz ligament unless the patient has already had the procedure done prior to CCRT. The jejunum is fixed onto the abdominal wall through two stitches of peritonization through strait needle and extra-corporeal fixation. A 12# Fr central venous catheter is placed into the lumen of jejunum and completed with two more stitches of peritonization (Fig. 17).

Completion of Procedure

Tri-incision

Following the thoracic procedure, the patient is placed into the supine or lithotomy position for both the abdominal and cervical procedures. The gastric conduit and cervical esophagus are anastomosed over the left cervical area through either posterior mediastinal or substernal route.

Ivor-Lewis

In the Ivor Lewis operation, we use a DST Series™ OrVil™ circular staple with the anvil introduced transorally to perform the intrathoracic oesophagogastrostomy (Fig. 18). While still open, the gastric tube is fixed with two retaining

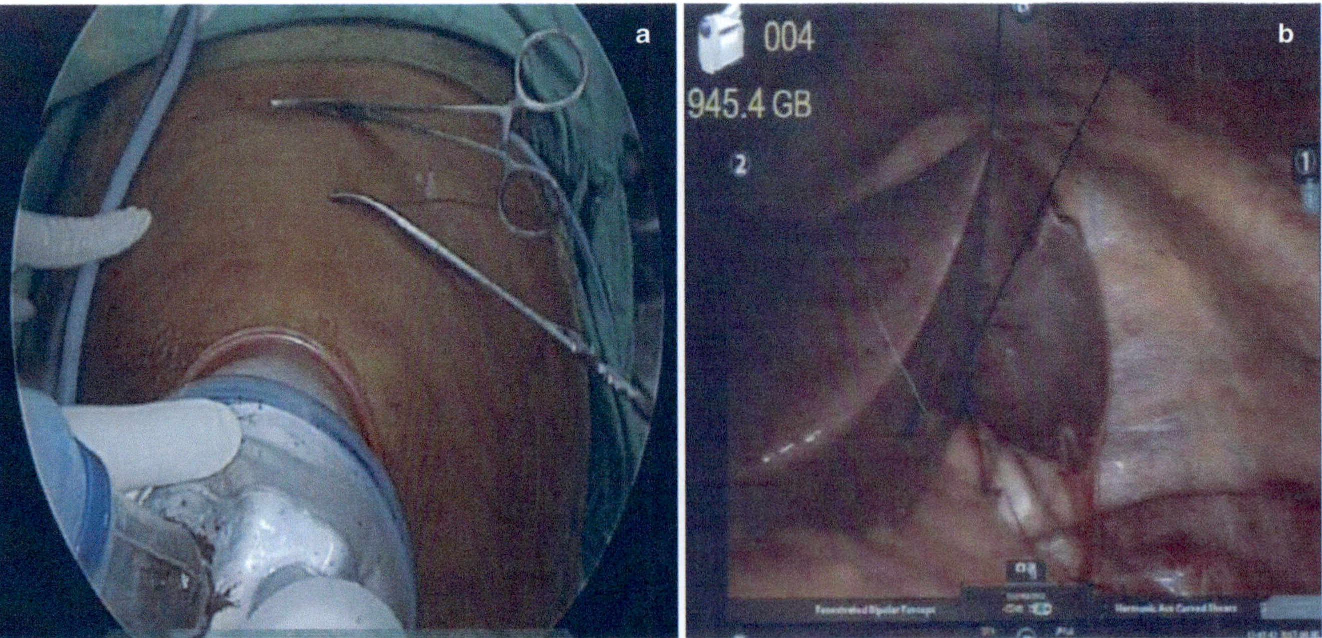

Fig. 15 (**a**) and (**b**). The liver is retracted with a self-retaining fixing stitch passed through the diaphragmatic hiatus and tightened extra-corporally

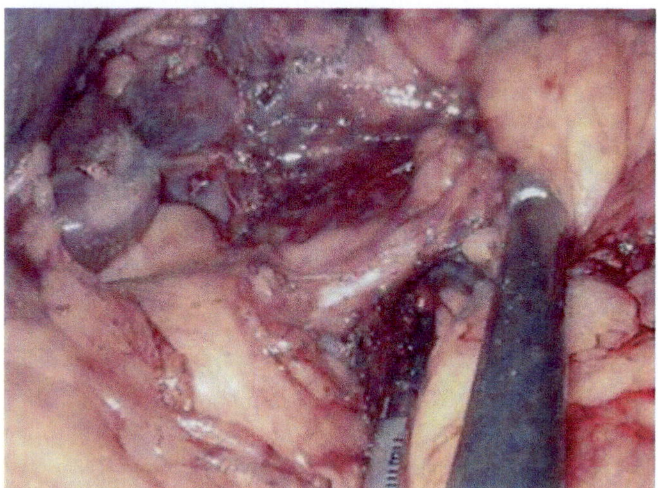

Fig. 16 Exposure of left gastric artery after lymphadenectomy in the hiatus, lesser curvature, left gastric artery and celiac trifurcation

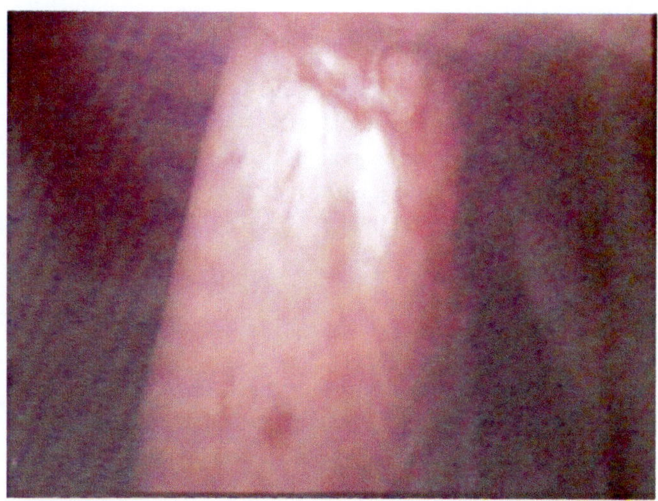

Fig. 17 Completion of laparoscopic jejunostomy by stitches of peritonization through strait needle and extra-coporial fixation. A 12# Fr central venous catheter was placed into the lumen of jejunum

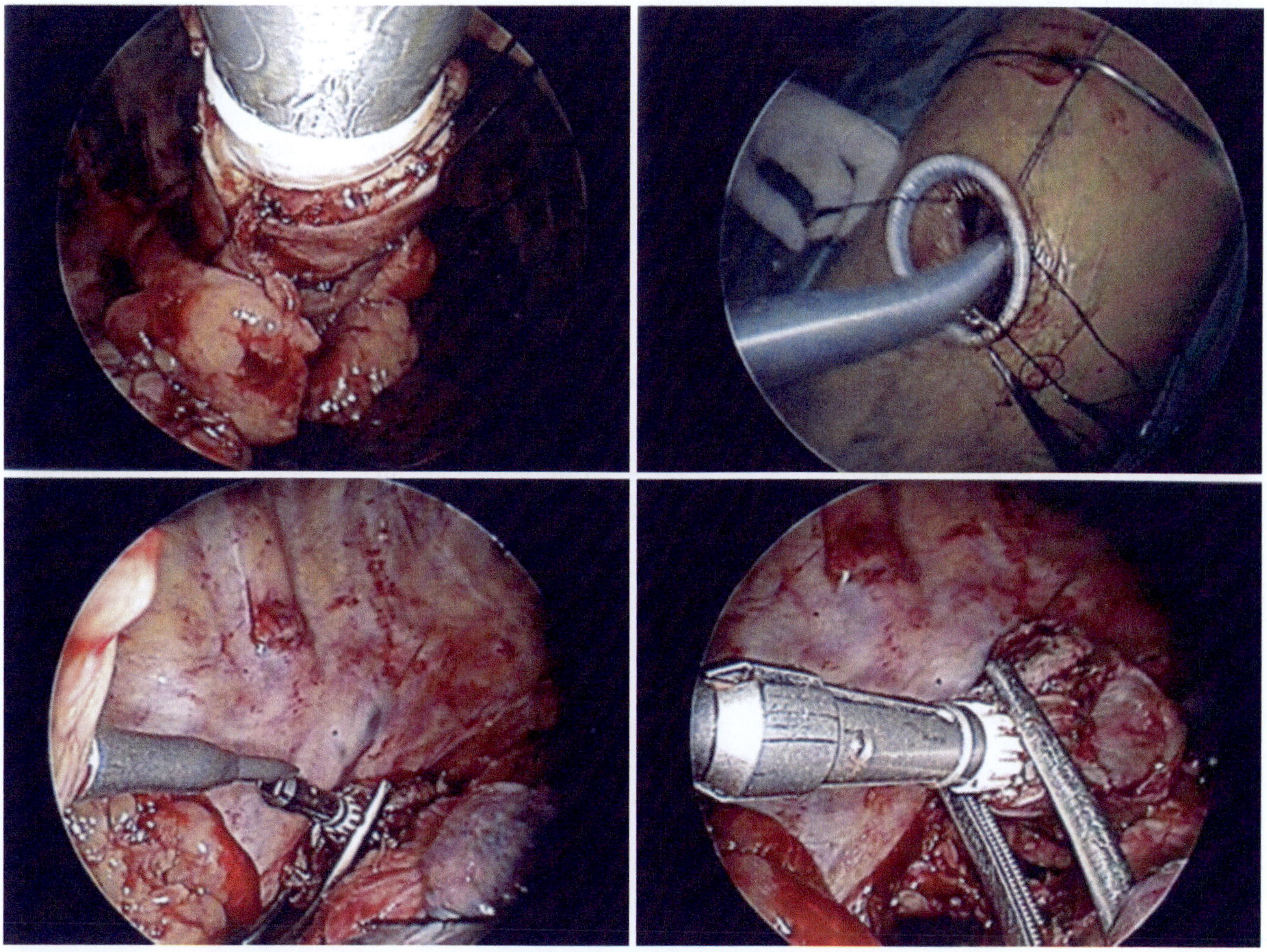

Fig. 18 In the Ivor Lewis esophagectomy, a DST OrVil circular staple with the anvil is introduced transorally to perform the intrathoracic oesophagogastrostomy. (Figure 18b, c and d) While still open, the gastric tube was fixed with two retaining stitches to allow the introduction of the PCEEA applier (18a)

stitches to allow the introduction of the PCEEA applier (Fig. 18). After completion of the esophagogastrostomy by approximation of both ends of PCEEA, the defect of gastric tube is closed with linear stapler. The sharp end of the staple lines on the stomach and esophagus is reinforced and inverted into the esophageal and gastric lumen to avoid dehiscence while resumption of oral intake.

Discussion

As our previously published results have shown, the number of dissected lymph nodes, the duration of postoperative critical care and the degree of postoperative complication from the minimally invasive single port approach is comparable to those associated with traditional MIE [17]. A later propensity-matched comparison study based on a larger patient population further demonstrated similar perioperative surgical results between the single and multiple-incision approaches in performing the thoracoscopic and laparoscopic procedures of MIE. Although, the pain scores were similar between the two groups of patients on the first day after surgery, however, the scores on the seventh day after surgery were significantly lower in the SIMIE group than in the multiple incision minimally invasive esophagectomy (MIMIE) group.

There is a concern for SIMIE which is the potential risk of incisional herniation along the peri-umbilical wound which might cause detriment to its cosmetic effect. In our series, there is two patients of incisional hernia (1/127, 1.5%) after SIMIE. An incidence of 2.9% has been found for the patients after various single-incision laparoscopic procedures [1], which might be attributed to a larger fascia defect created in the single-incision wound [1]. A careful physical examination is needed during each clinical follow-up for patients following single incision laparoscopic surgery.

In conclusion, MIE performed with a single-incision in both thoracoscopic and laparoscopic procedures is feasible and provides comparative perioperative results with those obtained by multi-incision approaches. The clinical value for the long-term outcome after surgery for esophageal cancer remained to be clarified in the future.

References

1. Agaba EA, et al. Incidence of port-site incisional hernia after single-incision laparoscopic surgery. JSLS. 2014;18(2):204–10. https://doi.org/10.4293/108680813X13693422518317.
2. Luketich JD, et al. Minimally invasive esophagectomy: outcomes in 222 patients. Ann Surg. 2003;238(4):486–94;discussion 494–5.
3. Smithers BM, et al. Comparison of the outcomes between open and minimally invasive esophagectomy. Ann Surg. 2007;245(2):232–40.
4. Palanivelu C, et al. Minimally invasive esophagectomy: thoracoscopic mobilization of the esophagus and mediastinal lymphadenectomy in prone position: experience of 130 patients. J Am Coll Surg. 2006;203(1):7–16.
5. Sutton CD, et al. Endoscopic-assisted intrathoracic oesophagogastrostomy without thoracotomy for tumours of the lower oesophagus and cardia. Eur J Surg Oncol. 2002;28(1):46–8.
6. Senkowski CK, et al. Minimally invasive esophagectomy: early experience and outcomes. Am Surg. 2006;72(8):677–83;discussion 683.
7. Nguyen NT, et al. Thoracoscopic and laparoscopic esophagectomy for benign and malignant disease: lessons learned from 46 consecutive procedures. J Am Coll Surg. 2003;197(6):902–13.
8. Nguyen NT, Schauer P, Luketich JD. Minimally invasive esophagectomy for Barrett's esophagus with high-grade dysplasia. Surgery. 2000;127(3):284–90.
9. Martin DJ, et al. Thoracoscopic and laparoscopic esophagectomy: initial experience and outcomes. Surg Endosc. 2005;19(12):1597–601.
10. Leibman S, et al. Minimally invasive esophagectomy: short- and long-term outcomes. Surg Endosc. 2006;20(3):428–33.
11. Shih CS, et al. Comparing the postoperative outcomes of video-assisted thoracoscopic surgery (VATS) segmentectomy using a multi-port technique versus a single-port technique for primary lung cancer. J Thorac Dis. 2016;8(Suppl 3):S287–94. https://doi.org/10.3978/j.issn.2072-1439.2016.01.78.
12. Wu CF, et al. Comparative short-term clinical outcomes of mediastinum tumor excision performed by conventional VATS and single-port VATS: is it worthwhile? Medicine (Baltimore). 2015;94(45):e1975. https://doi.org/10.1097/MD.0000000000001975.
13. Hsu PK, et al. Multiinstitutional analysis of single-port video-assisted thoracoscopic anatomical resection for primary lung cancer. Ann Thorac Surg. 2015;99(5):1739–44. https://doi.org/10.1016/j.athoracsur.2015.01.041.
14. Gonzalez-Rivas D, et al. Single-port video-assisted thoracoscopic anatomic segmentectomy and right upper lobectomy. Eur J Cardiothorac Surg. 2012;42(6):e169–71. https://doi.org/10.1093/ejcts/ezs482.
15. Jiang ZW, et al. Single-incision laparoscopic distal gastrectomy for early gastric cancer through a homemade single port access device. Hepato-Gastroenterology. 2015;62(138):518–23.
16. Khayat A, et al. Does single port improve results of laparoscopic colorectal surgery? A propensity score adjustment analysis. Surg Endosc. 2015;29(11):3216–23. https://doi.org/10.1007/s00464-015-4063-7.
17. Lee JM, et al. Single-incision laparo-thoracoscopic minimally invasive oesophagectomy to treat oesophageal cancerdagger. Eur J Cardiothorac Surg. 2016;49(Suppl 1):i59–63. https://doi.org/10.1093/ejcts/ezv392.

Part VI

The Future of Uniportal VATS

Non-intubated Uniportal VATS Major Pulmonary Resections

Diego Gonzalez-Rivas, Sonia Alvarado, and César Bonome

Abstract

Video-assisted thoracic surgery, initially developed and used only in minor procedures like biopsies or athipical resections, has been extended swiftly; and nowadays it is positioned as the first option for almost all procedures, like lobectomies or even pneumonectomies. In this field uniportal video-assisted thoracic surgery represents and excellent, minimally invasive strategy, allowing us to change our anesthesic management, evolving from the current standard management, which includes general anesthesia, intubation and one-lung ventilation, to spontaneous ventilation accompanied by different regional anesthesia techniques. We achieve with this new approach to reduce our patient's trauma and postoperative pain caused both by more aggressive surgical techniques and more invasive anesthesia approaches; without compromising efficiency.

Introduction

Nowadays we are witnesses to a constant evolution in thoracic surgery pursuing more secure surgical techniques for the diagnose and treatment of our patients, with the final purpose of reducing the trauma caused by these techniques without compromising its efficiency.

Electronic Supplementary Material The online version of this chapter (https://doi.org/10.1007/978-981-13-2604-2_35) contains supplementary material, which is available to authorized users.

D. Gonzalez-Rivas (✉)
Department of Thoracic Surgery, Shanghai Pulmonary Hospital, Tongji University School of Medicine, Shanghai, China

Department of Thoracic Surgery and Minimally Invasive Thoracic Surgery Unit (UCTMI), Coruña University Hospital, Coruña, Spain
e-mail: diego@uniportal.es

S. Alvarado · C. Bonome
Anesthesiology Department, University Hospital La Coruña, La Coruña, Spain

D. Gonzalez-Rivas et al. (eds.), *Atlas of Uniportal Video Assisted Thoracic Surgery*,
https://doi.org/10.1007/978-981-13-2604-2_35

In this context, VATS (video-assisted thoracic surgery) and more recently, thoracic surgery performed through a single incision (uniportal VATS) represents an excellent, minimally invasive strategy for major procedures, such as anatomical pulmonary resections (Fig. 1) [1]. The development of minimally invasive techniques allows us to change, in addition, the anesthetic management of these patients in order to minimize adverse effects due to our anesthetic approaches [2]. Our goal, should be to evolve from the current standard management, which includes general anesthesia, intubation and one-lung ventilation (OLV)—to spontaneous ventilation accompanied by different regional anesthesia techniques [3, 4].

Alternative or Recommendation: Advantages of Thoracic Surgery Without Intubation

Mechanical ventilation in thoracic surgery has a series of adverse effects such as barotrauma, volutrauma (due to lung overdistension), atelectrauma (due to the repetitive opening and closing of pulmonary alveoli), and biotrauma (due to the release of inflamatory mediators). Lung injury associated to mechanical ventilation is estimated around 4%, with a mortality of 25%. Nevertheless, subclinical lung injury is more frequent and it is related to post-operative complications [5, 6].

When the patient is anesthetized, in lateral position and under mechanical ventilation and OLV the upper lung does not ventilate, but it is still perfunded, leading to intrapulmonary shunt, worsening the ventilation/perfusion ratio (V/Q) [7]. Although perfusion in the upper, non-ventilated lung decreases, due to hypoxic pulmonary vasoconstriction (HPV), gravity, surgical interference and preexistent disease—hypoxemia is frequent.

In order to minimize mechanical ventilation's damage, we are provided with lung protective strategies, consisting of the usage of low tidal volumes, PEEP, low inspired oxygen concentrations, low ventilatory pressures, "permissive hypercapnia" and recruitment maneuvers [8].

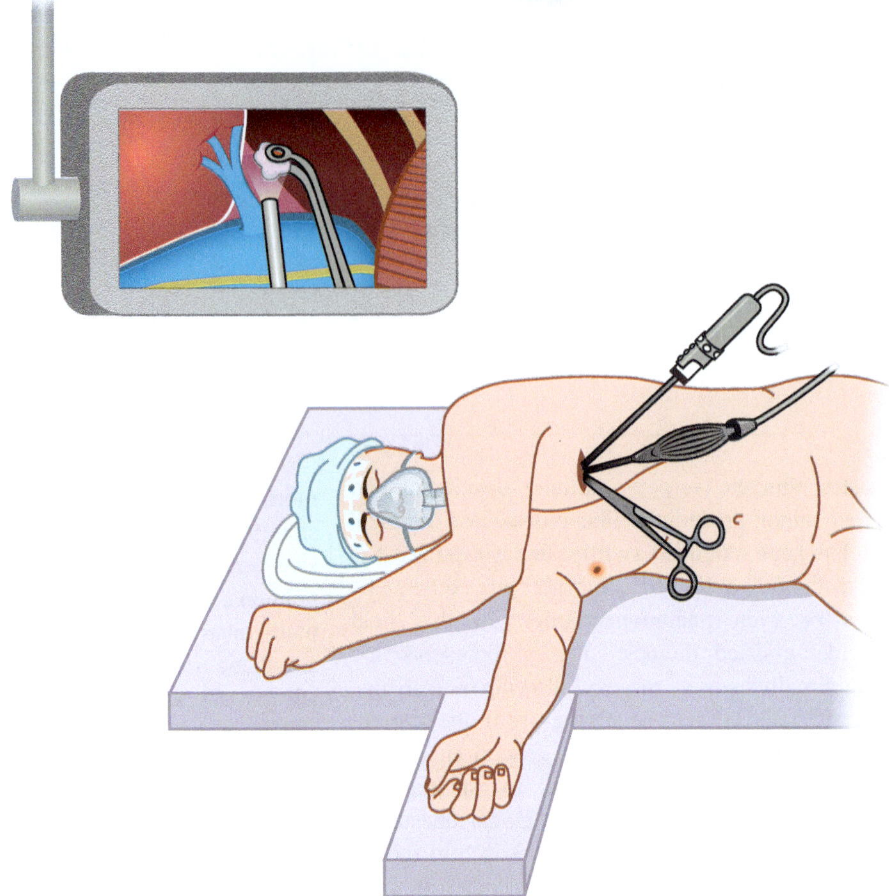

Fig. 1 Standard position for a non-intubated uniportal video-assisted thoracoscopic lobectomy

Some studies suggest that the use of this "permissive hypercapnia" can improve hemodinamics and V/Q ratio, and even have some protection effect over the inflamatory response [9]. In patients under spontaneous OLV, hypercapnia is not only possible, but frequent.

Nevertheless, hypercapnia is not free of risks for all patients, and it must be avoided in those presenting pulmonary hypertension, important alterations in heart rate or intracranial hypertension. In awake or sedated patients, with a normal right ventricular function, $PaCO_2$ levels should be easily tolerated until 70 mmHg [10].

Complications associated to orotracheal and endobronchial intubation must also be taken into consideration: pain, mucose ulceration, larynx and tracheal damage. Tracheobronchial rupture is one of the most feared complications [11].

General anesthesia itself, is also associated with a series of deleterious effects. Deep anesthesia, which is usually required for thoracic surgery, has been related with higher mortality rates and more postoperative cognitive impairment [12]. The use of muscle relaxants can cause diaphragmatic dysfunction, along with other complications derived from muscular residual blockade [13]. The use of opioids during general anesthesia is associated with hyperalgesia, vomit, nausea and respiratory depression, decreasing patient's satisfaction, and on the other hand increasing analgesic postoperative needs as well as hospital stay [14].

Anesthesia Management for Non-intubated Thoracic Surgery: From Theory to Practice

Performing thoracic surgery without intubation requires protocols to assess every indication and contraindication, exclusion criteria, patient's consent, the most adequate anesthetic technique considering the surgical procedure and the criteria to convert to general anesthesia.

Exclusion criteria, elaborated following our experience and the main research groups in thoracic surgery with non-intubated patients are shown in Table 1.

Inclusion criteria include every patient in whom these techniques reduce the morbidity derived from conventional thoracotomies and the risks of general anesthesia [4, 5, 15–18].

VATS in a non-intubated patient implies the use of thoracoscopic procedures with regional anesthesia techniques in patients in spontaneous ventilation and without manipulation of the airway. These regional techniques include local anesthesia, intercostal nerves blockades, paravertebral blockade and epidural anesthesia [19–21].

Monitoring

Standard monitoring must include electrocardiogram, non-invasive arterial pressure, pulse oximetry, respiratory rate and capnography.

The use of an anesthetic depth monitor is highly recommended if the use of intravenous sedation techniques is required.

Ventilation

Spontaneous ventilation in a non-intubated patient can be accompanied by supplementary oxygen support through nasal cannulas, facemask or even supraglottic devices, if sedation is profound.

Table 1 Exclusion criteria for non-intubated VATS

Difficult airway (Mallampati III–IV).
Hemodynamically unstable patients.
Obesity (BMI > 30).
Unexperienced or poorly cooperative VATS team.
Coagulopathy (INR > 1.5) or poorly respected antiagregation rules/ preanesthesia.
Persistent cough or secretions in upper airway.
High risk of regurgitation.
Neurological alterations (tumours, intracranial hypertension…).
Previous pulmonary resections.
Hypoxemia (PaO_2 < 60 mmHg) or hypercapnia (PCO_2 > 50 mmHg).
Central hypoventilation syndrome.
Contraindications for the use of regional anesthesia techniques.
Procedures that required lung isolation (bronchoalveolar lavage…).

A nasopharyngeal tube or Guedel cannula can be needed and/or recommended, because mild obstruction of the airway can increase expiratory positive pressure and therefore insufflate the collapsed lung.

A supraglottic device that can be useful in those groups starting out in non-intubating thoracic surgery is the laryngeal mask. It grants a permeable airway until the glottis, it allows spontaneous ventilation, preserve airway reflexes, allows to monitored pressure and ventilatory volumes, and it decreases the risk of aspiration in case of regurgitation (Fig. 2). Furthermore, in case of hypoxemia and hypercapnia, we can use a low pressure support ventilation (5–8 cmH20), which does not recruits the collapsed lung, but it increases the tidal volume in the decline lung [22].

Sedation

Sedation level is inversely proportional to the regional anesthetic technique being used. Techniques such as local anesthesia, intercostal or intra-pleural blockade need deeper sedation strategies than an epidural technique.

In VATS context, the term MAC (monitored anesthetic cares) is better than deep sedation because this term includes the possibility of using opioids for sedation as well as the use of supraglottic devices to improve ventilation and avoid airway obstruction [15, 17–22].

The combination of a hypnotic agent (propofol) and an short-acting opioid (remifentanil, sulfentanil) in continuous perfusion seems to be an advisable and easily applicable option for VATS surgery.

To monitor the anesthetic depth we generally use the quantification of the bispectral index. Recommended values are 50–60. In general, a remifentanil concentration of 3 ng/mL or sulfentanil concentration 0.3–0.4 ng/mL and a propofol concentration of 2–4 μg/mL in plasma is well tolerated and allows spontaneous ventilation.

Some groups reported the use of dexmedetomidine in continuous perfusion as a sedative drug (1 mcg/kg/h) to avoid the risk of respiratory depression associated to opioid agents. Anyway, this is a long-acting drug, and as such concentrations it increases the time of discharge at the reanimation unit. The use of lower doses (1 mcg/kg/h in initial sedation) is usually enough to achieve a long-lasting sedation,

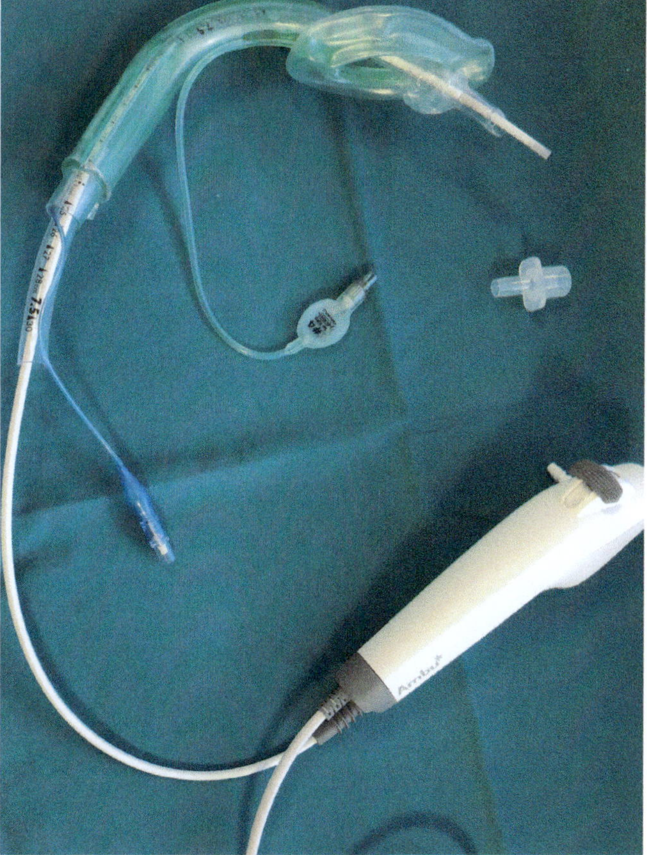

Fig. 2 Among the advantages of laryngeal mask, there is the possibility of intubation with fibrobronchosccope through it. In the photograph, a new model of laryngeal mask, the Ambu Aura-i (Ambu®)

aided by low doses of remifentanil without increasing the recovery time [23].

Regional Anesthesia Techniques

Local Anesthesia and Intercostal Blockade

Local anesthesia and intercostal blockade require deep sedation during thoracoscopic major pulmonary resections. In an uniportal VATS procedure, intercostal infiltration is usually enough for entering into the chest cavity and for postoperative analgesia. However it is not enough to control intraoperative stimuli caused by pleural manipulation and hilar dissection, therefore additional sedation and analgesia are required [19–22]. We initially use local anesthesia for skin incision, subcutaneous and intercostal space, and once the incision is opened, we blockade one or two intercostal spaces under thoracoscopic view (Fig. 3).

Paravertebral Blockade

Using this technique, we can block various intercostal spaces by administrating one dose of local anesthesia in levels T4–T5. Paravertebral technique avoids the patient's reaction to surgical incision and trocar introduction. Besides, a catheter can be placed in paravertebral space through this technique, in order to administrate further doses, if needed. The effectiveness of this blockade in thoracic surgery is excellent. However awake thoracic surgery without sedation has not been reported using this technique (Figs. 4, 5).

Epidural Anesthesia

This technique allows us, through a single puncture and the introduction of a catheter, to get a deeper, longer and wider

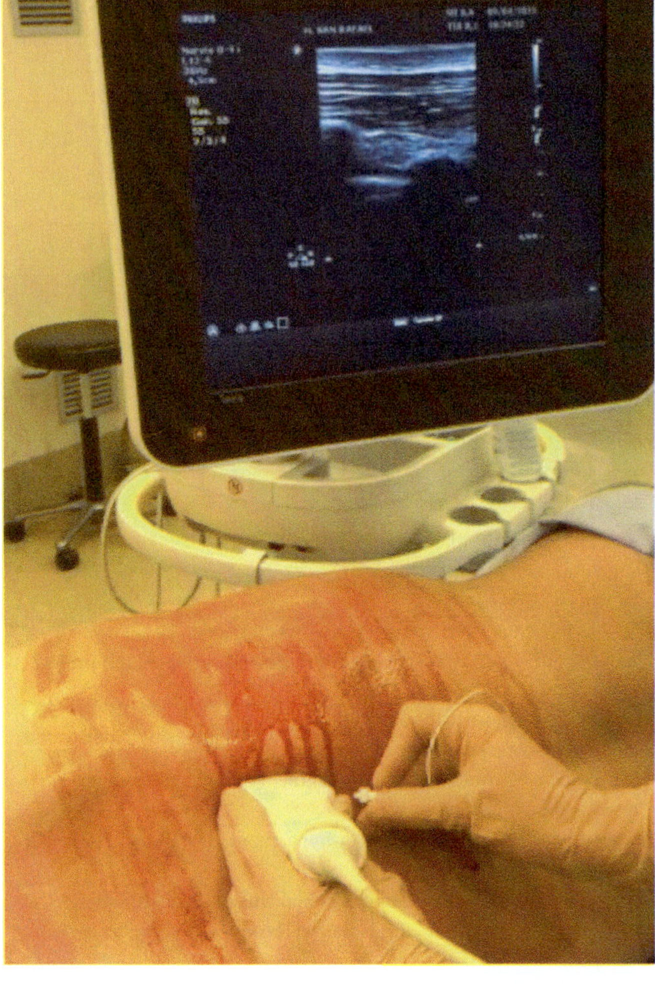

Fig. 4 Paravertebral blockade under ultrasound image

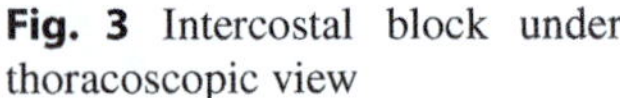

Fig. 3 Intercostal block under thoracoscopic view

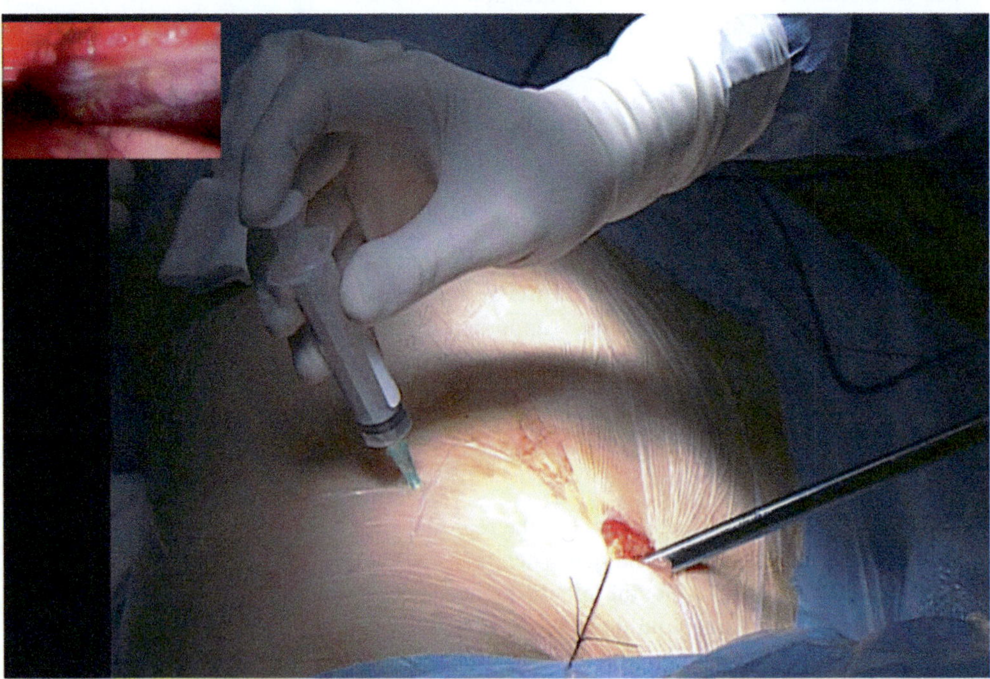

blockade. Its effectiveness depends on the level (usually T3–T5), dose and volume of the anesthetic agent being used [24, 25].

Epidural anesthesia does not block phrenic nerve (which provides motor and sensitive innervation to the diaphragm and mediastinum) or the vagus nerve (responsible for cough reflex) [20]. This is relevant as the bronchi and the trachea are deeply innervated and their manipulation can cause hemodynamic effects as well as cough reflex, which may obstruct surgery.

Vagus Nerve

One of the main difficulties when we want to perform non-intubated thoracic surgery is to control the stimulation of the vagus nerve, responsible for cough reflex [20]. Its blockade is of the upmost importance in VATS surgery in order to help the surgeon's work and avoid the need of reconversion into general anesthesia.

One way to avoid its stimulation is to achieve an adequate level of sedation. Other blockade strategies used by different groups include the direct infiltration of the vagus nerve during surgery. This blockade is easy to perform and it has few side effects [4, 15–17]. On right sided resections the vagus blockade is performed at the level of the paratracheal space (Fig. 6a, Video 1) and for left sided procedures at the level of the aortopulmonary window (Fig. 6b).

Another option, is the nebulization of lidocaine 2% about 30 min before surgery. There has been only one report concerning the blockade of stellate ganglion to avoid cough reflex. However this is not an accepted therapy for cough reflex, and may even trigger it [26].

From our point of view, and based on published studies, we show the different anesthesic possibilities for non-intubated thoracic surgery (Table 2).

The Video 1 shows an uniportal VATS anatomic right apical segmentectomy under spontaneous ventilation, by using

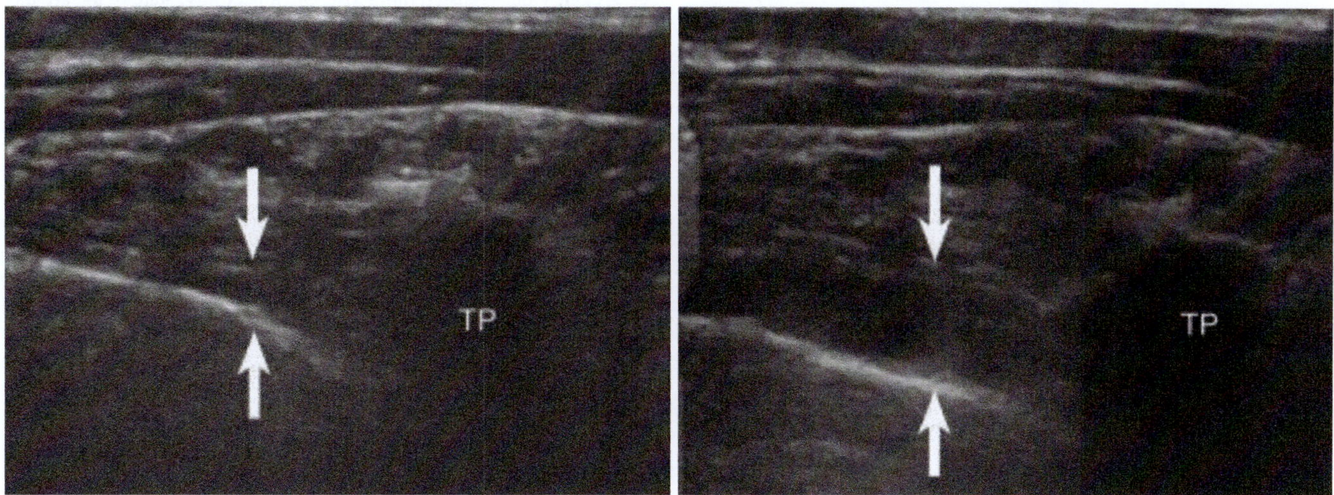

Fig. 5 Paravertebral blockade, ultrasound image, the white arrows are pointing the paravertebral space. Left before anaesthetic infiltration, right after anaesthetic infiltration. TP: Transverse process

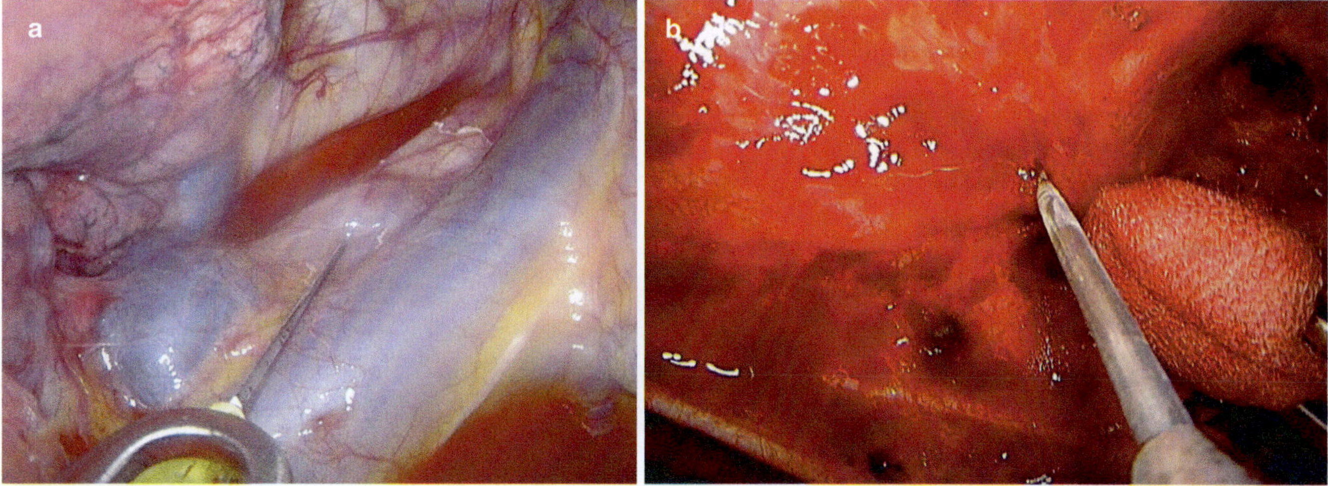

Fig. 6 Vagus blockade. (**a**) Paratracheal space. (**b**) Aortopulmonary window

Table 2 Anesthetic techniques for VATS

Anesthesic technique	Minor surgery	VATS multiportal	VATS uniportal
Local anesthesia – intercostal blockade			
Awake	+	–	–
Sedated	++	–	–
MAC	+++	++	+++
Paravertebral blockade			
Awake	+	–	–
Sedated	++	–	+
MAC	+++	++	+++
Epidural anesthesia			
Awake	++	–	–
Sedated	+++	+	++
MAC	+++	+++	+++
Epidural + vagus nerve blockade			
Awake	N	–	–
Sedated	N	+	++
MAC	N	+++	+++
Epidural + vagus nerve + phrenic nerve blockades			
Awake	N	¿?	¿?
Sedated	N	++	+++
MAC	N	+++	+++

(–) Not recommended, (+) possible, (++) technically feasible, (+++) recommended, (¿?) not proved, (N) not necessary, (MAC) monitored anesthetic cares

Table 3 Causes of conversion to general anesthesia

1. Surgical complications: major bleeding, pleural adhesions, large tumours…
2. Critical hypoxemia ($PaO_2 < 60\%$), hypercapnia, ($PaCO_2 > 80$) and acidosis (pH < 7.1).
3. Hemodynamic instability.
4. Persistent cough that impede the surgery.
5. Diaphragm's excessive movement.
6. Failure of regional anesthesia technique.
7. Inability to collapse the lung.

facial mask, intercostal block and vagus blockade. Sedation was accomplished with propofol and remifentanil in continuous perfusion.

Conversion to General Anesthesia

Intraoperative conversion to general anesthesia may be needed in some occasions, and the surgical team must have a plan to minimize patient's risk. Intubate a patient placed in lateral position is a challenge. The anesthesiologist must have the ability to choose the right airway device for the patient, considering the patient's airway, the time required to complete the surgery and which caused the conversion to general anesthesia (Table 3).

Conclusions

The tendency to a less aggressive thoracic surgery lead us to search minimal invasive surgical approaches and more secure anesthesic strategies, always trying to decrease secondary damage caused by general anesthesia, airway manipulation and mechanical ventilation.

Although long-term benefits are yet to be seen, this minimally invasive techniques are a very attractive alternative to general anesthesia for pulmonary resection procedures. Eventually, more groups are starting to use this procedures, which are also a perfect combination to fast-track programs in thoracic surgery [27, 28].

References

1. Shaw JP, Dembitzer FR, Wisnivesky JP, Litle VR, Weiser TS, Yun J, et al. Video-assisted thoracoscopic lobectomy: state of the art and future directions. Ann Thorac Surg. 2008;85(2):S705–9.
2. Kao MC, Lan CH, Huang CJ. Anesthesia for awake video-assisted thoracic surgery. Acta Anaesthesiol Taiwanica. 2012;50(3):126–30.
3. Chen KC, Cheng YJ, Hung MH, Tseng YD, Chen JS. Nonintubated thoracoscopic lung resection: a 3-year experience with 285 cases in a single institution. J Thorac Dis. 2012;4(4):347–51.
4. Gónzalez-Rivas D, Aymerich H, Bonome C, Fieira E. From open operations to nonintubated video-assisted thoracoscopic lobectomy: minimizing the trauma to the patient. Ann Thorac Surg. 2015;100(6):2003–5.
5. Della Rocca G, Coccia C. Acute lung injury in thoracic surgery. Curr Opin Anaesthesiol. 2013;26(1):40–6.
6. Schilling T, Kozian A, Huth C, Buhling F, Kretzschmar M, Welte T, et al. The pulmonary immune effects of mechanical ventilation in patients undergoing thoracic surgery. Anesth Analg. 2005;101(4):957–65.
7. Nagendran J, Stewart K, Hoskinson M, Archer SL. An anesthesiologist's guide to hypoxic pulmonary vasoconstriction: implications for managing single-lung anesthesia and atelectasis. Curr Opin Anaesthesiol. 2006;19(1):34–43.
8. Gothard J. Lung injury after thoracic surgery and one-lung ventilation. Curr Opin Anaesthesiol. 2006;19(1):5–10.
9. Laffey JG, Honan D, Hopkins N, Hyvelin JM, Boylan JF, McLoughlin P. Hypercapnic acidosis attenuates endotoxin-induced acute lung injury. Am J Respir Crit Care Med. 2004;169(1):46–56.
10. Feihl F, Perret C. Permissive hypercapnia. How permissive should we be? Am J Respir Crit Care Med. 1994;150(6):1722–37.
11. Fitzmaurice BG, Brodsky JB. Airway rupture from double-lumen tubes. J Cardiothorac Vasc Anesth. 1999;13(3):322–9.
12. Sessler DI, Sigl JC, Kelley SD, Chamoun NG, Manberg PJ, Saager L, et al. Hospital stay and mortality are increased in patients having a "triple low" of low blood pressure, low bispectral index, and low minimum alveolar concentration of volatile anesthesia. Anesthesiology. 2012;116(6):1195–203.
13. Welvaart WN, Paul MA, Stienen GJ, van Hees HW, Loer SA, Bouwman R, et al. Selective diaphragm muscle weakness after contractile inactivity during thoracic surgery. Ann Surg. 2011;254(6):1044–9.
14. Hausman MS Jr, Jewell ES, Engoren M. Regional versus general anesthesia in surgical patients with chronic obstructive pulmonary disease: does avoiding general anesthesia reduce the risk of postoperative complications? Anesth Analg. 2014;120(6):1405–12.

15. Vanni G, Tacconi F, Sellitri F, Ambrogi V, Mineo TC, Pompeo E. Impact of awake videothoracoscopic surgery on postoperative lymphocyte responses. Ann Thorac Surg. 2010;90(3):973–8.
16. Snyder GL, Greenberg S. Effect of anaesthetic technique and other perioperative factors on cancer recurrence. Br J Anaesth. 2010;105(2):106–15.
17. Yan TD. Video-assisted thoracoscopic lobectomy-from an experimental therapy to the standard of care. J Thorac Dis. 2013;5(Suppl 3):S175–6.
18. Lin XM, Yang Y, Chi C, Liu Y, Xie DY. Video-assisted thoracoscopic lobectomy: single-direction thoracoscopic lobectomy. J Thorac Dis. 2013;5(5):716–20.
19. Piccioni F, Langer M, Fumagalli L, Haeusler E, Conti B, Previtali P. Thoracic paravertebral anaesthesia for awake video-assisted thoracoscopic surgery daily. Anaesthesia. 2010;65(12):1221–4.
20. Rocco G, La Rocca A, Martucci N, Accardo R. Awake single-access (uniportal) video-assisted thoracoscopic surgery for spontaneous pneumothorax. J Thorac Cardiovasc Surg. 2011;142(4):944–5.
21. Inoue K, Moriyama K, Takeda J. Remifentanil for awake thoracoscopic bullectomy. J Cardiothorac Vasc Anesth. 2010;24(2): 386–7.
22. Katlic MR, Facktor MA. Video-assisted thoracic surgery utilizing local anesthesia and sedation: 384 consecutive cases. Ann Thorac Surg. 2010;90(1):240–5.
23. Hwang J, Min T, Kim D, Shin J. Non-intubated single port thoracoscopic procedure under local anesthesia with sedation for a 5-year-old girl. J Thorac Dis. 2014;6(7):148–51.
24. Macchiarini P, Rovira I, Ferrarello S. Awake upper airway surgery. Ann Thorac Surg. 2010;89(2):387–90;discussion 90–91.
25. Mineo TC, Pompeo E, Mineo D, Tacconi F, Marino M, Sabato AF. Awake nonresectional lung volume reduction surgery. Ann Surg. 2006;243(1):131–6.
26. Chen JS, Cheng YJ, Hung MH, Tseng YD, Chen KC, Lee YC. Nonintubated thoracoscopic lobectomy for lung cancer. Ann Surg. 2011;254(6):1038–43.
27. Gonzalez-Rivas D, Bonome C, Fieira E, Aymerich H, et al. Non-intubated video-assisted thoracoscopic lung resections: the future of thoracic surgery? Eur J Cardiothorac Surg. 2016;49(3):721–31.
28. Gonzalez-Rivas D, Fernandez R, de la Torre M, Rodriguez JL, Fontan L, Molina F. Single-port thoracoscopic lobectomy in a non-intubated patient: the least invasive procedure for major lung resection? Interact Cardiovasc Thorac Surg. 2014;19(4):552–5.

Subxiphoid Uniportal Video-Assisted Thoracoscopic Surgery

Diego Gonzalez-Rivas, Firas Abu Akar, and Jiang Lei

Introduction

The uniportal VATS technique is definitely a significant breakthrough in the field of minimally invasive thoracic surgery. In addition to the reduction of surgical trauma by reducing the number and the size of the incisions, the direct vision provided by the uniportal technique [1, 2], which coincides with the movement of the instruments in the same direction, and decrease the post operative pain and complications are the strongest factors in the success of this technique [3, 4]. This may have convinced many surgeons to adopt and practice the technique as a standard. There is no doubt that the subxiphoid technique is a further addition to the technology of uniportal VATS [5], which aims to reduce the surgical trauma more and more by entering the thoracic cavity through a nerve free zone, which may reduce the likelihood of chronic pain after the operation to nearly zero. The idea of employing the subxiphoid incision as an additional accessory incision was found more than two decades ago in approaching the thymomas and anterior mediastinal tumors [6, 7]. Since the first report on anatomical pulmonary resection through the uniportal subxiphoid approach in 2014 [8], some papers that describe the technique began to appear [9–12]. However this technique is still fresh, and all the reasonable theories which assume the odds of this technique are still needed to be evidence supported by randomized studies and scientific comparisons.

General Principles

The guiding principle that must be kept in mind when a surgeon considering utilizing the subxiphoid uniportal VATS technique in his practice is that previous experience in VATS is mandatory. In contrast to intercostal uniportal VATS technique, which can be learned and applied even if the surgeon is coming from the open surgery school [13], the learning of the subxiphoid technique requires a prior experience in uniportal VATS [10]. In addition, the right choice of cases that are facile to do with this technique is very important especially at the kickoff of the learning curve. Of particular significance is the availability of the instruments specially designed for this type of operation, which are long tools with a curved tip. In order to be able to practice this technique successfully, the availability of trained staff and especially the first assistant surgeon is strongly recommended, as his role during the surgery is very influential.

Patients Selection and Preoperative Assessment

As mentioned before, selecting the suitable cases is of great importance mostly at the beginning of the learning curve. During the initial experience, we encourage the surgeons to

Electronic Supplementary Material The online version of this chapter (https://doi.org/10.1007/978-981-13-2604-2_36) contains supplementary material, which is available to authorized users.

D. Gonzalez-Rivas (✉)
Department of Thoracic Surgery, Shanghai Pulmonary Hospital, Tongji University School of Medicine, Shanghai, China

Department of Thoracic Surgery and Minimally Invasive Thoracic Surgery Unit (UCTMI), Coruña University Hospital, Coruña, Spain
e-mail: diego@uniportal.es

F. A. Akar
Department of Cardiothoracic Surgery, Shaare Zedek Medical Center (SZMC), Jerusalem, Israel

Department of Cardiothoracic surgery, Makassed Charitable Society Hospital, East Jerusalem, Israel

J. Lei
Department of Thoracic Surgery, Shanghai Pulmonary Hospital, Tongji University School of Medicine, Shanghai, China

D. Gonzalez-Rivas et al. (eds.), *Atlas of Uniportal Video Assisted Thoracic Surgery*,
https://doi.org/10.1007/978-981-13-2604-2_36

choose the thin patients with low BMI. The process of creating the access port, identifying, dissecting and amputating the xiphoid cartilage is much easier in slim than in obese patients. In addition, the amount pericardial fat may be less when the patient is thinner, this facilitates access to the thoracic cavity. We note that the thoracic cavity in obese patients with high BMI is usually small in addition to the higher diaphragm level than in thin patients. This makes the process much more complex, especially when the lower lobectomies are performed.

Although all the lobectomies are feasible via subxiphoid technique, there is no wonder that the easiest lobes to be approached through the this technique are the right upper and middle lobes. This is because the angle of instrumentation and the insertion of staplers are straightway in the direction of the hilum and intersect with it by about 90 degrees. Therefore it's advised that the surgeons choose to deal with these lobes (preferably with complete or easy fissures) at the beginning of his subxiphoid experience.

It should be noted that dealing with the posterior areas of the thoracic cavity could be extremely difficult and tricky and that avoiding performing posterior resections via this approach may be justified and logical. Some authors considered some posterior segmentectomies like S2 and S6 to be a not suitable for this approach [10].

The sampling of mediastinal lymph nodes through the subxiphoid approach is not very difficult, but full lymph node dissection may require learning special methods and skills [14].

Patients with cardiomegaly or heart arrhythmia are not good candidates for this type of surgery. The large heart may block or obstacle the entry into the thoracic cavity (especially to the left side), this may oblige the surgeon to press the heart muscle for long periods of time during the operation which may cause a drop in blood pressure or may cause heart arrhythmias [10].

Operative Technique

Anesthesia Considerations

Standard methods for general anesthesia and single-lung ventilation are employed through either double lumen endotracheal tube or bronchial blocker. An arterial line is usually used for hemodynamic and arterial blood gas monitoring. Peripheral or external jugular intravenous line is employed for fluid and drug administration. Foley catheter for urine drainage and monitoring should be inserted as a routine. The epidural catheter, intercostal, or para-vertebral blocks are unnecessary in this approach. The anesthesiologist should be aware that in this approach, the compression and the friction with the pericardium which may cause irritation of the heart are not uncommon, and the patients may be exposed to changes in blood pressure or intraoperative arrhythmia up to 13% of the cases [10]. Therefore, keeping the patient well hydrated during the surgery may help to avoid these symptoms, with a caution that excessive fluid infusion during lung resections, especially pneumonectomy may have unfavorable effects.

Positioning

The patient can be placed in a semi-decubitus position (60–70° inclination) (Fig. 1). This position is more convenient for the surgeon and his assistant, so the movement of the instruments and hands will be more smooth and comfortable. In some cases, we found that putting the patient in full-decubitus position (90° lateral) may help to shift the heart to the contralateral side, which minimizes the interference with the instruments. In contrast to intercostal uniportal technique, the placement of a pillow under the axilla has no benefit in the wound creation process, and may even cause a bend of the xiphoid area, which may confuse the surgeon and lead to create the wound in the wrong and uncomfortable place. But the importance of placing the pillow under the axilla lies in relieving pressure on the shoulders and avoiding pain after surgery in this area. Therefore, the placement of the pillow is necessary, but the surgeon must mark the area of the xiphoid process prior to the positioning "when the patient lying on his back". When the purpose of the operation is resection of an anterior mediastinal mass or thymectomy, the patient is placed in the supine position (Fig. 2) with a roll placed beneath the thoracic spine in order to elevate the thoracic cage and to hyperextend the patient's neck.

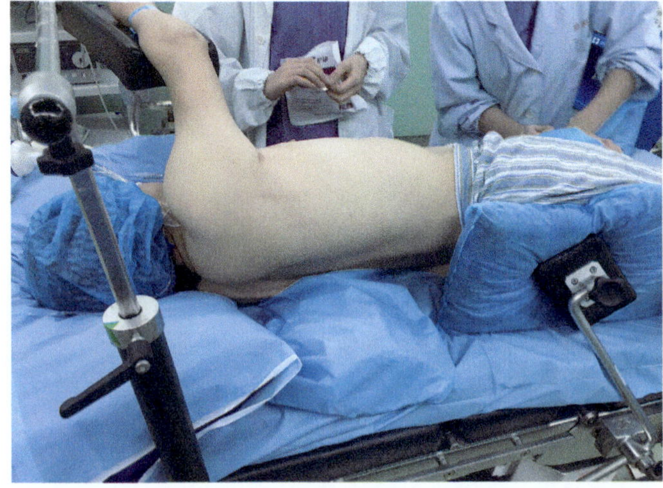

Fig. 1 Positioning for subxiphoid surgery semi-decubitus position 60–70° inclination "posterior view"

Creating the Wound and the Working Channel

The longitudinal incision (Fig. 3) is usually preferred, but in some cases, the transverse incision could be more convenient especially in approaching the anterior mediastinum and when the infrasternal angle (the angle between the two coastal margins) is more than 70°.

- After palpating the xiphoid process, a longitudinal mark is placed over its prominence, this must be done before the positioning (when the patient is in a supine position).

The patient is placed in the decubitus or semi decubitus position as previously mentioned and then after sterilizing and covering the skin, a longitudinal 3–4 cm skin incision is performed. The subcutaneous fatty tissue is then cut down in the same longitudinal direction until the xiphoid cartilage is reached. The xiphoid then detached from the linea alba and the rectus abdominis muscle from its anterior surface and lateral edges using diathermy. The Xiphoid is then picked up by Alice grasper and lifted anteriorly (Fig. 4a) to detach the posterior surface from its diaphragmatic attachment. After exposing the xiphoid

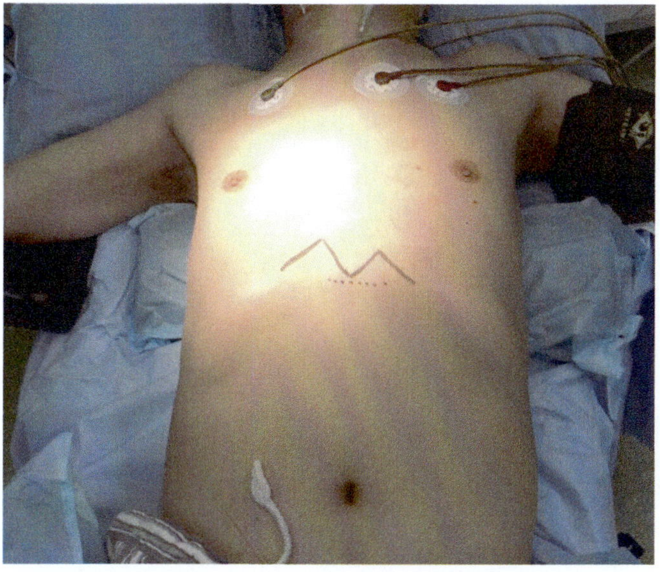

Fig. 2 Marking the skin for the incision before thymus surgery

Fig. 3 Longitudinal incision

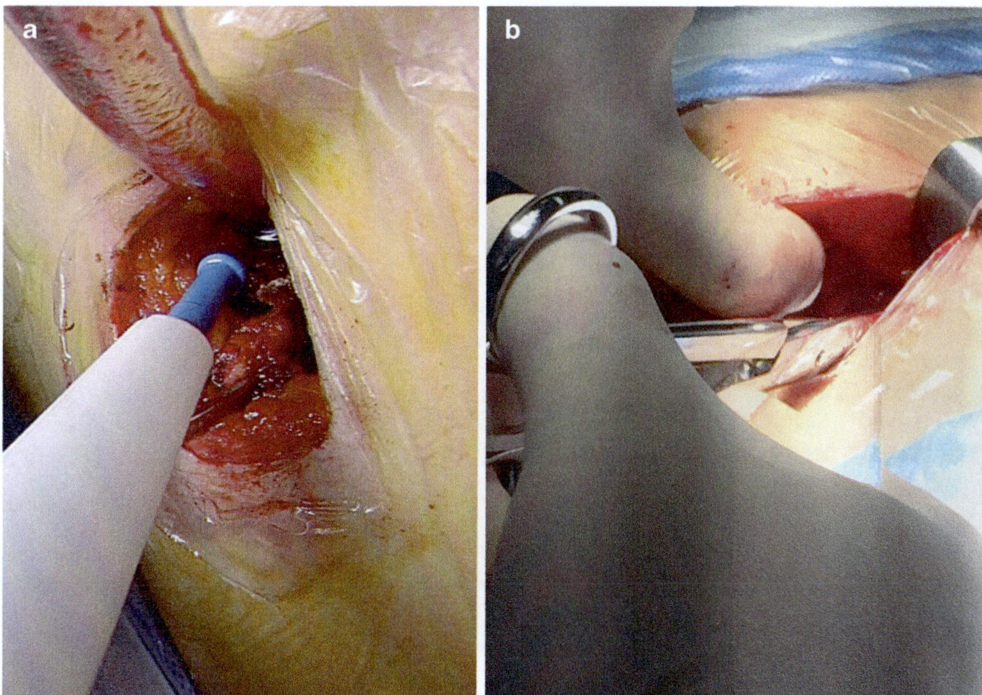

Fig. 4 (**a**) Grasping the xiphoid with an allis clamp before cutting. (**b**) Cutting the xiphoid process

process from all directions, it's disconnected from the sternum by a sturdy Mayo scissors (Fig. 4b). After the cut, the smoothness of the edges should be checked and any bump in the tip of the sternum should be removed so that the surgeon does not get injured and the rubbery wound protector does not tear easily during the procedure.

- Then the right and/or pleural or mediastinal space is accessed primarily through blind finger dissection guided by the internal surface of the chest wall or the sternum (Fig. 5a).
- The next step is to create the working channel for which the instrument is entered and the surgery is performed through: after the Xiphoid has been removed and the entrance to the channel is established, a wound protector is placed (Fig. 5b). Its functions are to facilitate the exposure significantly, maintaining the integrity of the wound and the cleanliness of the instruments during the procedure in addition to prevent the sowing of tumor cells to the wound during the surgery.

At this stage, the pericardial fat is removed (Fig. 6), which is a crucial step to facilitate the smooth Instrumentation during the surgery without disruption. Where at first the removal of the fatty tissue visible through the wound using

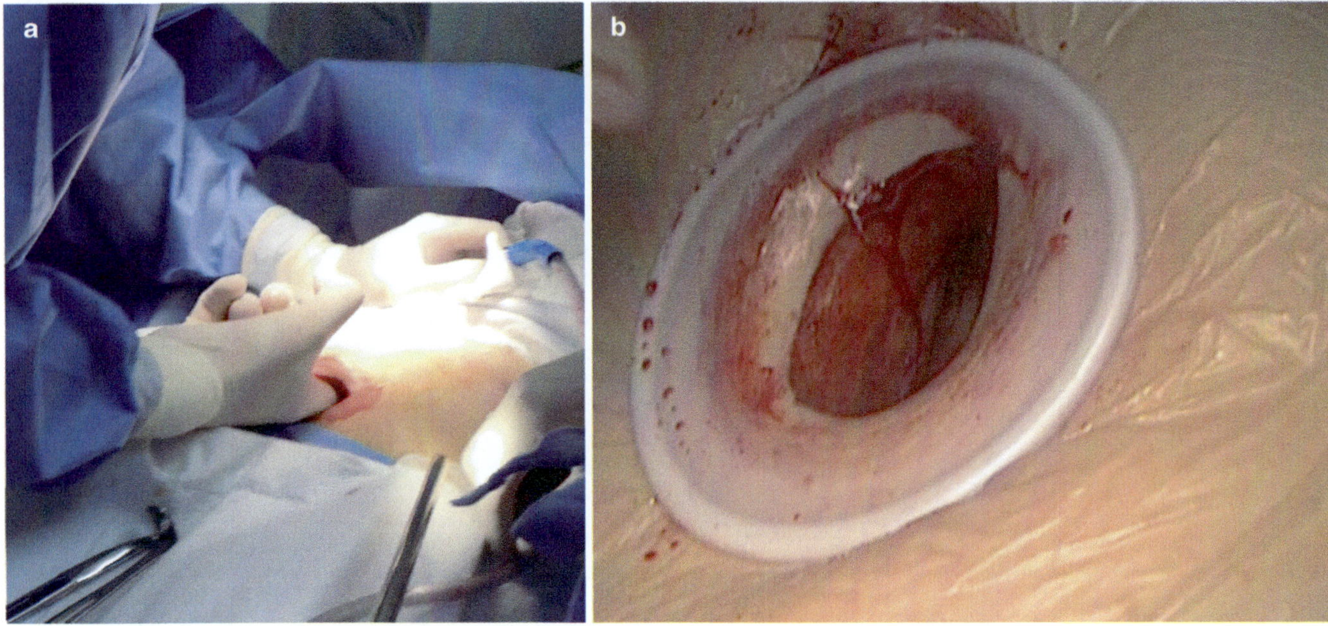

Fig. 5 (**a**) Creating a space behind the sternum by blunt digital dissection. (**b**) Wound protector

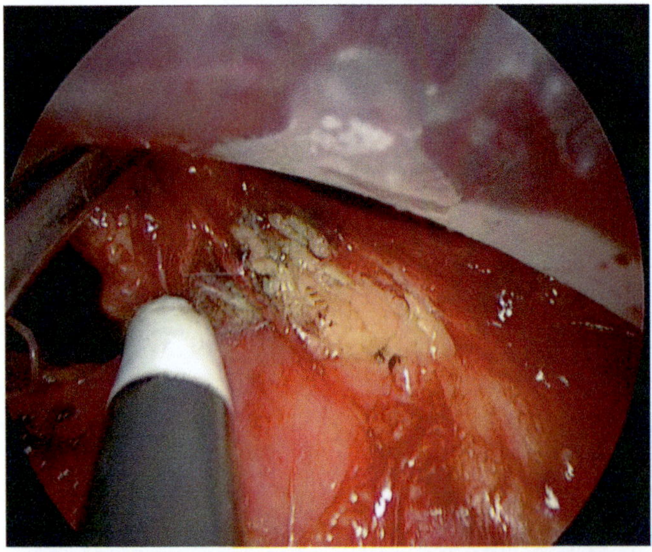

Fig. 6 Removal of pericardial fat

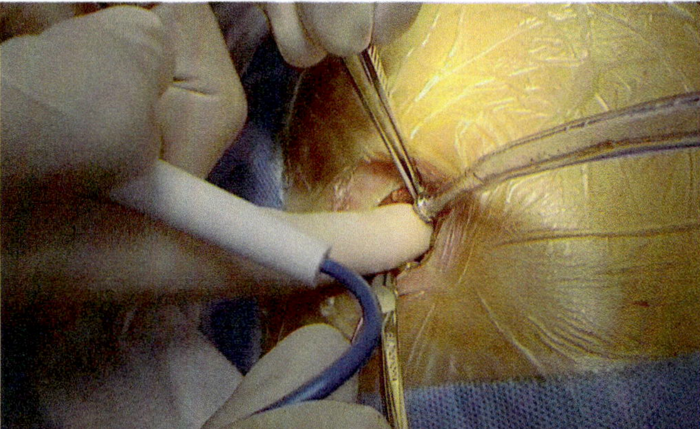

Fig. 7 Creation of subcostal access on the left side

a diathermy or energy device, the thoracoscope is then placed on the inferior edge of the wound to be able to see the deeper areas. The pericardial fat is removed as much as possible to make the path to helium free from obstructions.

The is an alternative way to create the subxiphoid access through the subcostal space (Video 1). In this kind of approach we don't need to remove the xiphoid process and also the pericardial fatty tissue. It is more suitable for the left side resections in order to diminish compression to the heart. Extra care must be taken during to avoid damage of the diaphragm (Fig. 7).

Basics of Instrumentation

When the incision is longitudinal, the curved suction is usually inserted first into the pleural or mediastinal space through caudal part of the wound, then the diaphragm or the pericardium is pressed gently to pave the way for camera insertion.

After that, the assistant surgeon carefully inserts the camera through the upper part of the wound with the tip of the camera pointing to the lateral part of the chest wall. After the insertion for several centimeters, the assistant surgeon guides the camera's tip to the hilum of the lung or to the area of interest, and at the same time stabilizes the shaft of the camera in the caudal part of the wound (Fig. 8a), allowing the main surgeon to insert other instruments into the upper part of the wound. In addition to avoiding contamination of the camera lens during the insertion, this method can avert any struggle or sword fighting between the thoracoscopic camera and the rest of instruments.

Coordination between the surgeon and his assistant are crucial in subxiphoid operations. The assistant should be placed in the back of the patient (Fig. 8b). Usually, the assistant surgeon has to hold and guide the camera in one hand most of the time during the operation, while the other hand holding the lung grasper in order to provide the countertraction necessary to enable the surgeon to conduct the dissection of the hilar structures.

The main surgeon usually uses his dominant hand to carry out the dissection or to perform movements that require precision, while using his other hand, mainly for support. The non-dominant hand usually controls the suction whose functions are to keep the surgical field clean of blood and smoke in addition to its benefit in obligating the retraction and tissue exposure in specific areas.

Subxiphoid Technique for Lobectomy

Right Upper Lobectomy (Video 2)

The authors believe that there is no oncological importance for a particular sequence of the division of the hilar structures, so we follow the dividing sequence which is appropriate to the situation. However, in the cases of upper lobectomies, it is more convenient to divide the lobar vein first. Once the thoracic cavity has been entered and explored, any adhesions in the way should be removed, a curved tip long ring forceps is used to grasp the right upper lobe at the area of S3 (Fig. 9a, b) and then retract the lobe posteriorly and inferiorly. This will expose the anterior-superior area of the right hilum. The right upper pulmonary vein identified, and the branch to the upper lobe is identified and distinguished from the branch to the middle lobe. The parietal pleura anterior to the vein is divided with caution not to injure the phrenic nerve which should be swept medially. Dissection of the hilar structures could be done using a long curved spatula, hook or energy device according to the preference of the surgeon while on the other hand the suction is used for assisting the dissection as discussed before. The dissection behind the vein is done by a right angle or an obtuse angle dissector. After the vein is encircled, a thread of silk or

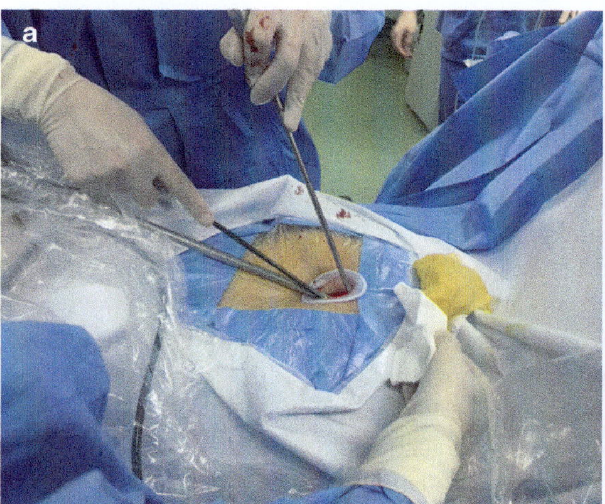

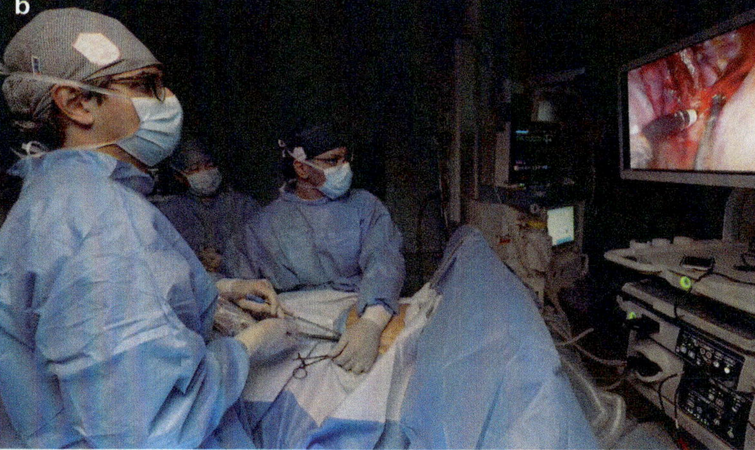

Fig. 8 (**a**) Instrumentation through longitudinal incision. (**b**) Position of surgeon and assistant during a right upper lobectomy

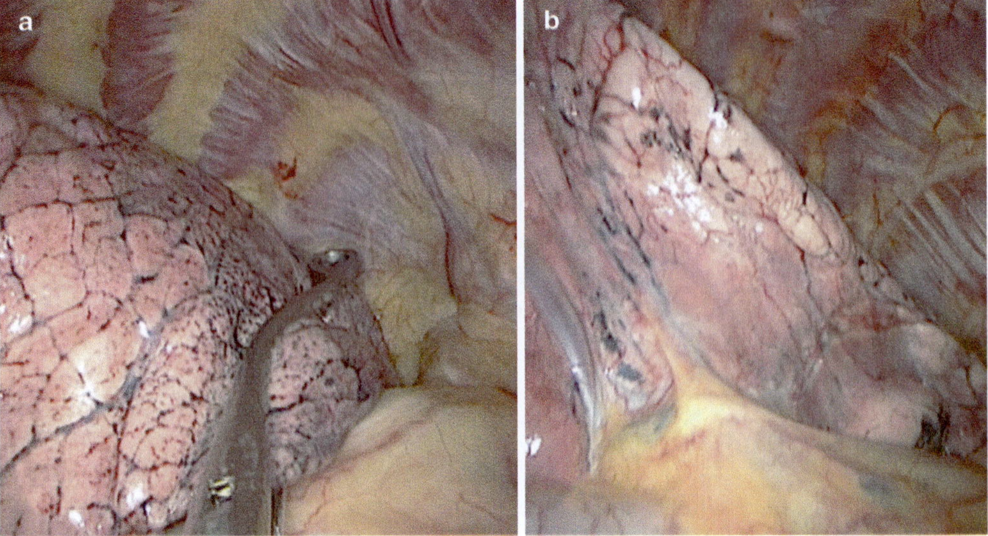

Fig. 9 (**a**) Grasping S3 during RUL lobectomy. (**b**) Retraction of S3 during RUL lobectomy

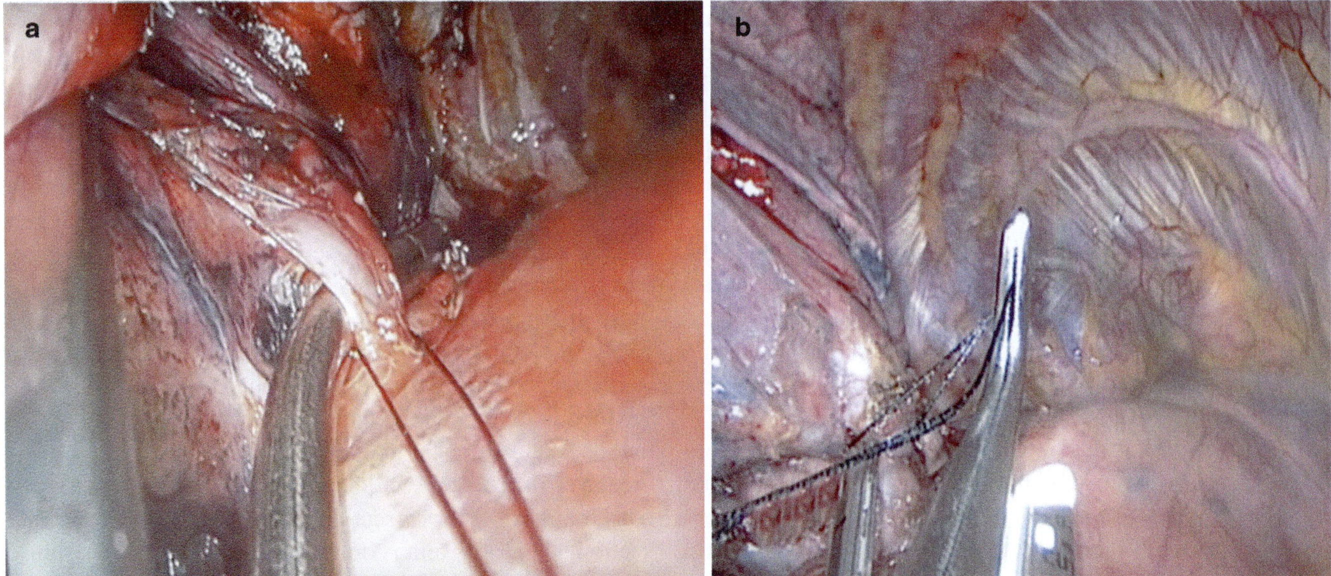

Fig. 10 Retraction of the right upper lobe vein to facilitate introducing the stapler by using a suction device (**a**) or by using a lateral traction with a silk thread (**b**)

rubbery vessel loop is placed around it (Fig. 10a). The vein then pulled slightly anteriorly to facilitate insertion of the stapler behind the vein. Alternatively, a curved-tip vascular stapler could be used to facilitate the passage around the structures. Another way to facilitate the passage of the stapler is to pass the curved suction first behind the vein (Fig. 10b) and then to turn it gently counterclockwise, this will provide a room for the passage of the stapler in addition to its usefulness to protect the artery from being injured during advancing the Stapler. After that, the truncus anterior branch (A1, A3) can be dissected in the same manner with the obtuse dissector and divided with the endo-GIA vascular stapler (Fig. 11a). The same dissector is used to dissect and encircle the bronchus to the right upper lobe. For better exposure in this stage, the traction grasper is moved to the area of S1 and then the lobe pulled inferiorly. Dissection around the bronchus should be far posterior as possible to avoid dissection within the parenchymal tissue. After encircling the bronchus, inflation test should be done as a routine then a bronchial stapler introduced in the same direction of the dissection (posterior as possible) (Fig. 11b). The posterior ascending artery (A2) then controlled and tied, clipped (vascular polymer clips) or stapled (Fig. 11c). This part could be the most dangerous and challenging part of the procedure and sometimes this branch could be identified at the crotch between the takeoff of the right upper lobe bronchus. In this case, it should be divided before dissecting and dividing the bronchus.

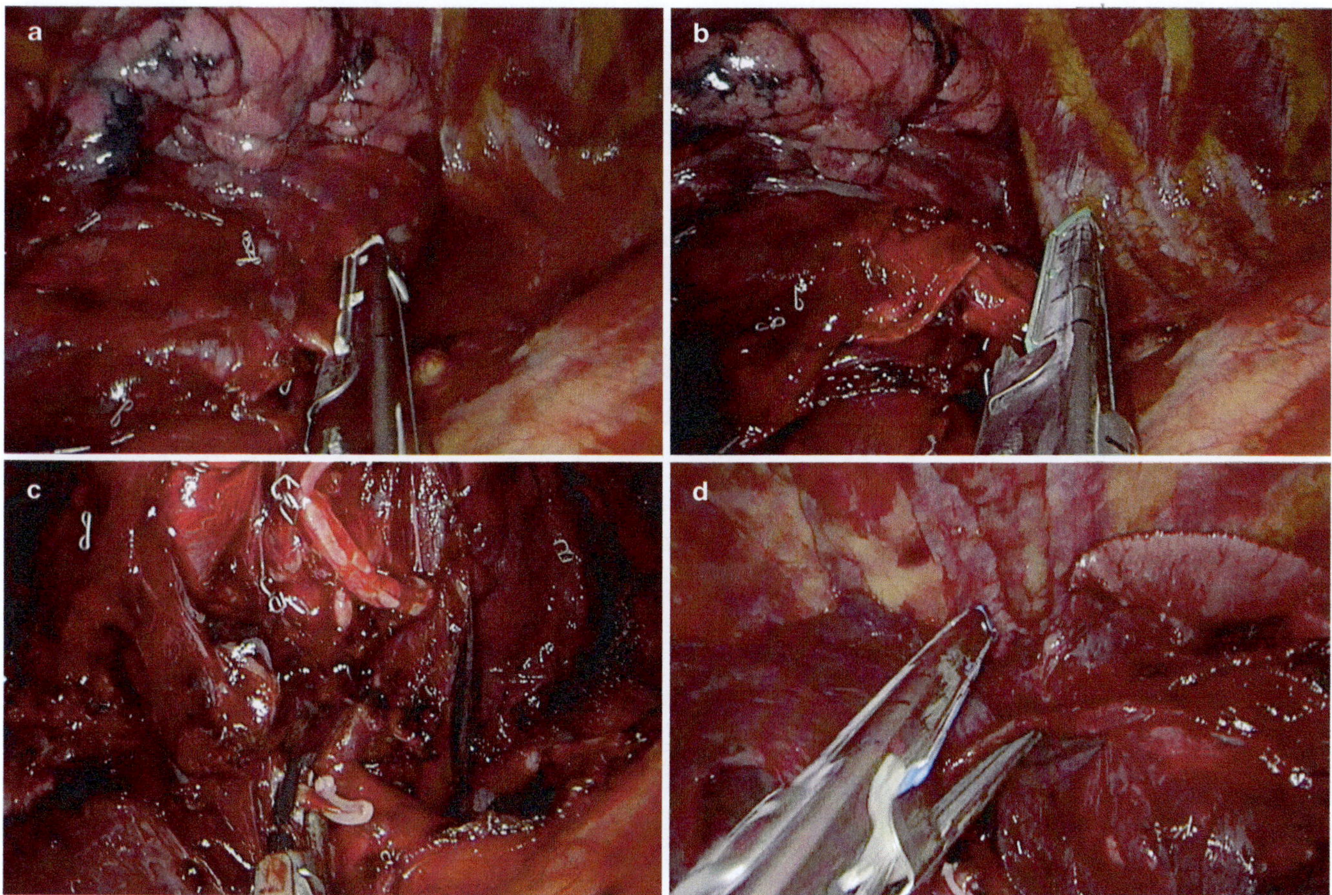

Fig. 11 (**a**) Division of truncus anterior during right upper lobectomy. (**b**) Oblique insertion of stapler for bronchial transection. (**c**) Division of posterior ascending artery with vascular clips for proximal control and energy devices for distal transection. (**d**) Completion of the posterior part of the fissure

In addition to all the mentioned above, the surgeon must be aware of the significant variations in the anatomy of the pulmonary artery, especially in the upper lobes. The upper lobes branches of the PA may vary from 2 to 5 branches in the right side and from 3 to 8 branches on the left-hand side.

The last step in the lobectomy is dividing the interlobar fissure (Fig. 11d). If the fissure is not well developed and its features are not clear, the distinctive mark of the border between the upper and middle lobe is the middle lobe vein. The lobe is grasped at the S3 area again and the fissure is then divided using multiple fires of endo-GIA reloads, starting from the anterior part of the fissure towards its posterior part, keeping in mind that the vein to the middle lobe is located inferior to the stapler while the distal stump of the bronchus and vascular structures are located superior to the stapler to be included in the resection. The specimen should be removed from the thoracic cavity using a protecting bag. Dividing the inferior pulmonary ligament is not a routine in the authors' practice, it could be performed if the surgeon noticed a large residual space by the end of the procedure.

Right Middle Lobectomy (Video 3)

It is probably the easiest major resection through the subxiphoid approach. The first step in middle lobectomy is the identification of the middle lobe vein which should be distinguished from the branches to the upper lobe. The lower lobe vein should be identified as well in order to exclude the presence of common venous trunk or any other abnormality (Fig. 12a). The middle lobe is then grasped and retracted posteriorly. This will expose the anterior aspect of the right hilum. The parietal pleura anterior to the vein is divided with caution not to injure the phrenic nerve which should be swept medially. The vein is dissected, encircled and divided using vascular endo GIA stapler. After that, the lobe should be retracted superiorly and the arterial branches to the middle lobe are approached through the fissure. A single dominant branch arises from the anterior surface of main PA, this branch could be found just inferior to the anterior part of the major fissure and it gives two short segmental branches (A4 and A5). Dividing the artery could be performed after dividing the bronchus in a case of undeveloped major fissure but if the fissure is well developed the author recommends dividing the artery before the bronchus using vascular endo-

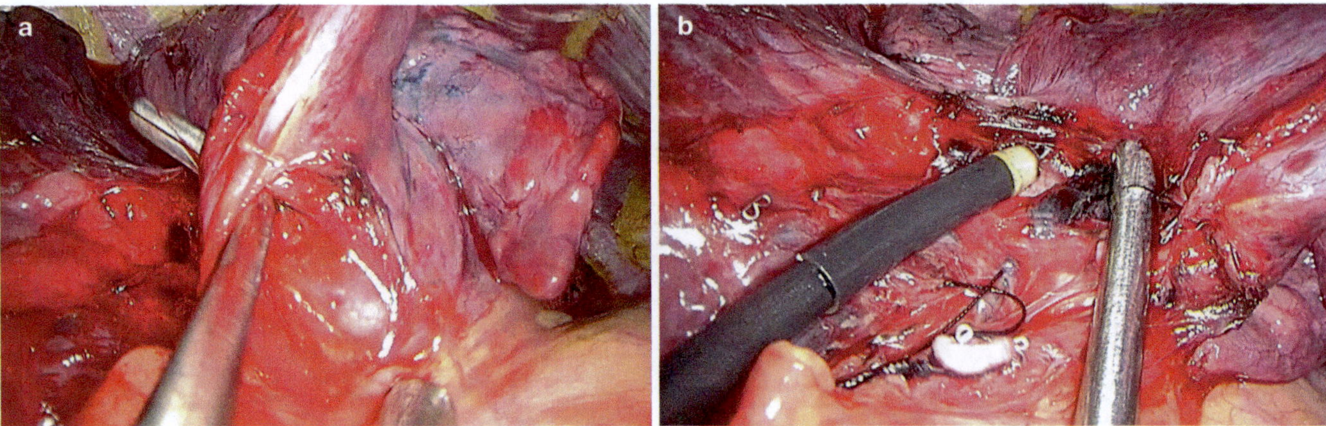

Fig. 12 (a) Retraction of middle lobe and dissection of middle lobe vein. (b) Dissection of lymph nodes is the fissure

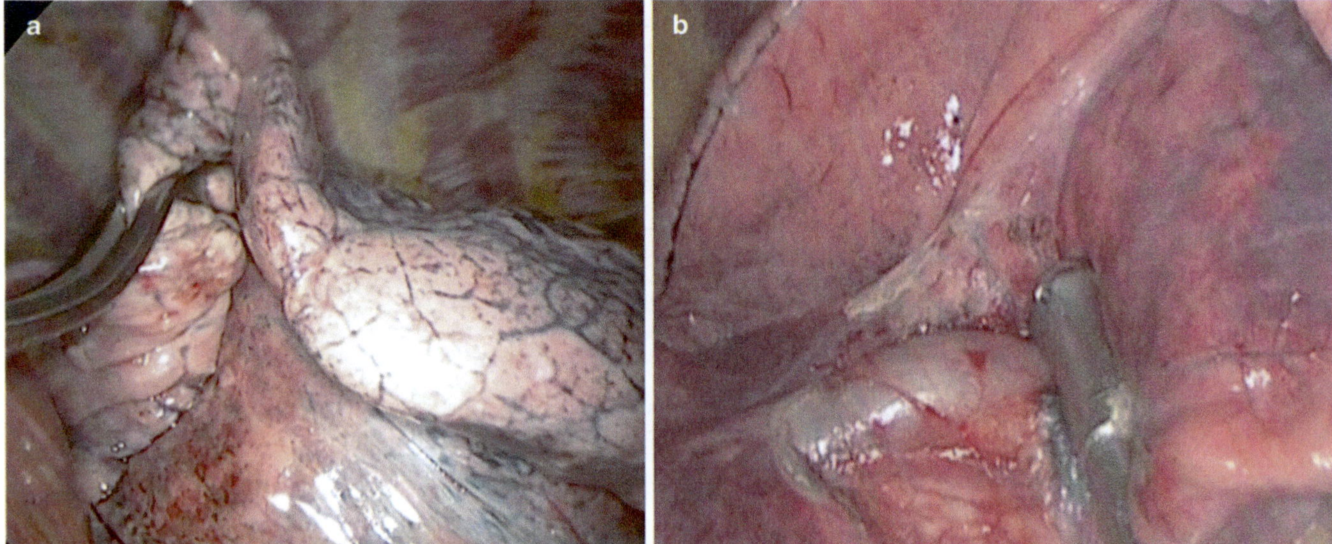

Fig. 13 (a) Grasping S8 during RLL lobectomy. (b) Exposing the artery during lower lobectomy

GIA reload. It is very important to remove the lymph nodes around the artery and bronchus to better define the anatomy (Fig. 12b). Alternatively, the arterial branches could be ligated or double clipped then divided with an energy device. The arterial anatomical variations are not uncommon in the middle lobectomy as well, separate segmental branches or multiple branches could be noticed in up to 50% of the cases of middle lobectomy [15, 16]. The lobe is then retracted posteriorly again in order to expose the middle lobe bronchus, which usually presents in-between the artery and the vein to the middle lobe. The bronchus is divided with an endovascular stapler. The parenchyma at the region of the minor fissure (between the middle and upper lobe) is then divided with an endo-GIA stapler according to its thickness. We must check that the distal stumps of the bronchus and vascular structures are above the stapler to be included in the resection. The specimen should be removed from the thoracic cavity using a protecting bag.

Right Lower Lobectomy (Video 4)

The sequence of steps for a right lower lobectomy usually begins with the dividing of the artery and then the bronchus and ends with dividing the vein. After grasping the lower lobe at the area of (S7–S8) and retract it caudally (Fig. 13a), we usually start by looking for the lower lobe artery inside the fissure that is dissected (Fig. 13b), encircled and stapled using vascular endo-GIA reload. Branch for the superior segment of the lower lobe (S6) should be identified and divided together with the basal trunk but alternatively, the two branches could be divided separately. Caution should be taken not to compromise the arterial branch to the middle lobe. The bronchus is then dissected, encircled and stapled using endo-GIA reload. It's important to make sure that the bronchus for the middle lobe is patent by performing the inflation test before firing the stapler. The inferior pulmonary ligament then transected and the inferior pulmonary vein

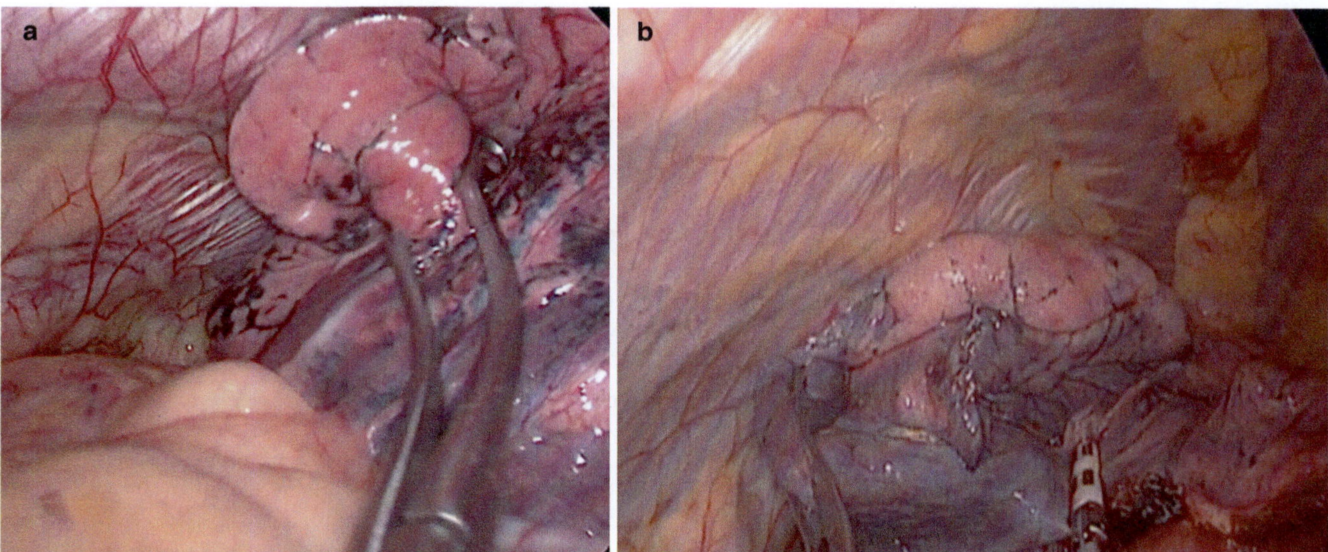

Fig. 14 (**a**) Grasping S3 during LUL lobectomy. (**b**) Retracting S2 anteriorly during LUL lobectomy

encircled and divided with vascular stapler when the fissure is fused, the fissureless technique could be done by starting from the bottom to top (from caudad to cephalad) i.e.: taking down the pulmonary ligament first then the vein is divided, the bronchus and finally the artery could be divided before dividing the parenchyma of the fissure. If the artery could be divided from the parenchyma, that would be ideal. Otherwise, and for safety manner, the artery could be stapled together with the parenchyma.

Often the diaphragm may be an obstacle for reaching the region of the inferior pulmonary ligament and the lower pulmonary vein. This problem can be overcome by changing the patient's position into (Anti-Trendelenburg) and compressing the diaphragm by the suction device during the procedure.

Left Upper Lobectomy (Video 5)

Anatomical wise, this lobectomy is the most complex among the five lobectomies. This mainly may be due to variations in the number and location of arterial branches. Approaching the left upper lobe via the subxiphoid approach may increase the complexity of the procedure. The presence of the heart on the left side may be an impediment to instrumentation which may be a challenge to the surgeon during the operation. The lobe grasped at the area of S3 and then retracted posteriorly and inferiorly (Fig. 14a). This will expose the anterior-superior area of the left hilum. The left upper pulmonary vein identified, encircled and divided first with vascular endo-GIA reload the curved tip staplers are very helpful in this step. This will expose the anterior and superior parts of the left main pulmonary artery. The upper lobe branches of this artery are dissected, encircled and divided sequentially and clockwise, starting with the truncus anterior which is usually the origin of two branches (A1, A3), then the feeding artery of the posterior segment (A2), ending with the feeder branches of the lingular segment (A4, A5). During the dissection of the posterior branch, the lobe is grasped at S2 area and retracted anteriorly (Fig. 14b), while during dissecting the lingular branches the lobe should be retracted superiorly by grasping the lingular from its edge at the fissure. The arterial branches could be divided by applying double clips or double ties on the proximal part of the branch and cut the distal part using an energy device. Alternatively, a vascular stapler could be used. The parenchyma then is divided and finally the bronchus. If the fissure is not well developed, "fissure-less" technique could be done by dividing the structures from top to bottom, leaving the posterior and lingular branches to the end just before completing the fissure.

Left Lower Lobectomy (Video 6)

The difficulty with this process lies in the fact that it is performed in the lower part of the left side. The heart and the diaphragm may be a serious obstacle to the procedure being performed comfortably. The authors advise the surgeons to have extensive experience in uniportal subxiphoid VATS before deciding to perform such a procedure. All heart diseases, especially CAD, heart arrhythmia, and cardiomegaly are absolute contraindication to perform left lower lobectomy through the subxiphoid approach. In addition, there are some relative contraindications such as excess obesity and COPD.

After entry to the left pleural space, the lower lobe grasped at the area of (S7–S8) and retract it caudally, we usually start by looking for the lower lobe artery inside the fissure that is dissected (Fig. 15a), encircled and stapled using a vascular stapler. Branch for the superior segment

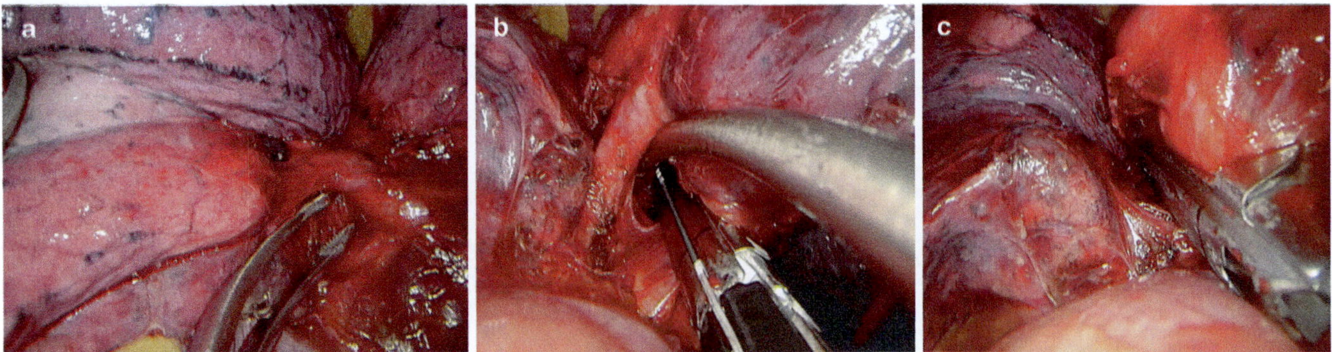

Fig. 15 (**a**) Dissection of basal trunk during RLL. (**b**) Division of inferior pulmonary vein. (**c**) Division of right lower lobe bronchus

of the left lower lobe (S6) should be identified and divided together with the basal trunk but alternatively, the two branches could be divided separately. Caution should be taken not to compromise the arterial branch to the lingular. The inferior pulmonary ligament is then transected and the left inferior pulmonary vein encircled and divided with vascular stapler (Fig. 15b). This step may necessitate some pressure on the pericardium and diaphragm. The bronchus is then dissected, encircled and stapled using the endo-GIA reload (Fig. 15c). When the fissure is fused, the fissureless technique could be done by starting from the bottom to top (from caudad to cephalad) i.e.: the lung grasped at the area of S8 and retracted cephalad. Taking down the pulmonary ligament first then the vein is divided, the bronchus and finally the artery before dividing the parenchyma of the fissure. If the artery could be divided from the parenchyma, that would be ideal. Otherwise, and for the safety manner, the artery could be stapled together with the parenchyma.

Thymectomy and Anterior Mediastinal Mass Resection (Video 7)

The subxiphoid approach is an excellent approach to perform surgery in both sides of the chest, therefore the resection of mediastinal masses is ideal with this technique. When the angle between the two costal margins is narrow (<90°) we preferred the vertical incision, while the transverse incision was chosen when the angle is wide (>90°). The subcutaneous tissue is dissected and the insertions of the rectus muscles to the coastal arches are divided along the midline. The cartilaginous xiphoid process is excised using surgical scissors. At this point, the collapse of the right lung is induced. The anterior mediastinum is opened from below, and a retrosternal tunnel is created by blunt digital dissection. A wound protector is applied through which the thoracoscope and all thoracoscopic instruments are introduced. In the vertical incision, in order to avoid crowding and instrumental interference, the video thoracoscope was placed at the most inferior part of the wound during the operation. Conversely, the video thoracoscope is alternatively placed at the two lateral angles when the incision is transverse. Most of the thymic tissue dissection is performed using a long endoscopic curved tip cautery in addition to energy devices and long curved tip instruments specially designed for subxiphoid procedures (Fig. 16). The mediastinal pleura is bilaterally cut near the sternal surface up to the level of the right internal thoracic vein. Bilateral opening the pleura from the start provide a great advantage of facilitating the exposure of the anterior mediastinum since it moves posteriorly giving wider space for instrumentation. The pericardial fat, the thymus gland, right and left epi-phrenic fat pads are dissected from the pericardium and diaphragm using a long curved spatula and ring forceps. Dissection proceeds cephalad under the thoracoscopic visualization in an en-bloc fashion. The phrenic nerves from both sides represent the lateral margins of dissection. The dissection proceeds superiorly until the left innominate vein is visualized. The most crucial part of this operation is the dissection of the adipose tissue from the innominate vein in order to expose the thymic veins. At this point, the operating table is rotated to the left side with the elevation of the right side, improving access to the innominate-cava angle thereby improving exposure and safety of the dissection. The right thymic horn is dissected and pulled to the left side by a ring forceps then divided at its most cranial point. The thymic veins (usually 1–4) are clipped and divided close to the left innominate vein using an energy device. At this point, the collapse of the left lung is induced while the right lung is re-ventilated. The left pericardial fat is dissected free from the pericardium while the adipose tissue is removed from the aorta-pulmonary window. The left thymic horn is dissected and divided in its most cranial point after retracting it caudally and to the right side. The specimen is extracted from the same incision after placing it in a retrieval bag. Hemostasis is ensured, and two 28 Fr chest tubes are inserted through the same incision while bilateral lung ventilation is resumed, and the wound closed in layers.

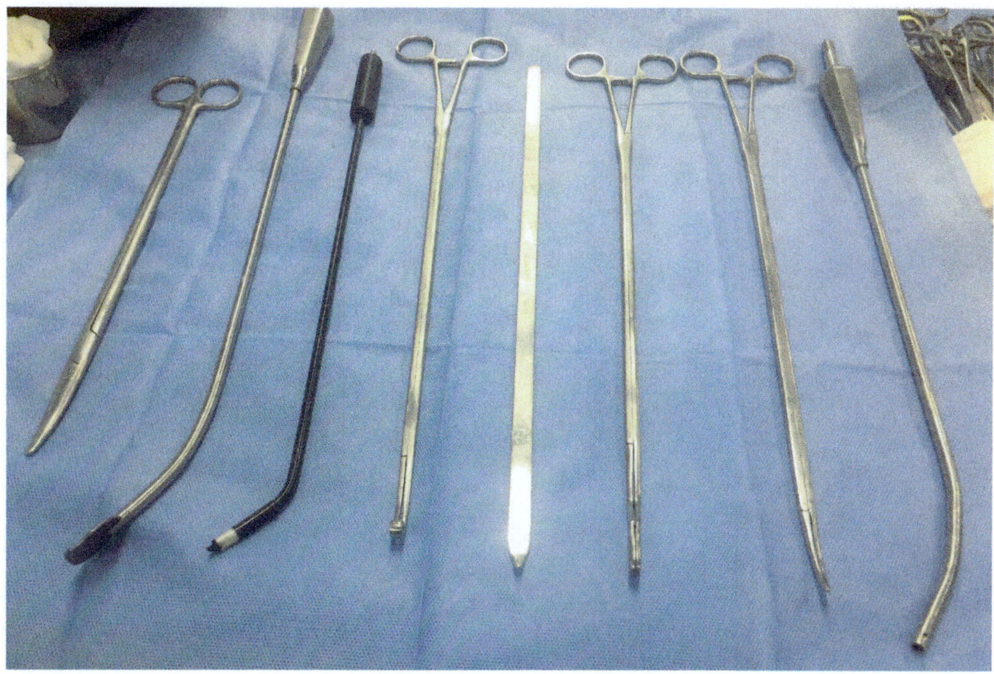

Fig. 16 Long and curved thoracoscopic Instruments for subxiphoid surgeries

Specimen Removal

For good oncological practice, each specimen must go out inside a protecting sack in order to prevent shedding of the cancer cells into the thoracic cavity or wound. The bag usually introduced through the same incision, and once it's inside the shaft of is fixed to the inferior part of the incision and the specimen and the sample pulled to be placed inside the bag using a thoracoscopic lung grasper (Fig. 17). When taking out the sample (especially large samples) through the subxiphoid incision, attention should be paid to the blood pressure of the patient and to be aware of the possibility of the impaction of the sample and compressing the heart causing a tamponade-like effect. When this occurs, the sample must be pushed back into the thoracic cavity immediately and think of another strategy for its removal, such as extending the wound; creating another opening or taking out the sample in stages after being divided inside the bag.

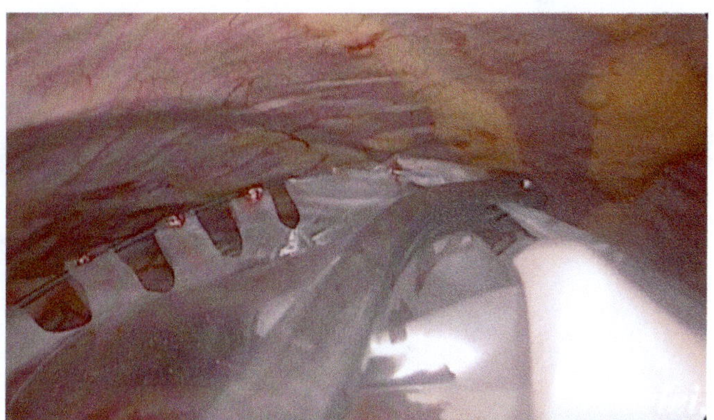

Fig. 17 Retrieval bag

Mediastinal and Hilar Lymph Nodes Dissection

The exposure in lymph node stations in subxiphoid approach is much more limited than the intercostal approach. All the lymph nodes stations could be dissected or sampled, but experience and special instruments designed for subxiphoid are the most important factors to ensure the success of the process. Experience in bimanual instrumentation and adequate manipulation of the lung is crucial for proper technique.

In the right side dissecting station 2–4 started after completion of the lobectomy. The upper lobe grasped at the area of S1 and retracted caudally. The pleura is open parallel with the azygos arch starting at the inferior aspect of the angle between the arch of azygos vein and the SVC which should be retracted laterally (Fig. 18), and the medial part of the azygos arch dissected from the underneath tissue. The azygos arch then retracted laterally using the suction device in order to facilitate the access to the paratracheal space. Alternatively, the azygos vein can be stapled. The dissection started then from caudal to cephalad using lymph node grasper and energy device to grasp the lymph node packet and separate it from the mediastinal structure. Station 4 and 2 packets could be removed en-bloc in between the anteriorly, trachea posteriorly, up to the right subclavian artery. Injury to the right recurrent laryngeal nerve, vagus nerve, and phrenic

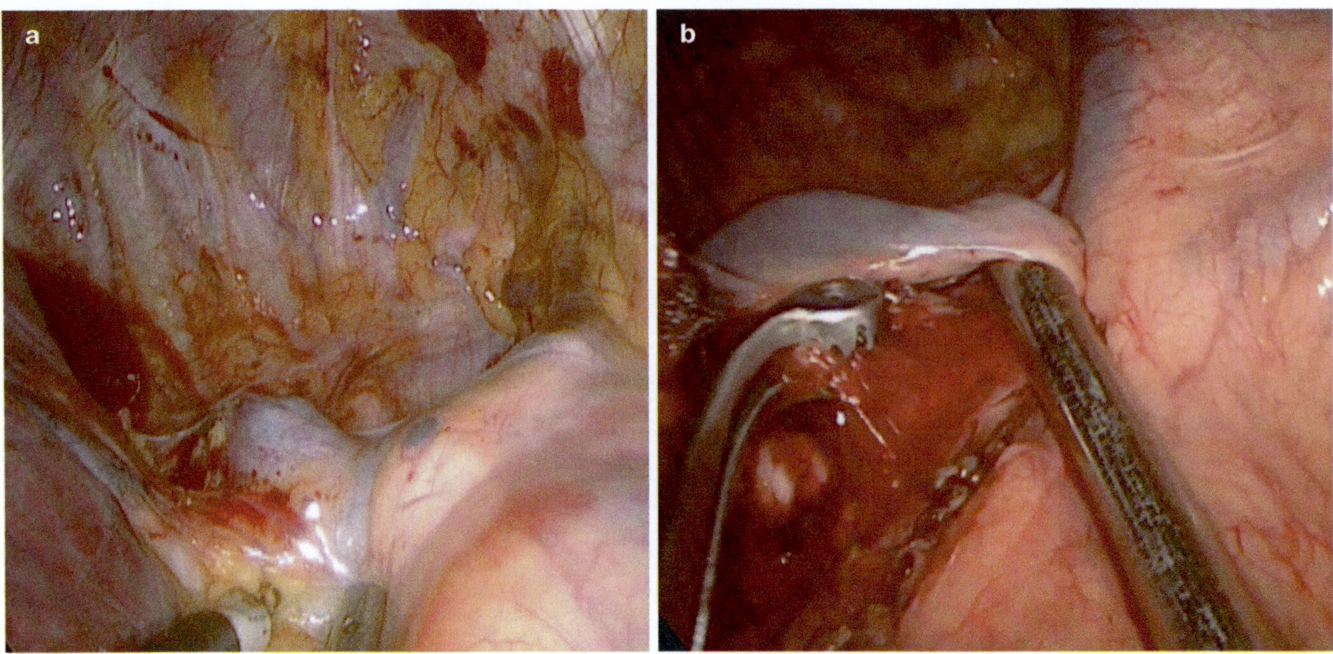

Fig. 18 (**a**) Starting LN dissection for station 4 at azygo-caval junction. (**b**) Retracting the SVC and grasping the node (station 4) during the lymph nodes dissection

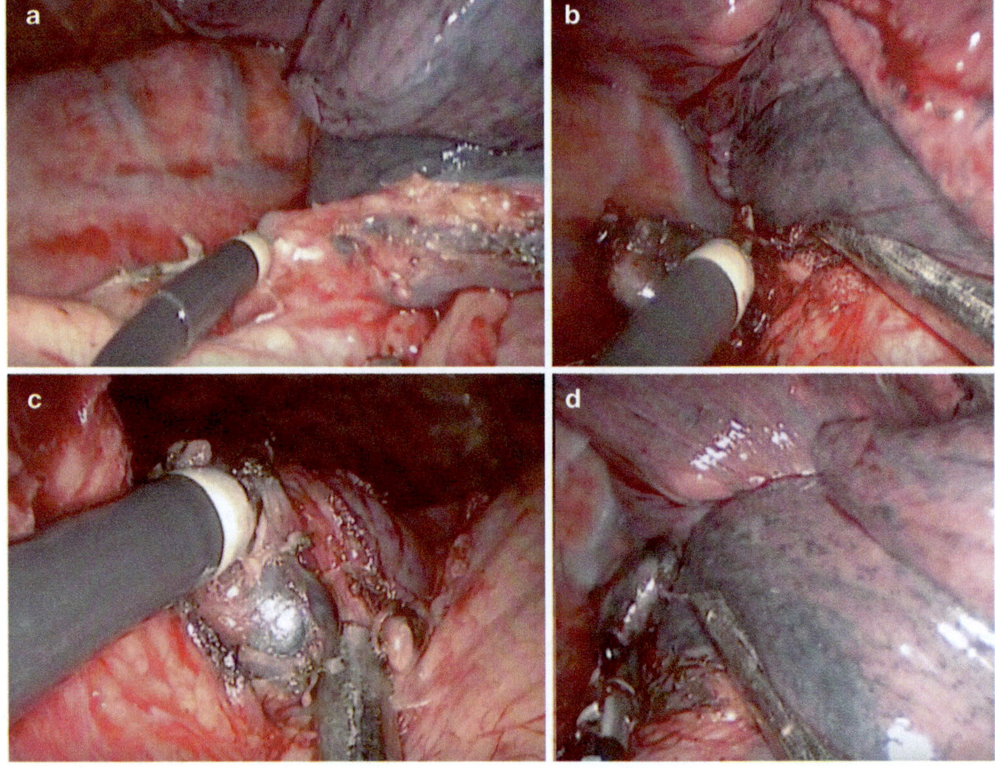

Fig. 19 (**a**) Station 7 lung retraction. (**b–d**) Dissection of lymph nodes station 7

nerve should be avoided during dissecting the superior part of the lymph node package. While esophageal, trachea, right PA, and pericardial injury should be avoided while dissecting the medial and inferior part of the packet. Exploring the area of dissection and meticulous hemostasis is of great importance after the lymph node dissection. Reaching the subcarinal space in order to dissect station [7] is quite challenging through the subxiphoid approach. If right the lower lobectomy did not performed, the lower lobe is grasped at the area of (S8) and retracted cephalad (Fig. 19a). The inferior pulmonary ligament is then divided in order to improve the exposure. The pleura is opened at the inferior border of the tracheal carina backward towards the esophagus, and the dissection of the lymph node packet is done from cephalad caudally until reaching the superior border of the left inferior pulmonary vein inferiorly and the pericardium medially (Fig. 19b–d).

In the left side, the dissection of stations 4–6 is even more challenging due to the proximity of the aortic arch, left PA, phrenic, vagus and left recurrent laryngeal nerves. The left upper lobe grasped (if didn't resected before) and retracted caudally, the dissection of lymph nodes stations are done with extra caution not to injure the surrounding structures. For dissecting station 7, the lung should be retracted anteriorly by grasping the area of (S2), achieving full lymph node dissection in this area is extremely difficult due to the limitation of the exposure and the length of left main stem bronchus.

Closure of the Wound

After hemostasis, one or two chest drain tube are inserted through the same port and fixed at the lateral part of the incision. In thymectomy cases, we usually put two drains, one in each pleural cavity and then we fix the tubes at both ends of the incision (Fig. 20) and we close the incision in layers.

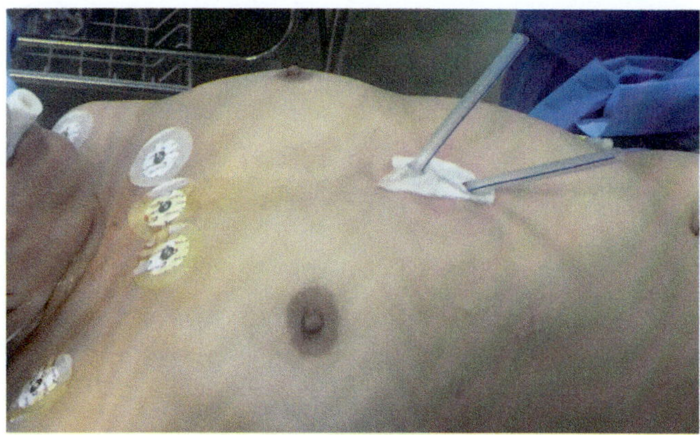

Fig. 20 Subxiphoid incision after closure with two chest tubes

References

1. Bertolaccini L, Viti A, Terzi A, Rocco G. Geometric and ergonomic characteristics of the uniportal video-assisted thoracoscopic surgery (VATS) approach. Ann Cardiothorac Surg. 2016;5(2):118–22.
2. Gonzalez-Rivas D. Keep calm and think uniportal. Video-assist Thorac Surg. 2016;1:15.
3. Akter F, Routledge T, Toufektzian L, Attia R. In minor and major thoracic procedures is uniport superior to multiport video-assisted thoracoscopic surgery? Interact Cardiovasc Thorac Surg. 2015;20(4):550–5.
4. Hao Z, Cai Y, Fu S, Zhang N, Fu X. Comparison study of post-operative pain and short-term quality of life between uniportal and three portal video-assisted thoracic surgery for radical lung cancer resection. Zhongguo Fei Ai Za Zhi. 2016;19(3):122–8.
5. Akar FA. Subxyphoid uniportal approach is it just a trend or the future of VATS. MOJ Surg. 2017;4(4):00076.
6. Zieliński M. Technique of transcervical-subxiphoid-VATS "maximal" thymectomy in treatment of myasthenia gravis. Przegl Lek. 2000;57(5):64–5.
7. Kido T, Hazama K, Inoue Y, Tanaka Y, Takao T. Resection of anterior mediastinal masses through an infrasternal approach. Ann Thorac Surg. 1999;67(1):263–5.
8. Liu CC, Wang BY, Shih CS. Ubxiphoid single-incision thoracoscopic left upper lobectomy. J Thorac Cardiovasc Surg. 2014;148:3250–1.
9. Hernandez-Arenas LA, Lin L, Yang Y, Liu M, Guido W, Gonzalez-Rivas D, Jiang G, Jiang L. Initial experience in uniportal subxiphoid video-assisted thoracoscopic surgery for major lung resections. Eur J Cardiothorac Surg. 2016;50(6):1060–6.
10. Hernandez-Arenas LA, Guido W, Jiang L. Learning curve and subxiphoid lung resections most common technical issues. J Vis Surg. 2016;2:117. https://doi.org/10.21037/jovs.2016.06.10.
11. Gonzalez-Rivas D, Lirio F, Sesma J, Abu Akar F. Subxiphoid uniportal video-assisted complex major pulmonary resections. J Vis Surg. 2017;3:93. https://doi.org/10.21037/jovs.2017.06.02.
12. Gonzalez-Rivas D, Yang Y, Lei J, Hernandez L, Jiang G. Subxiphoid uniportal video-assisted thoracoscopic middle lobectomy and anterior anatomic segmentectomy (S3). J Thorac Dis. 2016;8(3):540. https://doi.org/10.3978/j.issn.2072-1439.2016.02.63.
13. Aragón J, Pérez Méndez I. From open surgery to uniportal VATS: asturias experience. J Thorac Dis. 2014;6(Suppl 6):S644–9.
14. Guido Guerrero W, Hernandez Arenas LA, Jiang G, Yang Y, Gonzalez-Rivas D, Jiang L. Subxiphoid mediastinal lymphadenectomy. J Vis Surg. 2016;2:105.
15. Pearson FG, Cooper JD, Deslauriers J, et al. Anatomy of the lung. In: Thoracic surgery. 2nd ed. New York: Churchill Livingstone; 2002. p. 427–41.
16. Shields TW. Surgical anatomy of the lungs. In: Shields TW, LoCicero J, Ponn RB, et al., editors. General thoracic surgery. 7th ed. Philadelphia: Lippincott Williams & Wilkins; 2009.

Natural-Orifice Uniport VATS for Lung Resection

Ming-Ju Hsieh, Yen Chu, Yi-Cheng Wu, Chieng-Ying Liu, Tzu-Ping Chen, Yin-Kai Chao, Ching-Yang Wu, Chi-Ju Yeh, Po-Jen Ko, and Yun-Hen Liu

Introduction

Uniport video-assisted thoracoscopic surgery (VATS) was first reported in the mid-2000s. Since then, it has become an increasingly popular surgical technique for most thoracic surgery, and it has similar treatment outcomes that are comparable with those of traditional multiport VATS techniques. Unfortunately, postoperative wound discomfort and intercostal neuralgia have been found in a significant portion of patients [1–4].

Natural orifice surgery (NOS) is a surgical procedure that is performed through a natural orifice (the mouth, urethra, anus, or vagina) and avoids external skin incisions. NOS techniques offer several potential benefits that include less pain and improved cosmesis compared to thoracoscopic surgery [5–8]. The goal of this article is to provide a brief description of the development and potential future direction of natural-orifice uniport lung resection.

Historical Background

Kallo performed the first animal transgastric peritoneoscopy in 2004. All animals survived and gained weight until the end of the study. With the improvement of endoscopic instruments and surgical techniques, a variety of NOS in thoracic procedures has been described in porcine and canine models. These include transvesical, transgastric, transesophageal, transtracheal, transoral, and transumbilical approaches [9–17].

Electronic Supplementary Material The online version of this chapter (https://doi.org/10.1007/978-981-13-2604-2_37) contains supplementary material, which is available to authorized users.

M.-J. Hsieh · Y. Chu · Y.-C. Wu · C.-Y. Liu · T.-P. Chen
Y.-K. Chao · C.-Y. Wu · C.-J. Yeh · P.-J. Ko · Y.-H. Liu (✉)
Chang Gung Memorial Hospital, College of Medicine,
Chang Gung University, Taoyuan, Taiwan

Transvesical Approach

Lima and colleagues evaluated the feasibility of transvesical and transdiaphragmatic endoscopic approaches to access the pleural cavity and perform lung biopsies in six pigs. They described the feasibility of transvesical thoracoscopy via a 5-mm transvesical incision combined with a left diaphragmatic dome incision, and there were no complications [10]. However, no further work has provided new evidence to support the use of transvesicle thoracoscopy and whether it could be translated to clinical practice with benefits for patients.

Transgastric Approach

De Palma and colleagues reported the use of a transgastric approach to perform thoracic exploration and lung biopsy via gastric-wall and diaphragmatic incisions in four pigs. There were no adverse events during the peri- and postoperative periods, and they demonstrated the feasibility of transgastric thoracoscopy in a porcine model [11]. However, there have been no further larger animal series or human studies that specifically investigate transgastric thoracoscopy since the first report in 2010.

Transesophageal Approach

Fritscher-Ravens et al. first reported transesophageal NOS access to the mediastinum and pleural cavity in 2007 [18]. In 2011, the same group reported their experience with 12 pigs that underwent mediastinal lymph node resection with the transesophageal NOS technique (n = 46) and standard transthoracic VATS technique (n = 48). The authors determined that transesophageal NOS is a feasible approach for mediastinal lymph node resection without significant complications [19]. In 2012, Magno et al. reported that accessing the posterior mediastinum

D. Gonzalez-Rivas et al. (eds.), *Atlas of Uniportal Video Assisted Thoracic Surgery*,
https://doi.org/10.1007/978-981-13-2604-2_37

and thoracic vertebral bone biopsy were feasible and safe in a porcine model [20].

In another study, Moreira-Pinto et al. reported their experience with 14 pigs that underwent transesophageal pulmonary lobectomy. They demonstrated that right upper pulmonary lobectomy can be performed via transesophageal incision combined with a single transthoracic trocar incision. They concluded that transesophageal NOS may represent a step towards scar-free pulmonary lobectomy [21]. However, clinical application in humans has not started yet due to potential complications of tension pneumothorax caused by the injury of pleura and the lack of a device for secure esophagotomy closure.

Transtracheal Approach

Our teams have shown the feasibility of transtracheal endoscopic surgery in both canine and porcine models. In 2010, we reported the feasibility of evaluating the thoracic cavity and mediastinum using a single tracheal incision in two dogs [22]. In 2011, we reported experience with transtracheal thoracic exploration and pericardial window creation in 14 dogs. The results showed that transtracheal NOS is technically feasible but may be complicated by life-threatening lung injury and bleeding [13].

More recently, Khereba et al. reported the safety and feasibility of transtracheal pleuroscopy in eight swine without significant intraoperative complications. They used endobronchial ultrasound (EBUS) to locate a safe incision region in the trachea and avoid inadvertently perforating the vital mediastinal structures [23]. They reported that the trachea appears to be a safe port of entry for thoracic NOS in a swine model, but the technique is not yet ready for human trials.

Transoral Approach

In 2012, our team described experience with transoral surgical lung biopsy and pericardial window creation in canine models [17]. Later, we demonstrated the feasibility of using transoral incision to perform dorsal sympathectomy in the same model [24]. In 2013, we found that the transoral approach was comparable to conventional thoracoscopic surgery for small lung biopsy and pericardial window creation in terms of hemodynamic changes, inflammatory reaction, safety, and efficacy [25]. However, clinical trials in humans have not started yet due the small, limited workspace and small lung specimen removed via oral incision. It is necessary to collect more preclinical data before application in clinical practice.

Transumbilical Approach

Our team has investigated the feasibility of shifting the surgical wound from the standard intercostal space to the umbilical incision for thoracic surgery in canine models (Videos 1, 2, and 3). This technique has potential benefits of better avoiding of postoperative pulmonary complications and injury to the intercostal vessels and nerves. In 2013, we reported the feasibility of lung wedge resection using transumbilical incision in 12 dogs [15]. In 2014, we reported the feasibility of transumbilical lobectomy in 12 dogs, but the technique was associated with significant perioperative bleeding complications [26]. In 2016, we found that the transumbilical approach was comparable to conventional thoracoscopic surgery for lung wedge resection in terms of hemodynamic changes, inflammatory reaction, safety, and efficacy [27].

With growing experience, we completed a study on transumbilical segmentectomy in 10 dogs and demonstrated that transumbilical lung surgery can be completed with less postoperative morbidity and mortality (unpublished data). Regarding the clinical application of transumbilical thoracic surgery, Zhu et al. recently reported their experience with transumbilical thoracic sympathectomy in 148 patients with palmar hyperhidrosis. They concluded that transumbilical thoracic sympathectomy is a safe and effective alternative to conventional transthoracic thoracoscopic sympathectomy with less chest wall discomfort and better cosmetic benefits [28].

The major obstacle of the transumbilical approach in humans is the lack of long endoscopic instruments to reach the upper thoracic cavity. Another obstacle is the difficulty in evaluating the long-term sequelae of diaphragmatic incisions. Further studies are necessary to clarify the utility of the transumbilical approach in thoracic surgery.

Potential Future Direction

The development of NOS in thoracic surgery will primarily depend on the following factors. First, better health insurance payments and reimbursement policies are needed to facilitate the discovery of new diagnostic and therapeutic platforms for the treatment of thoracic disease. Second, investment in innovation is needed, including research and development on simple, safe, and convenient endoscopic instruments in industry. Third, collaboration in multidisciplinary teams is necessary, including scientists, researchers, and clinicians. Fourth, the anatomical and physical limitations of the human body should be addressed. For example, the long distance between the bladder and thoracic cavity is a major barrier to the transvesicle and transumbilical approach. Furthermore, the life-threatening complications, limited work-space, and lack of a simple device for NOS wound closure also lead to further restrictions of the transgastric, transesophageal, and transtracheal approaches.

With growing experience in both endoscopic and robotic operation, researchers in Korea have reported the feasibility of transoral robotic thyroidectomy in four patients [29]. Based on this report and the findings from our laboratory studies, we feel that robotic technology and the transoral periosteal approach may someday allow surgeons to perform simple thoracic procedures. However, further study is needed to prove the safety and efficacy of these methods.

References

1. Rocco G, Martin-Ucar A, Passera E, et al. Uniportal VATS wedge pulmonary resections. Ann Thorac Surg. 2004;77:726–8.
2. Gonzalez-Rivas D, Fieira E, Delgado M, et al. Uniportal video-assisted thoracoscopic sleeve lobectomy and other complex resections. J Thorac Dis. 2014;6(Suppl 6):S674–81.
3. Ocakcioglu I, Alpay L, Demir M, et al. Is single port enough in minimally surgery for pneumothorax? Surg Endosc. 2016;30(1):59–64.
4. Wang BY, Liu CY, Hsu PK, et al. Single-incision versus multiple-incision thoracoscopic lobectomy and segmentectomy: a propensity-matched analysis. Ann Surg. 2015;261:793.
5. Swanstrom LL, Kurian A, Dunst CM, et al. Long-term outcomes of an endoscopic myotomy for achalasia: the POEM procedure. Ann Surg. 2012;256:659.
6. Ujiki MB, Yetasook AK, Zapf M, et al. Peroral endoscopic myotomy: a short-term comparison with the standard laparoscopic approach. Surgery. 2013;154:893.
7. Lehmann KS, Ritz JP, Wibmer A, et al. The German registry for natural orifice translumenal endoscopic surgery: report of the first 551 patients. Ann Surg. 2010;252:263–70.
8. Chukwumah C, Zorron R, Marks JM, et al. Current status of natural orifice translumenal endoscopic surgery (NOTES). Curr Probl Surg. 2010;47:630–68.
9. Kalloo AN, Singh VK, Jagannath SB, et al. Flexible transgastric peritoneoscopy: a novel approach to diagnostic and therapeutic interventions in the peritoneal cavity. Gastrointest Endosc. 2004;60:114–7.
10. Lima E, Henriques-Coelho T, Rolanda C, et al. Transvesical thoracoscopy: a natural orifice translumenal endoscopic approach for thoracic surgery. Surg Endosc. 2007;21:854–8.
11. De Palma GD, Siciliano S, Addeo P, et al. A NOTES approach for thoracic surgery: transgastric thoracoscopy via a diaphragmatic incision in a survival porcine model. Minerva Chir. 2010;65:11–5.
12. Fritscher-Ravens A, Cuming T, Eisenberger CF, et al. Randomized comparative long-term survival study of endoscopic and thoracoscopic esophageal wall repair after NOTES mediastinoscopy in healthy and compromised animals. Endoscopy. 2010;42:468–74.
13. Liu YH, Wu YC, et al. Natural orifice transluminal endoscopic surgery: a transtracheal approach for the thoracic cavity in a live canine model. J Thorac Cardiovasc Surg. 2011;141:1223–30.
14. Liu YH, Wu YC, et al. Single-dose antimicrobial prophylaxis in transoral surgical lung biopsy: a preliminary experience. Surg Endosc. 2011;25:3912–7.
15. Lin TY, Chu Y, Wu YC, et al. Feasibility of transumbilical lung wedge resection in a canine model. J Laparoendosc Adv Surg Tech A. 2013;23:684–92.
16. Zhu LH, Chen L, Yang S, et al. Embryonic NOTES thoracic sympathectomy for palmar hyperhidrosis: results of a novel technique and comparison with the conventional VATS procedure. Surg Endosc. 2013;27:4124–9.
17. Ko PJ, Chu Y, Wu YC, et al. Feasibility of endoscopic transoral thoracic surgical lung biopsy and pericardial window creation. J Surg Res. 2012;175:207–14.
18. Fritscher-Ravens A, Patel K, Ghanbari A, et al. Natural orifice transluminal endoscopic surgery (NOTES) in the mediastinum: long-term survival animal experiments in transesophageal access, including minor surgical procedures. Endoscopy. 2007;39(10):870–5.
19. Fritscher-Ravens A, Cuming T, Olagbaiye F, et al. Endoscopic transesophageal vs. thoracoscopic removal of mediastinal lymph nodes: a prospective randomized trial in a long term animal survival model. Endoscopy. 2011;43:1090–6. https://doi.org/10.1055/s-0030-1256768.
20. Magno P, Khashab MA, Mas M, et al. Natural orifice translumenal endoscopic surgery for anterior spinal procedures. Minim Invasive Surg. 2012;2012:365814. https://doi.org/10.1155/2012/365814.
21. Moreira-Pinto J, Ferreira A, Miranda A, et al. Transesophageal pulmonary lobectomy with single transthoracic port assistance: study with survival assessment in a porcine model. Endoscopy. 2012;44:354–61.
22. Yang C, Liu HP, Chu Y, et al. Natural orifice transtracheal evaluation of the thoracic cavity and mediastinum. Surg Endosc. 2010;24:2905–7.
23. Khereba M, Thiffault V, Goudie E, et al. Transtracheal thoracic natural orifice transluminal endoscopic surgery (NOTES) in a swine model. Surg Endosc. 2016;30:783–8.
24. Yang C, Chu Y, Wu YC, et al. The lateral decubitus position improves transoral endoscopic access to the posterior aspects of the thorax. Surg Endosc. 2012;26:2988–92.
25. Chu Y, Liu CY, Wu YC, et al. Comparison of hemodynamic and inflammatory changes between transoral and transthoracic thoracoscopic surgery. PLoS One. 2013;8:e50338. https://doi.org/10.1371/journal.pone.0050338.
26. Yin SY, Chu Y, Wu YC, et al. Feasibility of transumbilical anatomic pulmonary lobectomy in a canine model. Surg Endosc. 2014;28:2980–7.
27. Lu HY, Chu Y, Wu YC, et al. Hemodynamic and inflammatory responses following transumbilical and transthoracic lung wedge resection in a live canine model. Int J Surg. 2015;16:116–22.
28. Zhu LH, Chen W, Chen L, et al. Transumbilical thoracic sympathectomy: a single-centre experience of 148 cases with up to 4 years of follow-up. Eur J Cardiothorac Surg. 2016;49(Suppl 1):i79–83.
29. Lee HY, You JY, Woo SU, et al. Transoral periosteal thyroidectomy: cadaver to human. Surg Endosc. 2015;29:898–904.

Natural Orifice Transluminal Endoscopic Surgery (NOTES) Uniportal VATS for Sympathectomy

Weisheng Chen

Abstract

Palmar hyperhidrosis (PH) is the symptom of excessive hand sweating caused by the erethism of the sympathetic nerve dominating the palmar sudoriferous. Compared to conventional thoracotomy, endoscopic thoracic sympathectomy has been recognized as the most effective way to treat this disease, as it achieves much improvement in minimizing the invasiveness. However, patients may partly suffer from chronic postoperative incisional pain, which is probably related to the stimulation of the intercostal nerve during the operation. To improve the situation, we introduced the concept of Natural Orifice Translumianl Endoscopic Surgery (NOTES), and carried out the experimental study of transumbilical thoracic sympathectomy. Furthermore, this surgical technique was applied to clinical treatment in April 2010 based on the great success of animal experiment. This surgical technique, which is mainly discussed in this chapter, has been proven to have advantages in reducing pain and improving cosmetic results after its application in nearly 200 clinical cases. The trial was approved by institutional review board of Fuzhou General Hospital, and informed consent was obtained from all participants and/or parents/LAR.

Inclusion and Exclusion Criteria

PH is an idiopathic disease featured by abnormal palmar sweating with no obvious cause, which exceeds normal physical need. Excessive palmar sweating that lasts for more than 6 months with the following two characteristics can be diagnosed as PH [1]: (1) bilateral and symmetrical; (2) symptoms with frequency of at least once a week; (3) age less than 25 years at the onset; (4) positive family history; (5) no hyperhidrosis during sleep; (6) affects daily life.

Inclusion Criteria

1. Diagnosed as PH;
2. Age between 12 and 50 years old;
3. Medium or heavy state according to the Lai scale [2];
4. Confirmation of the patient and family members to undergo the operation;
5. Willingness to undergo transumbilical endoscopic surgery after being informed of several other available surgical techniques.

Exclusion Criteria

1. Diagnosed as secondary hyperhidrosis;
2. History of thoracic or abdominal operation;
3. Previous history of thoracopathy such as pleural adhesions, pachynsis pleurae, or abdominal diseases such as peritonitis or intra-abdominal adhesions;
4. Bradycardia;
5. Coagulation disorders or cardiac, pulmonary, hepatic and renal dysfunctions, who could not endure conventional thoracic surgery.

Special Instruments and Equipments/Materials

Electronic gastroscope, ultrathin gastroscope, hot biopsy forceps and needle-knife for the ultrathin gastroscope. Self-made over-length trocar (Fig. 1): made of nontoxic/medical grade polyethylene by heating injection molding with a length of 50 cm, outside diameter of 6.5 mm, and inside

W. Chen (✉)
Department of Cardiothoracic Surgery, Fuzhou General Hospital, Fuzhou, China

D. Gonzalez-Rivas et al. (eds.), *Atlas of Uniportal Video Assisted Thoracic Surgery*,
https://doi.org/10.1007/978-981-13-2604-2_38

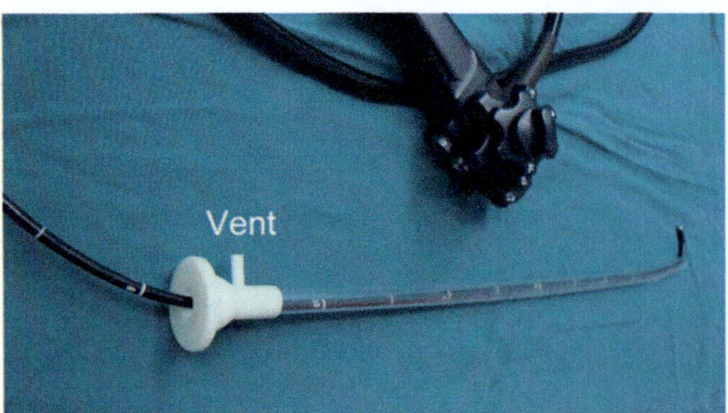

Fig. 1 Self-made over-length trocar

diameter of 5.5 mm. A 30 degree bend was made at the top of the trocar so that the bending of the gastroscope can be adjusted in the operation for better horizon.

Surgical Procedures

The supine position with upper limbs abducted (Fig. 2) and double lumen intubation were used for this surgery. After conventional disinfection and draping, a 5-mm arc incision is made along the inferior margin of the umbilicus, followed by the insertion of the special trocar through the incision. Carbon dioxide is injected through the trocar to establish pneumoperitoneum, with pressure stabilized between 8 and 12 mmHg using the pressure valve. The gastroscope can be inserted after all these procedures. The bare area of left diaphragm is chosen as the entry point of the thorax. A 5-mm incision is made on the left diaphragm using a needle-knife under the state of right side single lung ventilation (Fig. 3). Thus, the gastroscope can enter the left thoracic cavity through the incision on the diaphragm with the guidance of the needle-knife. The pneumoperitoneum is shut off after confirmation of pulmonary collapse. The sympathetic chain is identified along the neck of the ribs close to the costovertebral junctions, and the ganglions are localized in the corresponding intercostal space. Generally, the first rib is not visualized in the thoracic cavity, so the uppermost rib that could be seen is the second rib, followed by the third and fourth ribs (Fig. 4a). Hot biopsy forceps are used to grasp and ablate the T3 ganglia for palmar-only hyperhidrosis and to ablate the T3–T4 ganglias for combined palmar and axillary hyperhidrosis; the nerve of Kuntz and other branches was also interrupted (Fig. 4b). A palmar temperature increase of 1.5 °C confirmed adequate sympathectomy. Then the endoscope is recurved to check that no hemorrhaging had been caused by the incision in the diaphragm. The lung was fully re-expanded under the gastroscope, and the scope was pulled out from the thoracic cavity. The operating table was then tilted 30° to the left. Pneumoperitoneum was re-

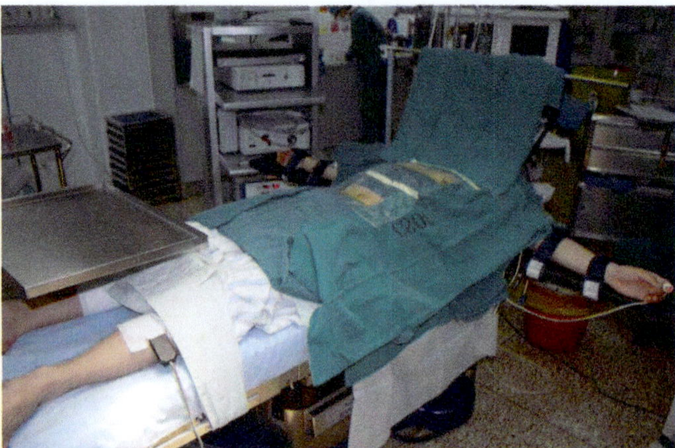

Fig. 2 Operative position

established with pressure stabilized between 5 and 8 mmHg using the pressure valve. Another incision is made on the right diaphragm under the state of left side single lung ventilation. Other procedures were the same to the left side after entering the right thoracic cavity. Bilateral lungs were expanded after removing the scope from the abdominal cavity. An aspirator is inserted through trocar to suck the gas left in the thoracic and abdominal cavity. The peritoneum and muscle was sutured, and the skin incision was close using tissue glue. Drainage tube for neither abdominal nor thoracic cavity was needed.

Postoperative Treatment and Care

Patients are sent in general wards after surgery, and chest X-ray was obtained after an hour. Patients with pneumothorax were monitored when lung compression was less than 30%, while closed thoracic drainage should be performed when lung compression is more than 30%. Patients with no obvious abnormity were allowed to be discharged on the second day.

Surgical Experience and Recommendation

Thoracic sympathectomy for PH treatment is often performed by a thoracic surgeon. The experience of operating a flexible endoscope for most thoracic surgeons is mainly acquired through the operation of the bronchoscope. Thus, less experience is acquired in gastrointestinal endoscopy, even some of the surgeon has never used a gastroscope. Therefore, the presence of a gastroscopy physician is suggested for guidance during the animal experiment stage and initial clinical application stage. It has been proven by the practice of our team that a thoracic surgeon with bronchoscope experience can operate the nasogastroscope to expertly complete the surgery

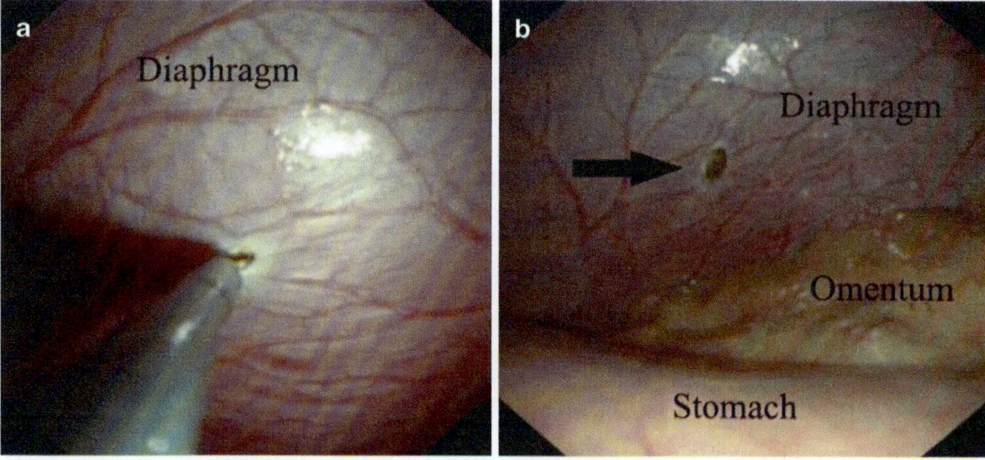

Fig. 3 Neostomy of the diaphragm under a gastroscope. (**a**) Made a 5-mm incision on the diaphragm with a needle-knife. (**b**) Position of the diaphragmatic incision

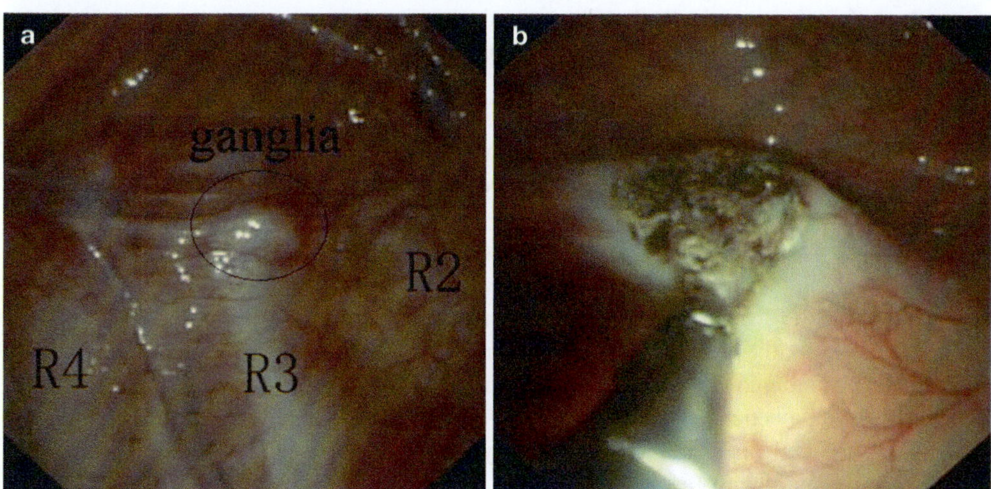

Fig. 4 Sympathicotomy under a gastroscope. (**a**) The ribs and the third ganglion. (**b**) Hot biopsy forceps is used to grasp and ablate the T3 ganglia

after 8–10 cases of animal experiments. However, some parts of the surgery still needs to be noted, as follows.

Umbilical Incision

Arc incision along the inner side of the upper margin of the umbilicus is suggested to obtain a better cosmetic result, which can be covered by the dropping abdominal adipose tissues. Thus, no scar can be seen. A conventional 5-mm trocar can be used first if the over-length trocar is difficult to be inserted, which can be switched after pneumoperitoneum is established.

Diaphragm Incision

Diaphragmectomy is the most important part of the surgery. The location of the neostomy is suggested at the superior border of the costal part of the diaphragm for several reasons. First, the heart, lung and other organs can be avoided at this part to ensure safety. Second, thick muscles in this place provide better healing after surgery. Third, a top-down view is offered when the gastroscope passes the incision, which is important for flexible endoscope without the support of a trocar. If the neostomy point is too low, the body of the gastroscope would go along the chest wall, providing a parallel view that is inconvenient for surgery.

The length of the needle-knife should be controlled well, since a long needle could directly impale the diaphragm, increasing the risk of lung or chest vessel damage; while a short needle cannot stab into the diaphragm deep enough, and will slide on the surface of diaphragm due to the contraction of the diaphragm stimulated by the electric current, causing a big incision or damage the visceral organs. Therefore, half of the needle is suggested. By holding the needle-knife against the diaphragm, the width of the neostomy can be controlled well. Locating with laparoscope for diaphragmectomy is suggested in the early stage of promoting the surgery for better image definition, in which the vessel distribution can be identified and hemorrhage is prevented. Small hemorrhages can be stopped using heating biopsy forceps during diaphragmectomy.

A small incision on the diaphragm which allows the gastroscope to barely go through is the best. A needle-knife can be used as a guidewire when it is difficult for the gastroscope to enter the incision. Hold the over-length trocar against the incision to maintain the incision at the extension state. Spin the scope body so that the scope can enter the thoracic cavity smoothly.

Intrathoracic Operation

Intrathoracic operation is a familiar procedure for thoracic surgeons, but its horizon is different from the thoracoscope due to different approaches. The thoracic sympathetic ganglion that needs to be burnt can be easily covered by the collapsed lung. It is our experience that the patient's position or operating table should be adjusted before the lung collapses. The right side operation can be performed in a dorsal elevated position slightly leaning to the left, while the left side operation can be performed in dorsal elevated position slightly leaning to the right. The visual operative field can be exposed well with the help of the gravity of the lung.

The first rib is mostly not visualized because it lies in a completely different plane and direction from the others. Thus, identification of the second and third rib was critical, which can be used to mark the ganglions. Location of interruption of sympathetic chain based on patient's distribution of sweating. T3 thoracic sympathetic ganglion is resected for single PH patients. For PH patients combined with axillary hyperhidrosis, T3 + T4 thoracic sympathectomy is performed.

Advantages and Disadvantages of This Surgery

Thoracoscopic thoracic sympathectomy is considered as one of the easiest thoracic surgery. Trauma of the thoracoscope is reduced due to the improvement of instruments and narrowing of the incision. But in the thoracoscope procedure, chest wall incisions can be associated with chronic neuropathic pain in up to 25% of patients [3]. Furthermore, a clinical study of 406 consecutive VATS sympathectomies reported that 93% of patients had wound pain at the time of discharge, 59.1% of patients experienced pain of more than 15 days' duration, and 15% of patients experienced dysesthesia [4]. A 4-year follow-up study of transumbilical and VATS thoracic sympathectomy patients was conducted by our team. Results showed in the tables (Tables 1 and 2) revealed that transumbilical thoracic sympathectomy is a safe and efficacious alternative to the conventional approach. This novel procedure can further reduce postoperative pain and chest wall paresthesia as well as afford maximum cosmetic benefits by hiding the surgical incision in the umbilicus [5]. However, it is undeniable that the operative time for transumbilical thoracic sympathectomy was longer than that of VATS thoracic sympathectomy. In addition, there is currently no effective device to deal with blood loss and pulmonary adhesions. As a result, patients with severe pulmonary or abdominal adhesions were not candidates for the procedure.

Table 1 Operative details

Demographics	E-NOTES (n = 148)	VATS (n = 44)	P-value
Level of sympathectomy, n (%)			
T3	81 (54.7)	23 (52.3)	0.77
T3 + T4	67 (45.3)	21 (47.7)	
Operating details, mean (range)			
Operating time, minutes	43 (39–107)	32 (25–43)	<0.001
Mean rise of palmar temperature, degrees	1.8 (1.5–4.1)	2.0 (1.5–4.5)	0.58
Postoperative hospital stay, days	1.4 ± 0.4	1.5 ± 0.4	0.44
Intraoperative complications, n (%)			
Bleeding	2 (1.4)	0 (0)	1.00
Complication immediately postoperatively, n (%)			
Pneumothorax	7 (4.7)	2 (4.5)	1.00

Table 2 Follow-up results

Demographics	E-NOTES (n = 148)	VATS (n = 44)	P-value
Pain score (visual analogue scale)			
Four hours after operation	1.7 ± 0.5	3.6 ± 0.7	<0.001
Eight hours after operation	3.5 ± 0.7	5.1 ± 0.8	<0.001
Twelve hours after operation	2.1 ± 0.8	4.6 ± 0.6	<0.001
Paresthesia: n (%)			
One day post-operation	31 (20.1)	17 (38.6)	0.017
One week post-operation	6 (4.1)	8 (18.2)	0.005
One month post-operation	0 (0.0)	4 (9.1)	0.002
Surgical results, n (%)			
PH complete resolution	145 (98.0)	43 (97.7)	1.000
AH complete resolution	50 (74.6)	16 (76.2)	0.885
PH recurred	2 (1.4)	1 (2.3)	1.000
Compensatory sweating, n (%)			
Mild	24 (16.2)	6 (13.6)	0.606
Moderate	6 (4.1)	3 (6.8)	
Severe	3 (2.0)	2 (4.5)	
Cosmesis: n (%)			
Satisfied	146 (98.6)	38 (86.4)	0.002
Fair	2 (1.4)	6 (13.6)	

PH: palmar hyperhidrosis; AH: axillary hyperhidrosis

Prospect

The evolution of NOTES and novel endolumenal techniques will be contingent on the development of the next-generation endoscope. Opportunities for advanced imaging technology, combined with multifunctional tools enabling retraction and triangulation within ergonomically engineered and precise systems, will advance both intralumenal and translumenal endoscopic procedures.

References

1. Hornberger J, Grimes K, Naumann M, et al. Multi-specialty working group on the recognition, diagnosis, and treatment of primary focal hyperhidrosis. Recognition, diagnosis, and treatment of primary focal hyperhidrosis [J]. J Am Acad Dermatol. 2004;51(2):274–86.
2. Lai YT, Yang LH, Chio CC, et al. Complications in patients with palmar hyperhidrosis treated with transthoracic endoscopic sympathectomy [J]. Neurosurgery. 1997;41(1):110–3.
3. Steegers MA, Snik DM, Verhagen AF, et al. Only half of the chronic pain after thoracic surgery shows a neuropathic component [J]. J Pain. 2008;9(10):955–61.
4. Rodrı'guez PM, Freixinet JL, Hussein M, et al. Side effects, complications and outcome of thoracoscopic sympathectomy for palmar and axillary hyperhidrosis in 406 patients [J]. Eur J Cardiothorac Surg. 2008;34(3):514–9.
5. Zhu LH, Chen W, Chen L, et al. Transumbilical thoracic sympathectomy: a single-centre experience of 148 cases with up to 4 years of follow-up [J]. Eur J Cardiothorac Surg. 2016;49(Suppl 1):i79–83.

Image-Guided Uniportal VATS in the Hybrid Operating Room

Ze-Rui Zhao and Calvin S. H. Ng

Abstract

The development of imaging technology has recently facilitated uniportal minimally-invasive thoracic surgery techniques. Cone-beam computed tomography (CBCT) shows promising results in visualizing the target lesion and its surrounding critical anatomy, with an average error of less than 2 mm. The hybrid operation room (OR), which integrates CBCT and the OR, is capable of providing unparalleled real-time imaging of the patient, which can be incorporated into electromagnetic navigation bronchoscopic marking of pulmonary lesion to reduce the likelihood of navigation tool malpositioning and, hence increase procedural accuracy. Furthermore, implantation of hookwires or microcoils that are widely used to localize pulmonary lesions can proceed in the hybrid suite, eliminating the common complications and discomfort associated with the conventional workflow carried out in the radiology suite. Implantation displacement leading to localization failure can also be reduced, and sublobar resection can be performed without resecting a larger area of parenchyma than desired. This hybrid OR provides a one-stop concept for simultaneously diagnosing and managing tiny pulmonary lesions.

Hybrid Theater and Its Preclinical Data

Preoperative adjunctive localization techniques including hookwire/microcoil placement or dye labeling conducted under computed tomography (CT) guidance play important roles in identifying pulmonary lesions during uniportal video-assisted thoracic surgery (VATS). However, these approaches may increase procedure-related complication and complexity of care. With the help of hybrid operating room (OR), lesser time for localization is needed, as well as a reduction in the rate of pneumothorax, metallic marker dislodgement, and dye diffusion (Fig. 1). As a result, surgeons could perform excisions precisely and safely, even for multifocal lesions, sparing pulmonary tissues [1].

Mobile cone-beam CT (CBCT) can provide sub-millimeter spatial resolution combined with soft tissue visibility even at a low radiation dose (~4.3 mGy/scan) [2]. However, with a significantly reduced contrast, the visibility of nodules in deflated lungs during surgery via CBCT can be challenging. In a pre-clinical study by Uneri and colleagues [3], the target registration error of CBCT in the anatomical targets was 1.9 mm and 0.6 mm for the model-driven and image-driven stage. Additionally, only a slightly increased dose (~4.6–11.1 mGy) is needed to visualize the collapsed lung tissue. As a result, clinicians would be aware of the potential anatomical characteristics of a lesion on imaging taken in the hybrid OR; for example, whether there is a direct endobronchial route for biopsy, or adjacent vessels to be aware of during metallic material implantation [4].

Structure of Hybrid Theater

In 2013, the first comprehensive hybrid suite (Advanced Multimodal Image-Guided Operating [AMIGO] suite) designed for general thoracic surgery was introduced by the Brigham and Women's Hospital for image-guided VATS (iVATS) [5]. The AMIGO suite has three separate but integrated compartments that incorporate magnetic resonance imaging, near-infrared imaging, CBCT, and positron emission tomography, providing excellent multidisciplinary radiologic support for a variety of surgical scenarios.

Electronic Supplementary Material The online version of this chapter (https://doi.org/10.1007/978-981-13-2604-2_39) contains supplementary material, which is available to authorized users.

Z.-R. Zhao · C. S. H. Ng (✉)
Division of Cardiothoracic Surgery, Department of Surgery, Prince of Wales Hospital, The Chinese University of Hong Kong, Hong Kong SAR, China
e-mail: calvinng@surgery.cuhk.edu.hk

D. Gonzalez-Rivas et al. (eds.), *Atlas of Uniportal Video Assisted Thoracic Surgery*, https://doi.org/10.1007/978-981-13-2604-2_39

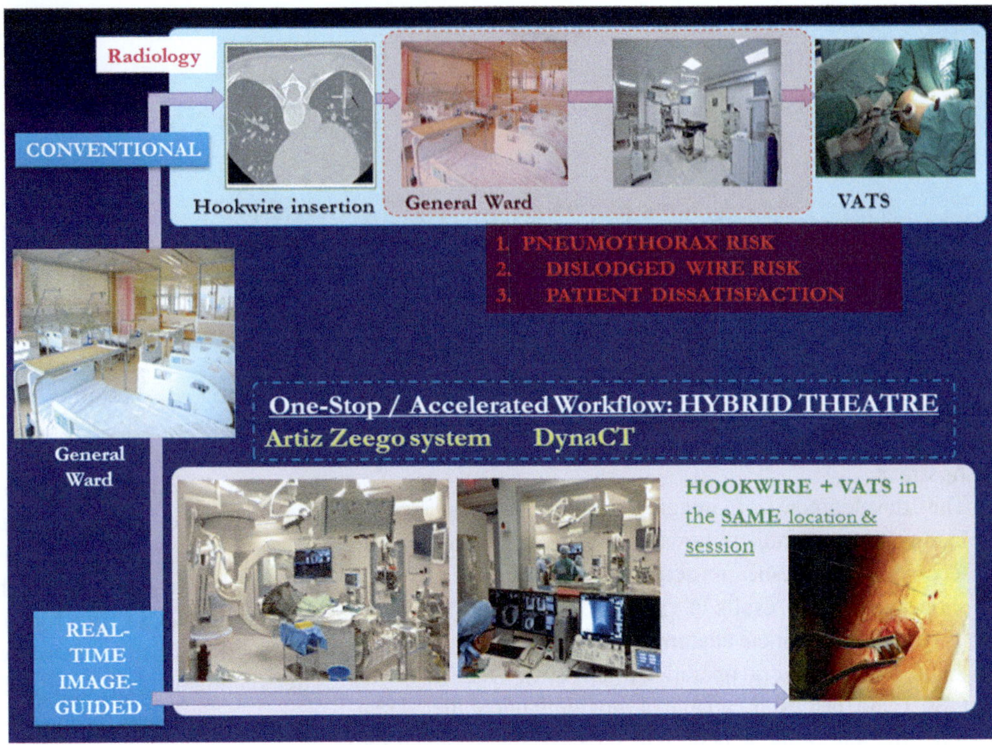

Fig. 1 Illustration of the pathways for hookwire localization followed by lung resection through a conventional approach requiring transfer and delays via the radiology department, and the hybrid one-stop approach

Table 1 Configurations of the hybrid operation room (OR) for image-guided thoracic surgery (Prince of Wales Hospital, Hong Kong)

Artis zeego multi-axis robotic imaging system (Siemens Healthcare AG, Forchheim, Germany)
Free-floating Artis OR table
Large display mounted on rails
syngo X Workplace (Siemens Healthcare AG, Forchheim, Germany)
Steris OR lamps
Dräger anesthetic workplace
Dräger Motiva supply unit
Olympus and Storz endoscopic systems
Medtronic superDimension™ navigation system (Covidien, Minneapolis, MN, USA)
2.5 m × 2.5 m (8.2 ft × 8.2 ft) laminar airflow field

A relatively smaller suite (approximately 760 square feet) was established in our hospital [6]. This suite also implemented a multidisciplinary design and is capable of image-guided electromagnetic navigation bronchoscopy (ENB) [7] and VATS procedures [6]. The floor-mounted CBCT has high flexibility and can be moved from a distant parked position to the surgical field without interfering with the laminar airflow in a short time. The detailed contents of the hybrid OR are described in Table 1 (Fig. 2).

Image-Guided ENB Diagnostic/Marking Procedure

As an advanced bronchoscopic technique, ENB utilizes electromagnetic sensor technology to ensure that the tip of the localization guide approaches the proximity of the lesion during the navigational phase. The extended working channel (EWC) is then locked onto the bronchoscope after withdrawing the sensor tip (Fig. 3). Clinicians are then able to deliver different tools for biopsy or markers for the lesion. The distance between the marked targets on the CT images and the registration points recorded by ENB, so-called the 'average fiducial target registration error' (AFTRE), represents the mean accuracy of the navigation system. Previous studies reported the average AFTRE to be 9 ± 6 mm in 92 cases [8]. More importantly, an AFTRE greater than 4 mm could lead to a significantly lower diagnostic accuracy (44.4% vs. 77.2%) [9].

Usually, fluoroscopy or radial probe endobronchial ultrasound (EBUS) is used as adjuvant means to indicate the position of the sensor tip in real time. However, such methods cannot solve the critical problem that leads to navigational error: whether the tip of the catheter is inside the difficult-to-reach lesion. If the EWC diverges from the target, continuous biopsy hits add limited value to histologic examination, leading to an 'all or none' phenomenon.

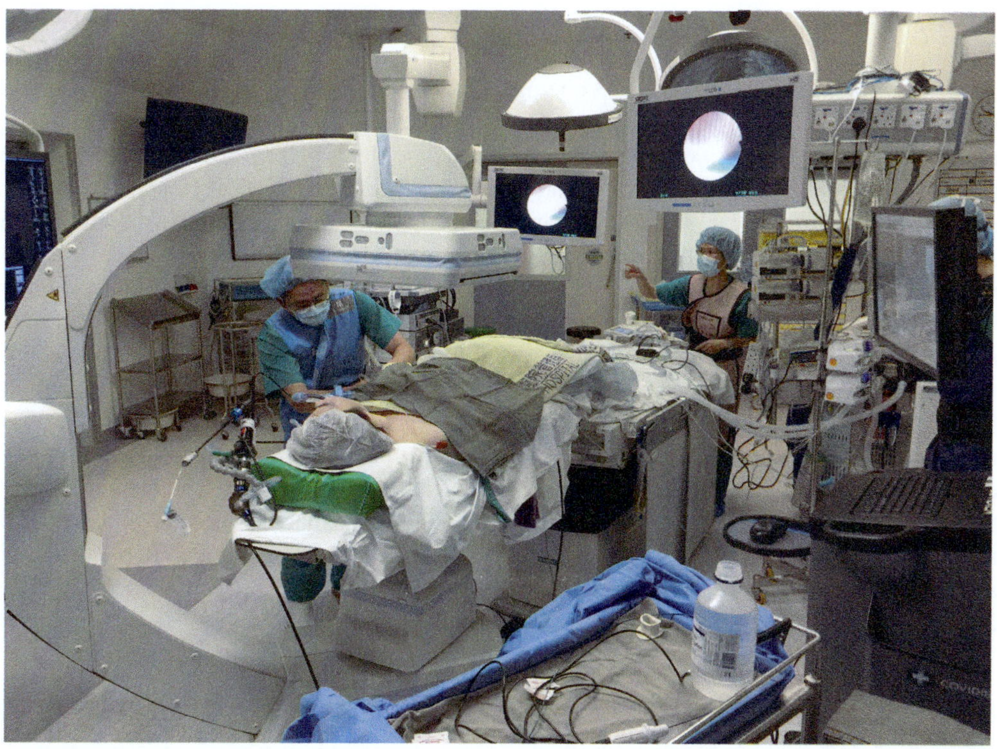

Fig. 2 The modern hybrid theatre layout with dynaCT and electromagnetic navigation bronchoscopy

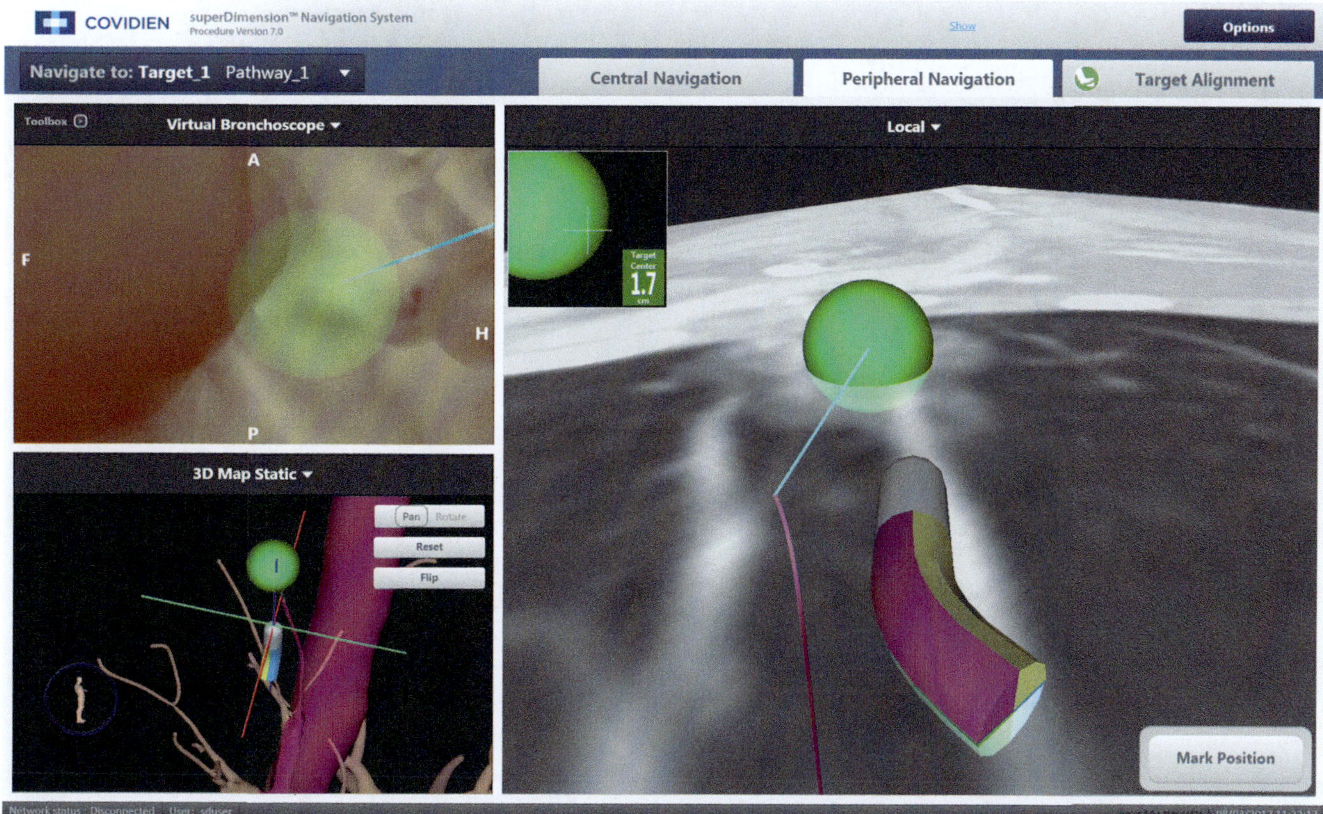

Fig. 3 Electromagnetic navigation bronchoscopy 3D virtual pathway showing successful navigation to the part GGO target lesion at the periphery

To further improve the accuracy and applicability of ENB technique, we described the use of integrated CBCT (syngo dynaCT; Siemens Healthcare AG, Forchheim, Germany) and ENB in a hybrid OR to guide and confirm the successful navigation as well as biopsy of an 8-mm lesion located in the right middle lobe [7]. In brief, after the EWC has been anchored according to the scheduled plan, the navigation system is switched off and then the Artis zeego multi-axis robotic imaging system (Siemens Healthcare AG, Forchheim, Germany) is moved to the working system without interfering the position of the patient. A 6-s suspension of ventilation allows the dynaCT to visualize the relative position between the current biopsy tool and lesion. During the scanning period, the bronchoscope is held by a non-metallic device mounted on the table. We recommend two intraoperative CBCT scans protocol before the biopsy: the first to identify potential minor misdirection of the instrument and the second to confirm satisfactory positioning of effector tool after any necessary adjustment has been completed. Two fluoroscopic images taken from different angles by the dynaCT can orientate the catheter after 2D/3D fusion with the preoperative CT data; hence, the radiation dose is further decreased and comparable to a preoperative percutaneous biopsy. It is logistic that the image from the dynaCT in the hybrid OR has superior accuracy over fluoroscopy or EBUS in revealing the direction of the catheter tip, as it provides the most direct evidence of whether the tip has reached the target lesion (Fig. 4). Thus, the navigational error can be decreased, especially when dealing with GGO lesions of small size.

Trans-bronchial injection of dye under ENB guidance also assist localizing pulmonary nodules during VATS sublobar resection. In our experience, we find that injection of 0.2 mL of methylene blue dye in the lesion is usually sufficient for localization. If the lesion is located deep in the parenchyma, an addition of 0.2 mL injected at the pleura is recommended to create the pleural dye marking seen during VATS. With the help of the hybrid technique, we have now been able to inject triple contrast mixture (0.2–0.5 mL) of

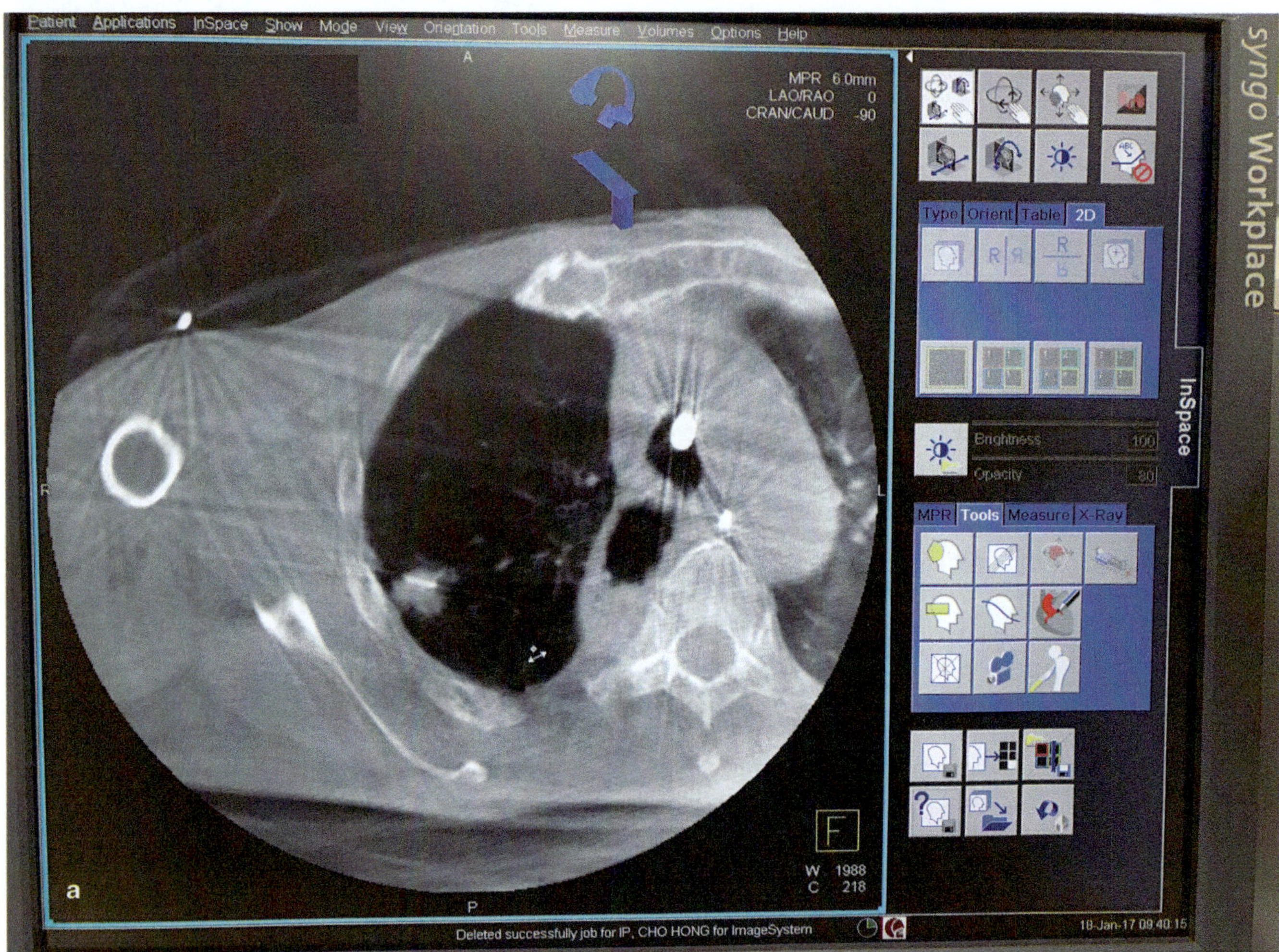

Fig. 4 DynaCT scan in hybrid operating room of right upper lobe small peripheral lesion following electromagnetic navigation bronchoscopy showing successful navigation and needle deployment; (**a**) axial, (**b**) coronal, (**c**) sagittal, and (**d**) digitally subtracted CT views

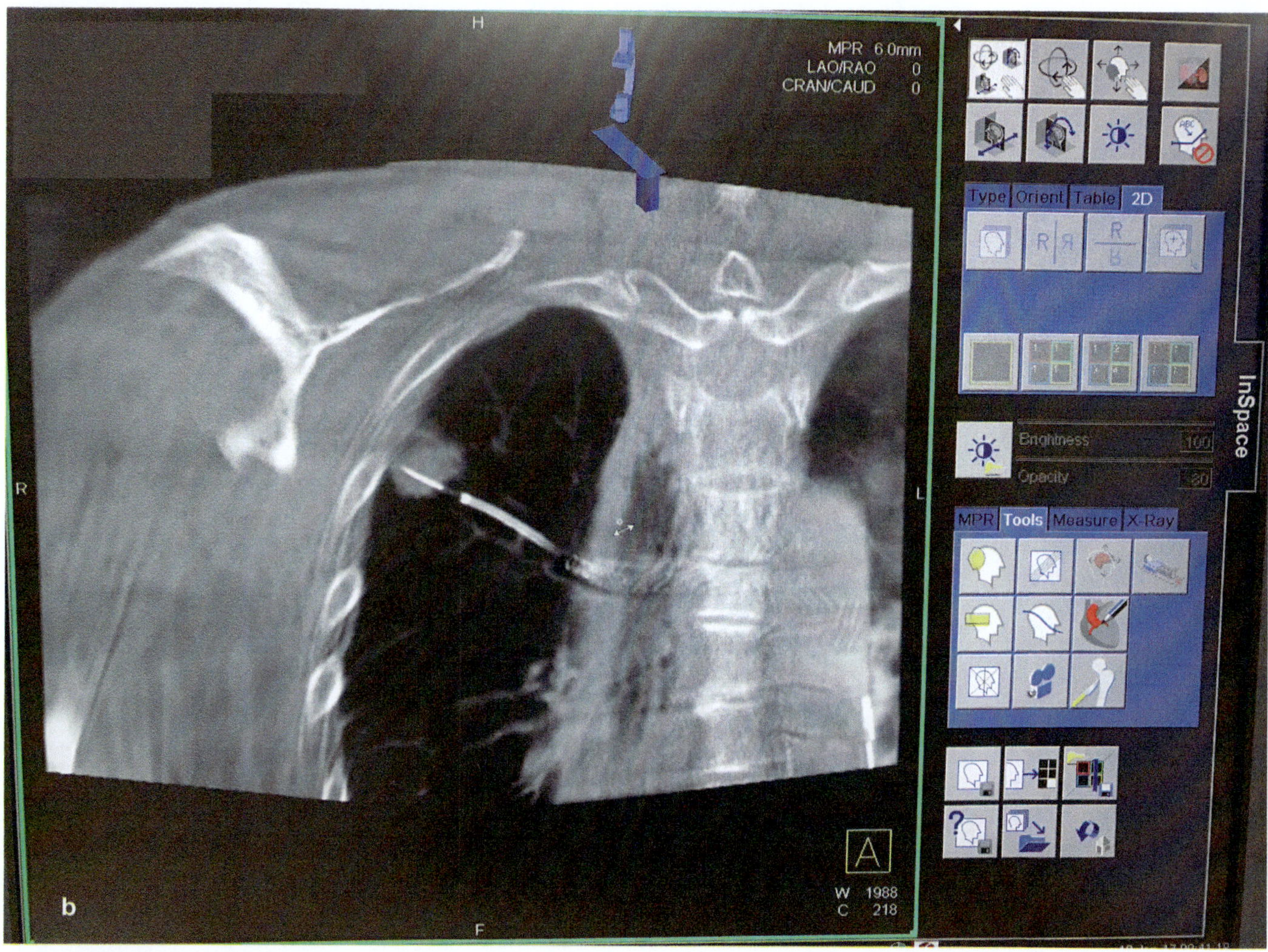

Fig. 4 (continued)

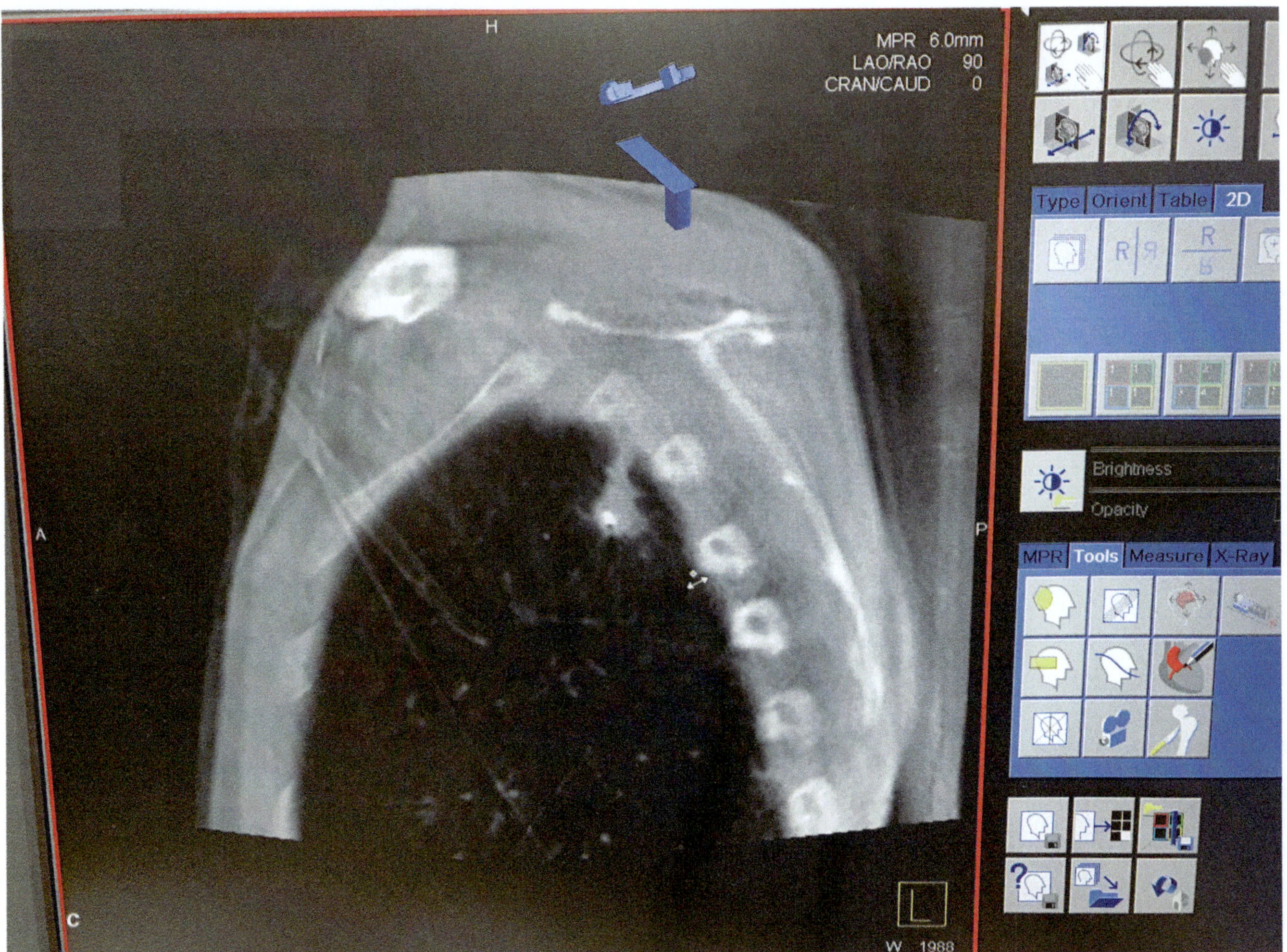

Fig. 4 (continued)

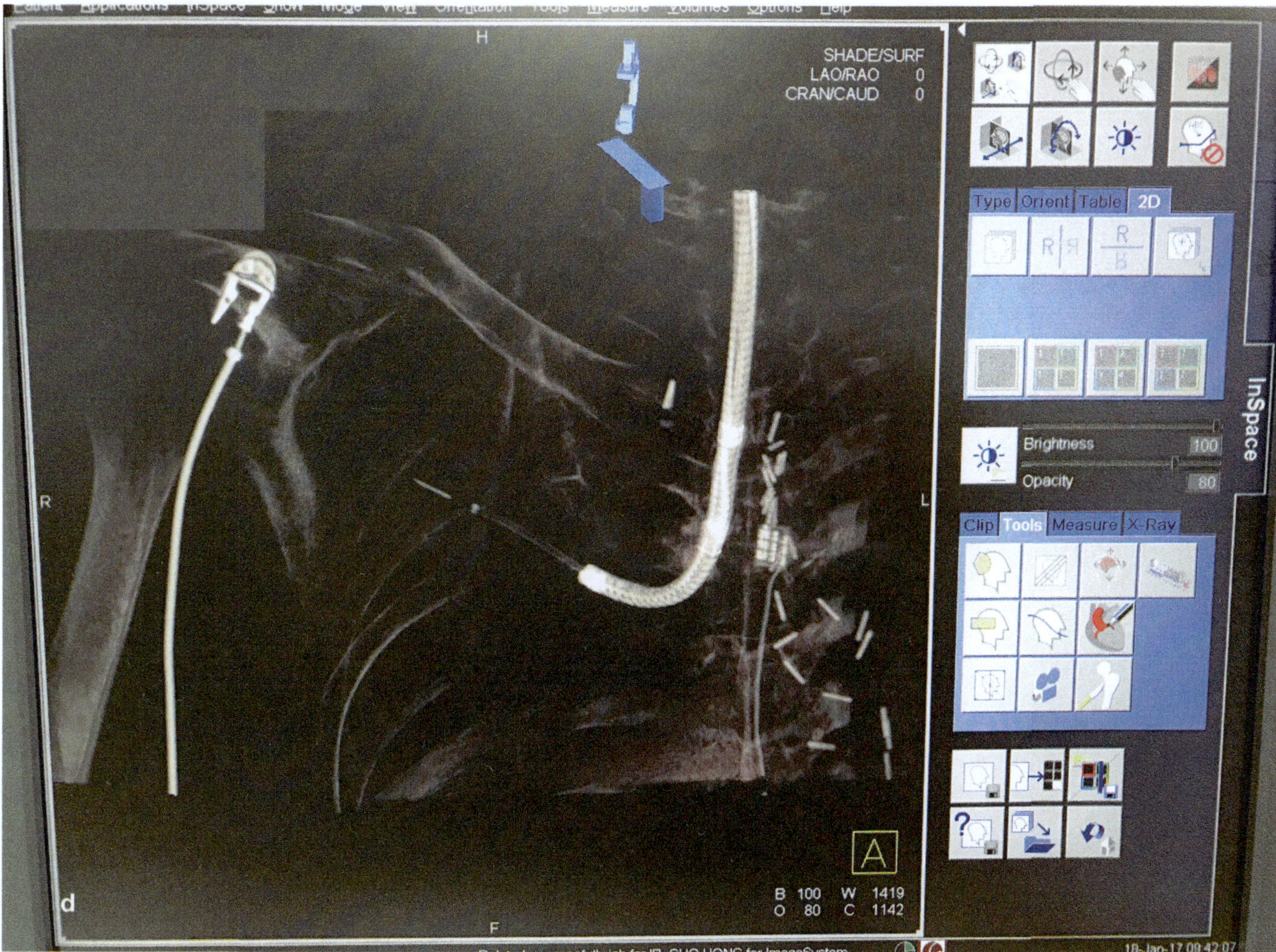

Fig. 4 (continued)

indocyanine green, methylene blue, and standard iohexol imaging contrast in the proximity to the target lesions to guide resection margin under uniportal VATS [10]. In detail, the fluoroscopic screening could monitor a clear blush of mixed contrast coming out of the injection needle of ENB (Video 1). A follow-up CBCT then provide exact information on the lung lesion and its relation to the dye contrast (Fig. 5). Uniportal VATS lung resection can visually identify the lesion stained with methylene blue (Video 2). If the methylene blue is unidentifiable due to dye dispersion, the marked area can be seen by near-infrared scope, thus allowing precise localization and accurate lung resection.

Image-Guided Metallic Implantation

Many thoracic surgeons would adopt metallic implantation such as hookwire or microcoil under CT guidance is given to its high efficacy of intraoperative localization (with a success rate of up to 94% and 100% for the hookwire and microcoil, respectively) [11, 12]. Generally, the techniques require localization to be performed in the radiology suite followed by surgery in the OR. However, the approach may result in patient discomfort and various complications such as pneumothorax or dislodgement of the localizing material during the period of transporting to the OR [13]. Nearly 24% of patients who undergo hookwire insertion would experience pneumothorax and chest tube drainage before surgery is required in 2–4% of them. Dislodgement from the mounting pleura leads to localization failure in 2–10% of the patients who undergo wire insertion, which is more frequent than for microcoil implantation (2.7%) [11].

As discussed, the hybrid OR provide a platform for simultaneous nodule localization with subsequent lung resection for thoracic surgeons. In the initial reports from the Brigham and Women's Hospital group, 23 pulmonary lesions of size 1.30 ± 0.38 cm underwent thoracoscopic surgery after fiducial placement under intraoperative C-arm CT [14]. According to their iVATS protocol, a 5-s end-inspiratory-hold 200° rotation with a 0.36 mGy/projection scanning for the field of

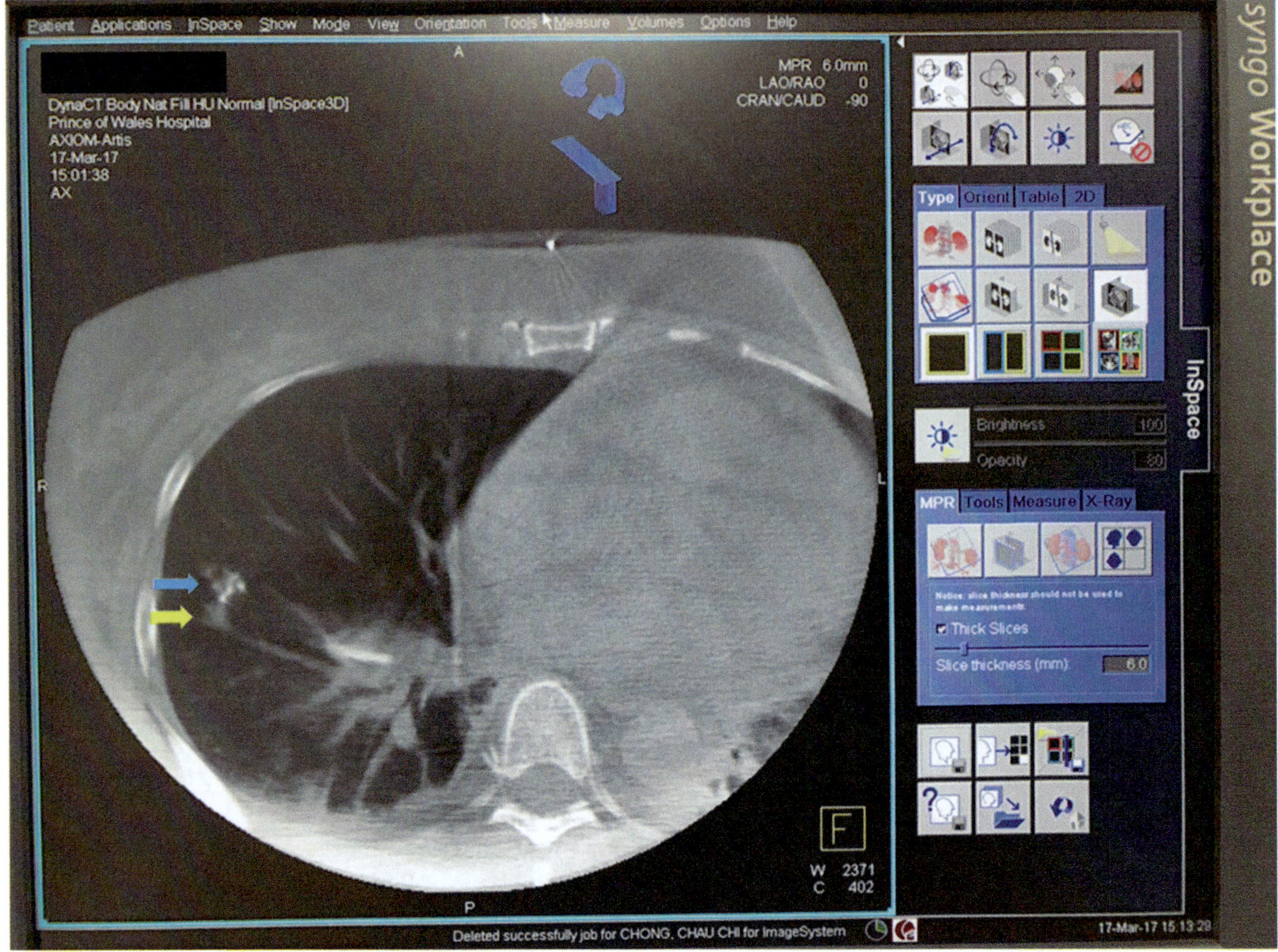

Fig. 5 DynaCT post-injection of methylene blue iodine contrast mixture showing a bright enhancing area representing the dye contrast (blue arrow) adjacent to the GGO pulmonary lesion (yellow arrow)

interest was enough to identify the lesions by CBCT. In their cohort, metallic implantations were successfully conducted in 20 (87.0%) cases, with a median procedure time of 39 min. Notably, no implantation-associated complication was found, compared with the traditional two-site approach. The average and total procedure radiation exposures were low (median: 1501 mGy × m^2; range, 665–16,326 mGy × m^2).

Our group also reported the single-port VATS (iSPVATS) major lung resection for a GGO nodule that underwent dynaCT-guided hookwire placement in the hybrid OR [6]. A slightly different workflow was introduced. We usually apply two fluoroscopic shots to ensure the lesion is in the isocenter of the CBCT. After obtaining the 3D real-time image of the thorax, the interventional radiologist deploys the hookwire to the chest and the position of the needle is further verified by dynaCT scans [1] (Fig. 6).

Approximately 30–40 min is needed to localize and place a hookwire before the incision making for uniportal VATS [15]. As the CBCT is capable of visualizing the anatomical structure in a deflated lung, re-localization of the nodule can be performed if dislodgement happens due to lung collapse under one-lung ventilation [3]. Our image-guided hookwire SPVATS technique would work perfectly for peripheral lesions of sub-centimeter size and may reduce the risk of complications associated with implantation. Moreover, precise localization of the lesion may reduce the chance of resecting excessive pulmonary tissue [15]. However, technical limitations inherent from this approach remain as nodules that are located near to the apex, great vessels, and diaphragm can be difficult to reach using the wire (see Chapter "Hookwire Localization of Pulmonary Nodules in Uniportal VATS").

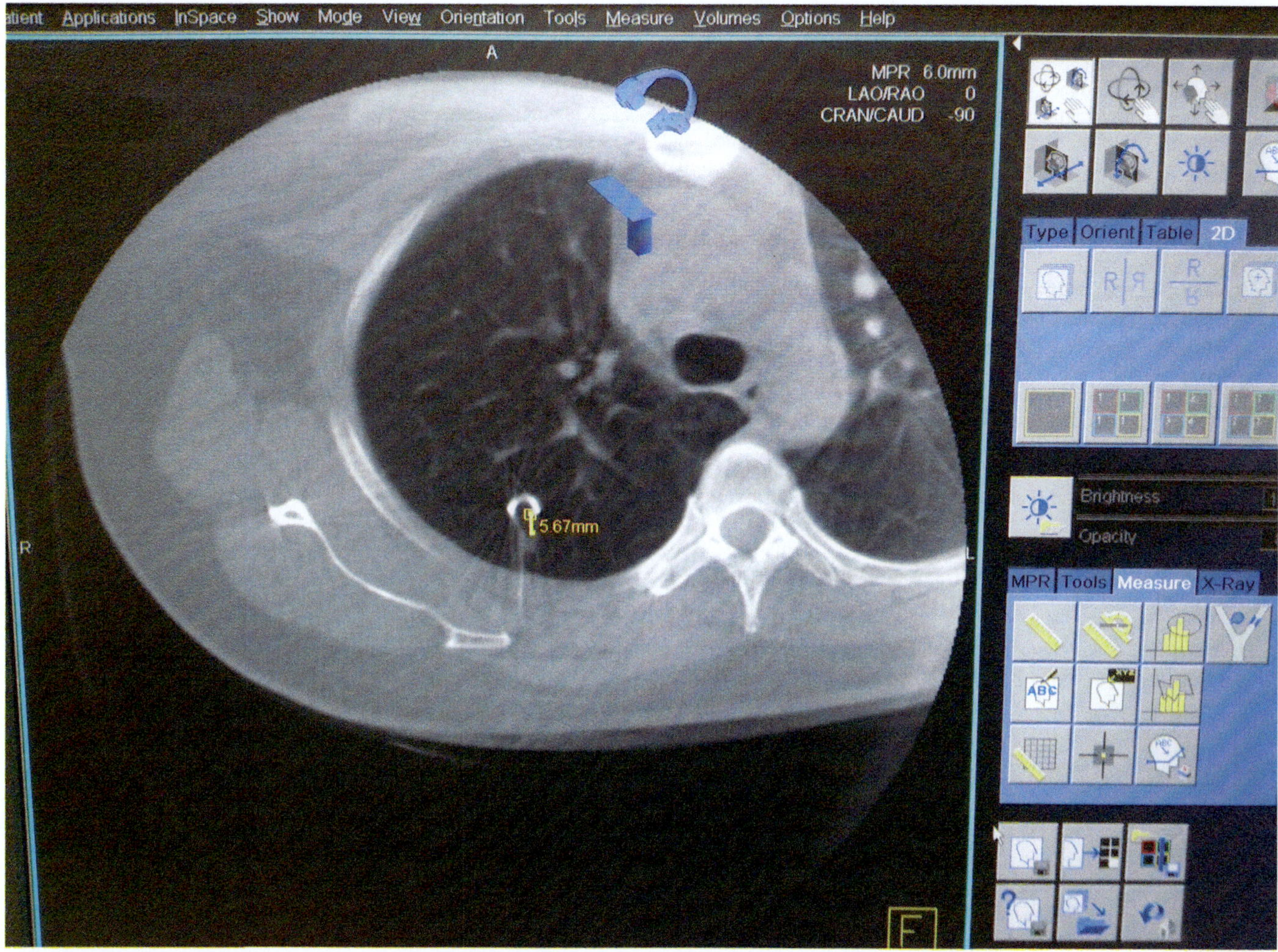

Fig. 6 Post hookwire insertion dynaCT in hybrid theatre showing wire just deep to the subcentimetre GGO lesion

Conclusions

Precise localization is critical in the management of small pulmonary lesions under uniportal VATS. Centralization of the diagnostic, localizing, and resecting procedures within a specially designed hybrid theater could enhance diagnostic accuracy as well as reduce the complications associated with the implantation of metallic markers. With real-time imaging guidance in the hybrid OR, ENB could become more accurate, thus may increase the true-negative rate during biopsy and, consequently, avoid unnecessary excision when treating multiple lesions [16]. Dye labeling under ENB may also obtain benefit from the hybrid strategy for not only confirming precision nodule marking, but also in providing additional information to the surgeon of the spatial relationship between dye and lesion to guide resection. The iSPVATS idea, using a hookwire/microcoil implantation, allows for a safer percutaneous procedure in the OR environment and minimizes the chance of dislodgement, which leads to failed localization.

Minimally invasive thoracic surgery is evolving from simply reducing the number of incisions to encompass a wider philosophy of performing more precise surgery, fast-tracking, and attempts to use tools such as non-intubated anesthesia to enhance patient recovery [17]. The hybrid OR may become increasingly prevalent in this progress as it establishes a cost-effective, one-stop procedural flow for image-guided thoracic surgery.

References

1. Zhao ZR, Lau RWH, Ng CSH. Hybrid theater and uniportal video-assisted thoracic surgery: the perfect match for lung nodule localization. Thorac Surg Clin. 2017;27:347–55.

2. Schafer S, Nithiananthan S, Mirota DJ, Uneri A, Stayman JW, Zbijewski W, et al. Mobile C-arm cone-beam CT for guidance of spine surgery: image quality, radiation dose, and integration with interventional guidance. Med Phys. 2011;38:4563–74.
3. Uneri A, Nithiananthan S, Schafer S, Otake Y, Stayman JW, Kleinszig G, et al. Deformable registration of the inflated and deflated lung in cone-beam CT-guided thoracic surgery: initial investigation of a combined model- and image-driven approach. Med Phys. 2013;40:017501.
4. Zhao ZR, Lau RW, Yu PS, Wong RH, Ng CS. Image-guided localization of small lung nodules in video-assisted thoracic surgery. J Thorac Dis. 2016;8:S731–7.
5. Advanced Multimodality Image Guided Operating (AMIGO). 2016. http://www.brighamandwomens.org/research/amigo/default.aspx. Accessed 1 Sep 2018.
6. Ng CS, Man Chu C, Kwok MW, Yim AP, Wong RH. Hybrid DynaCT scan-guided localization single-port lobectomy. [corrected]. Chest. 2015;147:e76–8.
7. Ng CS, Yu SC, Lau RW, Yim AP. Hybrid DynaCT-guided electromagnetic navigational bronchoscopic biopsy†. Eur J Cardiothorac Surg. 2016;49:i87–8.
8. Eberhardt R, Anantham D, Herth F, Feller-Kopman D, Ernst A. Electromagnetic navigation diagnostic bronchoscopy in peripheral lung lesions. Chest. 2007;131:1800–5.
9. Makris D, Scherpereel A, Leroy S, Bouchindhomme B, Faivre JB, Remy J, et al. Electromagnetic navigation diagnostic bronchoscopy for small peripheral lung lesions. Eur Respir J. 2007;29:1187–92.
10. Ng CSH, Zhao Z, Long H, Lau RWH. Electromagnetic navigation bronchoscopy triple contrast dye marking for lung nodule localization. Thorac Cardiovasc Surg. 2019 . doi: https://doi.org/10.1055/s-0038-1676964
11. Kidane B, Yasufuku K. Advances in image-guided thoracic surgery. Thorac Surg Clin. 2016;26:129–38.
12. Ng CS, Hui JW, Wong RH. Minimizing single-port access in video-assisted wedge resection, with a hookwire. Asian Cardiovasc Thorac Ann. 2013;21:114–5.
13. Zhao ZR, Lau RW, Ng CS. Hybrid theatre and alternative localization techniques in conventional and single-port video-assisted thoracoscopic surgery. J Thorac Dis. 2016;8:S319–27.
14. Gill RR, Zheng Y, Barlow JS, Jayender J, Girard EE, Hartigan PM, et al. Image-guided video assisted thoracoscopic surgery (iVATS) – phase I-II clinical trial. J Surg Oncol. 2015;112:18–25.
15. Yu PSY, Man Chu C, Lau RWH, Wan IYP, Underwood MJ, Yu SCH, et al. Video-assisted thoracic surgery for tiny pulmonary nodules with real-time image guidance in the hybrid theatre: the initial experience. J Thorac Dis. 2018;10:2933–9.
16. Ng CSH, Chu CM, Lo CK, Lau RWH. Hybrid operating room Dyna-computed tomography combined image-guided electromagnetic navigation bronchoscopy dye marking and hookwire localization video-assisted thoracic surgery metastasectomy. Interact Cardiovasc Thorac Surg. 2018;26:338–40.
17. Zhao ZR, Lau RWH, Ng CSH. Non-intubated video-assisted thoracic surgery: the final frontier? Eur J Cardiothorac Surg. 2016;50:925–6.

Development of 3D VATS

Jun Liu, Jingpei Li, Yidong Wang, Fengling Lai, Wei Wang, Guilin Peng, Zhihua Guo, Jiaxi He, Fei Cui, Shuben Li, and Jianxing He

Introduction and Development

To minimize surgical invasion and morbidity, video-assisted thoracic surgery (VATS) techniques, were developed and proven feasible and safe. Furthermore, long-term results proved comparable to thoracotomy, for resection of lung cancer [1], esophageal cancer [2], and thymic tumors [3], but with less morbidity. However, compared with thoracotomy, there is a steep learning curve with VATS because of poorer optics of the hilar structures and dissection planes that result from the two dimensional (2D) view.

The three dimensional (3D) display system was initially introduced into the field of surgery to perform cholecystectomy. Since then, surgeons have used this technology to perform general and urinary operations [4]. In the field of thoracic surgery, a 3D display system was not used until the introduction of the da Vinci robot surgical system [5]. The robotic surgical system has been reported to allow a more natural intrathoracic view and reduce the duration of postoperative hospitalization and even 30-day mortality [6], with oncologic results comparable to thoracotomy and VATS [7]. With these promising results and technical improvements, 3D-VATS has gradually been adapted in recent years.

Theoretically, 3D vision offers the advantage of improved depth perception and accuracy comparable to open operations [8] with amplified structure. It has been reported to allow improved discrimination and recognition of targeted organs, vessels and lymph nodes. Thus facilitating precise operation and shortening operative time [9–11]. Such advantages could presumably minimize intensive care unit lengths of stay and, finally, decrease hospitalization costs.

Current Status

Surgery

We first used the 3D system at our center in November 2013 for VATS pulmonary resection surgery [9]. Our surgeons reported experience of better depth perception and aided visualization of critical vascular relationships and multiple tissue layers, such as the bronchi, esophagus, lymph nodes and thoracic duct when using the 3D imaging system. In our operative experience conversion from the 3D to the 2D system was not necessary during any of the operations. We did not observe any significant adverse effects. There were no reports of nausea or headaches by surgeons. Pulmonary resection with the 3D VATS system was associated with significantly shorter operative time, but there was no significant decrease in blood loss, duration of chest tube drainage, length of hospital stays or postoperative complications [10]. Since the setting of medical price is controlled by the government in China, there is no difference between 2D and 3D VATS in terms of the costs of instruments. We believe that 3D VATS and 2D VATS lobectomy are both safe procedures.

The first report of a lobectomy for cancer using the 3D-VATS system wasn't until 2015 [11]. The same year, Li, Z et al. [12] reported the feasibility of 3D video-assisted thoracoscopic esophagectomy. Since the publication of these reports, we have routinely applied the use of the 3D system to perform all thoracic surgeries, pulmonary resection, esophagectomy, thymectomy, biopsy of chest wall, decollement of posterior mediastinal mass, and enucleation of

J. Liu · J. Li · W. Wang · G. Peng · Z. Guo
J. He · F. Cui · S. Li · J. He (✉)
Department of Thoracic Surgery and Oncology, The First Affiliated Hospital of Guangzhou Medical University, Guangzhou, China

Guangzhou Institute of Respiratory Disease & China State Key Laboratory of Respiratory Disease, Guangzhou, China

National Clinical Research Centre of Respiratory Disease, Guangzhou, China

Y. Wang · F. Lai
Department of Operation Room, The First Affiliated Hospital of Guangzhou Medical University, Guangzhou, China

D. Gonzalez-Rivas et al. (eds.), *Atlas of Uniportal Video Assisted Thoracic Surgery*,
https://doi.org/10.1007/978-981-13-2604-2_40

esophageal leiomyoma. To date, we have finished one thousand and five hundred 3D pulmonary resection surgeries, three hundred 3D mediastinal tumor resections and one hundred 3D esophagectomies.

Teaching

In our experience, another merit of 3D-VATS is that it greatly improves the assistant's performance during the operation. We believe that 3D certainly has a place for trainees for surgical skills as it reduces errors and time taken to complete tasks while increasing precision. However, there is presently limited reported evidence.

Issues and Concerns

Although the 3D system affords many advantages, the limitations of this technique include the need for extra polarizing glasses, and the surgeon to view the screen orthogonally to best observe 3D image. In addition the added weight of the 3D thoracoscope increases the difficulty of the scope-holder.

One of the other questions that needs to be answered is that of visual negative effects. Does this stereopsis technique (each eye being presented with a separate image) cause eye fatigue or visual inattention? However, current results are mostly subjective with further research to be done. More parameters for comparison are also needed in future study design.

One Step Ahead Glasses-Free 3D VATS

To be free from the polarizing glasses, we have designed a glasses-free 3D display system. With background computing, the screen can project a real-time 3D image to the surgeon with the help of pupils' detector (Fig. 1). Based on the detector and computing, the system can constantly regulate the image so that the optimum view is always seen by the surgeon. Without the polarization from the 3D glasses, surgeons can appreciate the same stereoscopic image with both eyes, however, the screen must be positioned at a distance of 1.8–2.2 m from the surgeon to view the glasses free 3D image.

This glasses-free 3D image is brighter than traditional 3D and provides more details of targeted structure and sensing of layers, such as vagina vasorum or mediastinal structures. However, there are still several unresolved issues. While a surgeon conducts an extensive operation, such as a quick movement of pulling the lung upwards or downwards, there may be a 1–2 s delay of the image. In addition as the scope is held by an assistant, not in a fixed position as it is on a robotic system, thus there is continuous intensive background computing because of any minor action of the assistant. As with the system, only the central half of the 3D image, or the area of the ongoing operation, is completely clear (Fig. 2). The peripheral circle, however, could be a bit blurred or twisted. It is possible, particularly when a scope-holder has little experience, that this could interfere with the surgery, however such issues can present themselves in any VATS operation. In addition, the image is specifically targeted at the operative surgeon, and the observation radius is only extended to 30 cm away from the surgeon's pupils. Because of this, most assistants must still observe the 3D image using the polarized glasses. Finally, if the environment is too bright, it is possible for the pupil detector to loose track of the surgeon's movement for this reason the lights are dimmed down during the operations.

Future

Tremendous improvements of surgical instruments come from surprising places. Virtual reality (VR) is currently extremely popular in the entertainment field. Recently, however, an Increasing number of training centers have reported the role of VR in surgical training [13, 14], with one report of it's use in an actual operation, with audiences using the VR technology to experience the operation from the surgeons view [15]. Many people are of the opinion that this technology will be of great value for surgical training and surgery in the future, though it is difficult to determine what that future will consist of in the field of VATS. However, we believe this technique will play a key role both in operations and the training field.

A couple other technologies may also have a promising future in the field of surgery. One such technology is an eye tracking system based on infrared radiation. The use of this technology in the glasses-free system could regulate the image to the surgeon's position, it would also allow movement of the scope with the help of a mechanical arm. This would free the scope holder and allow less background computing for a more steady image with less lag. Also of interest is the holographical 3D image technology that has been introduced into cardiac field. We believe this technology will be similarly promising in the field of thoracic VATS as a real-time 3D structure could better help surgeons locate lesions and identify the surrounding structures before surgery.

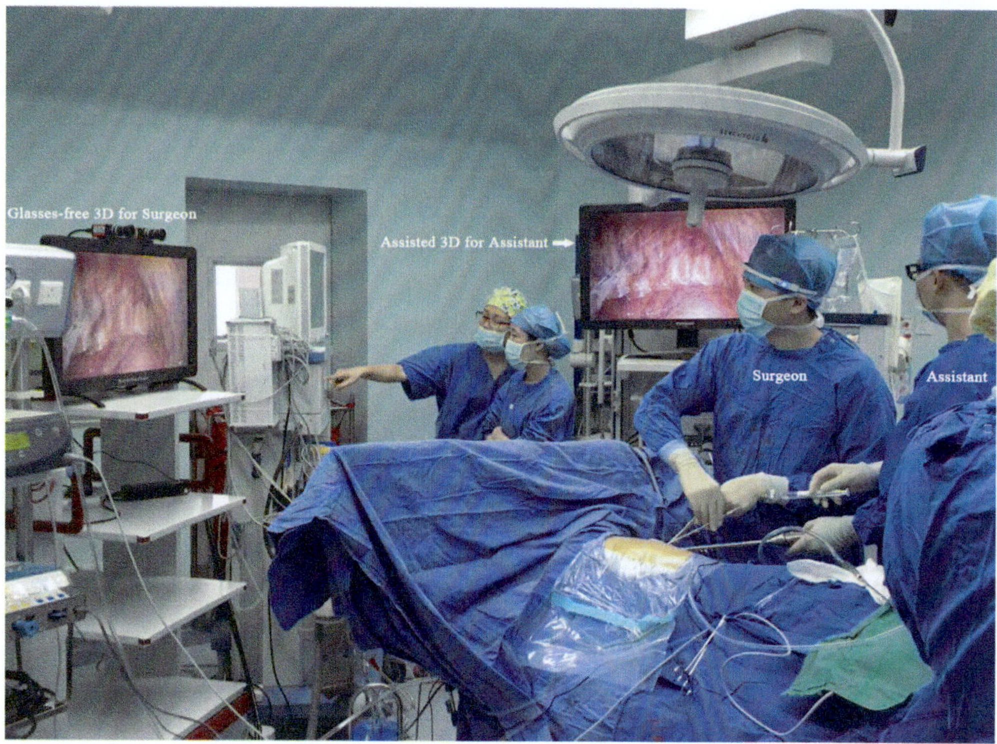

Fig. 1 The routine setting of glasses-free 3D VATS while assistant watching the assisted 3D display screen with extra polarizing glasses

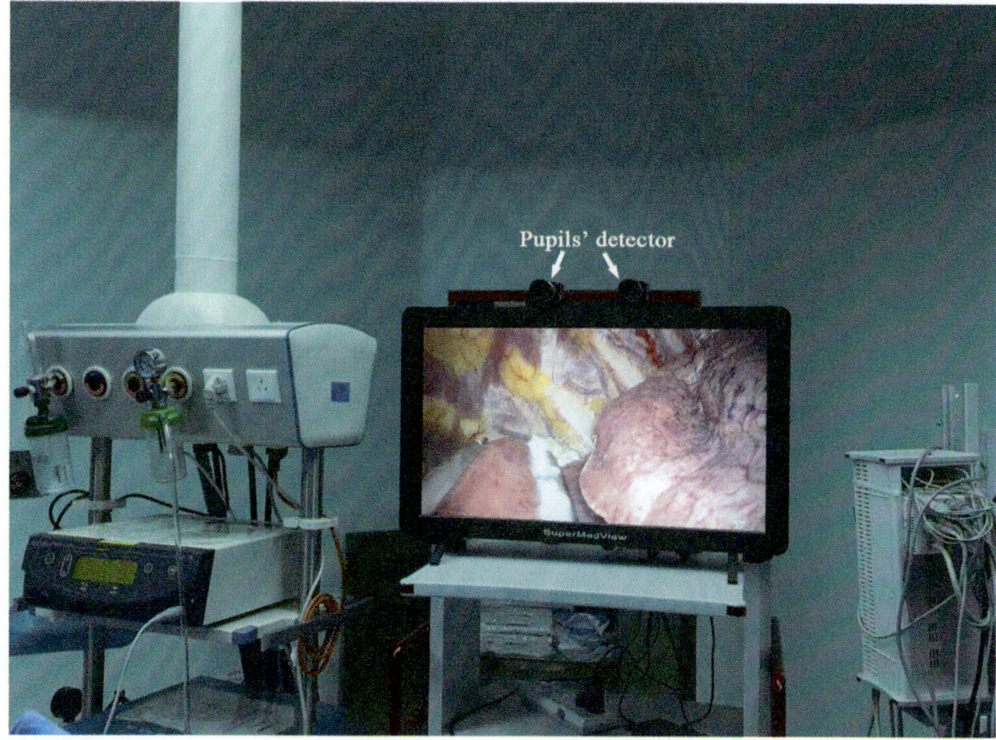

Fig. 2 The actual image of glasses-free 3D display screen with the pupils' detector

References

1. Falcoz PE, Puyraveau M, Thomas PA, et al. Video-assisted thoracoscopic surgery versus open lobectomy for primary non-small-cell lung cancer: a propensity-matched analysis of outcome from the European Society of Thoracic Surgeon database. Eur J Cardiothorac Surg. 2016;49:602–9.
2. Wang H, Shen Y, Feng M, et al. Outcomes, quality of life, and survival after esophagectomy for squamous cell carcinoma: a propensity score-matched comparison of operative approaches. J Thorac Cardiovasc Surg. 2015;149:1006–15.
3. Gu ZT, Mao T, Chen WH, et al. Comparison of video-assisted thoracoscopic surgery and median sternotomy approaches for thymic tumor resections at a single institution. Surg Laparosc Endosc Percutan Tech. 2015;25:47–51.
4. McLachlan G. From 2D to 3D: the future of surgery? Lancet. 2011;15(378):1368.
5. Ashton RC, Connery CP, Swistel DG, et al. Robot-assisted lobectomy. J Thorac Cardiovasc Surg. 2003;126:292–3.
6. Pardolesi A, Park B, Petrella F, et al. Robotic anatomic segmentectomy of the lung: technical aspects and initial results. Ann Thorac Surg. 2012;94:929–34.
7. Park BJ, Melfi F, Mussi A, et al. Robotic lobectomy for non-small cell lung cancer (NSCLC): long-term oncologic results. J Thorac Cardiovasc Surg. 2012;143:383–9.
8. Yamauchi Y, Shinohara K. Effect of binocular stereopsis on surgical manipulation performance and fatigue when using a stereoscopic endoscope. Stud Health Technol Inform. 2005;111:611–4.
9. Yang C, Mo L, Ma Y, et al. A comparative analysis of lung cancer patients treated with lobectomy via three-dimensional video-assisted thoracoscopic surgery versus two-dimensional resection. J Thorac Dis. 2015;7:1798–805.
10. Yang C, Wang W, Mo L, et al. Short-term outcome of three-dimensional versus two-dimensional video-assisted thoracic surgery for benign pulmonary diseases. Ann Thorac Surg. 2016;101:1297–302.
11. Bagan P, De Dominicis F, Hernigou J, et al. Complete thoracoscopic lobectomy for cancer: comparative study of three-dimensional high-definition with two-dimensional high-definition video systems dagger. Interact Cardiovasc Thorac Surg. 2015;20:820–3.
12. Li Z, Li JP, Qin X, et al. Three-dimensional vs two-dimensional video assisted thoracoscopic esophagectomy for patients with esophageal cancer. World J Gastroenterol. 2015;21:10675–82.
13. Jensen K, Ringsted C, Hansen HJ, et al. Simulation-based training for thoracoscopic lobectomy: a randomized controlled trial: virtual-reality versus black-box simulation. Surg Endosc. 2014;28:1821–9.
14. Jensen K, Bjerrum F, Hansen HJ, et al. A new possibility in thoracoscopic virtual reality simulation training: development and testing of a novel virtual reality simulator for video-assisted thoracoscopic surgery lobectomy. Interact Cardiovasc Thorac Surg. 2015;21:420–6.
15. https://www.theguardian.com/society/2016/mar/25/uk-cancer-surgery-live-streamed-virtual-reality.

Future Development and Technologies

Zheng Li and Calvin S. H. Ng

Abstract

Since its introduction in the beginning of this millennium, uniportal VATS has received great interests. Despite its advantages over conventional operations, uniportal VATS poses great challenges to the surgeon. This is mainly as a consequence of inserting and operating all the instruments via a small incision. In the uniportal VATS instruments have limited movement and instrument fencing is frequent with some haptic sensation loss. In addition, the vision is restricted as the endoscope is nearly parallel to the instruments. The advancement of technology has or will much alleviate these shortcomings. For example, wide-angled thoracoscope and flexible thoracoscope have to some extent lessen the fencing problem, and the wireless steerable endoscope system may further eliminate the instrument-endoscope fencing and provide panoramic view. New uniportal platforms derived from natural orifice transluminal endoscopic surgery (NOTES) and single-port access surgery approaches are on the horizon, which allows the uniportal VATS to be performed in a much easier way and via even smaller incisions. However, problems associated with provision of a steady platform, sufficient payload and applied force, tool change and equipment sterilization, haptic sensation, etc. remain to be solved. The diagnosis and intraoperative localization of small tumors can be challenging especially in uniportal VATS. Advanced multimodality image-guided operating room (AMIGO) and hybrid operating room can help in real-time diagnosis, localization and reduce the associated problems in patient transferring.

Z. Li
Department of Surgery, The Chinese University of Hong Kong, Prince of Wales Hospital, Hong Kong SAR, China

Chow Yuk Ho Technology Centre for Innovative Medicine, The Chinese University of Hong Kong, Hong Kong SAR, China

C. S. H. Ng (✉)
Division of Cardiothoracic Surgery, Department of Surgery, Prince of Wales Hospital, The Chinese University of Hong Kong, Hong Kong SAR, China
e-mail: calvinng@surgery.cuhk.edu.hk

Introduction

Uniportal video-assisted thoracic surgery (VATS) has a history of more than a decade. A uniportal VATS thoracic sympathectomy was first reported in 2000 [1], which ignites the enthusiasm of developing more complex uniportal procedures for a wide range of thoracic conditions. However, it is until recent years with the advancement of VATS equipment an increasing number of uniportal VATS procedures were reported. Surgeons show greater desire of further minimize the surgical access trauma, which in turn spurs the rapid development of uniportal VATS equipment. The potential benefits, e.g. better cosmesis, less pain, less complications, etc., together with patients' demand have driven uniportal VATS quickly spread across the world [2]. In uniportal VATS, all the instruments, including the endoscope, graspers, dissectors, staplers, etc., are inserted through the same small single incision. In executing the surgical tasks, the movement of the instruments are constrained and instrument fencing can often occur. The lack of angulation in the instruments also made the surgical operation cumbersome and prolong the procedure. The limited range and angle of vision provided by the thoracoscope made the operation even more difficult. In this chapter, we focus on a few areas of technological advancement, i.e., endoscopes and insertable operating platforms, of present and on the horizon that may help to overcome the aforementioned challenges. Also, advanced multimodality image-guided operating room that can help intraoperative diagnosis and localization is introduced.

Thoracoscopes

In uniportal VATS, the thoracoscope extends the human eyes into the chest cavity. Two key issues related to the endoscope are the image quality and the steerability. Commonly used thoracoscopes have a rigid shaft which embedded the rod lens inside. The viewing direction is normally in parallel

D. Gonzalez-Rivas et al. (eds.), *Atlas of Uniportal Video Assisted Thoracic Surgery*,
https://doi.org/10.1007/978-981-13-2604-2_41

with the rigid shaft and could be pre-modified by the bevel tip. To control the field of view (FOV), one could steer the endoscope shaft by pivoting around the incision port. The motion of the endoscope could interfere with the surgical instruments and increase instruments fencing. In addition, due to the small size of the incision port, the surgical instruments and the thoracoscope is nearly in parallel. This restricts the view of the surgical site and leads to more manipulations of the thoracoscope and intensify the instruments fencing. One approach to reduce the fencing is using thoracoscope with greater lens flexibility. One example is the EndoCAMeleon® by Karl Storz [3]. The wide-angled rigid thoracoscope allows vision between 0° and 120° through a rotating prism mechanism at the tip that provides variable views. The EndoCAMeleon is slightly wider than other video endoscopes for comparable visual resolution, hence occupying a larger portion of the single incision. Meanwhile, rotating and pivoting the shaft is still required, though with reduced frequency.

Another approach to reduce the frequency of endoscope shaft movement is using semi-rigid endoscope. The semi-rigid endoscope has a proximal rigid shaft and a distal flexible bending section, which is similar to the distal section of the flexible bronchoscope. The FOV could be controlled by either pivoting the shaft or bending the distal section without moving the shaft [4]. Two examples include the EndoEye from Olympus [5] and the cardioscope presented by Z Li, et al. [6]. In the EndoEye, the distal bending section could bend up to 100°, enabling the endoscope a wide FOV. However, the operation of the Endoeye is not as intuitive as the rigid endoscopes. The horizon of the video provided by the Endoeye changes with the bending of the flexible section. In addition, the length of the flexible bending section is constant, hence the bending trajectory is fixed. To change the viewing direction, the whole flexible section needs to deflect. The area swept by the tip bending motion is significant. This sweeping motion would obstruct the operation of surgical instruments. The cardioscope was designed based on the flexible mechanism proposed by Z. Li [6]. In the cardioscope, the flexible distal tip not only can bend to all directions but also change the length of the bending section. This provides the cardioscope the ability of avoiding structures and a wider FOV. More importantly, by adjusting the length of the bending section, the bending mode could also be controlled. This could save the space occupied by the flexible tip during bending. Figure 1 shows the cardioscope prototype and results in *ex-vivo* and *in-vivo* tests. Compared to the EndoEye, the cardioscope could better avoid instrument fencing but the image quality is lower. Further development is required to improve the image quality to match clinical requirement.

One common limitation shared by rigid endoscopes and semi-rigid endoscopes is that the shaft occupies space inside the surgical incision. Its movement interferes with other instruments despite strategies to limit this [7]. The ultimate design is perhaps a camera that does not need to occupy the surgical incision, does not interfere with other instruments and can provide multidirectional views. One promising design is the magnetically anchoring guidance systems (MAGS) [8]. Initially the MAGS are designed for single-incision laparoscopic surgery. However, MAGS may be more suited for operations in the chest cavity, e.g., uniportal VATS. The MAGS camera described by Cadeddu [9] has a camera viewing forward and two LED lights providing onboard illumination. It uses two permanent magnets for anchoring. A 14 gauge metal stem is used to secure the MAGS camera in place and assisting the anchoring. One

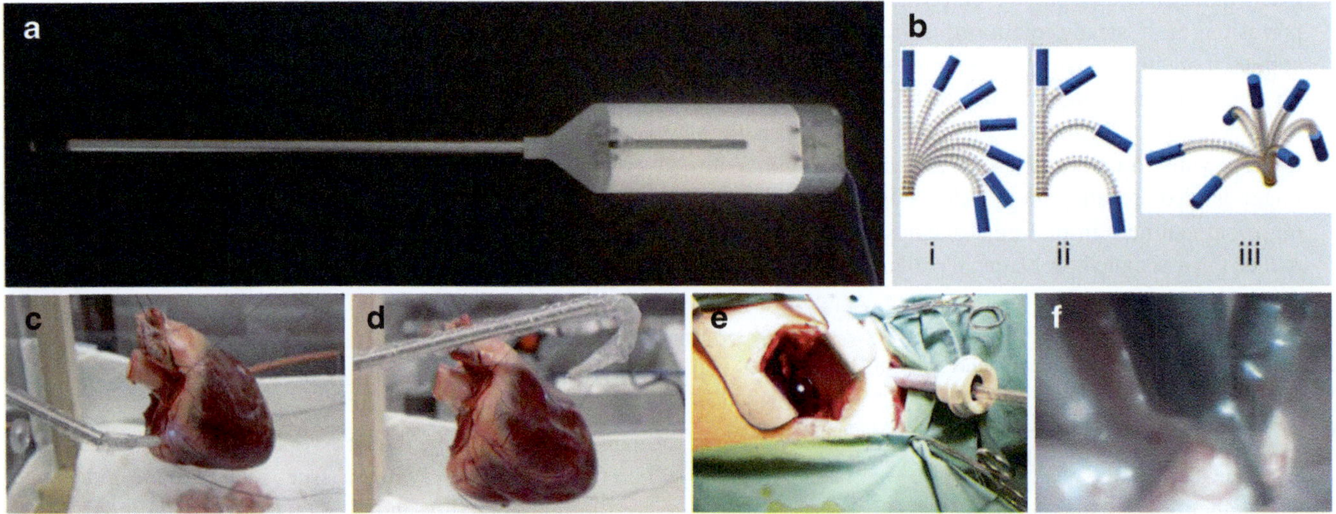

Fig. 1 The cardioscope: (**a**) the proof-of-concept prototype; (**b**) bending modes of the flexible tip; (**c**) operate with a short bending section; (**d**) operate with a longer bending section; (**e**) retroflexion in an animal model of thoracic surgery; (**f**) image provided by the cardioscope in guiding other operating tools during pig pleurectomy (Modified from figures in Ref. [12])

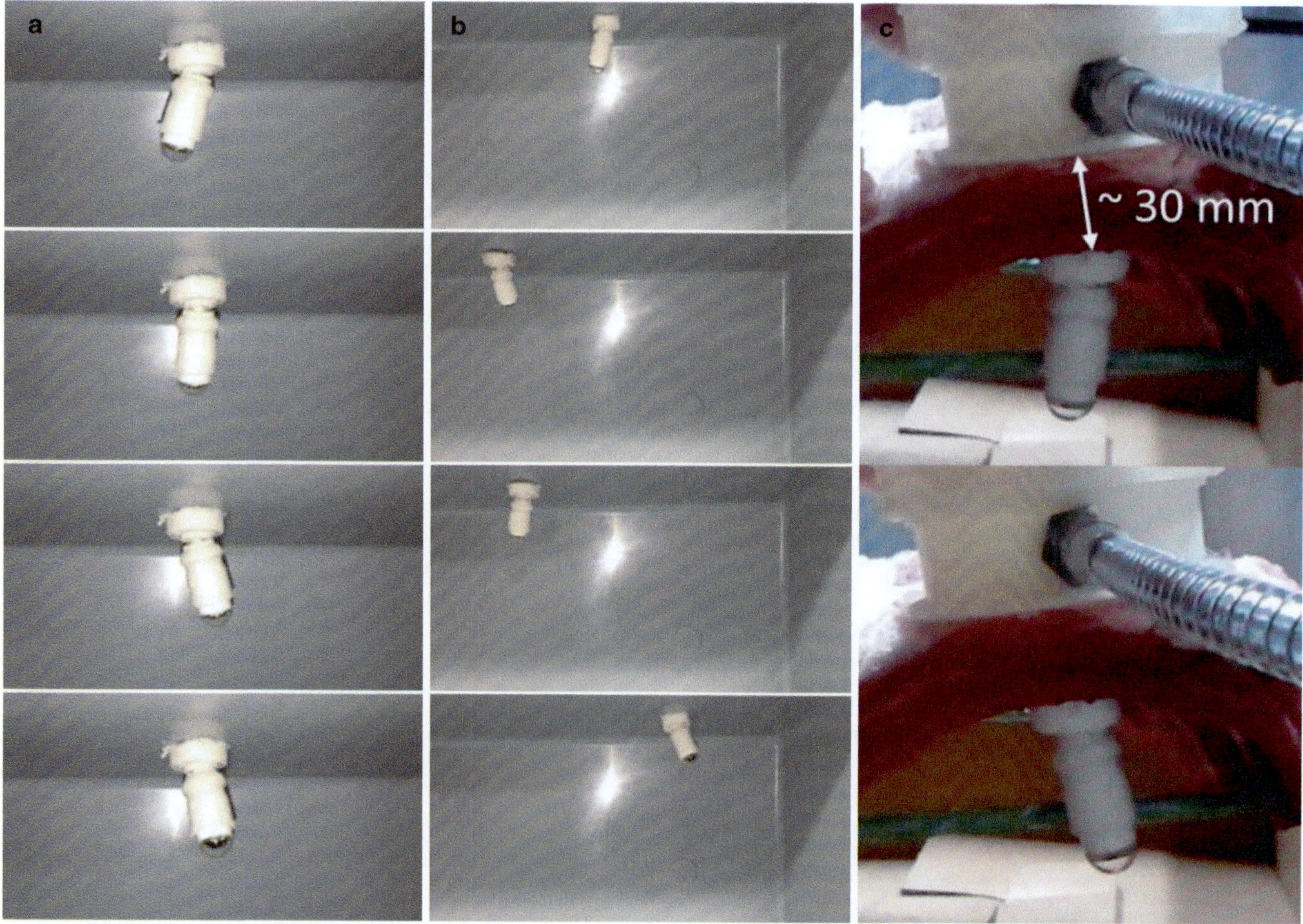

Fig. 2 Wireless steerable endoscope (WSE) prototype is steered counter gravity by a magnet: (**a**) adjustment of viewing direction *in situ*; (**b**) reposition by sliding movement; (**c**) maneuvering with the pig chest wall with 30 mm thickness (Modified from figures in Ref. [12])

shortcoming of this system is that the powering cable still occupies the space around the surgical incision and may entangle with the surgical operation instruments. Also, in uniportal VATS the viewing direction should be downward rather than forward. The authors proposed a remote wireless steerable endoscope (WSE). Before the operation, the WSE is inserted into the thoracic cavity through the incision and anchored to the internal thoracic wall with magnetic force. The video/image of the surgical site is transmitted to the monitor wirelessly and the FOV could be controlled by the external magnets. Compared to the aforementioned endoscopes, the WSE outperforms in omitting the cables associated with the endoscope, and does not interfere with instruments at the surgical incision [10]. The prototype of the WSE is shown in Fig. 2 [11, 12]. In the test, the wireless camera hangs onto the porcine rib cage, mimicking the chest wall. The anchoring distance covers the average thickness of chest wall. This prototype shows good performance of repositioning inside the chest cavity by sliding, changing the viewing direction and providing multiple views. Figure 2c shows the WSE operates with a 30 mm porcine rib cage. The WSE prototype could be maneuvered *in situ* as well as cross over the intercostal grooves effectively. Using this approach, the incision in the uniportal VATS could be potentially smaller as no space is required for the endoscope, or more space could be saved for the surgical instruments. Also, the instrument-endoscope fencing could be avoided since the WSE is away from the operating tools. At the present moment, this type of endoscope remains in the research labs. More efforts is needed to bring the WSE to clinical use.

Uniportal Platforms

Uniportal VATS is a kind of single port access (SPA) surgery, in which all the instruments share the same access port. In SPA surgery, the access port is made by surgical incision. When the port is a natural orifice, the surgery becomes the NOTES. Hence, platforms for uniportal VATS share a lot of similarities with that for SPA surgery and NOTES.

Platforms for NOTES could be categorized into two groups: one is flexible platforms and the other is miniaturized platforms [13, 14]. Table 1 summarizes some of the representative platforms for NOTES. Flexible platforms have a bendable shaft and a number of flexible arms at the distal tip. The shaft could be steered to conform to the lumen and delivery the arms to the surgical site. This type of platforms are currently the dominant platforms in NOTES applications. Examples include the Cobra produced by USGI [15], the Anuniscope developed by Karl Storz [16], the EndoSamurai presented by Olympus [17], the MASTER system invented by EndoMaster [18], the Flex system of Medrobotics [19] and the ESD robot prototyped in the Chinese University of Hong Kong [20]. For the flexible platforms, as the shaft is compliant, the positioning of the surgical arms is less accurate compared with the rigid counterparts, such as the da Vinci surgical system. Also, the base of the surgical arms is less steady. These are caused by the dilemma that the platform needs to be soft enough to navigate through the lumen while rigid enough to deliver the force. Therefore, controllable stiffness, such as shape lock, becomes necessitate for the flexible NOTES platforms. On the other hand, the surgical arms need to be dexterous enough and easily exchangeable via the working channel. In the examples, some have fixed arms at the tip that cannot be exchanged; others need to retract the entire endoscope to exchange. This would impede the further

Table 1 Examples of the NOTES platforms

Equipment/prototype	Figure	Advantages	Weakness
Cobra (USGI Medical) [15]		• Shape lock • Three independent arms	• Large diameter • Fixed tools • Difficult to manipulate • Low precision
Anubiscope (Karl Storz/IRCAD) [16]		• Two movable triangulating arms • Working channel for flexible instruments	• Limited triangulation • Limited maneuverability
EndoSamurai(Olympus) [17]		• Two bendable arms • Laparoscopic interface for bimanual coordination	• Require multiple operators • Limited maneuverability
MASTER (Endo Master) [18]		• Two 4-degrees of freedom arms • Standard dual-channel endoscope	• Large cap diameter • Fixed end-effector • Multiple operators
Flex System (Medrobotics) [19]		• High flexibility • Follow the leader • Two flexible arms	• Limited triangulation • Slow motion • Difficult to reposition
ESD Robot (CUHK) [20]		• Two flexible arms, 9 DoF in total • Compatible with TransPort®	• Difficult to change arms • Difficult to reposition accurately
Endoluminal Robotic Platform (Scuola Superiore Sant' Anna) [21]		• Reconfigurable inside the body • Save space	• Complex set-up • Tethered by wires for powering and image transmission

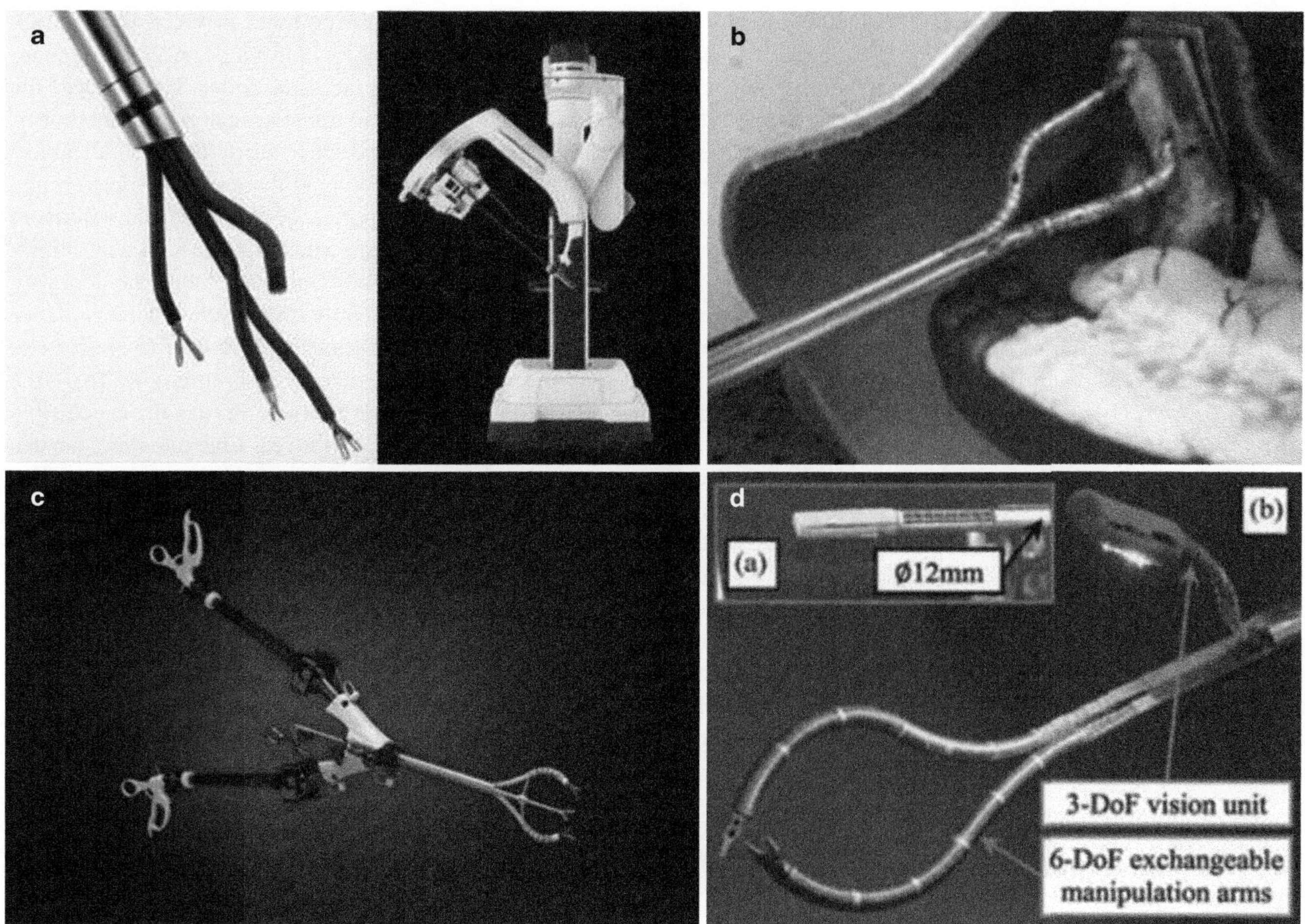

Fig. 3 Examples of single port access surgery platform. (**a**) da Vinci Single Port Robot [22]; (**b**) Titan Surgical Robot [23]; (**c**) Spider surgical system [24] and (**d**) SJTU unfoldable robotic system [25]

application of the platforms. In addition, the triangulation between the camera and the surgical instruments is important. In the current systems, this triangulation is limited due to the design is based on existing endoscopes or similar platforms. The other type of platform for NOTES is the miniature platforms. One example is the Endoluminal Robotic Platform by SSSA [21]. This type of platform does not suffer from the triangulation problem. Modules of the platform are inserted into the body cavity sequentially. Then, they are anchored and assembled at the surgical site. The miniature platforms could avoid tool collision, increase triangulation, and improve the dexterity of surgical arms. However, problems associated with these kinds of Platforms are poor payload ability, difficult to prototype, difficult to exchange tools, sterilization issue, etc. A promising approach would be to combine these two kinds of platforms. For example using the miniature device to provide imaging, illumination and assistance, while the main operation is performed by the flexible instruments.

In contrast to platforms for NOTES that has a flexible shaft, platforms for SPA surgery (including uniportal VATS) usually have a rigid shaft. Similarly, the distal end of the platform contains a number of dexterous arms for performing the surgery. Figure 3 listed some of the representative platforms, including the da Vinci single port robot produced by intuitive surgical Inc. [22], the SPORT surgical system made by Titan Medical Inc. [23], the SPIDER surgical system developed by TransEnterix [24] and the SJTU unfoldable robotic system (SURS) prototyped by Shanghai Jiaotong University [25]. In these systems, the flexible arms are positioned by the rigid shaft, which provides a steadier platform compared to the flexible NOTES platforms. The movement of the arms is typically controlled by the wires, cables and tendons, which transmits the motion of the motors. In these platforms, the distal surgical arm have more degrees of freedom compared to the arms in the flexible NOTES platform. As a result, the triangulation and dexterity are improved. The drawback is that, the backend actuation pack becomes more complex and heavier. Meanwhile, the payload ability of the arms remains limited. This is mainly attributed to the small size of the arms. To address this issue, novel flexible mechanisms that could provide sufficient workspace and dexterity while delivery sufficient force in a confined space are desired [26, 27].

In both NOTES and SPA surgery, electric cautery is commonly used for tissue dissection. The benefit is that the instrument could achieve hemostasis simultaneously. In addition, the instrument is less complex and lightweight. However, the smoke generated during the cautery would perfuse the confined surgical cavity and blur the endoscope view. Therefore, smoke evacuation should be considered in developing the platforms. Meanwhile, other smoke free methods, such as waterjet dissection could also be an option. Another common problem in the uniportal platforms is the sterilization of the surgical arms and endoscope. Each surgical arm contains multiple movable parts, which can make the sterilization difficult, costly and time consuming. Conventional sterilization methods, such as autoclave, would impair the mechanical strength of the driving cables inside the arms and damage the electronic components. The third challenge associated with the uniportal platforms is the exchange of surgical arms/instruments. Exchanging tools is inevitable in surgeries. In the robotic uniportal platforms, the instruments are driven by driving cables that transmit the motion from the motor pack. This requires the instruments be modular and be detachable from the motor pack as in the da Vinci surgical system.

Advanced Multimodality Image-Guided Operating Room

In uniportal VATS, intraoperative palpating and localizing tumors through the single small incision can be very difficult. Preoperative techniques, e.g., use computer tomography (CT) guidance and dye, contrast medium, radionucleotide labelling or hookwire/microcoil implantation are used to perform diagnosis and localization of the tumor. These preoperative techniques are conventionally performed in the radiology suite and the VATS is carried out in the operation room. This requires transferring the patients and may cause dislodgement of the hookwire, discomfort or complications.

Advanced multimodality image-guided operating room (AMIGO), or the hybrid operation room, has opened up new possibilities. The first report of the use of AMIGO in minimally invasive thoracic surgery (iVATS) was in 2013 by Prof. Raphael Bueno's group at Harvard University [28]. In the subsequent year, CUHK reported the first image-guided single-port VATS (iSPVATS) [29], in which the hookwire is placed under the guidance of Dyna-CT and single port VATS lobectomy is followed immediately. More recently, the CUHK group reported the first use of unparalleled real-time images from Dyna-CT to guide electromagnetic navigation bronchoscopy (ENB) in the hybrid operating room. This enables the identification of sub-centimeter lesion with high GGO content using ENB possible.

Benefits of hybrid operating room in VATS is threefold. Firstly, the hookwire insertion and uniportal VATS surgery can now be performed in the same room. This reduces the risks associated with patient transfer, such as pneumothorax, hookwire displacement and discomfort. This will also have benefits in cost and time saving as there are less transfers and less material usage, e.g. porter. Meanwhile, this will avoid the additional cost and time when there is hookwire migration or dislodge. In the hybrid operating room, the hookwire can be rapidly and conveniently reinserted with the guidance of the real-time on table scanner. Secondly, for lesions or regions where inserting a hookwire is infeasible (e.g., the lesion is too close to major thoracic vessels or inaccessible by a percutaneous approach), the real-time on-table scan can be used to localize the lesion for resection. Meanwhile, it can potentially provide additional information, e.g. resection margins. Thirdly, in the hybrid operating room information from different diagnostic modalities, e.g. CT and ENB, could be combined to improve the accuracy of the diagnosis. This would enable clinicians making more comprehensive intraoperative decisions and conduct operations more precisely.

It should be noted that, despite all its advantages, the widely adoption of hybrid operating room still relies on the fully trained multidisciplinary team of surgeons, radiologists and anesthetists.

Conclusion

To alleviate or solve the problems in uniportal VATS, technique efforts could be made from the endoscope, surgical platform and operating room. For endoscope, the wide-angled endoscope or flexible endoscopes such as Endoeye and Cardioscope can provide wider field of view for the surgeon, while reducing interference with other surgical instruments sharing the same incision. Wireless steerable endoscope systems may be the ideal solution for avoiding endoscope-instrument fencing, panoramic viewing of the whole operating space, and allowing further miniaturization of the surgical incision. The next generation of tools for performing uniportal VATS may be generated from the NOTES and SPA surgical platforms, which allows the eyes and hands of the surgeon to be inserted into the chest cavity and operate ergonomically and precisely. AMIGO is the future arena for surgeons to combat with thoracic diseases. It entails better intraoperative diagnosis, less cost and time. It also demands multidisciplinary clinicians working closely.

This chapter only touches handful aspects of the uniportal VATS technologies, while technology is evolving rapidly at an unprecedented pace. Regard to the future of uniportal VATS, any bold prediction today will turn out being conservative tomorrow. We believe much more complex procedures will be done through a single small incision, with greater patient safety and satisfaction, in the foreseeable future.

References

1. Nesher N, Galili R, Sharony R, et al. Videothorascopic sympathectomy (VATS) for palmar hyperhidriosis: summary of a clinical trial and surgical results [J]. Harefuah. 2000;138(11):913.
2. Ng CSH, Lau KKW, Gonzalez-Rivas D, Rocco G. Evolution in surgical approach & techniques for lung cancer. Thorax. 2013;68:681.
3. EndoCAMeleon® Hopkins® Telescope (visited on 2016, July 20), Available https://www.karlstorz.com/hk/en/cardiovascular-surgery.htm.
4. Ng CSH, Wong RHL, Lau RWH, Yim APC. Single port video-assisted thoracic surgery: advancing scope technology. Eur J Cardiothorac Surg. 2015;47(4):751.
5. Endoeye by Olympus (visited on 2015, October 24), Available http://medical.olympusamerica.com/products/endoeye.
6. Li Z, Oo MZ, Nalam V, et al. Design of a novel flexible endoscope—cardioscope [J]. J Mech Robot. 2016;8(5):051014.
7. Ng CSH, Wong RHL, Lau RWH, Yim APC. Minimizing chest wall trauma in single port video-assisted thoracic surgery. J Thorac Cardiovasc Surg. 2014;147(3):1095–6.
8. Park S, Bergs RA, Eberhart R, et al. Trocar-less instrumentation for laparoscopy: magnetic positioning of intra-abdominal camera and retractor [J]. Ann Surg. 2007;245(3):379–84.
9. Cadeddu J, Fernandez R, Desai M, et al. Novel magnetically guided intra-abdominal camera to facilitate laparoendoscopic single-site surgery: initial human experience [J]. Surg Endosc. 2009;23(8):1894–9.
10. Ng CSH, Rocco G, Wong RHL, Lau RWH, Yu SCH, Yim APC. Uniportal and single incision video assisted thoracic surgery – the state of the art. Interact Cardiovasc Thorac Surg. 2014;19(4):661–6.
11. Li Z, Ng CSH. Future of uniportal video-assisted thoracoscopic surgery—emerging technology [J]. Ann Cardiothorac Surg. 2016;5(2):127.
12. Zhao ZR, Li Z, Situ DR, et al. Recent clinical innovations in thoracic surgery in Hong Kong [J]. J Thorac Dis. 2016;8(Suppl 8):S618–26.
13. Ren HL, Lim CM, Wang J, Liu W, Song S, Li Z, Herbert G, Tse ZTH, Tan Z. Computer assisted transoral surgery with flexible robotics and navigation technologies: a review of recent progress and research challenges. Crit Rev Biomed Eng. 2013;4:365–91.
14. Vitiello V, Lee SL, Cundy TP, Yang GZ. Emerging robotic platforms for minimally invasive surgery. IEEE Rev Biomed Eng. 2013;6:111–26.
15. Bardou B, Nageotte F, Zanne P, de Mathelin M. Design of a telemanipulated system for transluminal surgery. In: Proceedings of the 31st annual international conference of the IEEE engineering in medicine and biology society. Minneapolis, MN, 2009. pp. 5577–5582.
16. Dallemagne B, Marescaux J. The ANUBISTM project. Minim Invasive Ther Allied Technol. 2010;19:257–61.
17. Spaun G, Zheng B, Swanström L. A multitasking platform for natural orifice translumenal endoscopic surgery (NOTES): a benchtop comparison of a new device for flexible endoscopic surgery and a standard dual-channel endoscope. Surg Endosc. 2009;23:2720–7.
18. Phee SJ, Kencana AP, Huynh VA, Sun ZL, Low SC, Yang K, Lomanto D, Ho KY. Design of a master and slave transluminal endoscopic robot for natural orifice transluminal endoscopic surgery. Proc Inst Mech Eng C J Mech Eng Sci. 2010;224: 1495–503.
19. The Flex Robotic System by Medrobotics (visited on 2015, October 24), Available http://medrobotics.com/gateway/flex-system-int/.
20. Lau KC, Leung EYY, Chiu PWY, et al. A flexible surgical robotic system for removal of early-stage gastrointestinal cancers by endoscopic submucosal dissection [J]. IEEE Trans Ind Inf. 2016;99:1–11.
21. Torora G, Dario P, Menciassi A. Array of robots augmenting the kinematics of endocavitary surgery. IEEE/ASME Trans Mechatron. 2014;19(6):1821–9.
22. Da Vinci Single Port Robot (visited on 2018, August 10), Available https://www.intuitivesurgical.com/sp/.
23. The SPORTTM Surgical System by Titan Medical Inc. (visited on 2015, October 24), Available http://www.titanmedicalinc.com/.
24. The SPIDER Surgical System by TransEnterix (visited on 2019, March 12), Available http://ir.transenterix.com/news-releases/news-release-details/transenterix-introduces-new-spider-surgical-system and https://www.sages.org/meetings/annual-meeting/abstracts-archive/single-port-cholecystectomy-with-the-transenterix-spider-a-single-institution-experience/.
25. Xu K, Zhao JG, Fu MX. Development of the SJTU unfoldable robotic system (SURS) for single port laparoscopy. IEEE/ASME Trans Mechatron. 2015;20(5):2133–45.
26. Li Z, Du R. Expanding workspace of underactuated flexible manipulator by actively deploying constrains. In: Proceedings of IEEE international conference on robotics and automation (ICRA 2014). Hong Kong, China, IEEE.
27. Li Z, Feiling J, Ren HL, Yu HY. A novel tele-operated flexible robot targeted for minimally invasive surgery. Engineering. 2015;1(1):73–8.
28. Gill RR, Zheng Y, Barlow JS, et al. Image-guided video assisted thoracoscopic surgery (iVATS)-phase I-II clinical trial [J]. J Surg Oncol. 2015;112(1):18–25.
29. Ng CSH, Chu CM, Kwok MWT, et al. Hybrid DynaCT scan-guided localization single-port lobectomy [J]. Chest J. 2015;147(3):e76–8.

The manufacturer's authorised representative in the EU is Springer Nature Customer Service Centre GmbH, Europaplatz 3, 69115 Heidelberg, Germany. If you have any concerns regarding our products, please contact ProductSafety@springernature.com

Printed and bound by CPI Group (UK) Ltd, Croydon, CR0 4YY
30/06/2025
01908363-0001